The Symptom and the Subject

The Symptom and the Subject

THE EMERGENCE OF THE
PHYSICAL BODY IN ANCIENT GREECE

Brooke Holmes

PRINCETON UNIVERSITY PRESS

PRINCETON AND OXFORD

Library of Congress Cataloging-in-Publication Data

Holmes, Brooke, 1976–
The symptom and the subject : the emergence of the physical body in ancient Greece /
Brooke Holmes.
p.   cm.
Includes bibliographical references and index.
ISBN 978-0-691-13899-2 (hardback : alk. paper)   1. Symptoms.   2. Medicine, Greek and
Roman.   3. Human body—Greece.   4. Greece—Civilization.   I. Title.
RC69.H6785   2010
616′.047—dc22   2009030026

British Library Cataloging-in-Publication Data is available

This book has been composed in Minion Pro

Printed on acid-free paper. ∞

press.princeton.edu

Printed in the United States of America

1   3   5   7   9   10   8   6   4   2

*To my mother and my sister,
and to the memory of my father*

————————————

Le symptôme, ce serait le réel apparent ou l'apparent réel.

Roland Barthes

CONTENTS

Some years ago I started thinking about the symptom and found I couldn't stop. I set out to write a dissertation about how literary representations of disease were affected by the shift to naturalizing interpretations of the symptom in fifth- and fourth-century medical writing. Yet the more I asked what defined those interpretations against other ways of understanding symptoms, the less satisfied I was with the answers. I got further into the medical texts, and the more I did, the stranger they seemed. What are these texts trying to see and to show? I read and reread the medical writers; I went back to the limited evidence we have for other ways of thinking about the symptom in early Greece to try to understand what was assumed about human beings and unseen threats. Eventually I came to conclude that the medical writers are seeing and showing the physical body, not as an anatomical object or a visible tableau, but as a largely hidden world of fluids, stuffs, flesh, bones, joints, and organs, loosely organized by what some of these writers call a *phusis*, "nature." As I will stress repeatedly, this body, which the Greeks call *sōma*, stands between what anyone can see or touch of a human being and a mostly submerged world created out of semiotic inference and imagination—hence, the central role of the symptom to the book.

The physical body is something new in the late archaic and classical periods. Of course, "new" is a loaded term when we talk about the Greeks. It lies at the heart of debates that go beyond questions of historical change and epistemic rupture to charged questions about whether the Greeks are like us or completely strange. The easy answer to such questions is that the Greeks are both familiar and foreign—but that answer fails to take us very far. In this book, I defend the idea that, through its emergence in the ancient Greek world as an object of investigation, the physical body comes to change how human beings can be imagined and how they can imagine themselves. I understand this transformation not in terms of a shift from superstition to sudden insight into biological reality. Rather, I see the physical body's emergence as generative because it encourages a way of thinking about people in physical terms. Much of this book explores the implications of this thinking both inside and outside medicine. These implications continue to be explored in the present, not only in the narrowly circumscribed arena of bioethics but also on the much more expansive ethical terrain that springs up around the problems posed by *having* a body to *being* human—hence, the importance of the subject to my project. I hope that this book, in its own way, contributes to these explorations.

This book belongs to a number of different disciplines or subfields, among them classical philology, history (ancient history, the history of medicine, the history of science, the history of ideas, the history of religion), literature and literary theory, philosophy, cultural studies, and anthropology. Its various affiliations can be credited in part to the questions it asks, in part to my own training as both a classicist and a comparatist. Interdisciplinarity is often praised, but it is hard to practice. Despite sea changes in the humanities and social sciences over the past thirty years, there is a lingering sense that "we must . . . be alert lest the crossing of disciplines involve a relaxing of discipline," as the 1975 Greene Report to the American Comparative Literature Association warned.[1] The anxious commitment to "standards" can still mask parochialism, a failure to recognize that the structure of the modern university does not neatly map onto historical evidence. But at the same time, disciplines, precisely because they are organized around ways of knowing, kinds of questions, and types of evidence, develop valuable strategies of inquiry and interpretation. They can thus help us find our way into distant cultures and texts, thereby making them generative for the present, without making these cultures and texts too familiar, thereby stripping them of disruptive force. In researching and writing this book, I have often crossed disciplines. But I have also tried to inhabit disciplines—some, of course, more than others—to pursue a set of questions about the physical body as a historical phenomenon, an object of conceptual and imaginative fascination, and the ground of lived experience. Even if these disciplines do not align with genres of knowing in the ancient world, working across and within them has driven home for me the truth that knowledge is, indeed, always situated.[2] I have also repeatedly become aware of the limits of my knowledge and my expertise. Nevertheless, this book is an attempt to tell a story that acknowledges the different ways of seeing the world that developed in classical Greece, as well as the ways we see today, without losing sight of a body whose power derives from its ambiguous position between physical object and ethical subject.

I have incurred many debts in writing this book. My debt is largest to Froma Zeitlin and Heinrich von Staden, who advised my dissertation, provided unflagging intellectual and emotional support, and have continued to be boundless sources of inspiration over the years. I also owe considerable thanks to Mark Buchan and Andrew Ford, not only for being such incisive readers but also for challenging my thinking along the way while remaining encouraging and good humored.

For years, I have benefited from correspondence and conversations with Jim Porter, who has shaped this project in countless ways. I am particularly grateful to him and to the anonymous reader for the Press for their detailed and insightful comments on an earlier version, which gave me the impetus and the tools I needed to undertake another revision to clarify my aims and ideas. Caroline Bynum not only provided enormously valuable feedback on drafts of the

[1] Bernheimer 1995.36.
[2] Haraway 1988.

introduction but also helped me see at several key points what really matters in intellectual work. Special thanks are due as well to Maud Gleason, who stepped in during the revision process and kindly convinced me to give the manuscript another go: the final product is much better as a result of her advice, though I am all too aware of how much room for improvement remains. Phiroze Vasunia generously helped the book find its way to a publisher, for which I am very grateful. And I am indebted to Joshua Katz for his careful reading of the first chapters, which saved me from many infelicities and errors. A number of other colleagues have offered valuable feedback on different chapters in the manuscript at its various stages or discussed key concepts, often graciously sharing their expertise to help me navigate new fields. I would like to thank, in particular, Hal Cook, Andrea Falcon, Chris Faraone, Barbara Kowalzig, Roy Laird, Jake Mackey, Ian Moyer, Kalliopi Nikolopoulou, Beate Pongratz-Leisten, Jutta Schicksore, and David Wolfsdorf. While I have not always succeeded in incorporating their suggestions or addressing their concerns, I have benefited enormously from these exchanges. For all the errors and omissions that remain, I take full responsibility.

I am pleased to have the opportunity to acknowledge the support of a number of institutions and foundations over the years of this project. My dissertation research was supported by the Center for Human Values at Princeton University, the Whiting Foundation, the Beinecke Scholarship Program, the Joseph E. Croft '73 Fellowship, and a Mary Isabel Sibley Fellowship from Phi Beta Kappa. Two Spray-Randleigh fellowships and an Arts and Humanities Research grant from the University of North Carolina, Chapel Hill helped me progress beyond the dissertation. And a year as a Mellon Fellow in the School of Historical Studies at the Institute for Advanced Study provided the ideal conditions to undertake the last round of major revisions; I gratefully acknowledge support from both the Institute and Princeton University during that year. The Magie Fund provided crucial support in the project's final stages.

Much of the support that made this book possible came from the communities of friends and colleagues of which I have had the opportunity to be a part over the years. My thinking and research were first fostered by my teachers at Columbia University, especially Nancy Worman and Gayatri Spivak. The Department of Comparative Literature at Princeton provided a thriving intellectual environment in my graduate years; I am especially grateful to April Alliston and Sandie Bermann and to Bob Fagles, whose presence is sorely missed. For friendship and discussion I thank Barry McCrea, May Mergenthaler, Masha Mimran, and especially Nick Rynearson. I continue to count on Jerry Passannante for always-inspiring conversations on all matters involving the materialist imagination. The warm welcome offered by my colleagues in the Department of Classics at UNC greatly eased my transition from student to faculty member, making it possible for me to continue expanding the project beyond the dissertation; special thanks, too, to Eric Downing, David Reeve, Patrick Miller, and Sarah Miller. My colleagues in the Department of Classics at Princeton have been an incredible source of support during a second transition and the final stages of the book. Audiences at Columbia, UNC, UC-Santa Barbara, the University of Southern California, Princeton, the University of Chicago, Harvard University, and the University of Pennsylvania have helped me shape this material, as have audiences in the ancient medicine community; I have benefited in particular from conversations with Paul Demont, Rebecca Flemming, Jennifer Clarke Kosak, and Ralph Rosen. I am also grateful to my editor, Rob Tempio, and my production editor, Mark Bellis, for all their help with seeing this book into print. I gratefully acknowledge my copy editor, Brian MacDonald, and Marcia Glass, Henryk Jaronowski, and Monica Boyer, for their assistance with the final preparation of the text. Finally, I would like to thank Joanna Ebenstein, who writes the wonderful blog Morbid Anatomy, for helping me find the image for the jacket.

None of this would have been possible without the love and support of my sister, my mom, and my grandparents. Miles Nelligan has endured this omnivorous project with pitch-perfect humor and encouragement: I can never thank him enough.

ABBREVIATIONS

EDITIONS, REFERENCE WORKS, AND JOURNALS

AJP	*American Journal of Philology*
AncPhil	*Ancient Philosophy*
Bertier	J. Bertier, ed. 1972. *Mnénisthée and Dieuchès*. Leiden.
BHM	*Bulletin of the History of Medicine*
BICS	*Bulletin of the Institute of Classical Studies*
Buchheim	T. Buchheim, ed. and trans. 1989. *Gorgias von Leontini. Reden, Fragmente und Testimonien*. Hamburg.
ClAnt	*Classical Antiquity*
CMG	*Corpus medicorum Graecorum*
CML	*Corpus medicorum Latinorum*
CP	*Classical Philology*
CQ	*Classical Quarterly*
CUF	Collection des universités de France
DG	H. Diels, ed. 1958. *Doxographi Graeci*. 3rd ed. Berlin.
Diels	H. Diels, ed. 1893. *Anonymi Londinensis ex Aristotelis Iatricis, Menoniis et aliis medicis eclogae*. Supplementum Aristotelicum III.1. Berlin.
DK	H. Diels, ed. 1951–52. *Die Fragmente der Vorsokratiker*. 6*th* ed., revised by W. Kranz. Berlin.
Edelstein	L. Edelstein and E. Edelstein. 1998. *Asclepius: Collection and Interpretation of the Testimonies*. 2 vols. Baltimore. Orig. pub. 1945.
FHSG	W. W. Fortenbaugh et al., eds. and trans. 1992–. *Theophrastus of Eresus: Sources for His Life, Writings, Thought, and Influence*. Leiden.
FGrHist	F. Jacoby, ed. 1923–58. *Die Fragmente der griechischen Historiker*. 3 vols. Berlin.
Garofalo	I. Garofalo, ed. 1988. *Erasistrati fragmenta*. Pisa.
Giannantoni	G. Giannantoni, ed. 1990. *Socratis et Socraticorum reliquiae*. 4 vols. Naples.
GRBS	*Greek, Roman, and Byzantine Studies*
G & R	*Greece and Rome*
Hordern	J. H. Hordern, ed. and trans. 2004. *Sophron's Mimes*. Oxford.
HSCP	*Harvard Studies in Classical Philology*
ICS	*Illinois Classical Studies*
IG	*Inscriptiones Graecae*. Berlin, 1873–.

JHM	*Journal of the History of Medicine and Allied Sciences*
JHS	*Journal of Hellenic Studies*
J.-V.L.	F. Jouan and H. Van Looy, eds. and trans. 1998–2003. *Euripide, Fragments*. CUF t. 8.1–4. Paris.
K	R. Kannicht, ed. 2004. *Tragicorum Graecorum fragmenta*. Vol. 5: *Euripides*. 2 vols. Göttingen.
Kannicht-Snell	R. Kannicht and B. Snell, eds. 1981. *Tragicorum Graecorum fragmenta*. Vol. 2. Göttingen.
Kühn	C. G. Kühn, ed. and trans. 1821–33. *Claudii Galeni opera omnia*. 20 vols. Leipzig. Reprint, Hildesheim, 1964–65.
Li	E. Littré, ed. and trans. 1839–61. *Œuvres complètes d'Hippocrate*. 10 vols. Paris.
LIMC	J. Boardman et al., eds. 1981–. *Lexicon iconographicum mythologiae classicae*. Zürich.
L-P	E. Lobel and D. Page, eds. 1955. *Poetarum Lesbiorum fragmenta*. Oxford.
Long-Sedley	A. A. Long and D. N. Sedley, eds. and trans. 1987. *The Hellenistic Philosophers*. 2 vols. Cambridge.
Martin-Primavesi	A. Martin and O. Primavesi, eds. and trans. 1999. *L'Empédocle de Strasbourg (P. Strasb. Gr. Inv. 1665–1666)*. Berlin.
Marx	F. Marx, ed. 1915. *A Cornelii Celsi quae supersunt. CML* I. Leipzig.
M-W	R. Merkelbach and M. L. West, eds. 1967. *Fragmenta Hesiodea*. Oxford.
Obbink	D. Obbink, ed. and trans. 1996–. *Philodemus, On Piety*. Oxford.
OSAP	*Oxford Studies in Ancient Philosophy*
PCG	R. Kassel and C. Austin, eds. 1983. *Poetae comici graeci*. 8 vols. Berlin.
PCPS	*Proceedings of the Cambridge Philological Society*
Pendrick	G. J. Pendrick, ed. and trans. 2002. *Antiphon the Sophist: The Fragments*. Cambridge.
Pfeiffer	R. Pfeiffer, ed. 1949–53. *Callimachus, Works*. 2 vols. Oxford.
PGM	K. Preisendanz, ed. 1973. *Papyri Graecae magicae*. 2 vols. 2nd ed. by A. Henrichs. Stuttgart.
PhR	*Philosophical Review*
PMG	D. L. Page, ed. 1962. *Poetae melici Graeci*. Oxford.
QUCC	*Quaderni urbinati di cultura classica*
R	S. Radt, ed. 1985–86. *Tragicorum Graecorum fragmenta*. Vol. 3: *Aeschylus*. Vol. 4: *Sophocles*. Göttingen.

Raeder	I. Raeder, ed. 1928–33. *Collectionum medicarum reliquiae Oribasii.* 4 vols. CMG VI.2.1–2. Leipzig.
RBPh	*Revue belge de philologie et d'histoire*
REA	*Revue des études anciennes*
REG	*Revue des études greques*
S-M	H. Maehler, ed. 1987–89. *Pindari carmina cum fragmentis, post B. Snell.* 2 vols. Leipzig.
TAPA	*Transactions of the American Philological Association*
van der Eijk	P. J. van der Eijk, ed. and trans. 2000–2001. *Diocles of Carystus.* 2 vols. Leiden.
von Staden	H. von Staden, ed. and trans. 1989. *Herophilus: The Art of Medicine in Early Alexandria.* Cambridge.
Waszinck	J. H. Waszinck, ed. 1962. *Timaeus a Calcidio translatus commentarioque instructus.* London.
W²	M. L. West, ed. 1989–92. *Iambi et elegi Graeci.* 2 vols. 2nd ed. Oxford.
West	M. L. West, ed. and trans. 2003. *Greek Epic Fragments.* Cambridge, Mass.
YCS	*Yale Classical Studies*
ZPE	*Zeitschrift für Papyrologie und Epigraphik*

Ancient Texts and Authors

Abbreviations for ancient sources follow H. G. Liddell, R. Scott, and H. S. Jones. *A Greek-English Lexicon* (with a Revised Supplement) (Oxford, 1996), except for the Hippocratic texts, for which abbreviations follow below, and Galen: abbreviations for Galen's texts follow R. J. Hankinson, ed., *The Cambridge Companion to Galen* (Cambridge, 2008), appendix 1, 391–97, which also includes information on modern editions. References to Galen also cite the volume and page number in the edition of C. G. Kühn, ed. and trans., *Claudii Galeni opera omnia*, 20 vols. (Leipzig, 1821–33; rep., Hildesheim, 1964–65).

Hippocratic Texts

For the Hippocratic writings cited in the text, I include the relevant page numbers from E. Littré, ed. and trans., *Œuvres complètes d'Hippocrate*, 10 vols. (Paris, 1839–61). I also cite the page and, where applicable, line numbers from the modern edition used, together with the abbreviation for the work. Information on English translations, when available, is also included. In cases where there are other modern editions, I provide additional bibliographic information. All modern editions of Hippocratic texts also appear in the bibliography for ease of reference.

A complete list of Hippocratic texts and editions with brief information on approximate dating and contents is available in appendix 3 of J. Jouanna, *Hippocrates*, trans. M. B. DeBevoise (Baltimore, 1999).

Acut.	*Regimen in Acute Diseases* (Li 2.224–377).
Joly	R. Joly, ed. and trans. 1972. *Hippocrate, Du régime des maladies aigués; Appendice; De l'aliment; De l'usage des liquides.* CUF t. 6.2. Paris.
	W.H.S. Jones, ed. and trans. 1923. *Hippocrates.* Vol. 2. Cambridge, Mass.
Acut. Sp.	*Regimen in Acute Diseases (Appendix)* (Li 2.394–529).
Joly	R. Joly, ed. and trans. 1972. *Hippocrate, Du régime des maladies aigués; Appendice; De l'aliment; De l'usage des liquides.* CUF t. 6.2. Paris.
	P. Potter, ed. and trans. 1988. *Hippocrates.* Vol. 6. Cambridge, Mass.
Aer.	*Airs, Waters, Places* (Li 2.12–93).
Jouanna	J. Jouanna, ed. and trans. 1996. *Hippocrate, Airs, eaux, lieux.* CUF t. 2.2. Paris.
	W.H.S. Jones, ed. and trans. 1923. *Hippocrates.* Vol. 1. Cambridge, Mass.
	H. Diller, ed. and trans. 1970. *Hippokrates. Über die Umwelt. (De aere aquis locis). CMG* I.1.2. Berlin.
Aff.	*On Affections* (Li 6.208–71).
Potter	P. Potter, ed. and trans. 1988. *Hippocrates.* Vol. 5. Cambridge, Mass.
Alim.	*Nutriment* (Li 9.98–121).
Joly	R. Joly, ed. and trans. 1972. *Hippocrate, Du régime des maladies aigués; Appendice; De l'aliment; De l'usage des liquides.* CUF t. 6.2. Paris.
	W.H.S. Jones, ed. and trans. 1923. *Hippocrates.* Vol. 1. Cambridge, Mass.
Aph.	*Aphorisms* (Li 4.458–609).
Jones	W.H.S. Jones, ed. and trans. 1931. *Hippocrates.* Vol. 4. Cambridge, Mass.
Artic.	*On Joints* (Li 4.78–327).
Kühlewein	H. Kühlewein, ed. 1894–1902. *Hippocratis opera quae feruntur omnia.* 2 vols. Leipzig.
	E. T. Withington, ed. and trans. 1928. *Hippocrates.* Vol. 3. Cambridge, Mass.
Art.	*On the Tekhnē* (Li 6.2–27).
Jouanna	J. Jouanna, ed. and trans. 1988. *Hippocrate, Des vents; De l'art.* CUF t. 5.1. Paris.

	W.H.S. Jones, ed. and trans. 1923. *Hippocrates*. Vol. 2. Cambridge, Mass.
	T. Gomperz, ed. and trans. 1910. *Die Apologie der Heilkunst. Eine griechische Sophistenrede des fünften vorchristlichen Jahrhunderts.* 2nd ed. Leipzig.
Carn.	*On Fleshes* (Li 8.584–615).
Joly	R. Joly, ed. and trans. 1978. *Hippocrate, Des lieux dans l'homme; Du système des glandes; Des fistules-Des hémorroïdes; De la vision; Des chairs; De la dentition.* CUF t. 13. Paris.
	P. Potter, ed. and trans. 1995. *Hippocrates*. Vol. 8. Cambridge, Mass.
	K. Deichgräber, ed. 1935. *Hippokrates über Entstehung und Aufbau des menschlichen Körpers: ΠΕΡΙ ΣΑΡΚΩΝ.* Leipzig.
Coac.	*Coan Prognoses* (Li 5.588–733).
Cord.	*On the Heart* (Li 9.80–93).
Duminil	M. P. Duminil, ed. and trans. 1998. *Hippocrate, Plaies; Nature des os; Cœur; Anatomie.* CUF t. 8. Paris.
Dec.	*Decorum* (Li 9.226–43).
Heiberg	I. L. Heiberg, ed. 1927. *Hippocratis opera.* CMG I.1. Leipzig.
	W.H.S. Jones, ed. and trans. 1923. *Hippocrates*. Vol. 2. Cambridge, Mass.
Dieb. iudic.	*Critical Days* (Li 9.298–307).
Ep.	*Letters* (Li 9.312–429).
Smith	W. D. Smith, ed. and trans. 1990. *Hippocrates, Pseudepigraphic Writings.* Leiden.
Epid. I	*Epidemics* I (Li 2.598–717).
Kühlewein	H. Kühlewein, ed. 1894–1902. *Hippocratis opera quae feruntur omnia.* 2 vols. Leipzig.
	W.H.S. Jones, ed. and trans. 1923. *Hippocrates*. Vol. 1. Cambridge, Mass.
Epid. II	*Epidemics* II (Li 5.72–139).
Smith	W. D. Smith, ed. and trans. 1994. *Hippocrates*. Vol. 7. Cambridge, Mass.
Epid. III	*Epidemics* III (Li 3.24–149).
Kühlewein	H. Kühlewein, ed. 1894–1902. *Hippocratis opera quae feruntur omnia.* 2 vols. Leipzig.
	W.H.S. Jones, ed. and trans. 1923. *Hippocrates*. Vol. 1. Cambridge, Mass.
Epid. IV	*Epidemics* IV (Li 5.144–97).
Smith	W. D. Smith, ed. and trans. 1994. *Hippocrates*. Vol. 7. Cambridge, Mass.

Epid. V	*Epidemics* V (Li 5.204–59).
Jouanna	J. Jouanna, ed. and trans. 2000. *Hippocrate, Epidémies V et VII.* CUF t. 4.3. Paris.
	W. D. Smith, ed. and trans. 1994. *Hippocrates.* Vol. 7. Cambridge, Mass.
Epid. VI	*Epidemics* VI (Li 5.266–357).
Manetti-Roselli	D. Manetti and A. Roselli, eds. and trans. 1982. *Ippocrate, Epidemie: libro sesto.* Florence.
	W. D. Smith, ed. and trans. 1994. *Hippocrates.* Vol. 7. Cambridge, Mass.
Epid. VII	*Epidemics* VII (Li 5.364–469).
Jouanna	J. Jouanna, ed. and trans. 2000. *Hippocrate, Epidémies V et VII.* CUF t. 4.3. Paris.
	W. D. Smith, ed. and trans. 1994. *Hippocrates.* Vol. 7. Cambridge, Mass.
Flat.	*On Breaths* (Li 6.90–115).
Jouanna	J. Jouanna, ed. and trans. 1988. *Hippocrate, Des vents; De l'art.* CUF t. 5.1. Paris.
	W.H.S. Jones, ed. and trans. 1923. *Hippocrates.* Vol. 2. Cambridge, Mass.
Fract.	*Fractures* (Li 3.412–563).
Kühlewein	H. Kühlewein, ed. 1894–1902. *Hippocratis opera quae feruntur omnia.* 2 vols. Leipzig.
	E. T. Withington, ed. and trans. 1928. *Hippocrates.* Vol. 3. Cambridge, Mass.
Genit./Nat. Puer.	*On Generation/On the Nature of the Child* (Li 7.470–543).
Joly	R. Joly, ed. and trans. 1970. *Hippocrate, De la génération; De la nature de l'enfant; Des maladies IV; Du fœtus de huit mois.* CUF t. 11. Paris.
	I. M. Lonie, trans. 1981. *The Hippocratic Treatises "On Generation," "On the Nature of the Child," "Diseases IV."* Berlin.
Glan.	*Glands* (Li 8.556–75).
Joly	R. Joly, ed. and trans. 1978. *Hippocrate, Des lieux dans l'homme; Du système des glandes; Des fistules-Des hémorroïdes; De la vision; Des chairs; De la dentition.* CUF t. 13. Paris.
	P. Potter, ed. and trans. 1995. *Hippocrates.* Vol. 8. Cambridge, Mass.
Haem.	*Haemorrhoids* (Li 6.436–45).
Joly	R. Joly, ed. and trans. 1978. *Hippocrate, Des lieux dans l'homme; Du système des glandes; Des fistules-Des*

	hémorroïdes; De la vision; Des chairs; De la dentition. CUF t. 13. Paris.
	P. Potter, ed. and trans. 1995. *Hippocrates.* Vol. 8. Cambridge, Mass.
Hebd.	*On Sevens* (Li 8.634–73).
Roscher	W. H. Roscher, ed. 1913. *Die hippokratische Schrift von der Siebenzahl in ihrer vierfachen Überlieferung.* Paderborn.
Hum.	*Humors* (Li 5.476–503).
Jones	W.H.S. Jones, ed. and trans. 1931. *Hippocrates.* Vol. 4. Cambridge, Mass.
Int.	*Internal Affections* (Li 7.166–303).
Potter	P. Potter, ed. and trans. 1994. *Hippocrates.* Vol. 4. Cambridge, Mass.
Iudic.	*Crises* (Li 9.276–95).
Liq.	*Use of Liquids* (Li 6.118–37).
Joly	R. Joly, ed. and trans. 1972. *Hippocrate, Du régime des maladies aigués; Appendice; De l'aliment; De l'usage des liquides.* CUF t. 6.2. Paris.
	P. Potter, ed. and trans. 1995. *Hippocrates.* Vol. 8. Cambridge, Mass.
Loc.	*On Places in a Human Being* (Li 6.276–349).
Craik	E. M. Craik, ed. and trans. 1998. *Hippocrates, Places in Man.* Oxford.
	R. Joly, ed. and trans. 1978. *Hippocrate, Des lieux dans l'homme; Du système des glandes; Des fistules-Des hémorroïdes; De la vision; Des chairs; De la dentition.* CUF t. 13. Paris.
	P. Potter, ed. and trans. 1995. *Hippocrates.* Vol. 8. Cambridge, Mass.
Mochl.	*Instruments of Reduction* (Li 4.340–95).
Kühlewein	H. Kühlewein, ed. 1894–1902. *Hippocratis opera quae feruntur omnia.* 2 vols. Leipzig.
	E. T. Withington, ed. and trans. 1928. *Hippocrates.* Vol. 3. Cambridge, Mass.
Morb. I	*On Diseases* I (Li 6.140–205).
Wittern	R. Wittern, ed. and trans. 1974. *Die hippokratische Schrift "De morbis I."* Hildesheim.
	P. Potter, ed. and trans. 1988. *Hippocrates.* Vol. 5. Cambridge, Mass.
Morb. II	*On Diseases* II (Li 7.8–115).
Jouanna	J. Jouanna, ed. and trans. 1983. *Hippocrate, Maladies II.* CUF t. 10.2. Paris.

	P. Potter, ed. and trans. 1988. *Hippocrates*. Vol. 5. Cambridge, Mass.
Morb. III	*On Diseases* III (Li 7.118–61).
Potter	P. Potter, ed. and trans. 1980. *Hippokrates. Über die Krankheiten III. CMG* I.2.3. Berlin.
	P. Potter, ed. and trans. 1988. *Hippocrates*. Vol. 6. Cambridge, Mass.
Morb. IV	*On Diseases* IV (Li 7.542–615).
Joly	R. Joly, ed. and trans. 1970. *Hippocrate, De la génération; De la nature de l'enfant; Des maladies IV; Du fœtus de huit mois*. CUF t. 11. Paris.
	I. M. Lonie, trans. 1981. *The Hippocratic Treatises "On Generation," "On the Nature of the Child," "Diseases IV."* Berlin.
Morb. Sacr.	*On the Sacred Disease* (Li 6.353–97).
Jouanna	J. Jouanna, ed. and trans. 2003. *Hippocrate, La maladie sacrée*. CUF t. 2.3. Paris.
	W.H.S. Jones, ed. and trans. 1923. *Hippocrates*. Vol. 2. Cambridge, Mass.
	H. Grensemann, ed. and trans. 1968. *Die hippokratische Schrift "Über die heilige Krankheit."* Berlin.
Mul. I	*Diseases of Women* I (Li 8.10–233).
Grensemann	H. Grensemann. 1982. *Hippokratische Gynäkologie. Die gynäkologischen Texte des Autors C nach den pseudohippokratischen Schriften "De muliebribus"* I, II *und "De sterilibus."* Wiesbaden.
	A. E. Hanson, trans. 1975. "Hippocrates: *Diseases of Women I." Signs* 1:567–84.
Mul. II	*Diseases of Women* II (Li 8.234–407).
Nat. Hom.	*On the Nature of a Human Being* (Li 6.32–69).
Jouanna	J. Jouanna, ed. and trans. 2002. *Hippocrate, La nature de l'homme*. 2nd ed. *CMG* I.1.3. Berlin.
	W.H.S. Jones, ed. and trans. 1931. *Hippocrates*. Vol. 4. Cambridge, Mass.
Nat. Mul.	*Nature of Women* (Li 7.312–431).
Bourbon	F. Bourbon, ed. and trans. 2008. *Hippocrate, Nature de la femme*. CUF t. 12.1. Paris.
Oct.	*On the Eight-Month Child* (Li 7.436–53, "On the Seven-Month Child"; Li 7.453–61, "On the Eight-Month Child").
Grensemann	H. Grensemann, ed. and trans. 1968. *Hippokrates. Über Achtmonatskinder. (De octimestri partu.) Über das Siebenmonatskind. <Unecht>. CMG* I.2.1. Berlin.

R. Joly, ed. and trans. 1970. *Hippocrate, De la génération; De la nature de l'enfant; Des maladies IV; Du fœtus de huit mois.* CUF t. 11. Paris.

Off. Med.   *In the Surgery* (Li 3.272–337).

Kühlewein   H. Kühlewein, ed. 1894–1902. *Hippocratis opera quae feruntur omnia.* 2 vols. Leipzig.

E. T. Withington, ed. and trans. 1928. *Hippocrates.* Vol. 3. Cambridge, Mass.

Oss.   *On the Nature of Bone* (Li 9.168–97).

Duminil   M. P. Duminil, ed. and trans. 1998. *Hippocrate, Plaies; Nature des os; Cœur; Anatomie.* CUF t. 8. Paris.

Prog.   *Prognostic* (Li 2.110–91).

Alex   B. Alexanderson, ed. 1963. *Die Hippokratische Schrift "Prognostikon."* Göteborg.

W.H.S. Jones, ed. and trans. 1923. *Hippocrates.* Vol. 2. Cambridge, Mass.

Prorrh. I   *Prorrhetic* I (Li 5.510–73).

Polack   H. Polack, ed. 1976. *Textkritische Untersuchungen zu der hippokratischen Schrift "Prorrhetikos I."* Hamburg.

P. Potter, ed. and trans. 1995. *Hippocrates.* Vol. 8. Cambridge, Mass.

Prorrh. II   *Prorrhetic* II (Li 9.6–75).

Potter   P. Potter, ed. and trans. 1995. *Hippocrates.* Vol. 8. Cambridge, Mass.

Salubr.   *On Regimen in Health* (Li 6.72–87).

Jouanna   J. Jouanna, ed. and trans. 2002. *Hippocrate, La nature de l'homme.* 2nd ed. CMG I.1.3. Berlin.

W.H.S. Jones, ed. and trans. 1931. *Hippocrates.* Vol. 4. Cambridge, Mass.

Steril.   *Sterile Women* (Li 8.408–63).

Grensemann   H. Grensemann. 1982. *Hippokratische Gynäkologie. Die gynäkologischen Texte des Autors C nach den pseudohippokratischen Schriften "De muliebribus" I, II und "De sterilibus."* Wiesbaden.

Superf.   *Superfetation* (Li 8.476–509).

Lienau   C. Lienau, ed. and trans. 1973. *Hippokrates. Über Nachempfängnis, Geburtshilfe und Schwangerschaftsleiden.* CMG I.2.2. Berlin.

Ulc.   *On Wounds* (Li 6.400–433).

Duminil   M. P. Duminil, ed. and trans. 1998. *Hippocrate, Plaies; Nature des os; Cœur; Anatomie.* CUF t. 8. Paris.

P. Potter, ed. and trans. 1995. *Hippocrates.* Vol. 8. Cambridge, Mass.

VC   *On Head Wounds* (Li 3.182–261).
    Hanson   M. Hanson, ed. and trans. 1999. *Hippocrates, On Head Wounds. CMG* I.4.1. Berlin.
                     E. T. Withington, ed. and trans. 1928. *Hippocrates.* Vol. 3. Cambridge, Mass.

Vict.   *On Regimen* (Li 6.466–663).
    Joly-Byl   R. Joly, with S. Byl, ed. and trans. 2003. *Hippocrate, Du régime.* 2nd ed. *CMG* I.2.4. Berlin.
                     W.H.S. Jones, ed. and trans. 1931. *Hippocrates.* Vol. 4. Cambridge, Mass.

Virg.   *Diseases of Young Girls* (Li 8.466–71).
    Lami   A. Lami, ed. and trans. 2007. "[Ippocrate], *Sui disturbi virginali*: testo, traduzione e commento." *Galenos* 1:15–59.
                     R. Flemming and A. E. Hanson, ed. and trans. 1998. "Hippocrates' *Peri Parthenion* ("Diseases of Young Girls"): Text and Translation." *Early Science and Medicine* 3:241–52.

VM   *On Ancient Medicine* (Li 1.570–637).
    Jouanna   J. Jouanna, ed. and trans. 1990. *Hippocrate, De l'ancienne médecine.* CUF t. 2.1. Paris.
                     W.H.S. Jones, ed. and trans. 1923. *Hippocrates.* Vol. 1. Cambridge, Mass.
                     A. J. Festugière, ed. and trans. 1948. *Hippocrate, L'ancienne médecine.* Paris.
                     M. Schiefsky, trans. 2005. *Hippocrates, On Ancient Medicine.* Leiden.

In an effort to address both specialists in the ancient world and a more general audience, I have adopted the following system. In the main text, I use Greek for block quotations and shorter quotations in parentheses. The most important words and phrases, as well as in-text references to the Greek primary texts, are transliterated and translated the first time they appear. One small idiosyncrasy: although I consistently use *sōma* and *psukhē*, especially in cases where I am discussing the semantic field of those Greek words, at times I use "body" (often qualified as "physical," to avoid the catchall feel of the phrase "the body" in contemporary scholarship) and "soul"; I prefer the transliterations because they make clear I am working with specific Greek terms, but I find the English words at times useful to remind the reader that we are speaking of evidence that deeply influences our own sense of "body" and "soul." (In my discussion of contemporary research on "the body," I naturally use the English terms.) I use Greek for the most part in the notes, retaining the most familiar transliterations from the main text. In nearly all cases, I have used Latinized forms of Greek proper names for the ease of nonspecialists.

Translations are my own unless otherwise noted, with the exception of block translations from Homer: these are drawn from R. Lattimore, trans., *The Iliad of Homer* (Chicago, 1961) and *The Odyssey of Homer* (Chicago, 1999).

The Symptom and the Subject

———————————

Symptoms and Subjects

Nothing drives us to ask why like the austere truth of human suffering. Hesiod, the first didactic poet in the Greek literary tradition, takes up the question on a grand scale early in the *Works and Days*, where we learn that conditions were not always bleak. In a past age, labor and suffering were unknown: the earth readily yielded food; men lived as companions to the gods. Everything changes when Prometheus, working on behalf of humankind, contests Zeus's omniscience with a ruse. Zeus, angered, takes fire away from people, only to have Prometheus steal it back in the stalk of a fennel plant. Zeus responds this time not by withholding gifts but by giving them: Pandora, the original woman, and the countless afflictions that scatter when she opens her infamous jar. From this time on, diseases have wandered the earth day and night. They overtake us in silence, because Zeus has taken away their voices. The stealth of their approach proves the poem's core axiom—"so it is in no way possible to escape the mind of Zeus" (*Op.* 105)—while the trauma they cause on arrival conflates the impossibility of escape with the inevitability of pain. In the world after Pandora, humans live and relive Zeus's decisive assertion of his power. Aeschylus will call this *pathei mathos*, knowledge through suffering (*Ag.* 177).

It is with a quite different view of the knowledge acquired through suffering that Plutarch, in the first centuries CE, comes back to Hesiod's explanation of disease and, more specifically, to the adverb on which it hinges: "silently."

> For all the diseases wander the earth not, as Hesiod says, "silently, since counselor Zeus has taken away their voice," but most of them have indigestion and sluggishness as their harbingers and forerunners and heralds, as it were. (*Mor.* 127D)[1]

In support of his point, Plutarch quotes from the *Aphorisms* of Hippocrates, still considered one of the foremost medical authorities of the day some five hundred years after his alleged floruit.[2] Plutarch is working with some assumptions that are absent from Hesiod's poem. Whereas, in the *Works and Days*, disease is a nebulous daemonic being, for Plutarch it is a process that unfolds

---

[1] οὐ γὰρ ἅπασαι κατὰ τὸν Ἡσίοδον ἐπιφοιτῶσιν αἱ νόσοι ʽσιγῇ, ἐπεὶ φωνὴν ἐξείλετο μητίετα Ζεύς,ʼ ἀλλʼ αἱ πλεῖσται καθάπερ προαγγέλους καὶ προδρόμους καὶ κήρυκας ἔχουσιν ἀπεψίας καὶ δυσκινησίας.

[2] *Aph.* II.5 (Li 4.470 = 108 Jones).

inside the hidden space of the body. And although the disease remains concealed, Plutarch believes that the pre-sufferings and pre-sensations produced by the body as it falls ill cue us to its presence. The disease that we fail to avoid thus holds different lessons for Plutarch. It proves that we have not been properly vigilant about what is happening inside us, while suggesting, too, that a body left on its own strays toward disaster.

Despite these differences, Hesiod and Plutarch are engaged in a similar task: each is trying to figure out where symptoms come from. For the purposes of this book, a symptom is a disruption—without obvious cause and often, though not always, painful—either to the experience of self or to the outward presentation of self. Insistently real, symptoms point to an imperceptible dimension of reality that cuts across the world that we do perceive. In one sense, this hidden world can be laid bare. After Athena lifts the mist from Diomedes' eyes in book 5 of the *Iliad*, for example, the gods on the battlefield are suddenly bathed in light. When, just after this revelation, Diomedes cuts the Trojan fighter Hyperion "beside the shoulder through the collar-bone with the great sword, so that neck and back were hewn free of the shoulder" (5.146–47), he confronts the inner body that will become so important to the learned Greco-Roman medical tradition and remains at the center of contemporary biomedicine. Yet symptoms reveal neither the "fictional" tableau of Greek gods nor the "real" mess of blood and flesh beneath the skin. Rather, for the ancients as for us, symptoms give rise to a way of seeing built on leaps, both logical and imaginative, into an unseen world—inferences about causes, reasons, and motivations. Like other spectacular anomalies, such as thunder or eclipses, symptoms demand interpretation. In fact, because they mark a catastrophic breach of the boundaries of a person, symptoms carry an unusually creative charge, asking us to imagine the nature and the limits of a human being and to "see" unseen agents and powers capable of causing harm. For this reason, I approach symptoms not as windows onto hidden worlds (innards or gods) but as phenomena that help to generate and sustain worldviews.

One such worldview, which had become entrenched by the time of Plutarch, is organized around what I will call the physical body. The central argument of this book is that this body, designated in Greek by the word *sōma*, emerges through changes in the interpretation of symptoms in the Greek world of the fifth and fourth centuries BCE. Beginning with Homer, moving through the fragments of the sixth- and fifth-century "physicists" and the classical-era medical treatises, and closing with the medical analogies of early philosophical ethics and the diseases of Euripidean tragedy, I analyze how, as the physical body "comes into the visible"—to adopt the medical writers' own language—it transforms the stories that can be told not only about human suffering but also about human nature.[3] The result, I argue, is a new kind of ethical subject.[4]

---

[3] ἐς τὸ φανερὸν ἀφικνεῖται (*Vict.* I 10, Li 6.486 = 134,12–13 Joly-Byl).

[4] By "ethical," I mean the human being as he (rarely she) is situated in a larger community that shares a set of values in relation to which judgments of praise and blame are made. The "subject" has been

The physical body on this account first materializes within what was called, at least by the end of the fifth century, the "inquiry into nature," which was advanced by a loose group of thinkers who attempted to conceptualize the forces underlying the visible world as impersonal.[5] The question of how human beings participate in this nonhuman web of power is taken up with particular vigor by the classical medical writers. What the early physicians "saw," as one medical writer succinctly declares, is that the things constituting the larger world "are inside a human being and they hurt him" (ἐν τῷ ἀνθρώπῳ ἐνεόντα καὶ λυμαινόμενα τὸν ἄνθρωπον).[6] This "inside" in Greek medicine is the physical body, where life processes take place and disease unfolds, often below the threshold of consciousness. Because this domain is largely hidden, most of what happens there can be detected only through symptoms, just as the unseen forces and stuffs in the inquiry into nature can be seen only "through the phenomena," as a famous dictum attributed to Anaxagoras states.[7] Symptoms thus work as springboards into an unseen world that has been adventurously reconceptualized. If Hesiod and other early poets plot the edges of a human being against an invisible realm of gods and *daimones*,[8] the medical writers encourage people to rethink that hidden realm in terms of powers like "the hot" and "the cold." At the same time, they extend this realm into the *sōma*, thereby redrawing the boundaries of the human.

an organizing idea in twentieth-century semiotics and critical theory: see Silverman 1983, esp. 3–53, 126–93. I adopt the term here in order to emphasize not only the conscious, rational aspects of a human being but also the nonconscious forces that work through him or her, forces that have figured prominently in recent critical theory. But rather than applying contemporary models of the subject, which are often developed in reaction to postclassical thinkers (e.g., Descartes, Kant), to classical antiquity, I am interested in how the very idea of nonconscious forces is conceptualized at a particular historical moment and applied to human nature. I have generally reserved "subject" for my discussions of the ethical implications of the physical body's emergence.

[5] "Inquiry into nature" (περὶ φύσεως ἱστορία): Pl. *Phd.* 96a8; cf. *Phdr.* 270a1 (μετεωρολογίας φύσεως πέρι); X. *Mem.* 1.1.14, with Leszl 2006.366–69. See also the references in late fifth-century medical texts, e.g., *Carn.* 15 (Li 8.604 = 197,26–198,1 Joly): φύσιν συγγράφοντες; *VM* 20 (Li 1.620 = 146,5 Jouanna): οἳ περὶ φύσιος γεγράφασιν. Aristotle will refer to those engaged in the inquiry as *phusiologoi* (e.g., *Metaph.* 990a3) and *phusikoi* (e.g., *Phys.* 184b17). But what the "inquiry into nature" encompassed continues to be a subject of debate: Laks 2006.7–12 identifies two basic characteristics—its totalizing ambitions, on which see also Long 1999b, and its focus on origins—while arguing that the identity of the earlier thinkers cannot be exhausted by the term "naturalistes" (2006. 18–21). Cf. Graham 2006, who makes an Ionian tradition of naturalizing explanation the backbone of early Greek philosophy. I discuss this debate in more detail in chapter 2. On the meaning of *phusis*, see further below, chapter 2, n.3.

[6] *VM* 14 (Li 1.602 = 136,9 Jouanna).

[7] DK59 B21a: ὄψις ἀδήλων τὰ φαινόμενα ("The vision of unseen things is through the phenomena").

[8] The divine and the daemonic (τὸ θεῖον . . . καὶ τὸ δαιμόνιον) are the two classes of explanation given by magico-religious healers, according to the author of *On the Sacred Disease* (1, Li 6.358 = 6,19 Jouanna). While the notion of a god is relatively clear, that of a *daimōn* or *to daimonion* is not. Throughout this book, I adopt the term "daemonic" to capture the uncertainty that characterizes responses to the symptom, the hostility believed to motivate that symptom, and the sense of the symptom as a disruption from another plane of reality.

In the second part of the book, I explore and defend the claim that the physical body plays a pivotal but unacknowledged role in ideas about the human in the fifth and early fourth centuries, as well as in the formation of a new kind of ethical subjectivity centered on practices of caring for the self. I explain the strength of its influence in terms of its dual identity. On the one hand, the physical body is a model of intelligibility: although its workings are hidden, a physician trained in the medical *tekhnē*, "science" or "art," may reconstruct them through reasoning. Doing so allows him both to intervene in disease and to manage health. On the other hand, that body is an untrustworthy and unfamiliar thing: it is prone to disorder, largely estranged from consciousness, and animated not by intentions but by impersonal, asocial powers. Its very strangeness, I argue, encourages ancient thinkers to take an increasing interest in the *psukhē* as the locus of the person.[9] The *sōma*, however, is not simply a foil to the *psukhē*. In its guise as an intelligible physical object, it is also its analogue, thereby contributing to the creation of the *psukhē* as an object of both knowledge and care in early philosophical ethics. Through these affinities with the *sōma*, the *psukhē* comes to be haunted by its daemonic energies, energies that also begin to infect tragic subjects in the latter part of the fifth century, particularly in the plays of Euripides.[10]

We continue to live with and in a body imagined as both an object of scientific knowledge and mastery and an unruly, threatening, inhuman thing. So entrenched is this body in modern Western culture that it is difficult to conceive of its absence. Yet it is precisely because medicine, biology, and the cognitive sciences increasingly inform so many of the stories we tell about ourselves that we must interrogate the body that these disciplines assume. In recent decades, path-breaking scholars have begun to piece together the history of the Western body. The body has also become increasingly visible in the practice of history itself, where it has come to serve as the primary locus for the imposition and expression of sociopolitical power: Michel Foucault, for example, famously describes the task of genealogy as the recovery of "a body totally imprinted by history"; cultural analysis informed by the theories of Pierre Bourdieu has probed how embodied practices embed us in social and cultural systems.[11]

---

[9] While the concept of the person has been historicized over the past century (see esp. Mauss 1985; see also Detienne 1973) and taken up as a specific category in contemporary philosophy (see C. Gill 1991), I use "person" in a loose sense to speak of the human being *qua* sentient, speaking, thinking being (and implicitly opposed to the impersonal).

[10] Other fifth-century genres, such as historiography and comedy, undeniably bear the imprint of medical ideas. Limits of time and space keep me from including them in this study. For an overview of the cultural influence of medical ideas in this period, see G. Lloyd 2003.

[11] A body imprinted by history: Foucault 1977b.148. In *Birth of the Clinic* (1973) and *Discipline and Punish* (1977a), the body materializes through institutions of power (the hospital and the prison, respectively) as an object of knowledge as well as an object of state regulation. For Bourdieu's use of the *habitus*, see Bourdieu 1977; 1990, esp. 52–79. For overviews of the role of "the body" in social and cultural analysis, see Lambek and Strathern 1998a.5–13; Joyce 2005.

Such work continues apace, even as its focus in some quarters has shifted away from the body's subjection to ideologies and institutions to lived experience.[12]

In ancient Greco-Roman studies, as in the humanities and the social sciences more generally, over the past few decades the body has been "a growth industry."[13] Yet, while we have compelling stories about how Christianity transforms classical concepts of the body, as well as ample evidence of the persistence of classical models, there is still little sense of how these concepts arise.[14] In neglecting this inquiry, we have left a larger question unexplored—namely, how the very concept of "the body" arises. J. I. Porter wrote a decade ago:

> But what about the category of "the body" itself? When does it come into existence? The issue has been discussed, mainly in speculative philological and philosophical contexts, but so far the nexus of problems implicating the results of Foucault-inspired research in more traditional problems of identity, likewise organized around the body, has not been addressed. As a result, the category of the body is generally assumed, not queried.[15]

Foucault himself, despite—or perhaps because of—his long-standing fascination with the making of the modern Western body, treats classical antiquity as the "before" to the "afters" that interest him (e.g., asceticism, psychoanalysis, biopower).[16] As a result, even his studies of ancient "techniques of the self" assume a body that is already given.[17] This book, starting from the assumption that the physical body is not given, aims to shed light on its emergence in classical Greek culture.

The idea that "the body" might not be given may seem strange. After all, the body would seem to have a good claim on always just being there. This, anyway, has long been the contention of those skeptical of Bruno Snell's striking claim that Homer does not have a concept of the unified, living body (*sōma*, on

---

[12] For a phenomenological approach to the body, see Merleau-Ponty 1962; 1968. See also, e.g., Csordas 1990, esp. 6–7; 1993; Mullarkey 1994; Joyce 2005; Young 2005.6–9.

[13] Growth industry: Stewart 1997.7. The first surge of interest in the body in classics accompanied the rise of gender and sexuality studies: see M. Katz 1989; Richlin 1997; Montserrat 1998; Wyke 1998; 1999. The introduction to Hopkins and Wyke 2005 indicates increasing interest in the lived body; this has been especially true in the study of material culture (e.g., Meskell 1996). Medical historians, however, have largely resisted the relevance of "the body" to their field: see, e.g., Nutton 2002.254; cf. G. Lloyd 1992.118–19.

[14] On the early Christian body, see P. Brown 1988; Rousselle 1988. On the Western medieval body: Bynum 1991; 1995.13–19. Laqueur 1990 begins his story with Aristotle, with a few references to the Hippocratics. For the humoral body in Western Europe, see, e.g., Duden 1991; Schoenfeldt 1999.

[15] Porter 1999b.3–4. See also Porter and Buchan 2004.9.

[16] See Porter 2005.

[17] For Foucault's work on the ancient world, see Foucault 1985; 1986; 1997.175–301; 2005. Cf. Hadot 1995.206–13, criticizing Foucault's work on freedom and self-fashioning in the first centuries CE as anachronistic. Post-Foucauldian work on biopolitics tends to begin with Aristotle without acknowledging his debts to physical and medical inquiry: see, e.g., Agamben 2004.13–16.

the few occasions that it does appear, is reserved for corpses).[18] Others, however, have thought that Snell is on to something important.[19] When we speak of "the" body, we imply that there is something of us that is not body: the person, the soul, or the mind. That we are not simply our bodies is a point that Socrates makes in *Alcibiades* I, probably one of Plato's earliest works, when he gets Alcibiades to agree that, because the *sōma* cannot use or rule itself, it must have a user and a ruler; Socrates calls this user and ruler *psukhē* and equates it with the person (130a1–c6). In the Homeric poems, though, we find no such duality. It is true that at the moment of death the hero splits into a corpse and a *psukhē*. Even then, however, the *psukhē* is merely a wraith that disappears to Hades, while the heroes themselves are said to remain on the battlefield.[20] *Sōma*, moreover, is not Homer's usual word for "corpse," as we will see. People, then, do not seem to "have" bodies in the Homeric poems, or at least the bodies they have in later Greek texts. So what does it mean to "have" a body?

This is not a question that interests Snell. Snell, in truth, cares little about bodies—his attention is focused on the soul. Once the Greeks discover this, or, rather, the distinction between body and soul, he speculates, they use *sōma* to cover everything that is not *psukhē*.[21] The integrated, living body thus falls back into just being there, as it has all along for Snell's critics, and Snell's dramatic gesture of withholding "the" body from the Greeks comes to a perfunctory end. While Snell's supporters have modified his claims over the years, they have concentrated on freeing Homeric disunity from the charge of primitivism and reframing it as "unity in multiplicity," leaving the fate of the body virtually untouched.[22] Neither Snell nor those sympathetic to his arguments have given much thought to how (what Snell sees as) the integrated, living body appears under the sign of the *sōma* in the late archaic and classical periods.[23]

---

[18] Snell 1953.1–22. Snell's views on this point are unchanged in the fourth German edition, published in 1975. On the meaning of *sōma* in Homer, see below.

[19] E.g., Dodds 1951.15–17; Vivante 1955; Koller 1958.276; Detienne 1973.46–47; Fränkel 1975.76; Laser 1983.3; Ferwerda 1986.111–12; Redfield 1994.175; Clarke 1999.115–19; De Hart 1999.357–58.

[20] See *Il.* 1.3–5. Vivante 1983 argues that one plausible candidate for describing the body in Homer is simply *autos*: what we call body is coextensive with the person until the moment of death.

[21] "Apparently [sc. *soma* and *psyche*] were evolved as complementary terms, and more likely than not it was *psyche* which first started on its course, perhaps under the influence of notions concerning the immortality of the soul . . . it may be inferred that, because the eschatological *psyche* had been correlated with the *soma* of the dead, the new *psyche*, the 'soul,' *demanding a body to suit it*, caused the term *soma* to be extended so that it was ultimately used also of the living body. But whatever the details of this evolution, the distinction between body and soul represents a 'discovery' which so impressed people's minds that it was thereafter accepted as self-evident, in spite of the fact that the relation between body and soul, and the nature of the soul itself, continued to be a topic of lively speculation" (Snell 1953.16–17, emphasis added).

[22] Homeric "unity in multiplicity": see Padel 1992.45–46 (the term is Norman Austin's). See also Bremmer 1983.66–69; Redfield 1985; Bolens 1999; 2000.55–59; Clarke 1999; Spatafora 1999. The thesis gains credibility from Jahn 1987. On the multiple "body" terms in Homer, see Vivante 1955.

[23] When Jean-Pierre Vernant, who accepts Snell's conclusions, speaks of the "discovery of the human body," he is referring to "a progressive conquest of its form . . . What is meant is evidently not a

Snell's controversial claims about the *sōma* are at once insightful and limited. Their limits are due, first, to the fact that the lexical evidence, albeit sparse before the fifth century, suggests that the word *sōma* had a wider semantic field than Snell allows. Limited, too, is the concept of the body that Snell declares missing in the Homeric poems, insofar as its absence denies a basic sense of self to the early Greeks.[24] By reopening the question of the body's historicity, we can move toward a more complex notion of what appears missing from Homer and other early Greek sources. Such an inquiry can, in turn, lead us to reconsider the role of the *sōma* not only in Snell's story but also in other genealogies of dualism that privilege *psukhē*. Such narratives largely concur in the assumption that the body is something self-evident that must be transcended. In contrast, I reject the idea of a self-evident, ahistorical body in order to explore the specific ways in which *sōma* is conceptualized in the classical period as a physical object that needs to be separated from the human and, more specifically, the ethical subject. By approaching the physical body not as something to be left behind but as an object of and an impetus to thought and imagination, we can begin to understand how it was generating ideas about the human in the fifth and fourth centuries. It is this conceptual productivity, together with its lasting consequences, that makes Snell's language of discovery insightful.

There are, of course, problems with Snell's model of historical change. Snell uses the trope of discovery to ground what he sees as the spiritual truth of the Western intellectual tradition—its grasp of the mind—in the Greek world, thereby making the Greeks our true ancestors. The teleology of his story now meets with a healthy distrust; the self he sees discovered in antiquity has been revealed to be an anachronistic projection, one that no longer even has a purchase on spiritual truth.[25] And yet, despite harsh criticism on a number of

---

question of the human body as an organic and physiological reality on which the self relies for its support" (1991e.159), though he elsewhere credits Greek medicine for contributing to the objectification of the body in anatomical and physiological terms (1991b.28; see also Detienne 1973.46). Bolens 1999 recognizes differing "logics of the body" in Homer and Plato but does not trace the relationship between them.

[24] That is, Snell fails to distinguish a basic human self-awareness from the specific kind of self-awareness that develops in certain quarters of the Greco-Roman world. For critical responses to Snell's argument that the early Greeks lack a unified sense of self, see the next note. The idea that all humans share a basic notion of mind-body (and/or soul-body) dualism has been defended in recent years on the basis of evidence from both anthropology (e.g., Lambek 1998) and cognitive psychology (e.g., Richert and Harris 2006, with further bibliography), though these accounts leave room for the cultural and historical factors that give different dualisms their specific shape (including what is often just called Western dualism, which on my argument requires the physical body).

[25] Half a century ago it was not uncommon for scholars to chart dramatic changes (usually "improvements") to the idea of the self between Homer and Plato without necessarily following Snell's route. See, e.g., Dodds 1951; Adkins 1960; Fränkel 1975. In recent years, however, part of the critique of Snell has involved downplaying or denying diachronic change: see, e.g., Halliwell 1990; C. Gill 1996a; Porter and Buchan 2004. See also Williams 1993, who calls Snell's general argument "a systematic failure" (28–29) but does see a difference between the concept of the subject found in Homer and tragedy and that found in Plato and Aristotle: the philosophers are distinguished by

fronts, Snell's presence is as strong as ever.[26] The questions he raises about the Greek subject do not go away. For, insofar as "the Greek past," as Bernard Williams once wrote, "is specially the past of modernity," these questions force us to keep surveying the ground on which we encounter the Greeks and reassessing what is at stake in that encounter for a present often impatient with history.[27] It is true that by asking the Greek past to tell us about ourselves we increase the risk of distorting it. But, when we insist too much on the Otherness of the Greeks, we run a similar risk of distortion. My aim here is to unsettle our sense of something so familiar that it has remained largely external to our critical apparatus, that is, the physical body. In so doing, I am neither defending that body as a found object, whether philosophical or scientific, nor casting it as the construction of culture. I prefer to see it, rather, as a uniquely powerful "conceptual object," a term I explain in greater detail below. By attending to the emergence of this object, we can perhaps recuperate some of the boldness of Snell's approach: his commitment to substantial changes in how subjectivity was imagined in the classical Greek world and his belief in the cascading implications of those changes for subsequent centuries, right up to the present.

I would like to stress again that what I am calling the physical body does not map onto the body that Snell thought was absent from the Homeric poems. The misalignment of these bodies is due in part to my interest in embedding the *sōma* more deeply in a history of ideas and practices. More fundamentally, however, I depart from Snell in my understanding of what it takes to "see" the body that comes to be taken for granted in the West, and here is where the symptom becomes central to this book. I thus use the rest of the introduction to explain in more detail what I am doing with the symptom and what I mean when I say that the physical body emerges at a specific historical moment. I begin by orienting my approach to symptoms in relationship to scholarship in the field of ancient medicine and science. I then briefly sketch how my project intersects with recent work on "the body" in classical antiquity. Finally, I return to Snell's claims about the *sōma* in order to set up a different framework for

---

their attempt to fit human ethical interests to the larger world. Williams nevertheless rejects narratives of change that privilege notions of agency, the will, or moral responsibility. For criticisms of Snell's view of the Greek self as anachronistic, see esp. Williams 1993.21–49 and C. Gill 1996a, who attributes to the Greeks a notion of identity in which psychological processes are seen as "functional components of an organic (or inorganic) system, and not as constituting a distinct category (that of the 'mental') as in Cartesian theory" (43, 34–41, on Snell's debts to Descartes, Kant, and Hegel). For other critiques of Snell along these lines, see Sharples 1983; Gaskin 1990; Halliwell 1990; Pelliccia 1995.17–27. Other scholars have defended the "fragmented" subject of Homeric poetry: see Padel 1992 and 1995, working from an anthropological perspective, and Porter and Buchan 2004, who, placing fragmentation under the sign of Lacanian psychoanalysis, argue that all but the fantasy of a unified self is foreclosed for both ancients and moderns.

[26] The final pages of Kurke 1999, for example, frame her ambitious project as a "materialist critique" of Snell's work. She argues that Snell's "seductive periodization" and belief in "authentic and pre-existent subjectivity" remain influential (335–36). See also Porter and Buchan 2004.7–8.

[27] Williams 1993.3. See also Snell 1953.258–63.

understanding the development of dualism by rethinking the problem of the *sōma* in the Homeric poems. Elaborating how the problem posed by the Homeric *sōma* becomes the problem not only of having a body but also of being an ethical subject is the task of the remaining chapters.

Seeing through Symptoms

The language of discovery is not Snell's alone. Discovery was for many years—and, in some circles, continues to be—a core motif in histories of early Greek science and philosophy. These histories followed how the Greeks succeeded in recognizing the nature of the physical world, long obscured by superstition and myth. In a similar vein, historians of medicine celebrated the authors of early medical texts for offering naturalistic explanations of disease without enlisting gods or *daimones*.[28] Rudolph Siegel, for example, in his account of "the evolution of the diagnostic art," credits the classical Greek medical writers with the discovery of the symptom, that is, "a phenomenon constituting a departure from a normal bodily constitution or function."[29] Because such a definition depends on the Greeks' knowledge of bodily constitutions and functions, it is not a stretch to place the physical body itself within the reality grasped through the "Greek miracle," whose history has been described by Karl Popper as "a splendid story . . . almost too good to be true."[30]

In recent years, however, the Greek miracle has, indeed, come to seem too good to be true, as we have become less comfortable conflating the ideas and

---

[28] The gods are never mentioned as causes of disease in the extant medical treatises. The author of *On the Sacred Disease* entertains the idea that one can be defiled *not* by a god but by "something else" (ὑφ᾽ ἑτέρου) and, hence, may require purification (1, Li 6.364 = 9,10–13 Jouanna). But it is not clear if he makes the claim in earnest or if it is part of his polemic against magico-religious healers. Moreover, he distinguishes defilement from disease and emphatically denies that a god or "something daemonic" can cause disease (1, Li 6.364 = 9,8–10 Jouanna; 11, Li 6.382 = 22,3–4 Jouanna); see also *Aer.* 22 (Li 2.80 = 241,5–9 Jouanna). Remarks that diseases are divine or might have "something divine" (τὸ θεῖον) in them do not imply agents. The gods are very rarely mentioned as potential healers: at *Vict.* IV 87 (Li 6.642 = 218,21–22 Joly-Byl), in addition to praying, one should also "help oneself"; *Morb. Sacr.* 1 (Li 6.364 = 9,13–15 Jouanna) implies that the gods should heal τὰ ἁμαρτήματα, "moral errors." Cf. *Virg.* 3 (Li 8.468 = 24,7–10 Lami), with Lami 2007.52–54: women wrongly thank Artemis for their release from the disease of virgins. On the place of the gods and the sacred in the *Oath*, see von Staden 1996; 2008, esp. 429–36. In short, while it may be true that "Hippocratic medicine does not rule out divine intervention" (Horstmanshoff and Stol 2004.6), the medical writers leave little room for it, "effectively, and in some cases deliberately, block[ing] any move to explain diseases—both particular types of diseases and individual incidences of them—by invoking divine or supernatural agencies" (G. Lloyd 1987.11); see also Hankinson 1998b.16–17, 34.

[29] Siegel 1964.299. Siegel takes his definition from the *New Century Dictionary* (London, 1927). For work in a similar vein, see, e.g., Riese 1944; Major 1957; Jandolo 1967. Cf. Joly 1966; Edelstein 1967d. "Whiggish" notions of medical history are now rare, but see von Staden 1992c and Flemming 2000.3–28 on other forms of presentism in the study of ancient science.

[30] Popper 1969.149.

practices associated with ancient inquiries into the natural world with those of early modern science and the present day. Scholars have shifted their focus from the physical theories of the early Greek philosophers to epistemology, politics, and ethics; they have paid more attention to the social and historical conditions of early Greek philosophy.[31] Historians of medicine have been engaged in what is arguably an even more sweeping intellectual renaissance. They have challenged the medical writers' grasp of anatomy and physiology, stressing instead continuities with older models.[32] They have highlighted the "divine" elements in ancient medicine and reevaluated the medical writers' self-distancing from traditional healers as a rhetorical stratagem in an agonistic "medical marketplace."[33] Such research has persuasively shown that the medical writers, while lively polemicists, in many cases provided new justification for conventional wisdom. The constructed and "fantastic" nature of what the medical writers believe about the body is particularly evident in their ideas about the female body, which dovetail neatly with long-held cultural stereotypes about female inferiority and women's childbearing function.[34] Even when these writers describe things that look familiar, such as the *facies Hippocratica* or "Hippocratic fingers," we are no longer confident that we see the same things as they did. Seeing in both cases is a highly motivated act that outstrips the phenomenon in the desire to grasp and manipulate an underlying reality.

Changes in the field of ancient medicine, as well as in the study of ancient philosophy more generally, have struck a serious blow to the once-celebrated positivism and secularity of the Greek miracle. Historians have thus been led to reexamine the ancient thinkers' methodologies for criteria to distinguish between a mythic worldview and one that, despite some modification, continues

---

[31] Long 1999b.5–10; G. Lloyd 2005.13–15; Naddaf 2005. Cf. Graham 2006, focused on the physical theories and unabashedly enthusiastic about miracles, intellectual leaps, and teleology (e.g., 2006.98, 106, 299). On social and political conditions, see below, n.76.

[32] This renaissance owes much to the work of G.E.R. Lloyd. Lloyd sees Greek medicine and science as distinct from magico-religious healing: see esp. Lloyd 1979; 1987. Yet he also challenges the notion of a rupture between two vast "mentalities" and seeks lines of continuity between the archaic and classical periods (Lloyd 1990). On these continuities, see also Joly 1966; Bratescu 1975; Jouanna 1988a; 1990a; von Staden 1992a; 1992b; Laskaris 1999; 2002; Hoessly 2001.247–313. For overviews of changes to the field, see G. Lloyd 1992, esp. 129–32; Nutton 2002; Horstmanshoff and Stol 2004.1–10; van der Eijk 2005b.1–8.

[33] On the divine in Hippocratic medicine: H. Miller 1953; Thivel 1975; Ducatillon 1990; Oberhelman 1990; Prioreschi 1992; von Staden 1996; Hankinson 1998b; Bratescu 2002; Collins 2003.24–26; van der Eijk 2004; 2005b.45–73. For the argument that medicine's success depends on the rhetorical skill of its advocates, see esp. A. Hanson 1991.81–87, emphasizing the fit between physical explanations and the ability of the Hippocratic physician to intervene. On medicine in relation to diverse healing practices, see G. Lloyd 1979.37–49; 1983.119–35; 1990.30–31; Nutton 1992 (introducing the term "medical marketplace"); 1995.

[34] On "fantastical" elements, see Joly 1966; G. Lloyd 1967.30–31; 1979.146–60; 1983; 1992.122–24. On medical representations of the female body, see below, pp. 185–87. See also Flemming 2000.3–9, cautioning that we cannot gauge whether ancient physicians had the same power to influence these stereotypes as their eighteenth- and nineteenth-century counterparts.

to be characterized as rational. Several factors have come to the fore: the use of proof, signs, and inferential reasoning in fifth-century authors; these authors' commitment to public argument and the criticism of opposing views; their concerns about epistemology and error; and their interest in systematization and explanation.[35] In this context, the medical writers have been deemed particularly relevant to the lively, cosmopolitan intellectual milieu of the classical Greek world—"too important to be left exclusively to the history of medicine."[36] One reason for their wider relevance lies in the use they make of symptoms. Indeed, the medical symptom has benefited considerably from the increased attention in recent years to methodological questions and sign reasoning, sometimes being pegged as an important precursor to the logico-inferential sign in Aristotelian semiotics.[37]

There are, however, several limitations to a strictly semiotic approach to the symptom. Reviewing these limitations will allow me to situate my approach to the symptom in relationship to recent work on the medical writers. First, such an approach has entailed a narrow focus on cases where the language of witnessing and proof—for example, *sēmeion/sēmēion*, "sign"; *marturion*, "witness"; and *tekmērion*, "proof"—is explicit. Yet, in practice, such language is quite rare.[38] In fact, the word *sumptōma*, "symptom," is not found in the extant fifth- and fourth-century medical texts, nor is there a word that "symptom" could be said to supersede when it does take on a medical cast in Hellenistic and imperial-age texts.[39] In most cases, the medical writers simply use demonstrative pronouns (τόδε, τάδε, τοῦτο, ταῦτα, τούτων τι) to refer to the bodily phenomena from which they build inferences. They are constantly creating inferences,

---

[35] For a definition of the rationality of Greek medicine in these terms, see van der Eijk 2005b.9 n.17. See also, on the rationality of early Greek philosophy, G. Lloyd 1967.32–34; Long 1999b.13–14; Graham 2006.10–13.

[36] Thomas 2000.24. See also Jaeger 1944, esp. 7–15. On the intellectual milieu of the fifth century, see esp. Thomas 1993; 2000, esp. 1–27, 249–69. On the public sphere of medicine, see Jouanna 1999.177–285; Craik 2001a.81–82; G. Lloyd and Sivin 2002.118–33; Schiefsky 2005a.5–71, esp. 38–46. Not every physician, of course, was interested in intellectual discourse or promulgated it. As social historians have stressed, the physician's status was often that of a simple craftsperson: see esp. Temkin 1953; Horstmanshoff 1990; Nutton 1992.

[37] See Diller 1932; Perilli 1991; 1994; G. Manetti 1993.70–91; 1994; Thomas 2000.168–212; Fausti 2002.

[38] Di Benedetto 1986.118 n.2; Langholf 1997–2004.914.

[39] The word appears once in the Hippocratic Corpus, at *Dec.* 6 (Li 9.234 = 27,14 Heiberg), but the treatise where it is used almost certainly dates from the late Hellenistic period. See also *Ep.* 16 (Li 9.346 = 72,19 Smith), another Hellenistic text. At *Flat.* 3 (Li 6.94 = 106,2–3 Jouanna), συμπτωμάτων (M) is a *varia lectio*: editors have almost uniformly adopted the reading of A, πάντων (Littré, Nelson, Jouanna; Ermerins emended to συμπάντων). The word πάθημα, particularly in the plural, comes closest to the later meaning of σύμπτωμα: it appears roughly sixty times in fifth- and fourth-century medical writing: see, e.g., *Epid.* I 2 (Li 2.606 = 182,1 Kühlewein); *Hum.* 8 (Li 5.488 = 78 Jones); *Mul.* I 1 (Li 8.10 = 88,12 Grensemann); *Prog.* 1 (Li 2.110 = 193,7 Alex). The plural ἀλγήματα can also denote the patient's sufferings: *Aff.* 27 (Li 6.240 = 48 Potter); *Flat.* 9 (Li 6.104 = 115,10 Jouanna).

turning the seen into knowledge about the unseen and using beliefs about the unseen to interpret the seen. But we miss out on much of this work if our criteria are lexical or if we limit ourselves to writers who are self-conscious about how they know what they know. Symptoms can serve as nodes of methodological reflection. Yet they also densely populate medicine's more mundane reaches.

A semiotic approach is also restricted in that it encourages scholars to analyze how the medical writers make inferences at the cost of neglecting what it is exactly that symptoms allow them to see. That the medical writers take such an interest in inferential reasoning is surely worth noting. But symptoms, precisely because they are perceived as alien without revealing the source of their otherness, provoke all kinds of inferences about invisible causes.[40] These inferences rely on both innate cognitive intuitions about causality and sociocultural and contextual frameworks of interpretation. In Peircean semiotics, they are classed as abductions.[41] Whereas in deduction, for example, each claim follows necessarily from prior claims, abduction involves a conjecture about the relationship of a particular event to a general rule.[42] Given that abduction involves an inferential leap, it is as possible for someone speculating about the hidden causes of disease to refer symptoms to unseen agents as it is for him or her to offer a naturalizing explanation.[43] Indeed, as recent cognitive-based approaches to religion have emphasized, the inference of agency is a likely response for people to have to symptoms and similar phenomena.[44] Moreover, as Elaine Scarry has argued,

---

[40] See further below, pp. 46–47, on the relationship between the perceptual indeterminacy of symptoms and inference.

[41] On Peirce, see Silverman 1983.14–25. See also G. Manetti 1993.48–51, discussing abduction in the medical writers.

[42] Peirce famously distinguishes deduction, induction, and abduction thus: in deduction, the rule is "all the beans from this bag are white," the case is "these beans are from this bag," which leads to the result, "these beans are white"; in induction, the case is "these beans are from this bag," the result is "these beans are white," leading to the rule, "all the beans from this bag are white"; in abduction, the rule is "all the beans from this bag are white," the result is "these beans are white," leading to the case, "these beans are from this bag."

[43] The anthropologist Alfred Gell defines an agent as "one who has the capacity to initiate causal events in his/her vicinity, which cannot be ascribed to the current state of the physical cosmos, but only to a special category of mental states; that is, intentions" (1998.19). On early Greek concepts of intention, see Williams 1993, esp. 21–55. Note that in conventional semiotics, symptoms are defined by the *absence* of intention: Sebeok 1976.124–27.

[44] The literature for cognitive approaches to religion is large and growing rapidly: for recent overviews, see Boyer 2001; J. Barrett 2007. I am not suggesting that abductions of agency, discussed further in the next chapter, are *more* natural, that is, more intuitive, than naturalizing explanations. Such a position threatens to reinstate a teleological account of the transition from religion (primitive) to science (intellectually complex). But, more important, it is an oversimplification. Recent research suggests—though the evidence is far from decisive—that, in the face of symptoms, people have a tendency to infer both unseen agents and natural causes (Keil et al. 1999). The activation of these inferential models depends not only on the symptoms (e.g., epileptic symptoms may be particularly conducive to agent-based explanations) but also on prevailing cultural frameworks. That is, *both* agent-based inferences and naturalizing ones are open to cultural elaboration, and that

one of the experiences that appears especially likely to make the mind imagine unseen agents and symbols of agency is pain.[45] Although we have only limited knowledge of magico-religious interpretations of symptoms in ancient Greece, the evidence that we do have exploits the explanatory force of gods, *daimones*, and heroes endowed with intentions, desires, emotions, and ideas about justice and purity—that is, social and ethical agents.[46] If we dismiss these agent-based explanations of symptoms as philosophically uninteresting (i.e., mere superstition) or turn them into sterile markers of Greek Otherness, we risk overlooking what gets lost when these explanations are challenged by new ways of imagining the unseen. Even more important, we fail to register the very strangeness of an unseen world understood in physical terms. Yet it may be because this world is not immediately intuitive in the cultural context of the mid- to late fifth century that the medical writers spend so much energy implicating it through inferential reasoning in the visible, tangible world.

One of the major claims of this book, as I have indicated, is that by explaining disease in terms of the physical body, rather than daemonic agents, medical writers and physicians are facilitating that body's emergence as a conceptual object. If we are going to see this process, we need to denaturalize the idea of natural causality. To this end, it is worth recalling Michael Frede's account of how the concept of a cause as "something which in some sense does something or other so as to produce or bring about an effect" develops in the ancient world.[47] Such a concept depends

> on the assumption that for everything to be explained there is something which plays with reference to it a role analogous to that which the person responsible plays with reference to what has gone wrong; i.e., the extension of the use of "*aition*" across the board is only intelligible on the assumption that with reference to everything there is something which by doing something or other is responsible for it.[48]

---

cultural work, in turn, determines specific acts of interpretation, perhaps overriding in some cases what may be more "implicitly" held theories of biological phenomena (Keil et al. 1999.289). On the cultural webs of meaning that inform the interpretation of symptoms, see also Good and DelVecchio Good 1981; Kleinman 1988.

[45] Scarry 1985, esp. 15–18.

[46] By "social," I mean these agents have intentions that are comprehensible within a human community; I use the adjective "ethical" to indicate agents (usually divine) who could be seen as upholding social norms and laws: though some notion of ethical is implicit in the idea of the social, there appears to be a difference between divine-daemonic agents who respond to transgressions against them and those divine-daemonic agents who are entrusted by the human community with upholding notions of justice and a social good. See, on social agency in Greece, Collins 2003.37–44. On social agency and intuitive psychology more generally: Gell 1998, esp. 4–11, 16–23; Boyer 2001.120–31.

[47] M. Frede 1987.125. Frede credits the Stoics with first theorizing the "active" cause. Vegetti 1999.276–79 makes the medical writers central to an earlier process of substituting impersonal causes for personal agents in the fifth century. See also Mansfeld 1980.379–81.

[48] M. Frede 1987.132.

Much depends here on the weight of the "thing" in Frede's "something." There are plenty of things in archaic poetry, both inside and outside the person, but they are deeply lodged in networks of intentionality, particularly when harm is involved. In medical writing, despite the remarkable variation in style, audience, and content we find under the rubric of the Hippocratic Corpus,[49] explanations of symptoms turn primarily on a struggle between different things inside the physical body, stuffs like "the sweet" or bile or "the hot," each capable of acting and suffering in a specific and strictly impersonal way (e.g., moistening, heating).[50] These things, together with the things outside the physical body, assume responsibility for causing damage. Reading the medical writers with care, we observe natural causality being put to work again and again.

It might not be so easy, however, for something to take over for someone. The difficulty is particularly acute when that someone is a god or a *daimōn*, agents whose intentions are uncommonly efficacious. Because gods and *daimones* achieve what they want so easily, their weapons are not so much instruments of power as symbols of unfettered agency, which mark "daemonic advantage over the human: that power to hurt, that aggressiveness."[51] What happens, then, when this power is vested in things? One possible answer is that it fragments. The result is that while disease continues to be objectified in medical writing— it is often closely associated with corrupted humors; it has a *phusis*—it is primarily understood as a process that is precipitated by external causes before taking hold within the physical body: what is passive in one encounter (e.g., tissue, bile) becomes, once damaged, part of the problem. The gods' "power to hurt" thus has to be built up through a series of events in which stuffs inside the physical body are systematically turned against life: daemonic agency breaks down into a series of mechanisms. This fragmentation, I suggest, frustrates the clean transfer of responsibility from the personal to the impersonal: cause is no longer synonymous with an intention but is distributed over a series of

[49] This variation has generated unease about lumping the medical texts together: see Laskaris 2002.2 n.5; van der Eijk 2005b.22–23. For an overview of attempts to organize medical writing according to genre and subgenre, see Wittern 1998.17–22. See also van Groningen 1958; Maloney, Potter, and Frohn 1979; Thivel 1981.119–51; Pigeaud 1988; Kollesch 1991; van der Eijk 1997. A. Hanson 1996, esp. 304–11, looks at the compositional contexts of the Hippocratic texts. Nevertheless, variation is a relative term: the perception of similarity is produced against the backdrop of what is different. For my purposes, it is often accurate to speak of medicine vis-à-vis magico-religious healing or the inquiry into nature or philosophical ethics. I consider internal diversity in the corpus in more detail in chapters 3 and 4.

[50] In addition to the extant texts and fragments, we have the Anonymous Londinensis papyrus, a doxography of late fifth- and fourth-century BCE medical opinions that was probably written in the first century CE and based on a fourth-century BCE Peripatetic history of medicine: see D. Manetti 1999 for further discussion. The author divides theories of disease into those that blame residues of digestion and those based on the idea that because our bodies are composed of a combination of elements, disease is "due to the elements" (4.26–28 = 6 Diels; 14.6–11 = 20–21 Diels). Extant treatises largely reflect the latter approach (though both theories assume that what *phusis* fails to assimilate becomes hostile). See also the disease theory outlined at Pl. *Ti.* 82a–86a.

[51] Padel 1992.152.

micro-events. Moreover, even if specific things are called *aitioi*, such as the brain in *On the Sacred Disease*, there is a sense that blame fails to stick to things whose antipathy toward the person at any moment is physical, rather than emotional and grounded in intersubjective relations.

The idea that the physical body both assumes causal responsibility for symptoms and yet deflects blame gives rise to another of this book's major claims—namely, that the physical body becomes an ethical responsibility for the embodied person or, more accurately, for persons believed to be capable of exercising mastery over themselves. What this means is that the emergence of the physical body, far from negating the moral framework of disease, as is sometimes supposed, transforms the field of social and ethical relations in which the person is embedded and, indeed, the very identity of the person as a social, ethical agent.

The importance of the person exposes one last limitation in strictly semiotic approaches to the symptom—namely, that these approaches have tended to downplay the fact that medical signs most often give access to the inside of a human being. By inside, I do not mean the place where a Homeric hero hides winged words, or even an anatomical cutaway. I am speaking, rather, of a space largely beyond what the physician can see and, crucially, below the threshold of consciousness, a space I refer to as the cavity.[52] The medical writers understand this as contained space, often designating it with the preposition "in" (ἐν) and putting weight on the related notions of surface, orifice, influx, efflux, concealment, and revelation. Even a cursory reading of the Hippocratic Corpus yields abundant evidence of these writers' fascination with the cavity's silent, automated workings.

It is both the silence and the automation of the cavity that makes it so uncanny. First, the silence of the physical body is the heir to the dangerous silence of the diseases unleashed when Pandora opens her jar. The reason symptoms feel daemonic even when they erupt from within us is that we are largely unaware of what goes on inside the cavity, allowing trouble to develop without our knowledge. Symptoms are always belated. They appear only after "the healthy" has been mastered by "the diseased," as we are told by the author of *On Regimen*, who claims to have invented the "pre-symptoms" wielded by Plutarch some centuries later in his argument against Hesiod.[53]

---

[52] "Cavity" roughly translates the medical writers' term κοιλίη, which is used of the whole chest cavity or, in a more restricted sense, of the belly: on both senses, see Jouanna 2003.258. I adopt it here to designate all of the *sōma*'s inner space.

[53] *Vict.* I 2 (Li 6.472 = 124,28–126,3 Joly-Byl); cf. III 69 (Li 6.606 = 200,28–32 Joly-Byl); *Art.* 11 (Li 6.20–22 = 238,15–20 Jouanna). The idea that symptoms are always belated, together with the idea of imperceptible inner space, is one of the main elements that distinguishes this book from Ruth Padel's excellent studies of interiority in the archaic and classical periods (1992; 1995). Padel writes, "That you could have a virus, or madness, and no one know, is not a concept available in ancient Greece" (1995.35; see also 43). For Padel, denying the modern notion of latency is one way to establish the historical specificity of ancient concepts of madness. Yet it is untrue that the concept of a hidden disease was not available to the ancient Greeks. Of course, we have to be wary of collapsing distinctions between, say, cancer cells and the things inside the body in the medical writers.

Symptoms are daemonic, too, because they are messengers from a foreign world, a world automated by forces that we are unable to control simply by intending or exhorting or supplicating: not only are we incapable of moving our heart in the way we move our legs, but we cannot check our bile as an Iliadic warrior can check his *thumos*. We can hardly be persuaded, as Aristotle observes, not to get hot or feel hunger (*EN* 1113b26–30). And while we may know intuitively how to cool or feed ourselves—though the physicians will contest this—in other cases we are subjected to symptoms precisely because we fail to understand their causes. If we were one day put in charge of our livers, Lewis Thomas once noted, we would soon be dead.[54] We need experts to interpret our symptoms and to counter the forces that produce them.

But however estranged we are from the cavity and all that it contains, we remain affected by it, bound by it, perhaps even created by it. Elizabeth Grosz writes:

> The body is a most peculiar "thing," for it is never quite reducible to being merely a thing; nor does it ever quite manage to rise above the status of thing. Thus it is both a thing and a nonthing, an object, but an object which somehow contains or coexists with an interiority, an object able to take itself and others as subjects, a unique kind of object not reducible to other objects. Human bodies, indeed all animate bodies, stretch and extend the notion of physicality that dominates the physical sciences, for animate bodies are objects necessarily different from other objects; they are materialities that are uncontainable in physicalist terms alone. If bodies are objects or things, they are like no others, for they are the centers of perspective, insight, reflection, desire, agency.[55]

The physical body is, thus, no ordinary object of inquiry, no neutral producer of signs. Rather, it is a privileged site for the translation of the inquiry into nature into human terms. On this terrain, the shift of responsibility from agents to things matters deeply. It matters not only because health and life are at stake but also because the things in question at some level *belong* to a person. But what is the proper place of the person in naturalizing explanations of the symptom? Where does he meet the physical body? These questions loom large as we explore what symptoms mean for the subjects through whom they occur.

Here, then, is the approach I adopt toward symptoms in naturalizing Greek medicine. I understand them, on the one hand, as a means of seeing that proceeds through inferential leaps from phenomena into an unseen world; and, on the other hand, as points of passage into an unseen world that has been reimagined and, more specifically, reimagined in relationship to the person. In other

---

Nevertheless, that wariness should extend in the other direction as well, as I have indicated: the danger of presentism finds its complement in the danger of establishing historical difference by simply negating the present.

[54] Cited in Leder 1990.48.

[55] Grosz 1994.xi.

words, what is seen is as important as how it is seen; the how of seeing is crucial to understanding the nature of what is seen.

So what is this unseen reality? In addition to macrocosmic webs of power, it encompasses tissues, bones, and sinews; the cavity; the things inside it; how and why they act and suffer; the overall nature of the physical body; and the concatenation of events that together represent the disease. I do not want to deny that Greek physicians, by thinking in these terms, are on to something fundamental about what I am happy to call the physical reality of disease. Yet I am not interested in defending a neopositivist position that naturalizing interpretations of the symptom are correct. I am advocating, rather, a third way between the old rationalizing histories and the more recent emphasis on the cultural provenance of corporeal signs. I argue that classical medical interpretations of symptoms allow physicians and their patients to "see" a cluster of things and ideas that constitute the physical body.

How should we understand this seeing? Scholars have challenged and complicated the idea of discovering the body, but they have not thrown it out altogether.[56] Snell believed that the mind needed to be discovered because it was immaterial, beyond the boundaries of the terrestrial world. The physical body, we might say, is largely submerged in the hidden regions of that world. What these regions look like and what goes on there can be glimpsed only through clues and fragments—effluvia, glimpses of the innards through wounds or lesions, sensations that communicate trouble imprecisely. Hence, the physical body is primarily seen through what one Hippocratic author calls the "vision of the mind" (ἡ τῆς γνώμης ὄψις, *Art.* 11, Li 6.20 = 237,11–13 Jouanna).[57] So crucial is this idea of mental seeing to the learned Greek medical tradition that even when, in third-century BCE Alexandria, physicians become better acquainted with the anatomical body through systematic human dissection, they often end up treating it as another surface concealing even smaller parts visible only to reason.[58] The prominence of mental seeing in the learned medical tradition

[56] Studies of the Hellenistic anatomists, for example, still acknowledge their contributions to modern models of the body: see von Staden 1989. Such work need not be incompatible with attention to historically embedded ways of seeing, as von Staden's scholarship amply demonstrates.

[57] Although significant for contemplative metaphysics, the idea of the vision of the mind seems to have first appeared in medical texts: see also *Flat.* 3 (Li 6.94 = 106,9–10 Jouanna); *Vict.* I 4 (Li 6.474–76 = 126,28–128,3 Joly-Byl). Cf. Democr. (DK68) B11, with the comments of Jouanna 1988b.178 on the fragment's relationship to *Art.* 11. Andrea Nightingale, seeking "the foundational construction of theoretical philosophy in its intellectual and its cultural context" (2004.7), neglects the medical writers, leading her to posit too strong a break between fourth-century philosophy and its predecessors. Certainly Plato will endow the concept of "seeing with the mind" with new meaning. Yet it is misleading to claim that, "There is no 'vision' of truth in . . . philosophical texts of the early period" (33). The importance of vision in Greek medicine is most apparent in a comparative context: see Kuriyama 1999, who draws a contrast with the significance of touch in ancient Chinese medicine. On visuality more generally in Greek culture, see Stewart 1997.14–23.

[58] On the "anatomical urge" in Greek medicine, see Kuriyama 1999.116–29. On the prehistory of systematic dissection, see Edelstein 1967e; G. Lloyd 1975a; Mansfeld 1975; von Staden 1989.141,

reminds us that the physical body is not a static, bounded object independent of a viewer and her (psychological, disciplinary, cultural) habits of seeing but, rather, a constellation of phenomena filtered through ideas about power, causality, and the unseen, phenomena that are often isolated in order to be investigated and manipulated.

Given both the thingness of the physical body and the nature of its materialization, it is perhaps best understood as a kind of conceptual object, an "epistemic thing," to adopt a term introduced by the historian of science Hans-Jörg Rheinberger.[59] We might see it as the prototype of a range of objects within the Western scientific tradition that flicker into perceptibility and are objectified against a horizon of expectations, then gain a foothold through textual transmission and institutionalized practices of inquiry and experimentation.[60] We must, of course, be cautious about projecting later conditions of seeing into the past. Words like empirical or experimental are often of limited usefulness— "experience" is a loaded term.[61] What interests me, in any event, is something very basic, something presupposed by scholarship on the later scientific tradition but downplayed in recent work on ancient medicine, with its focus on the divine and sociocultural context. It is simply this: the formation of a framework within which the *sōma* is described, explained, and manipulated *qua* natural thing, composite and changeable, yet sustained by the powers of heating, cooling, growing, disintegrating, absorbing, excreting—powers organized in the service of life. Many aspects of this body have always been available to the senses. Yet sensory perception alone has not determined its conceptual unfolding. It is

---

with n.6; 1992e; Annoni and Barras 1993. The idea of things "seen with the mind" is formalized in Hellenistic medicine as Erasistratus's τὰ λόγῳ θεωρητά (frr. 76–77 Garofalo).

[59] Rheinberger 1997.11–23, and esp. 28–31. See also Daston 2000 and J. Taylor 2005 (with further bibliography) on both contemporary Western and cross-cultural practices of materializing the body and other natural objects.

[60] For the importance of institutions to the survival of conceptual objects, see Latour 1999.145–73. On the generation of scientific objects, see also the comments at Csordas 1990.38.

[61] The debate over the empirical foundations of the inquiry into nature dates from Bacon's New Science. It culminated in the past century with the clash between Popper and Kirk, on which see G. Lloyd 1967; see also G. Lloyd 1979.129–46, reviewing the evidence for empiricism in the inquiry into nature. Some medical writers do develop the idea that knowledge ought to arise from and be tested against phenomena. Moreover, however theory-laden the concepts or however overriding the desire for coherence in medicine, the treatment of the physical body as a site of observation and praxis is crucial to how that body is conceptualized. At the same time, the desire of some medical writers to offer empirical evidence in support of their claims does not license us to collapse the difference between their practices of seeing and those of modern laboratories: see G. Lloyd 1979.146– 69, esp. 151: "The drawback, in this field of inquiry [i.e., empirical research], was that their investigations were not open-ended, but designed specifically to provide support for theories that appear to have been adopted usually on the basis of general, often philosophical, considerations and arguments." Lloyd does see a growing open-endedness in the Hellenistic and imperial periods. But cf. von Staden 1975.179–85 on the conditions that are conducive to experimentation at Alexandria: his analysis of the Empiricists' rejection of experimentation undermines teleological views of its history (185–93). For two recent discussions of the "scientific" nature of ancient science, see G. Lloyd 2004.12–23; Graham 2006.1–18, 93–106, 294–307.

precisely because the physical body is as much an object of mental vision as it is of the senses that it is itself so conceptually fertile, capable of producing new narratives and transforming existing ones.

The Physical Imagination

If this book departs from previous studies of the medical symptom because of its focus on the physical body and the embodied subject, it is the symptom, with its relationship to an unseen interior that distinguishes it from recent work on "the" body in classical antiquity. Scholarship on the ancient Greek body has been strongly influenced by research on the ideologies of the classical Greek city-states, especially Athens, as well as by the escalation of interest in the body and sexuality across the disciplines.[62] In his influential genealogy of the "democratic body," for example, David Halperin points to Solon's alleged elimination of debt bondage, as well as to cultural anxiety about passive homosexuality, in order to argue that the early Athenian *polis* used ideals of corporeal integrity and autarchy, rather than wealth or lineage, as the qualification for enfranchisement.[63] Halperin's claim is part of an influential line of research that has focused attention on how political actors in the classical period are defined through the gendered body: Froma Zeitlin's work on the performance and transgression of gender in tragedy and comedy; Nicole Loraux's studies of how the Athenian imaginary depends on a vulnerable, feminized body; the research of Leslie Kurke, Victoria Wohl, and others on the ways in which ideals of corporeal integrity operate at the juncture of aristocratic and democratic ideology.[64] Scholars

[62] On the latter, see, e.g., Halperin, Winkler, and Zeitlin 1990; Porter 1999a.

[63] Halperin 1990. See also Winkler 1990a; 1990b.45–70; Hunter 1992; Bassi 1998; Humphreys 1999; Sissa 1999. For the rights of the citizen vis-à-vis the *sōma*, see Dem. 22.55. The slave, conversely, is not master of his body: Ar. *Pl.* 6; neither is a woman: A. *Pr.* 859; E. *Med.* 232–34. These sources are all Athenian, but the concerns about autonomy they highlight surface in non-Athenian sources as well (e.g., Democritus: see below, chapter 5).

[64] See the works by Loraux in the bibliography, esp. Loraux 1995 and 1997. Loraux appropriates the psychoanalytic notion of the imaginary to describe the schemas and images mobilized by members of a given culture to organize their experience. Tragic bodies: Zeitlin 1996, esp. 123–284, 341–74. See also Loraux 1987; Murnaghan 1988; Faranda 1993; Serghidou 1997; Worman 1997; 1999; 2000; Bassi 1998; Hawley 1998; Cuny 2002; Rehm 2002.168–214; Crippa 2006; Holmes 2008. Comic bodies: Zeitlin 1996.375–416; Fletcher 1999; Foley 2000; Stehle 2002; Piqueux 2006. On embodied aristocratic ideals: Kurke 1999, esp. 142–51, 275–95; Wohl 2002; see also Hawhee 2004. On the semiotics of gendered bodies, see Worman 2002 and, for the imperial period, Gleason 1990; 1995. Although scholarship on the gendered body in the classical world predates Foucault, Foucault's argument that the categories "homosexuality" and "heterosexuality" are culturally constructed helped to popularize Kenneth Dover's division of bodies into penetrating (active) and penetrated (passive) and spurred new debate about gender and desire. For sympathetic readings of Foucault, see Halperin 1990 and Winkler 1990b; see also the essays in Halperin, Winkler, and Zeitlin 1990. Cf. Richlin 1993, challenging the idea of homosexuality as historically constructed; H. Parker 1997.60–63; J. Davidson 2001, who critiques the penetrated-penetrating binary. Feminists have

have also reevaluated the rise of naturalism in Greek art in the fifth century, historically framed as a sweeping transformation of the representation of the human body, in terms of the "parent culture's politics of truth."[65] It is difficult to overstate the importance of this work, which, in demonstrating the ways in which concepts of the body respond to sociopolitical factors and cultural norms, has eroded the assumption that bodies are given.

How does this work on the body relate to what I am calling the physical body? It may be useful here to reintroduce the category of the body. Doing so allows us to ask, Does "the democratic body" or the naturalistic body of early fifth-century sculpture or the gendered body describe the relationship that a citizen, or an idealized male subject, or a woman has to the *sōma*? Or is it our own rather slippery term "body" that organizes these topics?[66] If, indeed, *sōma* is the organizing term, is it informed by ideas about what we might call physicality, ideas essential to our own concept of the body? If so, where do these ideas come from and what role do they play in fifth-century Greek culture?

I raise these questions in part because the body has become broadly visible in both the humanities and the social sciences as a precondition of any self: it is now axiomatic that we must understand human beings as embodied subjects.[67] It is widely held that the body is engaged via a mental, albeit nonconscious, representation variably called a body schema or a body image. This schema, understood as an ahistorical, biological fact, allows our countless feelings and perceptions to be referred to a relatively unitary identity.[68] At the same time, the identity sustained by the body image is molded by stimuli and prone to fragmentation.

---

also criticized Foucault, pointing to the absence of women in his account of ancient sexuality: see Richlin 1991; 1998; Dean-Jones 1992; Greene 1996; Foxhall 1998, noting that many feminist ancient historians have nevertheless taken a "Foucauldian" approach to the female body (122). For a broad survey of Foucault's influence in classics, see the essays in Larmour, Miller, and Platter 1998.
[65] Stewart 1997.23. Cf. Elsner 2006, esp. 87, 92–95, privileging aesthetic form over political and social factors.
[66] As Caroline Bynum observed more than a decade ago, "There is no clear set of structures, behaviors, events, objects, experiences, words, and moments to which *body* currently refers" (1995.5, emphasis in original).
[67] Csordas 1993.135, drawing on the work of Merleau-Ponty, defines embodiment as "an indeterminate methodological field defined by perceptual experience and the mode of presence and engagement in the world" against the body understood as "a biological, material entity." See also Lambek and Strathern 1998a.13–19, treating embodiment as a category of sociocultural analysis; van Wolputte 2004 (with further bibliography).
[68] For overviews of body image, see Scheper-Hughes and Lock 1987.16–18; Grosz 1994.27–111, esp. 62–85. The neurologist Henry Head first developed the idea of a "postural schema." The concept was extended by Freud to describe the way in which the ego unifies the mass of our sensations to create the representation not of any anatomical "reality" but of a body shaped by the history of our libidinal investments, both pleasurable and painful, more or less intense, in its different zones (1923.25–26). What facilitates this imposition of unity in psychoanalysis is the child's perception of others' bodies as discrete and autonomous: see esp. Lacan 1977. For phenomenological approaches to body image, see Csordas 1993 (on "somatic modes of attention"); Mullarkey 1994.

Because body images not only shape but are also shaped by experience, one way of historicizing the body is by exploring how culture, ideology, visual media, religion, and science inflect embodied identities in different times and cultures as they are both lived and performed.[69] We can assume that body images responded to these various influences in ancient Greece as well.[70] What we cannot assume, however, is that identity thus formed was understood primarily in terms of the *sōma*.

The body may also be approached as a historically specific conceptual object used within a culture to express the unity of a human being (as a conscious field, as a discrete form) against internal and external worlds in flux. It can be used, too, to describe the part of a human being seen as the foil to something called the soul, the mind, or the person. If the *sōma* plays these roles in ancient Greece, it would seem to share conceptual ground with our own notion of "body" (without necessarily covering the same semantic field as "body" in contemporary scholarship). Do we find it used in these ways?

In a word, yes. In the fifth and fourth centuries BCE, I suggest, *sōma* can act both as a unifying term and as a foil to the person. Its capacity to fulfill these roles, however, is largely determined by its development into a physical object.[71] Consider, first, its relationship to the boundaries of a human being. In the archaic period, symptoms are commonly blamed on gods and daemonic agents capable of trespassing into the "felt" space of the self. If this felt space is contiguous with a daemonic world, we must conclude that it has boundaries that cannot be reduced to those of a "seen" three-dimensional object. I suggest, however, that, with the emergence of the physical body, the visible body acquires another dimension, namely a concealed inner space implicated in automatic physical processes. As a result, the skin, together with its orifices, becomes newly important as a barrier, attracting concerns about the opacity and the porosity of the self.[72] The self, in turn, is allied more closely with the body *qua* object.

---

[69] See, e.g., Young 1980; Butler 1993.57–91; Weiss 1999. Cf. Cheah 1996.112–21, critiquing the "hypertrophied" power attributed by Butler to the cultural and the historical as formative of bodies. On physical influences on the formation of body images, see Grosz 2005.4–7, 14–52; Lock 2007.275–79, developing the concept of "local biologies" to register the impact of environmental and genetic factors.

[70] The task of recovering historical body images, however, is particularly difficult for those working on the ancient world: see the methodological discussion in De Hart 1999. De Hart relates the new body image in classical Greek medicine to the "appearance of the new discrete citizen (*politēs*) in the city-state" (1999.359; cf. 369, 375–79). While I am in broad sympathy with De Hart's findings, I do not see the body image in medical writing as merely an effect of primarily political transformations (see further below, pp. 22–23).

[71] *Sōma* can stand for the person without a sense of physicality (as I have defined it) in some contexts, particularly in tragedy and the orators: see Hirzel 1914.8–28. But cf. below, n.119, where I argue against Hirzel's equation of the *sōma* and the person in Homer. (Hirzel's notion of person as a fundamental unity, moreover, does not always capture the nuances of the word's uses.)

[72] For evidence of how individual and cultural factors determine the skin's role as a "metaphysical boundary," see Knappett 2006.240–41, with further bibliography.

Second, as the physical body becomes increasingly important to accounts of human nature, it puts pressure on notions of the mind or the soul, precisely because it is conceptualized and imagined in such *impersonal, inhuman* terms. It has been argued that some form of mind-body dualism is part of the human condition.[73] What seems to distinguish the mind-body or soul-body problem in the West is "the sense of urgency regarding precise clarification of the points of separation or connection" between these two parts of a human being.[74] Traditionally, scholars interested in exploring how this problem takes shape in classical Greece have focused on changing ideas about the *psukhē*. I argue that we may better understand the defining urgency of Western dualism by exploring how *sōma* comes to be conceptualized in physical terms, thereby creating the need for an account of mind or soul in terms compatible with human experience and agency.

I do not wish to deny that there are areas of overlap between the semantic field of *sōma*, which I discuss below, and our notion of body that fall outside the domain of the physical body. Nevertheless, I suggest that as a conceptual object, the *sōma* is most coherent and most recognizable to us once it is endowed with a *phusis*. By refusing to take the "category" of the physical body for granted, we can begin to see in its emergence the potential for conceptual and cultural disruption.

It is worth asking anew, then, what seeing the hidden dimensions of reality in physical terms means for the concept of the *sōma*.[75] In focusing on this question, I depart from those approaches that inquire into the ideological or social pressures that shape the concept of the physical body; I do not try to reconstruct the historical context of the inquiry into nature itself.[76] The story I tell here goes in the other direction: from the question of how the physical body

[73] See above, n.24.

[74] Lambek 1998b.109.

[75] For interaction between the inquiry into nature and medicine, see Wellmann 1930; Jouanna 1961; Longrigg 1963; 1989; 1999; Vegetti 1976; 1998; Thivel 1981, esp. 338–57. See also Jouanna 1992, esp. 99–111, on moving beyond simple relations of influence to recognizing the interest in the physical body shared by physicians and those writing on nature in general.

[76] Previous decades have witnessed considerable speculation about the impact of social, political, and economic factors on the inquiry into nature and secular medicine in Greece. Vernant 1983.213–33, 385–97, 404 and, more recently, Naddaf 2005 have argued that philosophy has its roots in the birth of the *polis*. G.E.R. Lloyd, too, has focused on the (democratic) *polis* as a necessary condition for the rise of Greek philosophy and science. In the past twenty years, he has worked comparatively with evidence from ancient China: G. Lloyd 1990; 1996; 2002a; 2004; 2005; Lloyd and Sivin 2002. Cf. von Staden 1992c on the danger inherent in privileging politics when "most ancient Greek science was neither manifestly born out of Athenian democracy nor borne by it" (590). Seaford 2004.175–89 challenges the arguments of both Lloyd and Vernant; in his own account of philosophy's origins, he privileges the advent of monetization in eastern Greece (a factor discussed at Vernant 1983.390–94). See also the more sympathetic critique of Vernant's position in Laks 2006.86–99. Babylonian and Egyptian medical and philosophical traditions also remain highly relevant to speculation on the origins of Greek philosophy and medicine. For the connection with the Near

emerges within speculative and pragmatic inquiries into its nature to the impact of that body on ideas of the person in a broader cultural context. It is a story that not only explores the ways in which physicality was conceptualized, imagined, and investigated but also recognizes these processes as generative in their own right and, thus, capable of contributing to classical Greek notions of human nature.

One of the basic assumptions of the approach I adopt is that the inquiry into nature shares with other traditions of knowledge and praxis (e.g., the production of Attic tragedy, sculpture, the exegesis of oracles) a kind of internal momentum through which it acquires its own complex density.[77] G.E.R. Lloyd has written, "If the concepts of 'nature' and of 'causation' develop from certain implicit assumptions, those ideas had, again, to be made explicit and generalised. These conceptual moves sound simple: but they could not be made without allowing fundamental aspects of traditional beliefs to come under threat."[78] Not only traditional beliefs undergo change. Lloyd suggests that as concepts of "nature" and "causation" are made explicit and generalized as objects of inquiry and debate, they themselves begin to behave in different ways. By encroaching on the domain previously ceded to social agents, they encourage the conceptualization of new mechanisms of power to fill the space once occupied by the god's weapons or his intentions. Thus, while the inquiry into nature is undoubtedly not independent of a given historical and cultural milieu, neither that milieu nor, for that matter, an "enlightened" grasp of the physical world can account for its particular conceptual momentum. This momentum can, in turn, have an impact on other assumptions. For, as much as every genre or inquiry has its own internal momentum, there is also interaction between mutually implicated spheres. That is, concepts developed in one domain may gain sufficient traction in another to spark divergent inquiries or hybridize popular ways of thinking.[79]

The physical body, I suggest, is such a concept.[80] It first takes shape as part of a process through which sixth- and fifth-century physicists are rethinking the unseen world and the relationships of power behind phenomenal states and events. Indeed, fragments and testimonia indicate that many of these thinkers

---

East, see Burkert 1983; 1992; and the essays in Horstmanshoff and Stol 2004. For Egyptian medicine, see von Staden 1989.1–31, with further bibliography at 3 nn.8–10.

[77] G. Lloyd 2002b warns against assuming strict parameters of specialization before Plato. But cf. Laks 2006.63–81.

[78] G. Lloyd 1979.265. See also G. Lloyd 1987.1–49; 1991b.

[79] See the comments on "speciation" at Allen 2006.193–94.

[80] I do not assume, however, that the physical body had a uniform impact throughout the Greek world. We know little about its influence beyond an elite clientele, although *On Regimen* assumes both an audience of leisure and one of people who cannot devote themselves full-time to their health. Still, evidence from other periods suggests that ideas about the body in a lay public are slow to change: see Duden 1991.37, 179–84. It is likely, then, that the impact of the physical body on our textual record exaggerates its impact on the Greek world as a whole.

engaged questions of biology and physiology, presumably within a macrocosm-microcosm framework like the one found in Plato's *Timaeus*. Aristotle observes that the best physicists ended their studies with an examination of medical principles.[81] But the very fact that Aristotle classifies these principles as medical suggests that, at least by the fourth century, medicine had acquired a special purchase on the question of where the inquiry into nature intersects the human. It is possible, then, to see the physical body as a concept first developed as part of a larger inquiry into nature and elaborated under the rubric of medicine.

From where we stand, there are at least two reasons to privilege medicine in an account of the physical body's emergence. The first is practical. Regrettably, only fragments remain from those who wrote on nature, and much of this evidence has been compromised by its transmission.[82] Medical writing, on the other hand, represents one of the largest corpora from the classical period, with some sixty texts from the fifth and fourth centuries BCE attributed to "Hippocrates" extant, although it is certain that these texts are from multiple authors, none of whom can be reliably identified as the historical Hippocrates.[83] The sheer volume of evidence offered by the corpus makes it an obvious resource for anyone trying to investigate early Greek ideas about the nature of the *sōma*.

But it is not simply by default of textual survival that medical writing is so important to understanding the physical body. Evidence from the late fifth century confirms what Aristotle implies about medicine's special claim to the body—namely, that physicians were establishing a degree of independence vis-à-vis those studying "the things up above and the things below the earth" and, at least in one case, establishing that independence on the grounds that only through medicine can one investigate "what a human being is" (ὅ τι ἐστὶν ἄνθρωπος).[84] Medical treatises circulated widely; public debates on medical

---

[81] Arist. *Resp.* 480b26–30; *Sens.* 436a17–22. On biological and medical research in the inquiry into nature, see the overview in Jouanna 1999.262–68 and the relevant subchapters in Guthrie 1962–69.

[82] On the problems with the sources for early Greek philosophy, see Mansfeld 1999; Mejer 2006. For the use of the medical writers to make claims about Greek natural philosophy more generally, see G. Lloyd 1967.27–32; 1979.

[83] The earliest treatises of the Hippocratic Corpus are conventionally dated to the latter third of the fifth century: for the dating of individual treatises, see appendix 3 in Jouanna 1999. The prehistory of "Hippocrates" is a very old problem. The doxographers do not seem to have evidence for earlier medicine see, e.g., Plin. *NH* 29.1–2; Str. 14.2.19 for the later stories created to account for this lacuna. The author of the pseudo-Galenic *Definitiones medicae* appears to have been familiar with pre-Hippocratic texts but notes that they are few (Kühn 19.347). For references to earlier medical writings in works from the corpus, see *Acut.* 1–3 (Li 2.224–28, ch. 1 = 36,2–37,10 Joly); *Vict.* I 1 (Li 6.466–48 = 122,3–21 Joly-Byl). See also Jouanna 1974; W. Smith 1989.87–91. On the demise of the "Hippocratic Question," that is, the question of which treatises are by Hippocrates, see Edelstein 1967c; G. Lloyd 1975b. On the formation of the corpus in the Hellenistic period: W. Smith 1979.178–245.

[84] *VM* 1 (Li 1.572 = 119,7 Jouanna); 20 (Li 1.620 = 146,2 Jouanna). On "things up above . . . ," see Pl. *Ap.* 23d5–6.

topics were common.[85] Crucial to both the autonomy and the authority of medicine was its status as a *tekhnē*, that is, a corpus of knowledge that enables our active intervention in the world to make it more amenable to our needs and desires, achieves predictable outcomes, explains why those outcomes occur or fail to occur, and may be communicated to others.[86] When we acknowledge that physicians play an important role in the emergence of the physical body, we are also acknowledging that the contours of this body are in part determined by its position as an object of technical knowledge and manipulation.

Physicians secure their authority over the nature of the *sōma* in part by claiming to understand the causes of its sufferings. They are also fascinated, however, by the space in the relationship of causes to effects that is open to disruption and intercalation, what the early twentieth-century thinker Eugène Dupréel referred to as the interval.[87] We can understand this interval in two ways. On the one hand, the physician himself occupies the interval when he intervenes in the processes of disease and health. These processes are imagined to be internal to the nature of the *sōma*; the *tekhnē* enables the physician to manipulate them intentionally. The key term here is "intentionally," which signals the presence of an agent whose intelligence is in some sense discontinuous with both the *sōma*'s vital forces and the death drive of the disease. When the physician intervenes in the physical body, then, he is recuperating a place for agency within the cavity. In fact, in the classical period, the physician seems to represent a kind of idealized intelligent agency.[88] Such agency is then extended to the

---

[85] On the circulation of medical texts: X. *Mem.* 4.2.10. Aristophanes refers to a tribe of *iatrotekhnai* at *Nu.* 332. On public debates and sophistic discussions about *phusis*, see Gorg. *Hel.* 13; Pl. *Prt.* 315c5–6; and G. Lloyd 1979.87 n.146; Thomas 2000.249–57.

[86] In Herodotus, Darius refers to medicine simply as [the] *tekhnē* (3.129–30, cited at Thomas 2000.41). Predictable outcomes: *Art.* 4–7 (Li 6.6–12 = 227,6–232,11 Jouanna); explanatory work: Pl. *Grg.* 465a2–6; Arist. *Metaph.* 981a28–30; teachable: *Art.* 9 (Li 6.16 = 235,7–8 Jouanna); Arist. *Metaph.* 981b8–10. See further Reeve 2000; Nussbaum 2001.94–99; Schiefsky 2005a.5–18. Mastery and manipulation are also important to those who wrote "on nature." Heidegger's opposition between "mastering knowledge" and the "essential knowing" of a thinker like Parmenides (1992.5–6; cf. 53, 86–87, 128) is, thus, misleading for early Greek philosophy, given that a number of Presocratics treat knowledge as something that benefits the knower as an instrument of well-being: see Kingsley 1995.217–32, 335–47, on Empedocles and the Pythagoreans, in particular. Yet the idea of beneficial knowledge appears to have been most closely associated with medicine—hence, the importance of medical analogy. The idea that wisdom has no practical benefit is fully articulated in Aristotle (*Metaph.* 982b11–21); see Nightingale 2004.187–252.

[87] "There is always, between our two terms, a place for something intercalated, for the unexpected, for what is not given by the specific relationship of causality that links one term to the other" (Dupréel 1933.11, my translation). The interval, as Dupréel defines it, cannot be so small that there is no recognizable difference or threshold that distinguishes cause from effect or so large that there is no way to maintain a plausible connection between the two events. The concept of indeterminacy within causal series, and particularly microphysical contingency within living beings, was a popular subject of inquiry in the first part of the twentieth century: see Čapek 1992.

[88] See, e.g., Arist. *Metaph.* 1032b6–9, where the physician models the ability to reason inferentially and apply that reasoning to produce a desired result (i.e., health).

embodied patient through the practices of self-care (*epimeleia*) that flourish in the fifth and fourth centuries.

On the other hand, however, if physicians build the *tekhnē* on the idea that there is something to master, they also recognize that their quarry may at any moment slip away. Physicians face a number of obstacles in their attempts to bind effects to causes: the opacity of the *sōma*, the infinite variability of bodily constitutions, the fluid dynamics of the humors, and so on. Each body contains factors (existing levels of a humor, a patient's constitution) that help or hinder the disease. Interposed between catalyst and symptom, physical bodies are spaces of multiple possibilities that exceed what medicine can map. The *sōma* is, then, not simply an object of rational control but also something that evades control.

The *sōma* thus contributes to a concept of vulnerability that is different from that limned in Hesiod's *Works and Days*. It is not because of the god's anger or malicious *daimones* that we suffer—the world, it turns out, is rather indifferent to us. Our susceptibility to pain is due, rather, to the potentially harmful things unstably configured inside us; it is compounded by the fact we cannot see what is happening to us and, hence, avert disaster. While the *tekhnē* can manage these problems, it can also fail; and in failing, it challenges not only the physician's authority but also the capacity of embodied subjects to control their own physicality. In sum, the physical body materializes in medicine as an object of epistemic and technical control and yet is unstable, inhuman, daemonic. It may be because the narratives taking shape around the *sōma* in medical writing are so rich that it acquires such a powerful capacity for cultural provocation.[89]

The notion of cultural provocation raises the question of the impact of the physical body outside medicine. Earlier, I asked whether contemporary scholars are talking about *sōma* when they talk about the body in the ancient world; and if so, to what extent is *sōma* defined in physical terms. What I provisionally propose in response is this: to the extent the person in the classical *polis* is defined as an ethical subject through his proprietary relationship to his *sōma*, as Halperin and others have argued, this relationship is transformed by concerns about physicality in the latter part of the fifth century.[90] Consider, for example, the second book of Thucydides' *Histories*: the autarchic *sōma* (τὸ σῶμα αὔταρκες, 2.41), here with the sense primarily of person, features prominently in Pericles' praise of the Athenian citizen, only to resurface ten chapters later in the account of the plague as an ideal that fails to be upheld by doctors: "No

---

[89] Gillian Beer makes this point about nineteenth-century evolutionary theory: "The multiplicity of stories implicit in evolution was *in itself* an element in its power over the cultural imagination: what mattered was not only the specific stories it told, but the fact that it told many and diverse ones" (2000.106, emphasis in original). See also Kurke 1999.334: "It is the messiness of practice that gives it such power and endurance."

[90] Similar arguments have been proposed about Greek sculpture: representations of the human form (not necessarily identified as *sōma*) may have been influenced by emerging notions of the physical body in the fifth century: see Leftwich 1995; Métraux 1995.

sōma, strong or weak, showed itself autarchic in the face of the disease, which seized all alike, even those treated with every kind of regimen" (σῶμά τε αὔταρκες ὂν οὐδὲν διεφάνη πρὸς αὐτὸ ἰσχύος πέρι ἢ ἀσθενείας, ἀλλὰ πάντα ξυνῆρει καὶ τὰ πάσῃ διαίτῃ θεραπευόμενα, 2.51).[91] Thucydides here stages the collapse of the autarchic *sōma* from inside a worldview that has imbued concepts of the person with physicality. For, in pointing to the limits of medicine's power in the face of the plague, he is also acknowledging it, together with the body assumed by medicine.[92] In this context, Thucydides is interested in Athenian citizens, for whom the plague poses a specific and unexpected threat, realized through the physical body, to the ideal of autarchy. If we expand our focus, we find that the threat to autarchy could be attributed to the very nature of the *sōma*: by the late fifth century, the identities of those excluded from full personhood—women, slaves, barbarians—are being increasingly understood in terms of the difficulty or impossibility of mastering the daemonic tendencies in their bodies, while the identities of free men grow more dependent on their capacity for keeping the body under control. In order to understand the concerns about self-mastery that have been brought to light by much recent work in classics on the ancient Greek body, we need a better grasp of how these concerns are influenced by a concept of the physical body.

The body that slips away finds a natural home on the tragic stage. Tragedians necessarily rely on symptoms to realize pain and madness in dramatic space. Over the course of the fifth century, however, they expand the referential field of these symptoms to encompass not only a magico-religious worldview but the world of the physicians as well. This expansion is particularly evident in Euripides, who, I argue, turns symptoms in tragedies like the *Heracles*, the *Orestes*, and the *Hippolytus* into charged sites of overdetermination that attract explanations involving both daemonic agents and daemonic innards and natures. This is not to say that in Euripides "the gods have become diseases."[93] Rather, through stories of disease and madness, Euripides engages the implications of incorporating the daemonic into human nature alongside the implications of blaming our suffering on the gods. In doing so, he makes full use of the breadth of poetic imagination, its capacity to blur and entangle different versions of the real, and, most important, tragedy's drive to pursue the *meaning* of suffering in all its chaotic complexity.

The physical body assumes what is arguably its most tragic role not onstage but in an author whose suspicion of tragedy is widely known: Plato. In the *Timaeus*, usually placed among Plato's latest dialogues, the *sōma* is described as a composite thing, "always gaining or losing something," exposed to strong

[91] Loraux 1997.235 brilliantly equates this lost body with the hidden interior of the citizen body.
[92] Craik 2001b shows that, despite Thucydides' well-known skepticism about the causes of the Athenian plague, his description of it is shaped by humoral pathology. For references to regimen and mastery of the body, see Th. 6.15, 8.45. On Thucydides and Hippocratic medicine, there is a vast bibliography: see Craik 2001b.102–4 nn.1, 3–4.
[93] Carl Jung's complaint against modern literature, cited in Calasso 2001.169.

powers that "dissolve it . . . and make it waste away by bringing on diseases and old age," and necessarily subject to strong motions (perception, love, fear, anger), motions that must be mastered if our lives are to have value (33a2–6, 42a3–b2). Although it is a necessary condition of human life, the *sōma* is described by Plato as alien to our true nature, akin, rather, to what is feminine and bestial.[94] Its strangeness makes it an important resource as he tries to explain why humans fail to flourish, even as his commitment to the Socratic idea that we err through ignorance of the good leads him to develop an increasingly complex model of the *psukhē* and its diseases.[95]

Understood in terms of its threatening physicality, the body can seem remarkably familiar. It is not hard to see why. Plato, after all, is often placed at the origin of the body-soul problem and its close cousin, the mind-body problem, both problems we are still living with.[96] Yet it may be just because the Platonic body has had such a lasting impact on the Western philosophical and religious traditions that it has influenced the way we see the pre-Platonic world. Recall how easily the body falls into place in Snell's account of the discovery of the mind. Its anticlimactic arrival can be understood in part by the fact that there has always been a body waiting in the wings, not *the* body (timeless, real) but something like the body in Plato, or at least the body traditionally called Platonic. That is, if the body developed and transmitted by Plato's dialogues remains internal to our understanding of the body, it may have obscured its own historical emergence.[97]

It is Plato himself who models how to forget about the physical body. In the *Philebus*, another late dialogue, Socrates asks whether everything having to do with the *sōma* could ever just stop happening: no hunger and thirst, no pleasure and pain, no change at all (42d9–10). Protarchus, his interlocutor, can hardly imagine such a scenario, convinced as he is by the physicists that embodied life is nothing but flux. So Socrates finds another way out: everything in us might always be going "up and down," but this endless becoming will escape our notice if its peaks and valleys are leveled. It is possible, in other words, to cultivate a kind of *lēthē*, "amnesia," about the *sōma*.[98] But the very idea that the *sōma* could be forgotten in this way should flag our attention. For, by assuming that the body can be kept to a murmur largely submerged below the threshold of

---

[94] On the *sōma* as foreign to us, see, e.g., *Phd.* 114e1–3.

[95] Plato sometimes lays the blame for error and disorder on the *sōma*, sometimes on the lower parts of the *psukhē* ruled by appetite, pleasure, and pain: see below, chapter 5, n.31.

[96] E.g., Spelman 1982; Leder 1990.3; Grosz 1994.5. Carone 2005a.229, 231, with nn.7, 13, cites examples of this positioning of Plato within the analytic tradition. See also Dillon 1995 on the afterlife of Plato's ideas about the body in Platonism.

[97] It is worth noting that "Platonic dualism" is often an oversimplification. Plato's ideas about the body and the soul are fluid and complex: see the overview in T. Robinson 2000.

[98] The verb that Socrates uses to describe how a process like growth escapes the notice of the living being is λανθάνω (43b3). Cf. 33d2–34a5: in truth, Socrates says, this is not a kind of forgetting (λήθη), because one cannot forget what has never happened but, rather, insensitivity (ἀναισθησία) to the body.

consciousness, Plato shows himself to be already embedded in the conceptual-imaginative framework that I have been sketching. But because this framework has remained largely below the threshold of our own historical consciousness, what is needed is a process of *a-lētheia*, understood in the sense of non-forgetting, where it is not the "real" body brought to light but, rather, the physical body *qua* conceptual object.[99] The following chapters aim to contribute to this process. But before turning to them, I would like to circle back to Snell's account of the discovery of dualism to sketch an alternative framework for thinking about the respective roles of *sōma* and *psukhē* in this "discovery" and, specifically, the prehistory of *sōma*.

RETHINKING *SŌMA* AND *PSUKHĒ*

In *The Discovery of the Mind*, the *sōma* that appears when the mind is discovered is peripheral and inert. Snell is not the only scholar to have accorded the *sōma* so little importance, nor is his indifference a thing of the past.[100] Even for those who do not accept Snell's evolutionary tale, it has long been standard practice to give the development of the *psukhē* credit for the birth of philosophy's subject of reason or the flowering of the individual in the West. These genealogies have treated the *sōma* as virtually invisible. Nevertheless, as in Snell, they take a concept of the body for granted, insofar as they assume that a transformative notion of soul requires a robust concept of dualism.

The significance of dualism to changing concepts of the soul can be explained in part by recalling that, already in Homer, the *psukhē* is essentially born of a split: it flies away at the moment of death, leaving the corpse behind. But it is also true that scholarship on the archaic period is often shadowed by what lies ahead. A sense of teleology (material to immaterial, concrete to abstract) is particularly strong in narratives of the discovery of the soul, which, in anticipating the moment when the body-soul divide becomes "self-evident," approach the body as something to transcend.[101] In his first chapter, for example, Snell sets

---

[99] On *alētheia* and unveiling, see Heidegger 1992; Detienne 1996.

[100] Michael Clarke, for example, after a lengthy and sensitive study whose main premise is the absence of a body-soul distinction in Homer, concludes by following Snell in assuming that "the new category of 'soul' will march with a new category of 'body'" (1999.315). See also Williams 1993.26: "We do indeed have a concept of the body, and we agree that each of us has a body. We do not, *pace* Plato, Descartes, Christianity, and Snell, all agree that we each have a soul. Soul is, in a sense, a more speculative or theoretical conception than body." David Claus, to whose powerful suggestion that the body helps shape the soul through the figure of medical analogy I return below, writes that, "because ψυχή is the word that in time allows human life to be characterized as a composite of body and soul, its history is central to one of the most important and influential achievements of Greek thought" (1981.1). See also Laks 1999.253; Hankinson 2006.41.

[101] Self-evident: Snell 1953.17, cited above, n.21. Material to immaterial: e.g., Renehan 1980. Concrete to abstract: Onians 1954; Furley 1956.1–2. See also Nilsson 1941.1–2: "I cannot give up the historical development of humanity from lower to ever higher stages."

out to show that Homer "was *not yet* capable of understanding the soul as basically opposed to the body."[102] Homer, on Snell's reading, is hampered in two ways. Because he lacks awareness of the body and the soul as natural complements, he gives us heroes who are nothing but fragmented aggregates; however, if the definition of the soul requires us to recognize not-body, then "body" must be logically prior to soul: it is *all there is* before soul. Here, body describes not an organic unity but, rather, the corporeality that constrains Homer's understanding of the person. Bereft of a soul concept, Homer represents thought, emotion, and perception as continuous with other human faculties and experiences. Some scholars have taken this to mean that Homer's heroes are more, rather than less, unified.[103] For Snell, however, unity arises only when corporeality has been disciplined by being restricted to the body. The discovery of the mind thus imposes both an overarching unity on the aggregate of parts and a limit to the materiality of the self.

Snell's stance reflects a broader interest among historians in a soul defined against the material limits of the person. At least since Erwin Rohde published *Psyche: Seelencult und Unsterblichkeitsglaube der Griechen* in 1894, stories of how the pale Homeric soul is transformed from *Totengeist* to true self have foregrounded the transcendental aspirations of Orphism and Pythagoreanism.[104] Different scholars have stressed different factors associated with the mystery cults: a developed idea of personal survival after death, a heightened sense of moral accountability in the afterlife, an interest in purifying practices in life, and exposure to shamanistic techniques of mental dissociation.[105] Yet they largely concur that these cults privilege an ethereal soul and its life beyond death over embodied life. In what Rohde takes as a watershed passage in the history of the soul, Pindar describes the *sōma* as subject to overpowering death, while a "living *eidōlon* of life remains, for it alone is from the gods." During life, Pindar goes on, this *eidōlon*, "image," slumbers while the limbs are active and reveals the future during sleep (fr. 131b S–M). Moreover, many fifth-century thinkers associated with the inquiry into nature seem to have conceived of mind as uniquely fine and mobile stuff, qualities that imbue it with the capacity for intelligence and perhaps survival beyond death.[106] Empedocles, for example,

[102] Snell 1953.69, emphasis added.

[103] E.g., Clarke 1999.

[104] Rohde 1925 (English translation of the eighth edition). See also Hirzel 1914.29–30; Burnet 1916; Nilsson 1941; Jaeger 1947.73–89 (with the criticisms of Vlastos 1952.117–18); Dodds 1951.135–78; Furley 1956.4, 10–11; Burkert 1972.134 n.78, 136; Vernant 1983.381–85. A recent survey of mind-body dualism in Plato takes for granted the dominant "Orphic" genealogy of the Platonic soul, locating the care of the soul within this framework (T. Robinson 2000.37–38).

[105] On shamanism, see esp. Dodds 1951.140–56, with the cautionary remarks of Burkert 1972.164–65 and Bremmer 1983.24–39, 43–53.

[106] See Renehan 1980.111–27. Renehan disputes, however, that there is a genuine opposition between materiality (or corporeality) and immateriality (or incorporeality) in the Presocratics (and in all pre-Platonic thinkers) on the grounds that they lack concepts of body and matter as spatial extension (118–19, with n.33). Renehan's main target here is H. Gomperz 1932, who claimed to

makes reference to a holy *phrēn*, "mind," that survives multiple incarnations (DK31 B134).[107] Beliefs in the special nature of mind, such as we find in the fragments of Anaxagoras, have suggested to some that it might stand apart from the physical self—perhaps even in life—as easily as the *psukhē* distances itself from the corpse in the Homeric poems.

What is interesting, however, is that *psukhē* is not the standard term in these contexts: Pindar speaks of *eidōlon*; Empedocles, of *phrēn* and also *daimōn*; Anaxagoras, of *nous*. *Psukhē* does appear in relationship to metempsychosis, as well as in the fragments of Heraclitus, who uses it to designate that with which we grasp the *logos* of the entire physical world.[108] Nevertheless, we have very little evidence about the appearance of a new transcendental soul or mind concept in the late archaic period and even less evidence that it was identified with *psukhē*.[109] The standard story, then, according to which intuitions of the immateriality of the soul drive new concepts of the self, while the body is simply there, solid and passive, is largely speculative. This is not intended as an argument from silence: Plato's eschatological views, for example, undoubtedly owe much to the Orphic-Pythagorean tradition.[110] My claim, rather, is that the lacunose nature of our evidence has combined with preconceived ideas of corporeality and incorporeality—sometimes allied with the Cartesian opposition between *res extensa* and *res cogitans*, sometimes with Christian doctrines of resurrection and the intellectual puzzles to which they gave rise—to create a situation where the body-soul dualism that becomes dominant in the West, a dualism organized by concerns about materiality, is mysteriously discovered when history is not looking. This situation has kept us from investigating whether this dualism and the definitions of *sōma* and *psukhē* that it makes possible are part of a complex historical process for which we have more evidence

---

have found pre-Platonic uses of ἀσώματος with the sense of incorporeality: see esp. Renehan 1980.119–27; see also Huffman 1993.411–14, arguing that Philol. [DK44] B22, one of Gomperz's examples, is spurious.

[107] On Empedocles' relationship to mystery cults and Pythagoreanism, see Kingsley 1995.

[108] Metempsychosis: Xenoph. (DK21) B7, usually taken as referring to Pythagoras; see also Hdt. 2.123 and the discussion in Burkert 1972.120–36. For Heraclitus, see esp. DK22 B45; B85; B107; B115, with Nussbaum 1972. Two other Presocratic fragments featuring *psukhē* are problematic. Aristotle (*De an.* 405a19–21 = DK11 A22) attributes to Thales the idea that *psukhē* is a cause of motion (κινητικόν τι), but Clarke 1995.297–98 persuasively argues that Aristotle supplies *psukhē* where Thales refers to *theos*. The representation of *psukhē* as a hegemonic principle at Anaximenes (DK13) B2 is also suspect: see Claus 1981.122–25.

[109] The origins of the doctrines on reincarnation, for example, "are lost in obscurity" (Schibli 1990.107–8, with bibliography at n.10). See also Claus 1981.111–21, downplaying eschatological influences in the prehistory of Platonic dualism. There is a further question of how well eschatologically oriented theories of the soul articulated its relationship to the body: see Arist. *De an.* 407b15–26 (mentioning the Pythagoreans by name). The well-known σῶμα-σῆμα pun attributed to the Orphics by Plato (*Cra.* 400b9–c9; *Grg.* 493a1–3) gives little indication of how they might have specified the body's relationship to the soul.

[110] See Kingsley 1995.79–171, 328–30; Bernabé 2007. On Plato and Pythagoreanism more generally, see Burkert 1972.15–28, 83–96.

than we think. If we allow that the concept of the *sōma* has a history, we can see how the *sōma* itself helps to shape different ideas of what lies "beyond" its boundaries in the fifth and fourth centuries, and particularly the idea of a *psukhē* seen as the locus of reason, perceiving and sensing, emotion, desire, beliefs, value judgments, and intentional actions—in short, a *psukhē* understood as the locus of ethical subjectivity defined by the imperative to live well.

But how much history do we want to grant the *sōma*? After all, given the state of the evidence, it is hazardous to make claims about the meaning of *sōma* before the fifth century. Nevertheless, it is worth revisiting the debate about early concepts of the *sōma* if only to draw attention to an unexamined tension within its arguments that can shed light on later concepts of the *sōma*. Snell, we can recall, claims that, for Homer, *sōma* means corpse. His critics have countered that the idea of *sōma* as a (living) body "plain and simple . . . as bulk" or "as a lump" is, indeed, available to Homer; the poet, or, rather, the tradition, simply has no use for it.[111] They have asked how, if *sōma* does mean corpse in Homer, it could have migrated so easily into the sphere of life.[112] This last question is a good one. Yet it is hard to see how we get around the problem posed by *sōma*'s undeniably morbid connotations in the *Iliad* and the *Odyssey* by making "living body" a possible meaning of *sōma* for Homer. Rather, we will have only displaced the problem: *sōma* becomes a point of tension between life and death in our earliest evidence. In fact, on inspection, this seems to be the case.

Let us begin with the passages where Snell's critics have argued that *sōma* could mean living body. In one of these passages, from the *Odyssey*, Circe, explaining to Odysseus the treacherous passage past the Planktai, describes the sea as thick with the wreckage of ships and the *sōmata* of mortals. These *sōmata* might be alive. Yet, in aligning them with the planks of broken ships, the poet does little to suggest intact survivors.[113] We can better grasp the word's meaning by considering its two other appearances in the poem. In one case, *sōma* refers to the body of Elpenor, who, unbeknownst to his companions, falls off a roof to his death on Circe's island (11.53); in another, it refers to the suitors' unburied, unmourned corpses (24.187). These passages suggest that *sōma* is used of dead bodies that have been abandoned, forgotten, or are otherwise *akēdea*, "uncared for." It looks like a fitting term, then, for corpses lost at sea.[114]

---

[111] Bulk: Renehan 1979.278. Lump: West 1978.295. The philological critique is partly strategic, because no amount of ingenuity has made the one word that would decisively eliminate the fragmentation of the Homeric hero, that is, *psukhē*, mean "self" in Homer. Arguments focused on the mind-soul-self thus tend to reject lexical analysis: against Snell's strong "lexical bias," see Gaskin 1990.2–5; Halliwell 1990.37–38. Conversely, Renehan 1979.272 argues that a rebuttal of Snell's claims about *sōma* on philological grounds would weaken, if not refute, his entire argument about the fragmentation of the Homeric hero.

[112] Hirzel 1914.7; Herter 1957.209–10; West 1978.295; Renehan 1979.271.

[113] See *Od.* 12.67: πίνακάς τε νεῶν καὶ σώματα φωτῶν. Notice the parallel construction: noun plus dependent genitive. Cf. Koller 1958.277; Renehan 1979.272.

[114] On κῆδος in epic: Lynn-George 1996.

In a second passage whose meaning has been deemed ambiguous, this time from the *Iliad*, Menelaus comes upon Paris and rejoices like a lion happening upon a great *sōma*, a stag or a wild goat.[115]

> τὸν δ᾽ ὡς οὖν ἐνόησεν ἀρηΐφιλος Μενέλαος
> ἐρχόμενον προπάροιθεν ὁμίλου μακρὰ βιβάντα,
> ὥς τε λέων ἐχάρη μεγάλῳ ἐπὶ σώματι κύρσας,
> εὑρὼν ἢ ἔλαφον κεραὸν ἢ ἄγριον αἶγα
> πεινάων· μάλα γάρ τε κατεσθίει, εἴ περ ἂν αὐτὸν
> σεύωνται ταχέες τε κύνες θαλεροί τ᾽ αἰζηοί·
> ὣς ἐχάρη Μενέλαος Ἀλέξανδρον θεοειδέα
> ὀφθαλμοῖσιν ἰδών.

> (*Il.* 3.21–28)

> Now as soon as Menelaus the warlike caught sight of him
> making his way with long strides out in front of the army,
> he was glad, like a lion who comes on a mighty carcass,
> in his hunger chancing upon the *sōma* of a horned stag
> or wild goat; who eats it eagerly, although against him
> are hastening the hounds in their speed and the stalwart young men:
> thus Menelaus was happy finding godlike Alexandros
> there in front of his eyes.

Snell's critics, wondering why Paris would be likened to dead meat, have argued that the *sōma* here is still living. Yet the simile is primarily targeting affinities between Menelaus and the lion: bloodlust and unexpected good fortune in the hunt.[116] Although we cannot rule out the possibility that the felled stag or goat is still breathing, the most salient characteristic of *sōma* is that it is edible.

Edibility, like the idea of being "uncared for," may be more than incidentally important to the meaning of *sōma* in the Homeric poems. For the word does not simply denote "corpse," for which Homer overwhelmingly prefers *nekus* and *nekros*. Nor does *sōma*, which occurs only eight times in both epics combined, function as the natural complement of *psukhē*.[117] *Sōma* cues, rather, a world markedly indifferent to the human and defined, especially in the *Iliad*, by animality (*sōma*, but not *nekus* or *nekros*, is used of animals, as we have just seen).

---

[115] See also *Il.* 18.161; [Hes.] *Sc.* 426–28. Critics have wavered on whether the *sōma* here is alive or dead: see esp. Herter 1957. See also Redfield 1994.279 n.46: "*Soma* is used of a living body only when it is the prey of animals," with Koller 1958, who derives *sōma* from σίνομαι, "to plunder," and Merkelbach 1975.222.

[116] See Lonsdale 1990.50, emphasizing the repetition of ἐχάρη (23, 27).

[117] *Il.* 3.23, 7.79, 18.161, 22.342, 23.169; *Od.* 11.53, 12.67, 24.187. There are two passages where *sōma* and *psukhē* are found in close proximity (*Od.* 11.51–54, 24.186–91). In both cases, *psukhai* in Hades complain about their unburied *sōmata*: the stress here is on the denial of burial. Vernant's (1991c.63; 1991d.84) use of *sōma* as a generic term for corpse opposed to the *psukhē* in Homer or made into "the" body that is created at the moment of death is thus misleading.

Sōma is thus a charged term. Its force is perhaps most evident in one of the *Iliad*'s culminating scenes when Hector, mortally wounded, supplicates Achilles not to feed him to the dogs but to return his *sōma* to his parents (22.338–43). This request is remarkably foreshadowed in book 7. Proposing a duel to settle the war, Hector sets the following terms: if he should die, his opponent has the right to strip his armor, but he must return the *sōma* to the Trojans for a proper burial (7.76–80). Hector's words may have been deliberately jarring to the audience: this is the only time in the *Iliad*—with the notable exception of 22.342—that *sōma* is used of a dead human body. In any event, when Hector repeats the request in book 22, Achilles' shocking refusal brings out the word's dark undertones: "I wish only that my spirit and fury would drive me to hack your meat away and eat it raw for the things that you have done to me" (αἴ γάρ πως αὐτόν με μένος καὶ θυμὸς ἀνείη / ὤμ' ἀποταμνόμενον κρέα ἔδμεναι, οἷα μ' ἔοργας, 22.346–47).

Flesh denied burial is *the* raw nerve of the *Iliad*'s final books.[118] In exploring the idea of a death beyond a death—a death, that is, that comes from denying the hero the posthumous rites that memorialize his death and confer social recognition on it—the poet appears to accord *sōma* particular weight. Whereas the *psukhē* or the *eidōlon* preserves the visible identity of the person (but lacks solidity and density), *sōma* occupies the point when form is yielding to formlessness. It is closely related to the idea of flesh that passes into an animal economy (dogs, worms, birds, fish), an economy vividly described by Jean-Pierre Vernant:

> To hand someone over to wild animals does not mean only to deprive him of the status of a dead man by preventing his funeral. It is also to dissolve him into confusion and return him to chaos, utter nonhumanity. In the belly of the beasts that have devoured him, he becomes the flesh and blood of wild animals, and there is no longer the slightest appearance or trace of humanity: he is no longer in any way a person.[119]

The "utter nonhumanity" awaiting the corpse denied care is the fate of the *sōma*.

Both the corpse and the animal remain relevant to the semantic field of *sōma* in the later archaic and classical periods.[120] Yet this field appears messier as we accumulate evidence. The word *sōma* seems to lose its fraught relation-

---

[118] Segal 1971.36–41 notes the crescendo of animal images in book 22. See also Lonsdale 1990.90–102; Redfield 1994.167–69, 193–203; Bouvier 2005.

[119] Vernant 1991c.71–72. It is in the belly of the animal that the hero encounters the most radical version of the thingness that Simone Weil described as the product of force in the *Iliad*: "To define force—it is that *x* that turns anybody who is subjected into it into a *thing*. Exercised to the limit, it turns man into a thing in the most literal sense: it makes a corpse out of him. Somebody was here, and the next minute there is nobody here at all; this is a spectacle the *Iliad* never wearies of showing us" (2005.3, emphasis in original). Given these associations, it seems unlikely that *sōma* expresses personhood in Homer, as Hirzel 1914.5–8 argues.

[120] Animals (both dead and alive): e.g., A. *Pr.* 463; E. *Cyc.* 225; Hdt. 2.39–40; Pi. *N.* 3.47; S. *OC* 1568.

ship to the ritual recuperation of the dead person, readily designating what is covered by earth or burned on the pyre.[121] It is used in poetry and inscriptions as a foil to more ethereal and intangible entities: *psukhē*, but also *pneuma*, "air, breath"; *aretē*, "virtue"; and *noos*, "mind."[122]

There is, moreover, another, more serious challenge to the semantic boundaries of *sōma* that have been inferred from the Homeric evidence, a challenge that undercuts the diachronic orientation of Snell's account. Regardless of whether Homer can use *sōma* to designate the living body, Hesiod uses it in just this sense in the *Works and Days*, dated to the late eighth century BCE. He exhorts his audience to put on a cloak in the winter so that the hairs all over the *sōma* will not bristle, an exhortation found in a broadly "animalistic" context—Hesiod is talking about how various species withstand the winter cold—but one where animals are unambiguously alive.[123] In 1974, when the Cologne Epode, attributed to the seventh-century BCE poet Archilochus, was published, it offered further archaic evidence of *sōma* as living body (in this case as an object of the narrator's sexual predation).[124] Later material expands our sense of the living *sōma*. *Sōma* offers a surface for paint, oil, and perfume.[125] It drips with sweat.[126] It is endowed with strength and courage, gifts that flee in old age.[127] It can be embraced or struck.[128]

In these examples, *sōma* feels like a more ordinary word than it does in Homer. And the references to the living *sōma* in Hesiod and Archilochus should make us uneasy about creating a history of the word's semantic field on the

---

[121] For the *sōma* prepared for or associated with burial: And. 1.138; E. *HF* 703; *IT* 633; Hdt. 2.86, 4.71. On the pyre: E. *IT* 1155; *Supp.* 1019, 1211; Pi. *N.* 9.23; S. *El.* 758; *Tr.* 1197. See also the expression *nekrōn sōmata* at E. *Pho.* 1563; *Supp.* 358; *Tro.* 599. If the *sōma* is unburied (E. *Supp.* 62) or abused (S. *Ant.* 1198), it is explicitly identified as such.

[122] See Bacch. 3.91 (ἀρετή); E. *Supp.* 534 (πνεῦμα); fr. 734K (= *Temenos* fr. 7 J.-V.L.) (ἀρετή); and the epigram for the dead of Potideia (*IG* I³ 1179 II): αἰθὲρ μὲμ φσυχὰς ὑπεδέχσατο, σόμ[ατα δὲ χθὸν] τόνδε (the aether received the souls of these men, the earth their bodies). One of the earliest "mind-body" oppositions is found in the Theognidea, at frr. 649–50 (W²): ἆ δειλὴ Πενίη, τί ἐμοῖς ἐπικειμένη ὤμοις / σῶμα καταισχύνεις καὶ νόον ἡμέτερον (oh wretched Poverty, why lying on the shoulders do you shame our body and mind?). It is interesting to compare these lines to *Od.* 10.239–40, where Circe turns Odysseus's men into swine (οἱ δὲ συῶν μὲν ἔχον κεφαλὰς φωνήν τε τρίχας τε / καὶ δέμας, αὐτὰρ νοῦς ἦν ἔμπεδος [they had the head, voice, hair, and build of pigs, but the mind was firm]). That *nous* in the *Odyssey* passage is set against an aggregate (head-voice-hair-*demas*) lends support to the claim that Homer does not recognize *sōma* as an appropriate term for the living body. Clarke 1999.118 arrives at a similar conclusion.

[123] Hes. *Op.* 539–40; the *sōma* at [Hes.] *Sc.* 426 is also quite clearly alive. On clothing the *sōma*: e.g., A. *Pers.* 199; E. *Cyc.* 330; *El.* 544; Hdt. 7.61.

[124] Archil. fr. 196a.51 (W²). Merkelbach 1975 tried to adapt the idea of "prey" to the new Archilochean evidence. The result was an inadvertently feminist reading of the poem, in which the speaker's treatment of the girl turns her into a mere object (222). Slings 1975 is skeptical and takes the Archilochean passage as one of the oldest attestations of *sōma* as living body.

[125] Cephisod. fr. 3.1 (*PCG*); Hdt. 1.195, 4.191, 7.69.

[126] E. *Ba.* 620; Hdt. 3.125.

[127] Strength: E. *Rh.* 382; Hdt. 1.31; Th. 7.75. Loss of strength in old age: S. *OC* 610.

[128] Embrace: E. *El.* 1325; *Ion* 519; S. *OC* 200. Struck: A. *Th.* 896; Antiphon 3.4; Hdt. 6.117.

basis of the Homeric poems alone. What these poems give us, however, is the sense of coiled possibility inside the word *sōma*. They embed the *sōma* in a web of concerns—about formlessness and disintegration, vulnerability and our need for care, animality and interincorporation, and the "mute earth" (κωφὴ γαῖα, *Il.* 24.54) that swallows up the human—that may be more or less urgently expressed in other texts. In the classical sources, for example, *sōma* is often bound to the idea of life at risk. The threat may be external. But it may also arise from the nature of the *sōma* itself. In fact, I suggest that in the classical period, the physical body that emerges in biological and medical contexts realizes the semantic possibilities inherent in the Homeric usage while transferring the scene of their realization from the corpse to the living body.

From this perspective, we can imagine the world to which the Homeric *sōma* is condemned as a kind of precursor to the worlds described by the physicists, worlds populated by composite bodies caught up in intercorporeal flux. If, as I argue, the physical body emerges as the primary site through which human beings are *necessarily* implicated in such a world, then we can see that body as the site where the tension in Homer between the integrity of the person and the collapse into formlessness at death comes to be managed *in life*. Of course, in Homer, too, the living person is porous, caught in a field of forces trafficked between the mortal and immortal worlds; the self is forged in part through encounters with these forces, which are often expressed as daemonic intentions. It is therefore possible to understand the heirs to these intentions as the various stuffs and forces that impinge upon the physical body in medicine. Yet this is not the whole story. For, with the arrival of the physical body, the nonhuman abyss represented by the unburied corpse in Homer encroaches upon the living, not simply as a foreign element, but as the hollow, hidden core of the person. That is, the cavity becomes the ground of the physical body's ongoing struggle to maintain life against the constant threat of disorder, loss of self, and death, a threat posed not just by things coming into the cavity but by the things always inside it. Whereas the dead *sōma* in epic requires a single act of care to rescue it from disintegration, the physical body will demand constant attention in order to maintain its integrity. So great is its demand for care that it eventually comes to rival concerns about the wishes and the intentions of the gods.

If the physical body takes on elements of what Vernant calls "utter nonhumanity," it is not only the boundary between that body and the world that matters but also the boundary between the cavity and the sentient, thinking, social person. The medical writers routinely acknowledge this boundary in distinguishing between the *sōma* and *ho anthrōpos*, the "person" or "the human being." Yet, in their attempts to explain not only seizures and coughs but also cognition, emotion, and character in terms of the humors, they often treat that boundary as negligible. Perhaps because of the physicians' relative indifference to this boundary, thinkers outside medicine in the later fifth century begin to imagine an object of care that is both like and unlike the physical body. Some of them begin to call this part of a human being, responsive to words and images and subject to its own diseases, *psukhē*. Around this object a new kind of care begins to unfold in the late fifth century, catalyzed by a medical analogy that becomes integral to philosophical ethics in antiquity.

The medical analogy in one sense reverses the conventional arc of dualist genealogy by granting creative force to the physical body. The importance of that body has been stressed by David Claus who, having tracked the idea of the *psukhē* as "life-force" from Homer to Plato, concludes that the eventual understanding of the *psukhē* as an ethical-psychological agent may be indebted to "the development of an oblique analogy between body and soul by which rationalistic ideas of the body and its φύσις are transferred to the soul."[129] Yet because Claus remains focused on the soul, rather than the body, he does not elaborate this suggestion. As a result, the idea of the physical body as a generative concept vis-à-vis the soul remains a tantalizing hypothesis.

But analogy does not simply reverse the traditional story in which soul generates body. It also troubles the very notion of linear development by foregrounding the dynamic interaction of sameness and difference, rather than simple opposition, in the relationship between body and soul. Inquiries into the nature of the soul, undertaken in part to establish its difference from the body, end up restaging concerns about the fragility of the human in a physical world, thereby creating a renewed commitment to techniques of taking care. At the same time, such techniques help to delineate the body as a specific object of care. Even, then, as the emergence of the physical body encourages attempts to orient true human nature, that is, our social and ethical nature, around the soul, that body haunts us from within as a part of us that is both alien to the self and intimately implicated in it. I am thus interested both in how the physical body informs concepts of the soul (similarity) and in how it acts as a limit against which the human is formed (difference). Pursuing this approach, I hope, can shed new light on the knot of problems that first forms around the relationship between the body and the soul in the late fifth century.

TELLING STORIES

I begin this study by going back to the Homeric epics in an effort to deepen our sense of what is different about the physical body and the ethical subjectivity,

---

[129] Claus 1981.182; see also Vlastos 1945; 1946; 1952.121–23, on Presocratic naturalizing approaches to the soul. Claus decisively opposes his own approach to studies focused on the *psukhē* as transcendent: see esp. 1981.1–7; on the *psukhē* as a life-force or the emotional seat, see also Burnet 1916.253–56; Furley 1956.6–7; Darcus 1979a; Bremmer 1983.13–69 (on "body souls" that endow body with life and consciousness); Laks 1999.250–51; Lorenz 2003. In reaching his conclusions, Claus downplays the evidence from Heraclitus that suggests he saw *psukhē* as a rational agent (see esp. 1981.125–38). But this does not seriously affect Claus's claim about the role of "rationalistic" ideas about the body (which he himself does little to specify) in giving shape to psychic agency, only the historical priority he wishes to give to Socrates.

centered on practices of care, to which it gives rise. However wary scholars have become about using labels like "secular" and "rational" to describe Greek medicine in the fifth and fourth centuries, a shift from personal, daemonic explanations to naturalizing explanations remains basic to our understanding of learned medicine in this period and the medical tradition that unfolds from it. It is precisely because this shift remains so basic and, hence, unquestioned that I take the time to explore how daemonic explanations of the symptom work and the model of the person they assume. In so doing, I emphasize how important felt experience is to constituting the boundaries of a person in early Greek poetry. I am interested here in laying the groundwork for my argument that it is by acquiring an "objective" plane below the threshold of sensing that the physical body assumes much of the daemonic force behind the symptom. In the first chapter, I also focus on how the practice of referring symptoms to a divine-daemonic plane embeds them in a world populated by social agents and, thus, a web of emotions, moral expectations, and desires. I do not wish to set up an opposition between the whims of "personal" gods and naturalizing explanation. Rather, in following the emergence of the physical body, I want to think not only about what is gained for concepts of harm, healing, and the self but also about what gets lost—namely, an intuitively intelligible social framework for understanding suffering.[130] By taking seriously the social context of the symptom within a magico-religious model, we can better perceive that the physical body does not exist in isolation as an object of medical knowledge but demands to be reconciled with the socioethical domain.

In the following three chapters, I track the gradual emergence of the physical body by examining fragments from those working in the inquiry into nature and particularly the medical writings that we have from the classical period. Chapter 2 begins with a look at the broad shift from personal agents to impersonal causes within the inquiry into nature. I then consider how speculation about the physical world generates the idea of a community of composite objects joined together by the interchange of physical forces and stuffs, rather than by bonds of social or emotional reciprocity. One way—perhaps the dominant one—of conceptualizing these composite objects, I suggest, was as *sōmata*. The key term here is "conceptualize" because, as I have stressed, most of what happens to these bodies cannot be seen directly but only inferred on the basis of phenomenal evidence. By referring phenomena to the hidden depths of the *sōma*, these thinkers help establish it as the primary locus of our participation in the larger physical world.

In chapter 3, I explore in greater detail how ideas about the *sōma* take shape in medical writing around the figure of a concealed and dynamic cavity. I focus on the role played by symptoms in representing what happens in this space in the medical writers' field of vision and, thus, in enabling the physician to

---

[130] I do not mean to imply that suffering in the ancient world always made sense, only that the predominant cultural practices of interpretation referred it to agents with intentions and emotions.

exercise control over it. But I also consider the ways in which the hidden body acquires the characteristics that assimilate it to the daemonic realm: its opacity, its instability, the latent hostility of the humors, its impersonal automatism.

In chapter 4, I address the question of how this daemonic object is taken up as a part of the person. I begin by arguing that one way the medical writers make this connection is through the idea of an innate, vital force inside the *sōma*. This force not only stands behind the body's own efforts to fight disease but also turns out to guarantee the full range of phenomena and functions integral to both biological life and social and ethical life. At the same time, because this vital force, equated by some authors with the body's *phusis*, cannot secure human flourishing, there is a need for *tekhnē*. In the latter part of the chapter, I argue that the very untrustworthiness of the physical body requires the person *qua* technical agent to take responsibility for its flourishing, showing how it is precisely by taking or not taking care of the body (and, hence, exercising mastery over it) that free men are coming to be defined as ethical subjects at the end of the fifth century.

The final two chapters engage the problem of taking care not only of the body but also of a self more broadly understood. Chapter 5 looks at early versions of the medical analogy. The crux of my argument is that this analogy, centered on the idea of psychic disease, grows out of a desire to draw a line between the body and the person, understood as mind or soul, but ends up fostering a sense of urgency regarding the permeability of that line. In chapter 6, I argue that concerns about the fragility of the person understood in physical terms are, by the last quarter of the fifth century, coming to color tragic representations of disease, particularly in Euripides. I do not argue that these concerns displace the gods. Rather, I approach symptoms as spurs to test out different frameworks for interpreting daemonic interruptions in the self. Taking three of Euripides' tragedies—*Heracles*, *Orestes*, and *Hippolytus*—I show how the polysemy of the symptom works in practice. At the same time, I explore the tragic implications of approaching the symptom through the prism of contemporary medical and ethical ideas.[131]

---

[131] I see these studies taking up Padel's provocative claim that the conditions for the sporadic efflorescence of tragedy across two and a half millennia of Western history are found in cultures "poised on some momentary cusp between theological, or daemonological, and innovative scientific explanations for human pain. . . . Maybe," she goes on, "a medical and theological tug-of-war between religious and scientific explanation encourages an attention to madness as illustration of human suffering that is best expressed in tragedy" (1995.247). Padel thus treats the suffering subject in Attic tragedy as a historically contingent figure—a symptom of the friction in this period between religion and science, medicine and theology. Yet, in her own studies of tragic interiority, she tends to collapse distinctions. As Christopher Gill observes in a review, "One difficulty with this suggestion,"—that is, the importance of a "tug-of-war" between religious and scientific explanation—"as a way of summarizing her own approach, is that she tends . . . to present the fifth-century medical, religious, and tragic perspectives as (similar) aspects of a single thought-world, so that she provides little basis for seeing in Greek thought a transition from religious to scientific perspectives" (1996b.264).

I close with tragedy because its conceptual and imaginative space allows us to gauge the social and ethical complexity of what it means for human nature to be embodied and ensouled at the end of the fifth century. For the story of the physical body's emergence, haunted by fears of a daemonic space within the self, has a tragic streak: it is a story about pain more than about pleasure; and, insofar as it is about pleasure, it represents pleasure as a driving, disruptive force akin to the Furies that hound Orestes or Heracles. It is, of course, no secret that the physical body has had a bad reputation in the West since the Greeks. Part of the reason for its denigration may lie in the fact that it takes shape in large part as an object of medical knowledge and control, an object, that is, that is helpless but also dangerous when left on its own. It is perhaps the body's nimbus of vulnerability, together with its embeddedness in physical flux, that provokes so much hostility in Plato, the most influential early exponent of Western dualism. If we are to reverse some of this hostility, what we need is not a return to physicalism—though this has dominated the repudiation of Platonism and Cartesianism in recent years—but, rather, a rethinking of what it means to live in and through a body. One aspect of such a rethinking should be an investigation of the historical emergence of a body caught between technical mastery and daemonic unruliness.

From this brief survey, it is clear that this study treads a familiar path through archaic and classical Greek textual sources, one closely associated with the miracles and grand narratives that have been so important to claims of Greek innovation and exceptionalism.[132] But if a book about the symptom cannot escape ideas of rupture and historical difference, it is also the nature of the symptom to foster interpretive complexity: symptoms remind us that there is always something subjective about what counts as a rupture and how to make sense of it. Throughout this book, I have tried to incorporate this interpretive complexity into my story while keeping its central claims as lucid as possible. By enacting the emergence of the physical body in Greece as something real and imaginative, historical and timely, I hope to challenge the givenness of that body both in the Greek world and in our own. Although the terrain of the fabled Greek miracle is treacherous, the risks of revisiting it may be worth taking if we can make it unexpectedly generative within the present.

---

[132] For new perspectives on the "Greek miracle," see Goldhill and Osborne 2006; Osborne 2007. See also Laks 2006.107–22, on the figure of rupture in the history of early Greek philosophy. The concept of revolution has been problematized more generally in the history of modern science: see Osler 2000, who still stresses that in contextualizing the canon we need not deny historical change (8).

CHAPTER ONE

Before the Physical Body

ARISTOTLE DESCRIBED the *Iliad* as rich in suffering. It is likely that the poem's violence, together with its slow crescendo of grief, leaves most readers in agreement. At the same time, the epic celebrates the effulgence of the hero, which Jean-Pierre Vernant sees as a mortal's participation, albeit limited, in "that splendor that always clothes the body of a god."[1] The hero's fragility and his radiance meet at a point of great intensity in the poem. Achilles has killed Hector and stripped him of his armor:

> ἄλλοι δὲ περίδραμον υἷες Ἀχαιῶν,
> οἳ καὶ θηήσαντο φυὴν καὶ εἶδος ἀγητὸν
> Ἕκτορος· οὐδ᾽ ἄρα οἵ τις ἀνουτητί γε παρέστη.
> ὧδε δέ τις εἴπεσκεν ἰδὼν ἐς πλησίον ἄλλον·
> ʼ ὢ πόποι, ἦ μάλα δὴ μαλακώτερος ἀμφαφάασθαι
> Ἕκτωρ ἢ ὅτε νῆας ἐνέπρησεν πυρὶ κηλέῳ. ʼ
> ὣς ἄρα τις εἴπεσκε καὶ οὐτήσασκε παραστάς.

(*Il.* 22.369–75)

And the other sons of the Achaeans came running about him,
and gazed upon the stature and on the imposing beauty
of Hector; and none stood beside him who did not stab him;
and thus they would speak one to another, each looking at his neighbor:
"See now, Hector is much softer to handle than he was
when he set the ships ablaze with the burning firebrand."
So as they stood beside him they would speak, and stab him.

The Achaeans, awestruck, are compelled to look at Hector's *phuē*, his breeding or stature, and his *eidos*, his visible form. These terms, like *demas*, the "build" of the body, and *khrōs*, "skin, complexion, tint," focus on how the hero appears. The latter term, *khrōs*, however, is also the covering of the inner parts. This covering is not irrelevant to the scene of Hector's death. For the Achaeans are compelled, too, to pierce Hector's soft skin, thereby demonstrating how easy it is in the end to drive the bronze into a man whose brilliance, magnified by the firebrand, once made him appear invincible. Fascinated by the beautiful form, yet eager to violate its integrity, the Achaeans have a conflicted relationship to Hector's corpse that is not unlike the *Iliad*'s relationship to its mortal heroes.

---

[1] Vernant 1991b.36.

Yet, if the many wounds inflicted on Hector's corpse draw attention to skin that is neither stone nor iron (οὔ . . . λίθος χρὼς οὐδὲ σίδηρος, *Il.* 4.510), the other major death in the *Iliad*, that of Patroclus, reveals another kind of vulnerability. In the final moments of his *aristeia*, his "moment of glory," Patroclus is struck from behind by Apollo. His eyes spin, strength flows out of his limbs, and his armor falls to the ground, setting him up for a deadly human attack: the Trojan Euphorbus drives his spear into Patroclus before Hector steps in to deal the final blow. From one perspective, the Trojans' assault simply mimics the god's. Yet these attacks differ on a crucial point. Whereas the weapons of Euphorbus and Hector draw blood, Apollo's blow produces symptoms of hidden damage. Patroclus is thus vulnerable to the god in a way that he is not to his mortal enemies. If the skin is irrelevant in this scenario, it suggests that Patroclus has a second set of boundaries that can be transgressed. How are these boundaries constituted? How are they violated? If we are to understand what was different about medical interpretations of the symptom in the fifth and fourth centuries, we need to look at how discontinuities in the self are described and understood in our earliest evidence.

It is easy to comprehend how a spear pierces the flesh. It is more challenging to imagine how a god or a *daimōn* hurts a person. In this chapter, I try to make sense of magico-religious ideas about the harm caused by immortals by adopting two broad perspectives on the person: the "seen" and the "felt." In the category of the "seen," I include both of the ways in which Hector appears to the Achaeans after his death: as a three-dimensional, penetrable object; and as a human form, distinguished by its breeding, *phuē*, and a particular look, *eidos*. I use the category of the "felt" to refer to the conscious field that constitutes the unity of the self, as well as the daemonic energies that cut across it. I do not differentiate between "body" and "mind." For, while thinking about something is not the same as touching it, the distinction between physical and mental does not help with the questions that concern me here.[2]

By recognizing the seen and the felt as different dimensions of the person, I am trying to avoid privileging one of these dimensions at the expense of the other. More specifically, I am seeking an alternative to two of the more prominent approaches to Homeric "psychology" in the past few decades, one that emphasizes what I am calling the seen, the other what I am calling the felt. The first of these approaches has tried to correlate the rich vocabulary of human parts in Homer with an anatomical-physiological body that we are presumed to share with the early Greeks. Such an approach, I argue, neglects how important embodied experience is to ideas of the human being in early Greek poetry. We cannot assume, however, that what we consider to be embodied experiences are always seen this way by the Greeks. I am thinking here of the tendency in recent years to treat the gods as simple projections of what the person

---

[2] For the distorting influence of mind/soul-body dualism in Homeric scholarship, see Clarke 1999.39–49.

is feeling or thinking.[3] This second approach fails to give due weight to our evidence, which not only recognizes the presence of potentially seen agents in a world external to the self but also makes their actions central to human experience.

If these approaches are limited in their account of the person in Homer, alternatives cannot simply affirm the importance of the seen and the felt but must attempt to understand how they interact. For it is clear that these are not hermetically sealed categories but different, often complementary ways of experiencing and knowing: seeing, for example, has a felt dimension (the awe, for example, felt by the Achaeans when they gaze upon Hector's corpse); what one person feels is often accompanied by signs seen by others.[4] In this chapter, I try to trace how these modes of experience interact at the moment an immortal affects a mortal. I thus adopt the seen and the felt as necessarily imperfect categories in the interest of making an argument about what we can observe in our earliest evidence of the relationship between symptoms (what they feel like, but also how they register for others) and a potentially seen world of gods and daemonic agents that is rich in social meaning.

It might be argued that we cannot rely on the Homeric poems—or any other early Greek poetry—to tell us much about what people in the archaic period (or in earlier periods) truly thought about the gods' role in human experience.[5] It is true that these poems depict a rarefied world under unusually strong generic constraints. While Homeric scenes of wounding and death, for example, appear vividly real, we must also remember they are shaped by a poetic tradition from the level of the word to the unfolding of the theme.[6] Genre and theme exercise particular pressure on representations of disease in the poems. Scholars have often rightly observed that heroic epic, as a rule, has little interest in the kinds of diseases that the medical writers describe; even the two diseases most common in lyric poetry and tragedy, madness and *erōs*, are largely absent.[7]

[3] E.g., Gaskin 1990.11–12: "That Helen's passion is represented by the goddess Aphrodite should not of course deter us from ascribing it fully to Helen herself." See also Sharples 1983; Williams 1993.29–31.

[4] On the affective dimension of seeing: Onians 1954.15–22; Harrison 1960; Fränkel 1975.76–78. Critics in the past century often took the mingling of the affective and the cognitive as evidence for the "primitive" mind of Homeric people, although R. B. Onians rightly recognizes that "there is, perhaps, no such thing as 'un phénomène intellectuel ou cognitif pur' for us either" (1954.20).

[5] The problem, of course, is that historians have little else: Benveniste 1945 and Kudlien 1968 rely heavily on poetic sources. There is limited material evidence for Bronze Age and archaic medicine: see C. Warren 1970; Arnott 1996; 2004; Laskaris 1999; 2002.33–44.

[6] On the stylization of wounding scenes, see Loraux 1995.88–100; Salazar 2000.126–58; Saunders 2004.15–17; Holmes 2007. But see also van Wees 2004.153–65, 249–52, arguing that, in many respects, the epics do conform to what we know about early seventh-century BCE warfare.

[7] *Erōs* does surge up at crucial points, e.g., *Il.* 3.437–46, 14.153–360. On madness, see *Il.* 5.717, 831, 6.132, 200–202, 234, 389, 8.360, 15.128, 321–22; *Od.* 9.350, 11.537, with O'Brien-Moore 1924.67–74; Simon 1978.67–71; Mauri 1990; Padel 1995.25–26, 55–57; Hershkowitz 1998.125–60. On battle fury, see *Il.* 8.299, 9.239, 21.542, with Lincoln 1975; Dumézil 1983. Cf. Delcourt 1938, for whom

When disease does appear in the Homeric poems, it enacts broader thematic concerns. The larger plot of the *Iliad*, the wrath of Achilles, is anticipated, for example, by the plague that Apollo sends against the Achaeans in the first book as punishment for Agamemnon's folly.[8] In the *Odyssey*, too, people suffer in ways consistent with the poem's preoccupations. Anticleia in Hades tells her son that she was robbed of life by longing for him (11.203). And when Odysseus is tossed onto the shores of Scheria at the end of book 5, his joy mirrors the rejoicing of children whose father has just shaken off a wasting *daimōn* (394–97).[9] These diseases call to mind the spaces of wandering, waiting, and distress occupied by the *Odyssey's* characters. That both epics incorporate disease into a broader poetics of suffering would seem to confirm that they cannot be trusted as sources of historical information.

But we do not have to assume an opposition between the "real" world and a literary or imaginative one. We might instead see the epic poems as developing perspectives that conform to generic expectations, while still illuminating concepts or details that belonged to a more complex and pragmatic approach to disease in early Greece.[10] Epic, for example, tends to focus on divine or daemonic agents of harm. The attention to agents can be related to the genre's pronounced interest in efficient causes (who? what?) and final causes (why?) as opposed to instrumental ones (how?).[11] This interest can be understood, in turn, in light of epic's status as a narrative genre, whose commitment to plot can explain the heightened importance of reasons for actions. The poet's frequent attribution of cause to the gods may be explained further by the device of omniscient narration, which allows him to see into the divine world (though, of course, characters within the poems often attribute events to gods without knowing which god is involved). Other genres offer different perspectives. Seasonal causes of disease, for example, play a larger role in a text like Hesiod's *Works and Days*.[12] Lyric poetry tends toward fatalism and dwells on effects, as in Sappho's famously precise elaboration of the symptoms of *erōs* (fr. 31 L-P).[13] In the larger

---

even the plague does not qualify as a disease: she declares that "la notion même de *maladie* est rigoureusement exclue de la poétique épique" (23, emphasis in original).

[8] Holmes 2007.49–53. See also Blickman 1987 and, on wrath and disease, Austin 1999.

[9] The other reference to disease in the *Odyssey* is the "Zeus-sent disease" at 9.411, on which see Cordes 1991.115–16.

[10] Epic is a "secondary" speech genre, to adopt the terminology of M. M. Bakhtin. That is, its imaginative worlds, within which themes are developed, actions are taken, and events interpreted, open onto the "primary" worlds of its genesis (1986.61–62, 72–76, 98–99).

[11] For the interaction of these different aspects of cause in several contemporary African societies, see Sindzingre and Zempléni 1992; Samuelsen 2004.

[12] Hes. *Op.* 586–88 on the diseases associated with the rising of the Dog Star (though see also *Il.* 22.26–31). See also W. Smith 1966.550–52 on environment and health in epic.

[13] On the importance of *erōs* in lyric poetry, see Cyrino 1995. The fatalistic aspect of disease in early Greek culture is emphasized by R. Parker 1983, contesting Dodds's story of a transition from a "shame" to a "guilt" culture (adopted by Kudlien 1968). It is because fatalism is always a framework for interpreting disease, Parker argues, that the physicalist explanations advanced by the

context, then, an agent like the Apollo who sends down plague or strikes Patroclus looks particularly well suited to an epic poem.

But despite its particular generic focus, epic exhibits beliefs about the gods' power and unseen harm that resurface in a range of archaic and classical texts. The *Iliad* is a profound meditation on how a ruler's blindness can destroy his people; but the far-reaching consequences of a king's transgressions, as well as those of any member of a community, are assumed by Hesiod, Pindar, and Plato.[14] In the epics, the Olympian gods are infinitely attentive to human life; individual acts take on deep significance.[15] Yet everyday symptoms, too, can be traced to gods and *daimones*.[16] Crossing a river with unwashed hands incurs the gods' *nemesis* and future pain in Hesiod (*Op.* 741). In the Hippocratic treatise *Airs, Waters, Places*, Scythians attribute their impotence—mistakenly, in the author's eyes—to offenses against the gods (*Aer.* 22, Li 2.76 = 238,9–12 Jouanna). Freedom from suffering, bodily or otherwise, can be correlated with the absence of divine displeasure (Antiphon 5.81–83). In Plato's *Republic*, the assumption that the gods cause bad things to happen to people is standard (2, 379c2–7). When archaic poets relate afflictions, sensations, emotions, and mental states to divine and daemonic agents, this is not simply a poetic phenomenon.

Yet, if divine and daemonic agency is not a poetic phenomenon, what does it tell us about early Greek ideas not only about unseen harm but also about the person more generally? It is well known that early and mid-twentieth-century scholars such as Snell and Hermann Fränkel believed that when Homer ascribes sudden emotion, insight, or pain to the interference of the gods, he is reflecting a culture still incapable of understanding personal autonomy. They thus disqualified Homer's heroes as genuine agents.[17] Their critics have sought to overturn this conclusion by downplaying the gods' agency or even assimilating

---

Hippocratics are not opposed by theological prejudices (1983.256). This seems correct, insofar as interpretations of disease, whether magico-religious or naturalizing, are open to different inflections of blame. Yet I would argue that both fatalism and moralism are transformed by the emergence of the physical body, which makes having a body into an ethical problem.

[14] See Hes. *Op.* 242–43; fr. 30.15–17 (M-W); Pi. *P.* 3.34–37; Pl. *Leg.* 10, 910a7–b6; cf. *Od.* 19.109–14. On the relationship between the power to protect and the ability to rule, see Lynn-George 1993.199–201. On divine vengeance and disease, see, e.g., Hdt. 3.27–38, 6.75–84, and Dover 1974.77–78; Laser 1983.62–63; R. Parker 1983.235–56; Chaniotis 1995.325–26. See also A. *Eu.* 478–79, on the Erinyes' power to blight the land (cf. 921–25 on the power to make it fertile).

[15] It is sometimes argued that epic and tragedy are misleading genres for this reason: not every cough was blamed on daemonic agents: see G. Lloyd 1987.12. The problem with this claim is that it implies the gods or, perhaps more accurately, a daemonic or spirit world, was somehow separate from everyday life and, thus, "supernatural." Yet, in contemporary cultures structured around a spirit world, the division between the natural and the supernatural "often fails to resonate with local worldviews" (Samuelsen 2004.90). Scurlock 1999 deftly shows how that division has led scholars astray in their reconstruction of the relationship between healing professionals in ancient Assyrian medicine.

[16] See R. Parker 1983.243–44.

[17] Snell 1953.29–31; see also 103–8, 122–23 (making the decision the distinguishing feature of tragedy); Fränkel 1975, esp. 80–81.

it entirely to motivations and forces within the person. But if this corrective has helped discredit the marionette model of the early Greek person advanced by Snell and Fränkel, it has also produced its own distortions. When we treat the gods as metaphors for "real" psychological elements, we ignore the historical process through which the very concept of psychology, especially moral psychology, becomes possible. We cannot understand that process without giving the gods' social and ethical agency due weight.

I am by no means advocating a return to the marionette model. Rather, building on scholarship that has challenged the polarity between agency and passivity, I reexamine the dynamics of interaction between gods and people. In the introduction, I argued that because symptoms are particularly indeterminate sensations, they support a range of inferences or abductions about hidden causes. In the ancient Greek world, these abductions, as with abductions provoked by a wide spectrum of unusual events in archaic and classical texts, habitually involve gods and *daimones*.[18] They thus belong to what the anthropologist Alfred Gell has called "the abduction of agency."[19] There is, of course, space for these inferences to be wrong. Not every bird means something, as one suitor in the *Odyssey* says (2.181–82); although, if he were to realize he was in the *Odyssey*, he might be less blasé. Nevertheless, in archaic Greece and throughout the ancient Mediterranean, there is widespread evidence that people were receptive to potential signs and ready to trace unusual events to the gods and other daemonic agents.[20] The tendency within archaic Greek culture to infer the presence of gods behind unusual phenomena presumably contributed to the belief that discontinuities in the self indicated a divine presence.

Symptoms are characterized by another kind of indeterminacy. Although I have associated them most closely with dramatic ruptures in experience, in some cases it is less clear whether a phenomenon counts as a disruption at all: experiences of otherness are often imprecise and, thus, subjectively and culturally determined. Given how fuzzy the line between the symptom and the feeling of a self can be, it may be useful to think of a culturally specific continuum traversing both the person and the terrain of the divine and the daemonic. This continuum would determine not only how perceptions and sensations of otherness are interpreted but also when perceptions and sensations register as

---

[18] See Csordas 1990.8–10, 16–17, 22–23, 38–39; 1993.148–53, reading the relationship between perceptual indeterminacy and the divine through Merleau-Ponty's notion of the preobjective. See also Lambek 1998.112–18. Versnel 1987 shows how imprecise the stimuli associated with Greek ideas of *epiphaneia* could be.

[19] Gell 1998. See also Bird-David 1999. It is not only contemporary anthropologists who are interested in the abduction of agency. Democritus and later ancient thinkers located the origins of religion in false inferences of agency in response to meteorological events (DK68 A75 = S. E. *M.* 9.24). See further Henrichs 1975.96–106.

[20] The abduction of agency is cross-culturally widespread. For speculation on why this is so, see Boyer 1996 and the recent research cited in J. Barrett 2007. See also Fadiman 1997 for a specific and enlightening cross-cultural perspective on daemonic or spirit-based agency.

other in the first place.[21] If Odysseus's *thumos* counters what Odysseus (however we understand the referent of the proper name) thinks is the best course of action, this situation is perfectly consistent with how Greeks in the archaic and classical periods envisioned decision-making.[22] If an idea appears through the agency of a god, we sense both the intimacy of the human and the divine and the potential tension between them—think, for example, of Agamemnon's deceitful dream.[23] Finally, in a trauma like the plague or cases where normally tractable parts of the self gain unexpected autonomy, the difference between the self and a daemonic other comes into sharp relief. At this end of the continuum, then, we could locate the scene in the *Odyssey* where Athena causes the suitors to laugh with "alien jaws" (γναθμοῖσι γελώων ἀλλοτρίοισιν, 20.347). The goddess's appropriation of a part of the self is powerful enough to sever it from the proper name altogether.

Thus, if the poet or a character infers that a god or another daemonic agent is acting on himself or another person, we should not conclude that we are dealing with a primitive or incomplete notion of subjectivity. Such abductions illustrate, rather, a fluid, experiential relationship between what is objectified as the self and what is objectified as other, as well as the role of culture in determining how this otherness is interpreted. It can be hard for modern readers, who tend not to see gods behind surges of strength or sudden pain, to recognize the complex conditions under which an event or feeling would have encouraged a Greek of this period to infer the intentions of a god. Yet these difficulties should lead us neither to dismiss the gods' agency as a turn of phrase, nor to equate the possibility of that agency with the necessity of referring everything to gods, nor to deny human desires, intentions, and deliberations.[24] If we recognize that the boundaries of the hero are, in fact, strengthened by the alien intentions and forces that traverse him, we can stop worrying that the Homeric hero is less than a person, while leaving open the possibility that these boundaries can be rethought.

In sum, then, I approach the Homeric poems and other poetic sources as evidence for a magico-religious framework for interpreting symptoms that, far from denying the boundaries of a self, helps to constitute them. I try to keep in mind the caveats set out above regarding the use of literary evidence in making historical claims. At the same time, I believe we also need to consider that literature and art do not simply reflect cultural assumptions and practices but also sustain and

---

[21] Csordas 1990.13–23 discusses such a continuum in the context of contemporary Charismatic Christianity: see his comments on "the transgression or surpassing of a tolerance threshold defined by intensity, generalization, duration, or frequency of distress" (15–16).

[22] Fränkel 1975.78–79; Simon 1978.63–64; Gill 1996a.41–93; Clarke 1999.63–66. See also the comments at Williams 1993.30–31.

[23] *Il.* 2.23–34. Ideas appear through the god: *Od.* 2.124–25, 19.10, 138, 485. See further Pelliccia 1995.92–98, 250–68.

[24] The person's own actions can always be part of the causal picture. The locus classicus for the idea of self-inflicted suffering is *Od.* 1.32–34, where mortals gain pains in excess of what is fated through their own folly (σφῇσιν ἀτασθαλίῃσιν).

shape them. From this perspective, a genre such as epic, like ritual practice, lends support to a magico-religious worldview. Indeed, it is precisely because Plato assumes, in the *Republic*, that epic has so much cultural capital that he wants to appropriate its power to give a different account of human suffering.[25] Plato's explanation of suffering in that text turns out to be strongly influenced by contemporary medical explanations of disease. And the medical writers, too, are encroaching, more or less aggressively, on existing cultural narratives about suffering to show how things inside the body, not gods, hurt a person.[26] Before considering their accounts in detail, however, I would like to look more closely at the narratives whose authority they are seeking to arrogate, closing with a brief examination of how magico-religious explanations of disease inform ancient healing practices.

DAEMONIC VIOLENCE

Barely ten lines into the *Iliad*, a terrifying disease strikes. The priest Chryses, having failed to ransom his daughter from Agamemnon, urges Apollo to "let the Danaans pay for my tears with your missiles" (τείσειαν Δαναοὶ ἐμὰ δάκρυα σοῖσι βέλεσσιν, 1.42); the god obliges:

ὣς ἔφατ' εὐχόμενος, τοῦ δ' ἔκλυε Φοῖβος Ἀπόλλων,
βῆ δὲ κατ' Οὐλύμποιο καρήνων χωόμενος κῆρ,
τόξ' ὤμοισιν ἔχων ἀμφηρεφέα τε φαρέτρην·
ἔκλαγξαν δ' ἄρ' ὀϊστοὶ ἐπ' ὤμων χωομένοιο,
αὐτοῦ κινηθέντος· ὁ δ' ἤϊε νυκτὶ ἐοικώς.
ἕζετ' ἔπειτ' ἀπάνευθε νεῶν, μετὰ δ' ἰὸν ἕηκε·
δεινὴ δὲ κλαγγὴ γένετ' ἀργυρέοιο βιοῖο·
οὐρῆας μὲν πρῶτον ἐπῴχετο καὶ κύνας ἀργούς,
αὐτὰρ ἔπειτ' αὐτοῖσι βέλος ἐχεπευκὲς ἐφιεὶς
βάλλ'· αἰεὶ δὲ πυραὶ νεκύων καίοντο θαμειαί.

(*Il.* 1.43–52)

So he spoke in prayer, and Phoebus Apollo heard him,
and strode down along the pinnacles of Olympus, angered
in his heart, carrying across his shoulders the bow and the hooded
quiver; and the shafts clashed on the shoulders of the god, in anger
moved. He came as night comes down and knelt then
apart and opposite the ships and let go an arrow.
Terrible was the clash that rose from the bow of silver.
First he went after the mules and the circling dogs, then let go
a tearing arrow against the men themselves
and struck. The corpse fires burned everywhere and did not stop burning.

---

[25] See Allen 2000.

[26] Given the debate about the "secularity" of medicine, I stress that what matters here is the gods *qua* causes, not the validity of ritual or the existence of the gods more generally.

The representation of Apollo's action displays several striking tensions. First, consider its adverbs and prepositions: Apollo descends, like night, from Olympus to the plains of Troy.[27] Yet, once he is in the vicinity of the ships, he sits down apart from (ἀπάνευθε) them. The image of the god striding down anticipates the impending interference of the divine world in the human, but these worlds touch without overlapping. What crosses the last stretch separating the god and the army is the arrow. The god's anger cuts to the heart of the camp, yet he himself remains outside it.

Second, these arrows provoke all kinds of noise for the listener of the poem: they clash on Apollo's shoulders as he moves; the bow gives forth a terrible clang with their release. But the enjambment in the final line suggests that the attack arrives for the army much as the verb *ball(e)*, "he struck," does for the listener: abruptly and without forewarning. Despite the fact that the animals succumb first—an omen of trouble—the account of the attack captures something central to symptoms, namely, that they appear from left field, from a place that you can neither see nor strike back at. Unlike the bellowing of the wounded Ares, which causes a shivering to take hold of both armies (5.862–63), the noisy quiver only acquaints *us* with the god's weapons. For the Achaeans, Apollo's baneful presence is announced not by the arrow but by the disease.

Throughout antiquity, our sources understand the onset of plague in terms of Apollo's archetypal weapon.[28] Arrows sent by Apollo and his sister, Artemis *Toxodamnos*, "arrow-conquering," can also deliver sudden death, as they do to the children of Niobe.[29] Another powerful daemonic agent, Erōs, is closely associated with the bow and arrow in tragedy and vase painting in the fifth century.[30] But why are arrows so important to concepts of illness and godsent suffering? One way of starting to answer this question is by recognizing that they call up a specific set of spatial and visual relations, as we saw in the description of the plague's arrival. By drawing a line from the hidden god to his unsuspecting victim, arrows make painfully evident a gap in the latter's field of vision.

Because the archer commands a visual advantage over his victim, he is an ambiguous figure in the symbolic world of epic and in Greek warfare more

---

[27] On the relationship between the swiftness of Νύξ and the presence of a god, see Clarke 1995.311–12.

[28] G. Lloyd 1966.206–7; Faraone 1992.59–61, with appendices I and II. On arrows and sickness generally, see Bremmer 1983.43–46; Padel 1992.152–53; and the discussion of the extensive cross-cultural evidence on the relationship between disease and godsent arrows in Eliade 1968.463–65. Macr. *Sat.* 1.17.9–30 maps the complex relationships among Apollo, sickness, arrows, and healing: see also Farnell 1896–1909, 4:233–41, 408–11 nn.208–20; Bernheim and Zener 1978, for speculation on Sminthian Apollo.

[29] τοξόδαμνος: Diph. fr. 29.3 (*PCG*); E. *Hipp.* 1451; Lyc. *Alex.* 1331. *Il.* 21.489–96 makes a mockery of this title. On the arrows of Apollo and Artemis as envoys of sudden death, see *Il.* 6.205, 427–28, 21.482–84, 24.605–6; *Od.* 11.171–73, 15.407–11. Apollo and Artemis are the archers from whom one cannot hide in Sophocles' *Niobe* (fr. 441aR). Zeus "bends his bow" against Paris at A. *Ag.* 362–66.

[30] E. *Hipp.* 530–32; *IA* 548–51; *Med.* 633–35; fr. 850K, with Pearson 1909. On early representations of the personification Erōs with a bow, see Cohen 1994.698.

generally. For, at least in theory, epic rules of engagement assume face-to-face combat.[31] The relationship between the combatants, described by verbs prefixed by *anti*-(ἀντιάζω, ἀντιβολέω, ἄντομαι), "opposite," entails reciprocal seeing (ἄντα ἰδών, e.g., 13.184, 17.305), as well as the public, ritualized exchange of weapons and words.[32] The ideal of frontal engagement is further supported by the shame that comes with a wound in the back, which is interpreted as a mark of flight.[33] However unreal such an ideal was, epic poetry, and the archaic and classical ideology of warfare more generally, appears uncomfortable with the idea that the enemy might be behind you.

This is not to say that the poet of the *Iliad* refuses to recognize that an enemy might approach or attack unnoticed. The Trojan warrior Dolops is killed, for example, when Menelaus, coming up from the side unobserved (λαθών), hits him with a spear from behind (15.540–42). In this instance, however, the stealth of the attack appears to indict its perpetrator Menelaus, never known for his warcraft, more than its victim. Hector, facing Ajax in single combat, boasts, "but I have no wish to strike you, great as you are, by stealth, watching for my chance [λάθρη ὀπιπεύσας]" (7.242–43), implying that such a strategy would diminish his stature. The adverb *lathrēi*, like the verb *lanthanō*, marks an inequitable distribution of knowledge: this is how gods move among men and couple with women (13.352, 16.184), or how Aegisthus kills Agamemnon (*Od.* 4.92). It is not, however, how you should kill your opponent in epic warfare, at least under normal conditions. Menelaus's attack, then, appears compromised by its adverb. In the case of Dolops, we are dealing no longer with a warrior facing a stronger opponent but with a warrior who is vulnerable because he cannot see his attacker.

Menelaus is fighting with the spear, but it is primarily the archer who gains his advantage by striking from outside his victim's field of vision and whose own vision is often stressed.[34] Harpalion retreats "glancing warily in all directions [πάντοσε παπταίνων], lest someone should wound him with a bronze" (*Il.* 13.649). But he cannot, for all his caution, see the arrow of Meriones coming to kill him. Arrows deliver two of the most important and unexpected plot developments in Homeric epic. When the archer Pandarus takes aim at Menelaus as the two armies are negotiating a truce in book 4 of the *Iliad*, his arrow comes

---

[31] The encounter is both specular and erotic. On the erotic overtones of the encounter (ὀαριστύς) between warriors, see *Il.* 13.291, 17.228, and esp. 22.126–28, with Vermeule 1979.101, 157–59; Monsacré 1984.63–77; Loraux 1995.80–81. Van Wees 2004.160–61, 165 stresses that face-to-face combat is an ideal, observing that it is far more common in the *Iliad* for warriors to attack one another without warning. Nevertheless, the single-combat duel, as the ideal, is a natural counterweight to the symbolic role of archery.

[32] Words: Bassi 1998.55–63.

[33] For wounds in the back, see, e.g., *Il.* 5.55–57, 65–67, 11.446–49, 12.43–44, 15.341–42, 20.413–18, 487–89. For the importance of this motif to a code of heroic conduct, see *Il.* 8.94–95, 13.288–91, 22.283–85; Tyrt. frr. 11.17–20, 12.25 (W²), with Salazar 2000.156 (216–17 on the motif in later literature).

[34] See, e.g., *Il.* 5.95, 8.269, 11.581, 12.389; *Od.* 11.606–8.

out of left field for all involved. Odysseus, still in the guise of the beggar, takes his first step toward reclaiming Ithaca by shooting an arrow at Antinoös as he is about to take a sip of wine, when "in his heart there was no thought of murder" (*Od.* 22.11–12). The audacity of Odysseus's plan lies in the fact that instead of assuming a space of rule-governed combat where the arrow appears as the interloper, it puts the archer front and center and exploits the suitors' belief that they lie outside the boundaries of the game.[35]

Like a sophistic argument, archery permits the weaker to tackle the stronger. Diomedes, hit by Pandarus's arrow, asks Athena to "grant that I might kill this man and come within spearcast, he who struck me first [ὅς μ᾽ ἔβαλε φθάμενος]" (*Il.* 5.118–19), where the verb *phthanō*, "to get in front of" or "to be first," expresses the archer's visual advantage. Diomedes' scorn comes out in the open later, when, after a second arrow wound, he calls the arrow the weapon of a "nobody, a man lacking fighting power" (ἀνδρὸς ἀνάλκιδος οὐτιδανοῖο, 11.390), a charge that dogs the bowman throughout antiquity.[36] When blame is attributed to the archer, it is, in turn, deflected from the victim. In an anecdote related by Thucydides, an Athenian ally taunts a prisoner of the battle of Sphacteria that the true Spartans were those who fell in combat. The prisoner replies that arrows would be worth a lot if they could pick out the brave from the cowardly. Thucydides' gloss is, "those killed were the ones who happened to encounter [ἐντυγχάνων] stones and arrows" (4.40). Here, where the missiles become blows of chance, the conditions of praise and blame are nullified.

It is precisely the archer's exemption from fair play that assimilates him to the gods. For the gods, too, regularly violate the rules of visual reciprocity, often with equally damaging results. The similarities between the archer and the god are brought out neatly in book 15, where we can observe nested layers of visibility. Teucer, aiming his arrow at an unsuspecting Hector, cannot escape the shrewd mind of Zeus (ἀλλ᾽ οὐ λῆθε Διὸς πυκινὸν νόον, 461), who overrides the archer's intention by breaking his bowstring and striking the arrow aside. Hector uses the strange event to rally his troops, claiming that he has witnessed the arrows of his opponents frustrated by Zeus—perhaps naming Zeus in order to appropriate sovereign power for his own plan to take the offensive in battle.[37] Teucer's brother, Ajax, simply credits god, *theos*; Teucer himself blames *daimōn*

---

[35] The bow is the instrument that enables the transition from the game (ritualized or symbolic combat) to "real" violence: Odysseus becomes like an avenging Apollo (Nagler 1990.348–56). Apollonius appropriates the arrow in the *Argonautica* to shift the course of his epic toward *erōs* (3.275–87).

[36] Geometric art does suggest that archers can be seen as independent, full-status fighters in the eighth century (van Wees 2004.166–67, 251–52). But the bow is less popular in archaic and classical art, where it comes to be associated with the barbarian: Cohen 1994; van Wees 2004.167–71, 175. For the barbarian associations, see also A. *Pers.* 147–49; S. *Aj.* 1120–23. Salazar 2000.220–21 discusses the denigration of the archer in later literature.

[37] See also Collins 1998.54–67, esp. 65: Hector reads the event as an indication that Zeus is on his side.

for cutting short his plans (15.468).[38] Each explanation responds to the unexpected eruption of a different order of causality within the world of combat: it is because the event has no obvious cause—Teucer pointedly remarks that he had just that morning bound his bow with a fresh-twisted sinew—that its witnesses infer divine or daemonic agency. Though the concept of *daimōn* is difficult to determine in Homer, it appears to be associated with sudden and uncanny incursions of divinity into the observable order, especially those which bring about good or ill fortune: a daemonic world "crackl[es] with temperamental, potentially malevolent, divinity."[39]

The nature of the daemonic is expressed with particular clarity by the arrow and the visual asymmetries it exposes. But daemonic attack may take other forms, as we see in another crucial instance of Apollo's aggression in the *Iliad*: the death of Patroclus. In narrating the god's attack on Patroclus, the poet adapts the tropes that we saw earlier in relation to the plague to the idiom of close combat, while also proleptically tracing the fatal arrow wound that the *Iliad* does not describe, that of Achilles.[40] Like Achilles, Patroclus is a remarkably proto-tragic hero, pushing beyond what is fated (16.707). As he charges a fourth time against the Trojans, the narrator equates him with a *daimōn* (δαίμονι ἶσος, 16.786; cf. 705), marking the tension between the more-than-human warrior and the all-too-human victim of the gods.[41] This tension breaks through in the apostrophe of the next line: "There, Patroclus, the end of your life was shown forth" (ἔνθ᾽ ἄρα τοι Πάτροκλε φάνη βιότοιο τελευτή, 16.787), a line that is, of course, unheard by Patroclus, just as the end of his life, coming into our view, cannot be seen by him.

It is within this proto-tragic framework that the poet stages Patroclus's encounter with Apollo. But "encounter," perhaps, is the wrong word. For the *anti*-verbs of face-to-face engagement that appear (ἤντετο, 788; ἀντεβόλησε, 790)

---

[38] Homer does not strictly distinguish *daimōn* from *theos*: see Untersteiner 1939; Herter 1950.139–40; Wilford 1965; Tsagarakis 1977.98–116; Brenk 1986.2071–82, with an overview of previous scholarly literature. Jörgensen 1904 pointed out that it is almost always characters who refer to *daimōn* in Homer, although this turns out to be truer of the *Odyssey* than of the *Iliad*. The difference, rather than implying a historical development—the poets gradually carving up and naming the numinous, a thesis critiqued by J. Smith 1978—may be explained by the role of the omniscient narrator in the respective poems: see Dodds 1951.10–13. While *daimōn* can be held responsible for negative outcomes (see, e.g., *Od.* 10.64, 24.149, with Dodds 1951.11–12; Tsagarakis 1977.105–12; Brenk 1986.2073–74, 2082–83), it is not strictly evil, as in the early Christian period: in Hesiod, for example, *daimones* are good (ἐσθλοί, *Op.* 122–23).

[39] Padel 1992.140. See also Fränkel 1975.70–71; Padel 1992.114–61.

[40] At *Il.* 21.278, Achilles predicts that he will be killed by Apollo's missiles; see also Pi. *Pae.* 6.78–86 and *LIMC* s.v. Achilleus. It is generally agreed that Patroclus's death anticipates Achilles' own: see, e.g., Nickel 2002.230–31; Allan 2005b.13. For Patroclus as a sacrificial substitute for Achilles, see Lowenstam 1981.126–77.

[41] The motif of a triple assault repulsed by a god on the fourth attempt first appears at 16.702–4, where the hand of Apollo pushes Patroclus back. The only other triple assaults are at 5.436–39 (Diomedes) and 20.445–48 (Achilles), and these three warriors alone are called δαίμονι ἶσος. See also *Od.* 21.125–29 (Telemachus tries to string his father's bow).

are quickly undercut by clues of the relationship's true asymmetry. After all, how does one meet in combat (ἀντιβολέω) the one who strikes from afar (ἑκατηβόλος)?[42] Shrouded in a deep mist, Apollo moves through the crowd unnoticed by Patroclus before coming to stand behind him (στῆ δ' ὄπιθεν, 791). As in the account of Apollo's attack in book 1, there is a highly effective enjambment in the narration of Apollo's arrival: "Phoebus came against you in the strong encounter, terrible" (ἤντετο γάρ τοι Φοῖβος ἐνὶ κρατερῇ ὑσμίνῃ / δεινός, 788–89). By the time we hear the word *deinos*, "terrible," the god is already upon Patroclus. Moreover, like the plague victims, Patroclus cannot see what hit him. Struck on the back by Apollo's downturned hand (χειρὶ καταπρηνεῖ, 792), his eyes spin—a rare anticipation of one of tragedy's most important symptoms of inner crisis—*atē* seizes him, and he is left dazed and naked before Euphorbus's spear.[43] And if, when the far-shooter strikes from up close, he strikes from behind, it appears necessary that Euphorbus's attack come from the same place, despite the fact that we are not told how Patroclus has been turned around.[44] It comes as no surprise that Euphorbus, slinking away, looks as cowardly as an archer.

Patroclus, it would seem, is struck quite literally by Apollo. Dramatic symptoms are, in fact, frequently expressed, from the archaic period onward, not only in terms of arrows but also in terms of daemonic blows or seizures. The Chorus in Sophocles' *Ajax* wonders about the blow (πληγή) from heaven that has felled their leader (278–79); while, in Aristophanes' *Birds*, someone out at night runs the risk of meeting the hero Orestes—heroes were among the agents that could be blamed for symptoms—and being struck (πληγείς) by him all

---

[42] The epithet has also been interpreted as "he who shoots at will," based on the "gloss" provided by Hera at *Il*. 21.484 (referring to Artemis). See Faraone 1992.71 n.58. Willcock 1970.9 n.21 argues that Apollo "acts at one remove from reality" when he strikes Patroclus, and, in fact, gods never kill humans directly on the battlefield (Ares is an exception: see *Il*. 5.842–44, with Kirk 1990.147). I would say, rather, the gods act on a different but nevertheless very real dimension of the hero.

[43] στρεφεδίνηθεν δέ οἱ ὄσσε anticipates Aeschylus's στροφοδινοῦνται (*Ag*. 51; see also *Pr*. 882: τροχοδινεῖται δ' ὄμμαθ' ἑλίγδην). As Janko 1992.412 notes, elsewhere in epic, turning eyes indicate *good* vision (*Il*. 17.679–80, ὄσσε φαεινώ / πάντοσε δινείσθην; cf. *h. Herm*. 45). Janko contrasts the death of Patroclus with 13.434–40, where Poseidon paralyzes Alcathous on the battlefield, arguing that in that case, the god interferes "directly with his mind"; Patroclus, on the other hand, is never represented as insane (1992.413–14). It is hard to know how to understand this claim. Phrases like τὸν δ' ἄτη φρένας εἷλε (16.805) and στῆ δὲ ταφών (806) are clearer than anything in the Alcathous passage regarding the god's interference with cognitive functions. See Lowenstam 1981.82, who connects the two passages, and Hershkowitz 1998.151–52, 157–58: "The uncanny events which compose Patroclus' death . . . all contribute to an atmosphere which in a post-Homeric epic context would be defined by madness" (157). Derek Collins argues that Patroclus is possessed from the moment he puts on Achilles' armor (1998.35–42), but this reading removes the sense that there are different gradations of possession.

[44] The omission has troubled commentators. Janko 1992.408–9 infers that Apollo's blow makes Patroclus turn around; see also 414. How warriors get wounded in the back was a problem for scholiasts as well: see 278 on the death of Cleitus.

along his right side (1490–93).[45] In the *Homeric Hymn to Demeter*, the goddess declares she will protect the infant Demophoön against magical attack (ἐπηλυσίη) and the "under-cutter" (ὑποτάμνον, 228–30), probably a kind of *daimōn*.[46] The shadowy figure of Ephialtes is held responsible for nightmares characterized by sudden, suffocating attacks and strong fevers: later popular etymology derives his name from the verb *ephallomai*, "to spring" or "to attack."[47] The mad are "struck aside" (παράκοπος, παραπεπληγμένος).[48]

In these cases of attack, as in arrow attacks, the assailant often exploits a visual advantage over his victim. On vases and gems, gods and *daimones* are often depicted assaulting from above or behind.[49] *Atē*, the godsent folly that leads one astray and the ruin that follows, walks with delicate feet on the heads of men (*Il.* 19.91–94).[50] It is in part because *daimones* or gods see all while acting, like Apollo, clothed in mist, that they can disrupt human lives at will.[51] "Who," asks Odysseus, "could see with his eyes a god not wishing to be seen as he goes here or there?" (τίς ἂν θεὸν οὐκ ἐθέλοντα / ὀφθαλμοῖσιν ἴδοιτ᾽ ἢ ἔνθ᾽ ἢ ἔνθα κιόντα, *Od.* 10.573–74).

---

[45] See also Ar. *Av.* 712 and *Ach.* 1166, with Brelich 1958.228 n.5. The verb πλήσσω, "to strike," also gives rise to the adjectives ἀπόπληκτος and ἔκπληκτος, "to be struck dumb, dazed, or mad": see Ar. *V.* 948; Hdt. 2.173; Men. *Dysc.* 312; fr. 348 (*PCG*); S. fr. 248R. The terms continue be used in medical contexts: *Aph.* II.42 (Li 4.482 = 118 Jones), VI.57 (Li 4.578 = 192 Jones); *Coac.* 157 (Li 5.618); *Flat.* 13 (Li 6.110 = 120,12–121,5 Jouanna). The language of "blows" is found in Latin too; e.g., Lucr. *DRN* 6.805, describing the effect of wine on a fever. For heroes or daemonic agents as envoys of disease, see Ar. fr. 322 (*PCG*); Ath. 11, 461c; Babr. 63; D. L. 8.32; Men. fr. 348 (*PCG*); Philostr. *Her.* 18.1–6; with Julius Tambornino 1909.55–62; Rohde 1925.134–36; Herter 1950.125–27; W. Smith 1965.406–13; Lanata 1967.28–37; R. Parker 1983.243–44; Brenk 1986.2070–71; Dunbar 1995.453, 692–93; Jouanna 2003.61. Pan and the nymphs, too, can be blamed for sudden attacks and disease, as at Men. *Dysc.* 309–13: see Roscher 1900.76–82; Julius Tambornino 1909.58, 66–67; Borgeaud 1988.88–118, with 239 nn.2–4; Faraone 1999.46 (on erotic "seizures").

[46] Cf. *h. Herm.* 37; Pollux 4.187, where ἐπηλυσία appears in a list of diseases between pleuritis and strangury. At Nonn. *D.* 14.328, it describes the assault of a god in battle. Other daemonic "assault" words: ἔφοδος: A. *Eu.* 370; E. *Ion* 1048–49; προσβολή: A. *Ch.* 283; Ar. *Pax* 39. On the "under-cutter" and the "wood-cutter" in the next line, see Faraone 2001, arguing that these are the names of demons who attack teething children.

[47] For the *daimōn*, see Phryn. Com. frr. 1–5 (*PCG*); Sophron frr. 67–68 (Hordern). The word ἐφιάλτης is glossed as a fever with shivering fits (ῥιγοπύρετον) in the *Suda*. On Ephialtes and other fever and nightmare demons, see Roscher 1898.178–80; 1900; Herter 1950.126; Johnston 1995.383. On the Babylonian night-terror demon, see Stol 1993.38–42.

[48] E.g., A. *Eu.* 329; *Pr.* 581; Ar. *Lys.* 831; E. *Ba.* 33, 1000; *HF* 935; *Hipp.* 38, 238. On madness terms with παρα-, see Mattes 1970.104–6; Borgeaud 1988.122; Padel 1992.117–19; 1995.21–22, 120–23; Byl 2006, on the Hippocratic Corpus.

[49] On the visual characteristics of *daimones*, see Roscher 1900.29–38, 52–53; Padel 1992.125–32 (esp. 129–32, on winged adversaries), 157–59; Johnston 1995.371–79 (esp. 374–75, on winged figures).

[50] Blindness—mental or physical—is not the "original" meaning of *atē*, as, for example, Doyle 1984 would like: see Padel 1995.167–69, 184 n.43. Nevertheless, blindness is certainly at the center of its semantic field. On *atē*, see also Dodds 1951.1–27; Padel 1995.167–96, 246–59. On the related concept of *atasthaliai*, see Hooker 1988; Padel 1995.170.

[51] Clothed in mist: see, e.g., Hes. *Op.* 255: ἠέρα ἑσσάμενοι; *Il.* 9.571: ἠεροφοῖτις, with Hainsworth 1993.137–38.

These descriptions of daemonic aggression are no doubt familiar to readers of Greek poetry. One might extend that familiarity to the Greeks, arguing that, at least by the classical period, these expressions were largely "metaphorical." Yet the Hippocratic writings themselves preserve evidence that daemonic violence was, in the classical period, still a persuasive explanation for symptoms, particularly spectacular ones, and worthy of energetic rebuttal. The most detailed attack in the corpus on those who would explain illness—here, epileptic seizure—in terms of the daemonic and the divine sheds some light on what these explanations might have looked like:[52]

ἴσως δὲ οὐχ οὕτως ἔχει ταῦτα, ἀλλ᾿ ἄνθρωποι βίου δεόμενοι πολλὰ καὶ παντοῖα τεχνῶνται καὶ ποικίλλουσιν ἔς τε τἆλλα πάντα καὶ ἐς τὴν νοῦσον ταύτην, ἑκάστῳ εἴδει τοῦ πάθεος θεῷ τὴν αἰτίην προστιθέντες. οὐ γὰρ ἐναλλά[ξ, ἀλλὰ][53] πλεονάκις γε μὴν ταὐτὰ μεμίμηνται· ἢν μὲν γὰρ αἶγα μιμῶνται κἢν βρύχωνται κἢν τὰ δεξιὰ σπῶνται, Μητέρα θεῶν φασιν αἰτίην εἶναι· ἢν δὲ ὀξύτερον καὶ ἐντονώτερον φθέγγηται, ἵππῳ εἰκάζουσι καί φασι Ποσειδέωνα αἴτιον εἶναι· ἢν δὲ καὶ τῆς κόπρου τι παριῇ, ὃ πολλάκις γίνεται ὑπὸ τῆς νούσου βιαζομένοισιν, Ἐνοδίης θεοῦ πρόσκειται ἡ ἐπωνυμίη· ἢν δὲ πυκνότερον καὶ λεπτότερον οἷον ὄρνιθες, Ἀπόλλων νόμιος· ἢν δὲ ἀφρὸν ἐκ τοῦ στόματος ἀφιῇ καὶ τοῖσι ποσὶ λακτίζῃ, Ἄρης τὴν αἰτίην ἔχει· οἷσι δὲ νυκτὸς δείματα παρίσταται καὶ φόβοι καὶ παράνοιαι καὶ ἀναπηδήσιες ἐκ τῆς κλίνης καὶ φεύξιες ἔξω, Ἑκάτης φασὶν εἶναι ἐπιβολὰς καὶ ἡρώων ἐφόδους. (*Morb. Sacr.* 1, Li 6.360–62 = 7,17–8,13 Jouanna)

Perhaps things are not this way; rather people in need of an income concoct and devise many and varied fictions, about this disease as about other things, laying the blame for each expression of the affection upon a particular god. For it is not sometimes one thing, sometimes another that the patients imitate, but they are often the same things. If he imitates a goat, if he grinds his teeth, or suffers convulsion on the right side of his body, they say that the Mother of the Gods is responsible. If he utters a piercing, loud cry, they liken him to a horse and say that Poseidon is responsible. If he also passes some excrement, which often happens to those overpowered by the disease, the name of the goddess Enodia is supplied. If he utters a sound[54] that is more frequent and thin, like that of a bird—Apollo Nomios. If he foams at the mouth and kicks, Ares holds responsibility. For those who suffer night terrors and fears and delirium and leap from their beds and run out of doors, they say that these are the assaults of Hecate and the attacks of the heroes.

These interpretations of symptoms share a number of similarities with the diagnostic paradigms found in early Mesopotamian evidence.[55] They also mobilize

---

[52] For discussion of the passage, see W. Smith 1965.405–10; Lanata 1967.57–60; R. Parker 1983.244–45; Faraone 1992.44–45.

[53] ἐναλλάξ, ἀλλὰ Jouanna: ἐν ἀλλὰ M: ἄλλα θ. See Jouanna 2003.56–57.

[54] Supplying φθέγγηται from line 6 (see Jouanna 2003.59–60).

[55] For example, "if, at the time it overcomes him, his limbs are dissolving, his innards seize him time and again, his bowels move: Hand of a Spirit" (Stol 1993.61). See Geller 2004 and Heeßel

symbolic associations familiar from Greek cult.[56] This passage indicates that an etiological paradigm committed to daemonic and divine agency was no conceit of poets or painters. Our evidence about how symptoms were interpreted within a magico-religious framework is remarkably consistent in its emphasis on external attack, whether through arrows, blows, or seizures, and on the agents held responsible. This model is an important foil to medical explanation, even in cases where it is not targeted for rebuttal.

If the modus operandi of divine assailants overlaps in significant ways with that of the mortal archer or the stealth fighter, what does this mean? Is Euphorbus imitating Apollo when he retraces the god's blow with visible, "real" weapons? Or is it Apollo who is acting like a human combatant, and a cowardly one at that? The god, like Euphorbus, exploits Patroclus's blind spot. Yet, although Apollo's encounter with Patroclus appears staged in the "real" space of the battlefield, there are, as it were, *too many* references to blindness: why does Apollo, already shrouded in mist, need to strike Patroclus from behind? These multiple cues suggest that something more is going on here—that, despite Apollo's apparent spatial proximity, his blow is more like his arrow in its ability to bypass the skin and strike Patroclus's core forces directly.

We might understand Apollo's attack as straddling two dimensions of reality. That is, the attack appears choreographed in such a way as to map the basic epistemic asymmetry between mortals and immortals onto how bodies relate to one another on the battlefield, and specifically how they move in and out of fields of vision: knowing is expressed through seeing; seeing represents knowing.[57] Apollo is thus exploiting *two* related types of vulnerability. On the one hand, he commands a simple power advantage over his victim—like a lion or a spear, he has the capacity to cause serious harm. On the other hand, as a god, he has an excess of knowledge or sight.[58] At the moment he strikes Patroclus, Apollo uses this twofold power to translate Patroclus's defenselessness vis-à-vis the gods into his exposure, expressed through both blindness and nakedness, on the

---

2004, esp. 108–10. See also the text on epilepsy in Kinnier Wilson and Reynolds 1990; Stol 1993. On the Assyrio-Babylonian model of "if p, then q," see G. Manetti 1993.6–13. There may also be vestiges of archaic Greek diagnostic strategies in the Hippocratic passage, as R. Parker 1983.210 suggests. The correlation of symptoms with specific gods or daemons, however, is widespread: see Csordas 1990.14–15 on a similar diagnostic model among contemporary Charismatic Christians.

[56] Jouanna 2003.8 n.3, 57–61. On the attacks of Hecate, see also E. *Hel.* 569; *Trag. Adesp.* 375 (Kannicht-Snell).

[57] I am not saying that knowing can *only* be acquired through seeing in Homer, but, rather, that knowledge is particularly implicated in sight in contexts focused on asymmetries of power. Von Fritz (1943.88–91; 1945) and Snell (1953.13, 136–39) understand knowledge in Homer as largely dependent on sense perception, especially sight, a claim that plays a significant role in their respective claims about the development of abstract knowledge and logical thought. (A more extensive bibliography on this argument can be found at Lesher 1994.2 n.4.) Cf. Hussey 1990.13–14, pointing to instances in Homer where knowledge is not derived through sense perception, though he acknowledges the close relationship between knowing and seeing; Lesher 1994.6–7.

[58] For a discussion of gods primarily in terms of their (strategic) epistemic advantage, see Boyer 2001.150–67.

battlefield. A pair of mortal heroes then takes advantage of Patroclus's vulnerability as we shift from the logic of the symptom to the logic of the wound.

Although we have been focusing on the relationships between mortals and immortals, the gods, too, turn out to be immune neither to epistemic asymmetries nor to the vulnerability they create. If the wounds of Ares and Aphrodite in *Iliad* 5 prove that divine skin can be violated,[59] Hera's deception of Zeus in *Iliad* 14 illustrates how gods can harm or incapacitate other gods by exploiting their blind spots. Her mission relies on the aid of Hupnos, the personification of sleep. His power, in turn, requires that *he not be seen* by Zeus, a condition here, as in *Iliad* 16, that is marked by the poet. Arriving "before the eyes of Zeus alight on him" (πάρος Διὸς ὄσσε ἰδέσθαι, 14.286), Hupnos positions himself up *above* the god atop the highest tree on Mount Ida, up in the aether. There, hidden by the branches, he assumes a bird disguise like those used by gods when they intervene in mortal affairs.[60] Zeus, trusting in his power, believes that not even sharp-eyed Helios will be able to see through (διαδράκοι, 344) the cloud that he draws around himself and Hera to conceal their lovemaking. That very cloud, however, becomes the deep sleep that Hupnos pours out to block the god's vision. The cloud recalls the wave of *erōs* that has already enveloped Zeus's *phrenes* (ἀμφεκάλυψεν, 294). Both sleep and desire thus translate Zeus's visual disadvantage vis-à-vis the personified Hupnos into a more disabling blindness that allows Hera to aid the Greeks. This is as close to a breakdown in Zeus's defenses as we get: because he has already secured his hegemony in the *Iliad*, there is no Euphorbus waiting in the wings. Those who die as a result of his blindness are, rather, his mortal protégés.[61] Nevertheless, Zeus does have blind spots, and these are correlated with his occupation of space in human-like form. That is, it is his embodiment that creates the potential for infinite nesting: just as the archer Teucer can be seen and, hence, controlled by an unseen Zeus, so Zeus himself can be seen and controlled by Hupnos (who himself might be seen by another god). Nested visual asymmetries correspond to a continuum of ever more efficacious agency, which is as dependent on position—Zeus, for example, can become subject to Hupnos—as it is on a fated apportioning of power.

When the poet choreographs Apollo's attack on Patroclus or describes the "meeting" of Hupnos and Zeus, he would seem to be anthropomorphizing his divine actors—that is, projecting the human onto the nonhuman. In a canonical article, T.B.L. Webster made bodily appearance one of the three major aspects of personification in the Greek world, together with physical life and movement and mental power and feelings.[62]

---

[59] See Loraux 1986; 1995.93.

[60] Gods appearing as birds: *Od.* 3.372, 22.239–40. Cf. *Il.* 5.778, 13.62–64, 15.237–38 (gods are like birds).

[61] Compare Agamemnon's etiology of *atē* at *Il.* 19.95–133, where Heracles suffers from Zeus's blindness. On Zeus's hegemony in the *Iliad*, see Slatkin 1991.

[62] Webster 1954.10. See also G. Lloyd 1966.200–202; Stafford 2000.1–44. On different ways of projecting the human, see also Boyer 1996.89–92.

But we might wonder what motivates the poet to endow the gods with bodies in the first place. They do not seem to need them in order to act: Zeus breaks Teucer's bowstring without any mention being made of how this happens. Hupnos describes himself "being poured" (ἀμφιχυθείς, 14.253) over the god's *noos*, rather than acting on him *qua* embodied agent.[63] In fact, even actual contact between bodies does not tell us much about how a god exercises his power. If we look closely, when Apollo hits Patroclus "with downturned hand" (χειρὶ καταπρηνεῖ, 16.792), he directly damages the flashpoints of Patroclus's agency: his limbs, his eyes, and his *phrenes*. The expression "with downturned hand" occurs in only one other place in the Homeric epics, in *Odyssey* 13: Poseidon strikes the ship of the Phaeacians "with downturned hand" in order to petrify it (164).[64] These attacks assume total susceptibility to a god's power, a power that in the *Odyssey* example is entirely unlike the power involved in mortal-on-mortal violence. They thus warn against applying our realism and its laws to Apollo's assault on Patroclus.[65]

Moreover, despite the fact that Apollo's slap is *like* an arrow or a blow from behind, it leaves neither a wound nor a bruise: the violation does not involve the skin.[66] To understand what is going on here, we need to take a closer look at two ways of imagining the integrity of the person. I begin by sketching this integrity in neutral terms, but it will become increasingly clear that I am particularly interested in how it is violated and how violations are explained. I then return to the question of why human-like bodies are used to conceptualize divine and daemonic aggression.

The Seen and the Felt

The crippling impact of Apollo's slap would seem to confirm Fränkel's well-known claim that the Homeric subject is an open force field (*offenes Kraftfeld*).[67] On the basis of this claim, Fränkel draws a conclusion that dovetails with those

---

[63] In Greek art, Hupnos *is* represented as an embodied agent who often stands in miniature form on top of his victims: see Vermeule 1979.145–54; Mainoldi 1987.39–45; Shapiro 1993.132–58.

[64] See also *h. Ap.* 334, where χειρὶ καταπρηνεῖ is used of Hera calling upon the chthonic gods. Lowenstam 1981.68–73 discusses all three examples and concludes that the phrase is used only under conditions where a concealed god strikes a destructive blow. He persuasively argues that the blow to the ship is a displacement of the blow that Poseidon desires to deliver to Odysseus (1981.90–96). On the related phrase χερσὶ καταπρηνέσσ', which appears in relationship to thigh-slapping, see Lowenstam 1981.31–67.

[65] See Padel 1992.33–44; 1995.169.

[66] Compare the marvelous blinding of Epizelus during the Battle of Marathon at Hdt. 6.117: he loses his sight suddenly, "though neither struck nor wounded on any part of his body" (οὔτε πληγέντα οὐδὲν τοῦ σώματος οὔτε βληθέντα). At *Il.* 24.757–59, one killed by Apollo's gentle arrows shows no trace of a wound. But see below, p. 136, on the "stricken" (βλήτοι), who do have mysterious bruises on their flanks.

[67] Fränkel 1975.80–81. See also Dodds 1951.13–18; Snell 1953.29–31.

of Snell: "It is meaningless to ask where [the hero's] own force begins and that from outside ends ... our own basic antithesis between self and not-self does not yet exist in Homeric consciousness."[68] Yet the idea of a *Kraftfeld* need not foreclose the integrity of the subject in Homer. Indeed, the spectacular loss of control that we have just witnessed in Patroclus makes sense only if the poet already has a working idea of the centripetal force of identity over and above the pressures of the external world. If a Homeric hero infers the presence of something daemonic—barring cases such as *atē*, where the knowledge of the daemonic blow is conferred retroactively—it is precisely because he has a finely calibrated awareness of norms both in himself and in the world around him: recall Teucer's pointed remark about the fresh sinew on his bow. The sense of self is not so much challenged by perceptions of otherness as *built* out of such perceptions.

The sensed boundaries of the self are just one means of drawing up a person in Homer. The person also has a visibly unified form and structure, an *eidos* and a *demas*. He is a three-dimensional object covered by the *khrōs*, whose violation can cause the innards to fall out; he is a locus of internal dialogue severed from the public domain by the "wall of teeth." He is the center of intentions, a synthesis of energies directed outward through the limbs, *melea* and *guia*.[69] He is bound together by forces, concentrated in the knees and limbs, that flow away if he is struck by fear or injured—indeed, death from one perspective is simply a loosening of the bonds that hold the person together.[70] Boundaries within the person, though less fixed, are important, too. When the *phrenes* contain the *thumos*, a person thinks clearly.[71] Andromache's *ētor*, usually somewhere in the chest, rises to her mouth when she learns of Hector's death (*Il.* 22.451–53).

For the purposes of this chapter, I would like to narrow these ways of thinking about the boundaries of the self to two, one corresponding to violations via the weapon, the other implicated in daemonic-divine attack. The first set of boundaries concerns what I call the seen, that is, primarily the structure of the person and the skin, as well as the flesh and bones revealed by a deep wound; the second concerns the felt, that is, the cognitive-affective dimension of the person: surges of strength, emotions, thoughts, breath, and so on.[72] The seen and the felt are, in essence, different perspectives on the person. The *phrenes*, for example,

---

[68] Fränkel 1975.80. At the same time, Fränkel holds that "Homeric man" feels himself to be "a unitary being" (76).

[69] On the intentional body, see Merleau-Ponty 1962, esp. 112–77.

[70] E.g., *Il.* 21.114; *Od.* 4.703, 23.205. Bolens 2000 argues that "le corps chez Homère est *un tout articulé* ... organisé selon une logique définissable, une logique de rapports et de jonction" (56, emphasis in original). On death as a loosening of the bonds of self: Bolens 2000.43–46. On the rehearsal of this loosening in syncope, see Nehring 1947.

[71] See Caswell 1990.43–44; see also 52: "The relationship of θυμός to φρήν/φρένες is that of content to container." I do, however, think that this conceptual model risks falling back on the idea that *thumos* can be localized in an anatomical sense and that its primary "reality" is spatial.

[72] See also the discussion in Holmes 2007.54–57.

are both something that comes out on the tip of a spear (*Il.* 16.504) and a locus of feeling, pain, and thought. The limbs and knees may be enlivened by an influx of *menos* (*Il.* 5.122), unnerved by desire (*Od.* 18.212), or weighted down by hunger (*Il.* 19.165–66).[73] Yet they are also integral to the visible morphology of the person, as the *phrenes* are not. Neither of these ways of knowing gives access to a single "real" body onto which every kind of perception can be mapped. That is to say that *no* objective perspective, whether "anatomical" or "culturo-historical," captures the subjective experience of embodiment. Each perspective is informed by both nature and culture; each is governed by its own logic.

If the poet describes a spear entering the side of the nose, passing between the teeth and through the tongue, and coming out behind the angle of the jaw on the other side of the neck (*Il.* 5.290–93), he is assuming a person comprising both seen parts and potentially seen parts. By drawing a line between two points, the spear emphasizes the continuity of inside and outside: what enters this three-dimensional object passes through localizable parts and reemerges at a predictable point. Although the person's fleshy innards are revealed only at the moment of death, the anatomical knowledge informing the description of this moment is always available to the poet.[74] In fact, because it is through identifying with the target of his weapons that the hero maps his own points of weakness, that knowledge is available in some sense to the warrior, too.[75] Battle is an education in the topography of an object that can be wounded in many different ways.

In contrast, Homer's descriptions of, say, the *thumos*, assume a felt relationship to a self whose boundaries are more difficult for us to reconstruct, though no less real. For the self does not simply occupy space in relation to other objects. It is also a conscious field.[76] Guillemette Bolens has persuasively suggested that this integrated, *felt* awareness of the self is the primary meaning of *thumos*.[77] In truth, the domain of the felt covers a whole complex of things that have been the object of prolonged and vexed study by modern scholars, not

[73] On the limbs: Bolens 2000.19–59.

[74] Homer's anatomy is often admired, although its precision is debatable: for attempts to gauge its accuracy, see Saunders 1999; Friedrich 2003. On anatomy, the symbolic topography of the warrior's body, and the stylization of wounds, see above, n.6. Vermeule 1979.96 picks up on the poetic potential of anatomical detail ("There is an almost baroque magnificence in the physical ruin of Homer's heroes").

[75] On a warrior's knowledge of his opponent's body, see, e.g., *Il.* 4.467–68, 22.321. See also Daremberg 1865.75–76; Marg 1976.10; Grmek 1989.28.

[76] The continuities within this conscious field are captured by the idea of a "dialogue" between parts of the self, discussed in C. Gill 1996a. Gill, however, argues that there is nothing in Homer's psychological terminology to distinguish unconscious and conscious thought processes and dismisses the idea that thought is conscious as Cartesian (1996a.43–45, 58–60). Yet there is no reason to assume a notion of nonconscious thought; consciousness, moreover, appears to designate the space of the self. The emergence of the physical body, I suggest, creates the possibility of nonconscious space, which is then taken up in complex ways in relationship to the soul.

[77] Bolens 2000.50.

only *thumos* but also *ētor, kēr, kradiē, phrēn/phrenes, prapides,* and sometimes *menos, noos,* and *psukhē.* Part of the trouble in these studies is the tension they perceive between the spatial qualities of (most of) these entities—things are located *in* them, they are subject to attack, they at times appear to have definite coordinates inside the person—and their role as faculties. Much energy, moreover, has been devoted to determining their anatomical referents. The very difficulty of reconciling Homer's innards with our understanding of the body can explain why so many of these studies feel inconclusive.

One strategy for avoiding some of these problems has been to jettison the principle of difference within this field of terms altogether and to focus on the collective behavior of the various parts. Thomas Jahn has argued that the terms *ētor, kēr, kradiē, thumos, phrēn/phrenes,* and *prapides* are basically interchangeable in Homer insofar as their psychological function is concerned, concluding that the use of individual terms is largely determined by metrical convenience.[78] Developing the implications of Jahn's findings, Michael Clarke has attributed thoughts and emotions in Homer and other archaic poetry to a single psychological "apparatus," which any single term may invoke.[79] Whereas scholars seeking to define and identify each member of what Clarke calls the "*thumos-*family" have tended to see the Homeric self as fragmented, Clarke concludes that the very difficulty of assigning functions to individual "organs" confirms that we are dealing with a single apparatus.[80]

Both Jahn and Clarke, however, continue to work with a basic notion of physical location in opposition to mental function.[81] Thus, despite the fact that all the parts work together, they are still parts, whose identities are secured through anatomical or physiological difference. The commitment to the underlying corporeal reality of the Homeric self has proved tenacious. R. B. Onians's identification of *thumos* with breath, for example, continues to look attractive to scholars.[82] Yet, even if this identification captures something of the mobility and the ephemeral nature of *thumos,* it nevertheless risks mistaking *thumos* for

[78] Jahn 1987.

[79] Clarke 1999.61–126. See also Halliwell 1990.37–42; Padel 1992.12–48 ("innards"); C. Gill 1996a.41–93, 175–239; Spatafora 1999.12.

[80] Clarke 1999.64. The tendency to work through these terms and assign each entity a clear identity is well represented in Böhme 1929, which Clarke locates at the end of a long tradition of German Homerists (1999.64 n.11). The methodology lives on in individual treatments of members of Clarke's *thumos*-family, such as the studies of S. Darcus (1979b; 1980; 1981), later publishing as S. D. Sullivan (1983; 1987; 1988; 1994a; 1994b; 1995; 1996); see also Bolelli 1948; Cheyns 1980; 1985; Claus 1981.11–47; Caswell 1990.

[81] Jahn sees *ētor, kēr, kradiē, phrenes, prapides,* and *thumos* as *Körperteile* with interchangeable psychological meanings (1987.9–17). Clarke has recourse to the idea of "intangible mental activity" in seeking to account for the identity of the *thumos*-complex in nonanatomical terms (1999.79); elsewhere, he speaks of an "abstract" sense of force (1995.302 n.27).

[82] See Onians 1954.44–50 and Clarke 1999.75–83. See also Justesen 1928.17–32; Larock 1930, esp. 381–84; Caswell 1990.7; Padel 1992.27–30. Cf. Bolens 2000.48–51, stressing the limitations of the physiological reading.

an ahistorical, physical stuff. As Onians himself observes, *thumos* "expressed a much richer concept for the Homeric Greeks than our 'breath' or mere outer air received and expelled."[83] *Thumos* is as much defined by its power to impel a warrior to battle as it is through its warmth or its vaporous nature. Moreover, its warmth and its cloudiness are gauged from a primarily subjective viewpoint that treats *thumos* within the person, not in terms of our notion of breath, but as something both gaseous and liquid—"breath related to blood" we might say; Homer says simply *thumos*.[84] Breath and *thumos*, then, share some properties but not others. Those properties we do not recognize are not cultural additions to a physical reality. Rather, they register what it feels like to inhabit a body at a particular cultural and historical moment as much as how a body is seen.

Similar caveats are worth keeping in mind when we deal with the *phrenes*. On the basis of their later identification with the diaphragm in medical writing, some scholars have assumed they have the same meaning in earlier literature; others, arguing that the language Homer uses to describe the *phrenes* suggests containing structures—the plural is more common—probably fitted around the heart, have equated them with the lungs.[85] Once this identification is in place, the frequent description of the *phrenes* as dark can be referred to the fact that "the adult lung is bluish grey"; another common adjective, *pukinos*, "close, dense," but also "wise," is explained by the "multitude of branching passages and veins within each lung and the intricate tracery, the polygonal lobules of the outside."[86] Yet, what does it mean to identify the *phrenes* with the lungs? If, for example, the epic poets say that wine "holds" or "goes around" or "weighs down" the *phrenes*, are they making a mistake?[87] Onians thinks that the *fact* that the lungs do not receive wine is irrelevant to an investigation of ancient belief (a tacit acknowledgment that he believes the ancients are, indeed, mistaken on this point).[88] In fact, the emergence of the use of physiological facts in arguments about reality is deeply relevant to ancient beliefs about the person. Consider the Hippocratic treatise *On Diseases* IV, whose author firmly believes that it is erroneous to say the lungs, here identified as *pleumones*, are

---

[83] Onians 1954.46.

[84] "Breath related to blood": Onians 1954.48. On *thumos* as both gaseous and liquid, see also Padel 1992.29, 89; Clarke 1999.79–92.

[85] *Phrenes* as lungs: Justesen 1928.4–16; Onians 1954.23–43; Clarke 1999.77–79. As diaphragm: Böhme 1929.3–9; Larock 1930.385–88. Others have seen the *phrenes* as a group of organs in the chest or something indeterminate: see Ireland and Steel 1975, esp. 194; Cheyns 1980, esp. 167; Sullivan 1988.21–29. See also Darcus 1979b; Padel 1992.20–26. The *prapides* are sometimes seen as synonymous with *phrenes*, but cf. Sullivan 1987; Spatafora 1999.12. For the *phrenes* holding the heart: *Il.* 16.481; the liver: *Od.* 9.301.

[86] Onians 1954.28. But not all scholars who grant *phrenes* an anatomical meaning read every appearance of the word in this light: see Ireland and Steel 1975.187–88, critiquing Onians's "literalism."

[87] E.g., *Od.* 9.362, 18.331, 19.122. See also Alc. fr. 347 (L-P), with *pleumones*, and the examples at Onians 1954.36.

[88] Onians 1954.35–36.

moistened by wine.[89] His perception of error is founded on a view of anatomical and physiological reality not unlike the view we use to gauge the archaic poets' mistake: he refers, among other things, to the softness and delicacy of the lungs, and the idea of the lung as hollow, resonant space.[90] Yet we cannot assume the anatomical and physiological reality of the lungs is the touchstone of truth in the Homeric poems. This is not to say what we call anatomy or physiology has nothing to do with archaic views of the person. Rather, human beings are simply not imagined in these terms. In Homer, *phrenes* are just *phrenes*: they turn (*Il.* 6.61) and flutter (*Od.* 22.298); they are deceived by love (*Od.* 15.421), bitten by words (*Il.* 5.493), and maddened by wine (*Od.* 21.297).[91] The fact that we have bodies would seem to bring us closer to Homer. But by assuming anatomy as the "real" that we share with Homer, we risk forgetting the historical, cultural, and scientific schemas that mediate our own embodied experience and encounters with the innards.

What happens when the flesh is cut open in Homer? The *phrenes*, we have seen, can exit the chest on a spearhead.[92] Does the cut establish a continuum between the felt and the seen? As it turns out, whatever appears through the cut seems to belong to the register of the visual and *its* laws, losing any relationship to cognition and emotion. In fact, epic poetry associates the revelation of innards with the moment of death, when the warrior is on his way to becoming a corpse and, hence, no longer animated from within.[93] Only with the inquiry into nature and the subsequent changes to medicine does the inside of the living body come to be imagined primarily as *potentially seen*, a historical shift that culminates with the desire of Hellenistic physicians to bear witness to the inner life of the body through vivisection.[94] In that intellectual climate, an epic poet might mime an anatomist: in charting the workings of the Erotes inside Medea, Apollonius describes a terrible pain smoldering through her flesh, going on to map its path onto the structures (e.g., the nerves) discovered by his contemporary Herophilus (3.762–63). In Homer, by contrast, the world of the felt is not referred back to an anatomical substratum; limbs and organs and skin

---

[89] See Onians 1954.37–40, on the relationship of *phrenes* and *pleumones*. Onians thinks the words are used interchangeably until *phrenes* is appropriated for the diaphragm in the classical period.

[90] *Morb.* IV 56 (Li 7.604–8 = 119,18–122,3 Joly). See Lonie 1981.361–63 for the controversy about lungs and liquid in later centuries.

[91] On "turning," see Spatafora 1999.42–48.

[92] Note that *menos, noos, psukhē,* and *thumos* are never wounded or seen.

[93] It is at this point, too, that the hero finally sees himself from outside, assuming the form of the *eidōlon* who stands over and mourns the corpse. For representations of *eidōla* on vase paintings, see Siebert 1981; Shapiro 1993.136–37, nos. 70–71.

[94] One of the arguments against the practice in antiquity, however, was that the anatomical eye always arrives too late: the moment the cut is made, there is no longer anything left of life to see (Cels. *De med.* procem. 42–43 = 24,4–14 Marx). For the evidence on vivisection, see Herophilus frr. 63a–c, 66 (von Staden), with the judicious discussion in von Staden 1989.144–53, 234–36, who concludes that vivisection was probably practiced on humans in Hellenistic Alexandria.

are not viewed primarily as objects.[95] The world of the felt has its own boundaries, and these boundaries are crossed in specific ways.

THE BOUNDARIES OF THE FELT

It has become clear that a daemonic force like *hupnos* does not so much violate the boundaries of the seen as bypass them altogether to produce an unmediated effect on the felt. How should we understand this effect? We can start to answer this question by exploring the flow of forces in and through the felt. First, felt forces participate in the dynamics of wind and water, best expressed in the surging and turning of the sea.[96] Thoughts whirl in the chest (*Od.* 20.217–18). *Thumos* moves like rushing winds and tempests.[97] Anguished deliberation is as tumultuous as a blizzard or a rainstorm (*Il.* 10.5–10). In objectifying inner turmoil in words, the epic poet draws on a natural world that is both seen and felt: the idea of the troubled sea, for example, may assume not only the spectacle of waves but also the feeling of being at sea in a storm. Whereas, for a Hippocratic author, wind is "invisible to sight, visible to reason" (*Flat.* 3, Li 6.94 = 106,9–10 Jouanna), wind in Homer is not the opposite of the seen but describes another mode of experience.[98]

Thumos not only behaves like wind but is also affected by it; if a swelling sea is like an unsettled person, it may also provoke those unsettling feelings.[99] That there are continuities between forces outside the person and inside the person does not mean, however, that it is useless to distinguish between not-self and self, as Fränkel asserted, for the reason that boundaries are perceived in relation to a unified conscious field.

Moreover, the person is not simply aware of this felt domain of the self but exercises a degree of intentionality over the stuffs-forces found there, such as *penthos*, "grief"; *kholos*, "anger"; and *thumos* itself. A warrior "remembers" or "is mindful of" his *alkē*, "strength."[100] Conversely, he can check these energies. Peleus advises Achilles as he sets out for Troy: "My child, Athena and Hera will give you power, if they wish, but you check the greathearted *thumos* in your chest (τέκνον ἐμόν, κάρτος μὲν Ἀθηναίη τε καὶ Ἥρη / δώσουσ', αἴ κ' ἐθέλωσι,

---

[95] This does not mean that epic poetry does not imagine feelings are caused by concrete stuffs inside the body. Rather, it places more emphasis on what these things feel like than on locating them on an anatomical map.

[96] What Michel Serres has called *la belle noiseuse* (1995, esp. 13–14). On the dynamics of these forces: Caswell 1990.51–61; Padel 1992.78–98; Clarke 1999.79–115; Spatafora 1999. Marine turbulence is an idea with a long afterlife, elaborated in tragic ideas about the mind, the medical imagination of fluxes, and philosophical ideals of calm.

[97] See esp. Padel 1992.96–97; see also Kuriyama 1999.233–70.

[98] The *unseen* is, rather, closely related to the idea of gods moving through the world cloaked in mist, as Renehan 1980.108–9 observes.

[99] On continuities between the natural world and persons, see Clarke 1995.308.

[100] See, e.g., *Il.* 4.418 and 6.112, with Collins 1998.78–125.

σὺ δὲ μεγαλήτορα θυμὸν / ἴσχειν ἐν στήθεσσι, *Il.* 9.254–56). In other relationships, the direction of power appears fuzzier. If Bellerophon gnaws at his *thumos*, for example, we are led to imagine inner turmoil, rather than fully intentional action.[101] The innards can themselves act on a person. Nevertheless, in practice these distinctions appear to matter little. The poet moves easily between expressions like Achilles nursed his anger (*Il.* 4.513) and those like "anger seized her" (*Il.* 4.23) or "came upon them" (*Il.* 9.525). Innards are responsive to the person in a way that humors will not be, creating a dynamic and continuous field of experience.[102]

Peleus's advice to Achilles assumes that he is not the only agent whose intentions affect the domain of the felt: what Hera and Athena want (αἴ κ᾽ ἐθέλωσι) also determines what happens there. Peleus describes an overlap or perhaps even a fusion of intentionality. It is often the case that when the hero does what he most strives to do or acts in the most praiseworthy way, he senses the gods in his act. Insofar as his aims and actions are derived from, and take on value in relationship to, a set of ideals shared by his community, what matters is not where the reasons for action "originate," that is, inside or outside the self, but what they achieve. It is that achievement which confers honor on the hero, whose success is never his alone.[103]

In other contexts, however, the presence of the divine or the daemonic is perceived through a rupture or discontinuity within the conscious field of the self. Consider an example from *Iliad* 19, where Odysseus is urging Achilles to allow the troops to eat:

οὐ γὰρ ἀνὴρ πρόπαν ἦμαρ ἐς ἠέλιον καταδύντα
ἄκμηνος σίτοιο δυνήσεται ἄντα μάχεσθαι·
εἴ περ γὰρ θυμῷ γε μενοινάᾳ πολεμίζειν,
ἀλλά τε λάθρῃ γυῖα βαρύνεται, ἠδὲ κιχάνει
δίψα τε καὶ λιμός, βλάβεται δέ τε γούνατ᾽ ἰόντι.

(*Il.* 19.162–66)

For a man will not have strength to fight his way forward all day
long until the sun goes down if he is starved for food. Even
though in his heart he be very passionate for the battle,
yet without his knowing it his limbs will go heavy, and hunger
and thirst will catch up with him and cumber his knees as he moves on.

Earlier, we saw the adverb *lathrēi* used of stealth attacks and the movement of gods among mortals. Here it signals a gap between the warrior's outward-directed attention and his awareness of his own limbs. It is this gap that allows hunger and thirst to creep up and harm his powers. Odysseus's language suggests

---

[101] E.g., *Il.* 6.202: θυμὸν κατέδων. Eating or gnawing the *thumos*: Spatafora 1999.17–39.
[102] On the fluid relationship between acting and being acted upon, see esp. Clarke 1999.66–73. See also Pelliccia 1995, esp. 52–77.
[103] See C. Gill 1996a, esp. 10–13.

that he understands hunger not as a void, as will be the case in the medical writers, but as an agent like sleep. The verb *kikhanō* means something like "to meet with" or "to overtake": a spear might "catch" you (*Il.* 10.370); death can "run you down" (*Il.* 11.451); one warrior might overtake another (16.342). Hunger itself is elsewhere described as something to ward off or flee.[104] Odysseus's language casts hunger as stealthy, invasive, and daemonic. He correlates this invasiveness with a felt sense of otherness or discontinuity.

There are a number of experiences that are sufficiently discontinuous or disruptive to invite the abduction of daemonic-divine agency. One well-known example is the sudden influx into the hero of *menos*, a force that also courses through rivers, fire, and the sun.[105] *Menos* is innate in the warrior, yet it can also be bestowed by the gods, who place it (βάλε, *Il.* 5.513) in a warrior's chest, breathe it into him (ἐμπνεύσῃσι, *Il.* 15.60), or just give it to him (δῶκε, *Il.* 5.2). Surges of strength can thus be perceived by the warrior as signs of a divine presence. When, for example, Poseidon adopts the form of Calchas to rouse the Aiantes to battle in *Iliad* 13, he fills them with *menos* by striking them with his staff and making their limbs, feet, and hands light (13.59–61; cf. *Il.* 5.122). It is through the eagerness in his *thumos* and the lightness of his limbs as much as by the traces "of feet and of legs" left by the departing Poseidon, that Oïlean Ajax recognizes the presence of a god. Telamonian Ajax seconds the feeling: his hands rage, his *menos* increases, his feet rush to take him into battle—tangible evidence of the god's solicitude (13.66–80). Poseidon acts as easily on the strength of the Aiantes as he will on the Achaean wall after the fall of Troy (*Il.* 12.13–26). The former action is neither metaphorical nor abstract. It is registered by the warriors themselves as something unusual, like a flash of lightning in a blue sky (*Il.* 8.68–77).

The domain of the felt is thus contiguous with the gods' power and desires. I am not denying that the spatial, visible body and its orifices offer an intuitive model for thinking of relationships between self and other in terms of inside and outside.[106] Nevertheless, that model cannot adequately account for the kinds of contact that we have been examining. If *erōs* is "curled up" (ἐλυσθείς) under the *kardia*, as in a poem by Archilochus, a spear thrust through the chest would not reveal its presence.[107] Similarly, when Homer has Hupnos say he is

---

[104] E.g., *Od.* 5.166; Hes. *Op.* 647, with Jouanna 1983a.24; Laser 1983.69–70. On hunger as a *daimōn*, see Roscher 1898.186–87.

[105] E.g., *Il.* 6.182, 12.18, 23.190. *Menos* covers what is for us a range of feelings, not only strength and lightness on the battlefield but also, for example, the sharp tingling in the nose that Odysseus feels upon reuniting with his father (*Od.* 24.318–19). For discussions of *menos*, see Böhme 1929.11–19; Dodds 1951.8–9; Giacomelli 1980; Bremmer 1983.57–60; Monsacré 1984.55–57; Jahn 1987.39–45; Vernant 1991b.39–41; Padel 1992.24–26; Redfield 1994.171–74.

[106] As Gell 1998.132–33 argues. Cf. Bolens 2000, arguing that Homer has no sense of the body as a "container" or "envelope." But Bolens neglects the importance of the seen body in Homer, making her contrast between an "articulated" body and a "contained" one too rigid.

[107] See fr. 191 (W²). On the localization of *erōs* in the person in lyric poetry, see Sullivan 1983.

poured over Zeus's *noos*, he captures sleep both as an agent interacting with Hera and as an event. G.E.R. Lloyd argues these perspectives must be treated as "*complementary*, rather than as *alternative*, conceptions of the same phenomenon."[108] So, although the lyric poets readily ascribe mischief and sadism to the personification Erōs, the force *erōs* is presumably not playing knucklebones after it settles in the chest, just as sleep, once drifted over the eyes, is no longer imagined to be brokering deals with Hera. There are no entities like *erōs* or sleep independent of the typed scenarios in which some properties (e.g., human-like form, possession of intentions and desires) are activated and others (e.g., qualia) disappear according to a kind of Heisenberg uncertainty principle for daemonic forces.[109]

This "principle" can shed light on why our archaic and classical Greek sources do not seem to work with the model of possession by indwelling demons that becomes popular in later antiquity and the medieval period.[110] For if cultures have differing assumptions about how the boundaries of the person are constituted, we might expect that they also conceptualize the interactions between the person and a daemonic world in different ways. If, in later periods, people begin to think about demons in terms of bodily habitation, a mind-set that is perhaps clearest in the medieval "physiology" of possession, the shift may be due in part to a historical process by which the insides of the person come to be defined primarily as potentially seen, anatomical space bounded by skin and accessed through orifices: it is interesting that when, in the second century CE, Lucian speaks of an indwelling demon, he sees that demon as entering a *sōma*, a word that in this period is firmly tied to the physical body.[111] In the earlier

---

[108] G. Lloyd 1966.202 (emphasis in original).

[109] This holds true for the two instances in the *Iliad* where it might be said a god enters a warrior. At 17.210–12, Ares "enters [Hector] . . . and his limbs are filled inside with *alkē* and *sthenos*" (δῦ δέ μιν Ἄρης / δεινὸς ἐνυάλιος, πλῆσθεν δ᾽ ἄρα οἱ μέλε᾽ ἐντὸς / ἀλκῆς καὶ σθένεος); at 9.239, Diomedes says that strong *lussa* has entered Hector. In both cases, there is no question that there is an influx of divinized force into the hero. But these instances differ only slightly from other examples of *menos* flooding the warrior. It is not the god *qua* embodied and intentional agent that enters the warrior: Ares is the Olympian capable of functioning as depersonalized force (e.g., *Il.* 13.444, 14.485). Cf. Collins 1998.17–34, arguing for a stronger view of possession in this passage.

[110] See esp. W. Smith 1965, arguing that bodily possession is unknown in pre-Christian Greece, becoming widespread only after the influx of "orientalist" ideas in the late Hellenistic and Roman imperial periods; see also Faraone 1999.45–49, esp. 47 n.34; Kotansky 1995. Many scholars of Greek religion and magic now accept that the "indwelling" demon is Semitic: see Kotansky 1995.246–48, with n.7, 273–77. It may be, however, that the indwelling demon takes root in the Greek-speaking world not only through cultural contact but also because of changing ideas about the inner body as habitable space. Earlier work on possession tends to simply assume an indwelling model: Julius Tambornino 1909, esp. 75–91; O'Brien-Moore 1924.82–86; Dodds 1951.71–72; Mattes 1970.41–42. Padel 1983.12–14 defends this tradition against Smith, but her evidence is limited: still, see, e.g., Sophron frr. 3–9 (Hordern), with discussion in R. Parker 1983.222–24. Faraone 1992.45–46 and Kotansky 1995.254–57 look more generally at "flee" formulas in the classical and Hellenistic Greek worlds.

[111] *Philops.* 16. On the physiology of possession in Medieval Europe, see Caciola 2000.279–85, who shows that medieval practices of exorcism assume a body that can be sealed against demonic incursion (289–90, 303 n.66).

texts, however, daemonic agents do not occupy inner space as much as they affect the felt domain directly.

The exception that would seem to prove the rule against indwelling demons, at least in the classical period, is the shadowy *engastrimuthos* or *engastrimantis*, "belly-talker" or "belly-diviner," who has a *daimōn* that prophesies from his belly. The belly-talker offers a rare case where the *daimōn* retains its own voice, a key index of personal identity in Greek culture. In the parabasis of the *Wasps*, for example, Aristophanes playfully compares himself to the speaking *daimōn*, saying he slipped "into other people's stomachs" (εἰς ἀλλοτρίας γαστέρας ἐνδύς, 1020) before he was old enough to stage his own comic production.[112] It may not be an accident that a speaking *daimōn* is located in the belly, a likely container given its association with the womb.[113] When Zeus incorporates Metis in the *Theogony*, for example, he places her in his *nēdus*, "belly" or "womb," where she devises good and evil for him (886–901).[114] Greek sources often associate daemonic penetration with women and the dark, mysterious inner space that characterizes them.[115] The conventions of revelation for male and female seers reflect these conceptual habits. Whereas Calchas and Tiresias have insight into the motivations of the gods, seers like Cassandra and the Pythia are represented as conduits for Apollo's word, expressed as a generative, divine breath that remains alien to its vessel.[116]

Breath, however, with its mysterious passage *through* the person, also represents the boundary between self and daemonic other as more ambiguous.[117] When Hesiod, for example, says the Muses breathed (ἐνέπνευσαν, *Th.* 31) a divine voice into him, this inspiration fuses imperceptibly with the poet's own

---

[112] See also *Epid.* V 63 (Li 5.242 = 29,3 Jouanna; cf. *Epid.* VII 28 [Li 5.400 = 69,17 Jouanna]) and Pl. *Sph.* 252c2–9; J. Katz and Volk 2000 make a compelling case for a reference at Hes. *Th.* 26–28. That the *daimōn* was itself named the ἐγγαστρίμυθος underscores the strong notion of possession operative over and above "inspiration." For Near Eastern examples, see J. Katz and Volk 2000.125–27.

[113] On the womb as a container, see Manuli 1980.399; duBois 1988.110–29; Sissa 1990a.155–67; A. Hanson 1992b.38–39; Dean-Jones 1994.65; H. King 1998.33–35.

[114] See also Call. *Del.* 86–93, 188–90, where Apollo prophesies from the womb, and *PGM* VIII 1–2, "come to me, Lord Hermes, as babies come to the bellies of women" (ἐλ[θ]έ μοι, κύριε Ἑρμῆ, ὡς τὰ βρέφη εἰς τὰ[ς] κοιλίας τῶν γυναι[κ]ῶν). I owe these references to an oral presentation by Sarah Iles Johnston and Adria Haluszka.

[115] Padel 1983. For cross-cultural claims about women and spirit possession, see Maurizio 1995; Caciola 2000. On the idea of the wandering womb, where the womb itself can be seen as a kind of *daimōn*, see below, chapter 4, n.161.

[116] For the relationship between breath and procreation, see A. *Ag.* 1206–7; *Supp.* 17, 40–45, 577. Various classical writers on biology physicalize this dynamic by making πνεῦμα a major component of semen: see *Genit./Nat. Puer.* 12 (Li 7.486–88 = 53,1–55,3 Joly); Pl. *Ti.* 91b2–4; Arist. *GA* 736b35–737a1. On Cassandra, see Barra 1993, esp. 29–43. On the Pythia, whom Longinus describes as pregnant with divine vapors exhaled by the earth (*De subl.* 13), see Sissa 1990a.9–70, 168–70, although most of her evidence is late. See also Maurizio 1995.81–83, 85–86 on the "randomizing devices" that signal the Pythia's message is uncontaminated by human intentions.

[117] On the ambiguity of breath, see esp. Padel 1992.89–98. See also Caswell 1990.52–56.

capacity to transmit epic memory.[118] The influx of divine breath in this context gives rise to a performance that seems to express the person's own character, skills, and intentions. *Menos* works in a similar way: when Poseidon bestows it on the Aiantes, for example, he stirs them to battle without compelling specific acts. The complicated afterlife of a god's touch in a person can create a kind of "double determination," particularly in the case of proto-tragic actions.[119] Early in the *Iliad*, for example, Andromache tells Hector, "your *menos* will destroy you" (φθίσει σε τὸ σὸν μένος, *Il.* 6.407; cf. 22.459), her emphasis on "your" drawing our attention to the tangled relationship between Hector's own desire for glory and his fated death. This relationship reminds us how fluid the boundary between self and other can be, both in the domain of the felt and in explanations of what people suffer and what they do. It is difficult for us not only to know where to draw the line between self and others in foreign cultures. Even within those cultures, the perceived transgression of that line is subtle, context-bound, and open to dispute.

FEAR AND THE VISUAL FIELD OF THE SELF

One of the phenomena most conducive to understanding the person as a space of passage and transformation between daemonic force, on the one hand, and symptoms and actions, on the other, is fear. In the *Iliad*, both *deos*, "terror," and *phobos*, "fear" or "flight," are divinized forces that seize (ἔλλαβε, *Il.* 11.402; ᾗρει, *Il.* 7.479) the warrior.[120] At the same time, how a warrior responds to fear's attack reveals something about him. For, while the Homeric hero is trafficked by a range of fluid forces, it is also true that a warrior's *menos* or *thumos* must be unflinching in battle.[121] If a warrior fails to stand firm, that failure, while motivated by an onslaught of daemonic fear, publicly testifies to his lack of *aretē*.

The idea of publicly staged *aretē* requires some modification of the binary felt-seen model. Up to now, I have focused on how daemonic presence is felt

---

[118] The idea of inspiration is developed at length by Plato in the *Ion*; see also *Cra.* 396d1–397a2; *Phdr.* 265b2–c3; Democr. (DK68) B18. It is hard to know whether the model is original to him. For analyses of the archaic and classical evidence for inspiration, see Dodds 1951.80–82; Tigerstedt 1970; Murray 1981; J. Katz and Volk 2000.127–29.

[119] On double determination, see esp. Dodds 1951.1–27 and Lesky 1961; 1966. See also Adkins 1960.10–25; Harrison 1960.77–79; Fränkel 1975.64–75; Janko 1992.3–7. Decisions are also "doubly" determined, but where the god offers good reasons that lead the hero to perform actions—Athena's persuasion of Achilles to spare Agamemnon's life is a classic example (*Il.* 1.207–14)—there is far less tension between the gods' presence and the hero himself. Indeed, the gods' presence confirms their solicitude for the hero and thus elevates his status.

[120] See also *Il.* 8.77, 17.67; *Od.* 11.43, 633, 12.243, 22.42, 24.450, 533. For the (possible) personification of *phobos*, see *Il.* 4.440, 5.739, 11.37. At *Il.* 13.298–300, Phobos is the son of Ares. For *phobos* as flight, see, e.g., *Il.* 5.252, 8.139.

[121] *Il.* 5.126, 254, 527, 17.157, 20.372; *Od.* 21.426.

from within. Yet that presence often registers in a shared perceptual field. Surges of *menos*, for example, not only are subjectively sensed but also transform how the warrior appears to others: Hector rages across the battlefield with "the eyes of a Gorgon or man-destroying Ares" (*Il.* 8.349); elsewhere, his eyes glitter and he foams at the lips (*Il.* 15.605–10); Achilles, his eyes glowing, gnashes his teeth in his murderous rage (*Il.* 19.365–66).[122] The very strangeness of these phenomena is gauged against how these characters normally appear, that is, against a public, seen identity. What I have been calling the seen, then, encompasses not only skin that can be penetrated but also skin understood as a visible surface rich in information about character, mood, and intentions.[123] Whereas a warrior scanning the skin for points amenable to the spear views his opponent simply as a penetrable object, the Achaeans thrusting their spears into Hector's corpse are noticing, too, his breeding and his heroic appearance.

Indeed, what someone can and will do in Homer is thought to be largely predictable on the basis of how he appears, at least in the *Iliad*; in the *Odyssey*, appearances are more likely to deceive. Thersites, the *porte-parole* of the common warrior, is deformed (*Il.* 2.216–18), while the cowardly Dolon, though swift of foot, is ugly with respect to his *eidos* (*Il.* 10.316). At the other end of the spectrum, Priam says of Agamemnon that he "looks like a kingly man" (βασιλῆϊ γὰρ ἀνδρὶ ἔοικε, *Il.* 3.170), while Ajax is second only to Achilles in his appearance, *eidos*, and his deeds, *erga*, the two qualities mirroring and confirming each other in a public field of vision (*Il.* 17.279–80). Far from challenging this model, a character like the wily Odysseus only underscores its presence.[124]

Given that the surface of the person can express so much meaning, it is ideal for the visible realization of cultural values such as *aretē*. The "heraldic" function of the skin is particularly important in the case of fear, as is made evident through Idomeneus's barbed praise of Meriones in *Iliad* 13:

> οἶδ᾽ ἀρετὴν οἷός ἐσσι· τί σε χρὴ ταῦτα λέγεσθαι;
> εἰ γὰρ νῦν παρὰ νηυσὶ λεγοίμεθα πάντες ἄριστοι
> ἐς λόχον, ἔνθα μάλιστ᾽ ἀρετὴ διαείδεται ἀνδρῶν,
> ἔνθ᾽ ὅ τε δειλὸς ἀνὴρ ὅς τ᾽ ἄλκιμος ἐξεφαάνθη·
> τοῦ μὲν γάρ τε κακοῦ τρέπεται χρὼς ἄλλυδις ἄλλη,

---

[122] For flashing eyes, see also *Il.* 12.466, 19.16–17. Eyes as a channel between inside and outside: Padel 1992.59–63; Lateiner 1995.43.

[123] See Worman 2002.41–107 on this visible surface in archaic poetry. See also Innocenti 1970; Vernant 1991c; Treherne 1995; Bassi 2003.33–37.

[124] For Odysseus, see *Il.* 3.191–224; cf. *Od.* 8.176–77, 17.454, with Bassi 1998.118–40; Worman 2002.12, 90–101. It is not so much that Odysseus confounds the system with his body. Rather, the difficulty of assigning him a permanent corporeal type is tied to the very flexibility of his modes of thought. To the extent that we are speaking of heroic type, we are speaking of male bodies; female bodies are much less transparent: see Worman 2002.86–89, 101–6 on Helen; Zeitlin 1996.53–86 and H. King 1998.23–27 on Pandora. See also Thgn. frr. 965–67 (W²) for anxiety about the transparency of character in the high-stakes world of the archaic elite.

οὐδέ οἱ ἀτρέμας ἧσθαι ἐρητύετ᾽ ἐν φρεσὶ θυμός,
ἀλλὰ μετοκλάζει καὶ ἐπ᾽ ἀμφοτέρους πόδας ἵζει,
ἐν δέ τέ οἱ κραδίη μεγάλα στέρνοισι πατάσσει
κῆρας ὀϊομένῳ, πάταγος δέ τε γίγνετ᾽ ὀδόντων·
τοῦ δ᾽ ἀγαθοῦ οὔτ᾽ ἂρ τρέπεται χρὼς οὔτε τι λίην
ταρβεῖ, ἐπειδὰν πρῶτον ἐσίζηται λόχον ἀνδρῶν,
ἀρᾶται δὲ τάχιστα μιγήμεναι ἐν δαῒ λυγρῇ·
οὐδέ κεν ἔνθα τεόν γε μένος καὶ χεῖρας ὄνοιτο.

(*Il.* 13.275–87)

I know your *aretē* and what you are. Why need you speak of it?
If now beside the ships all the best of us were to assemble
for a hidden position, and there man's courage is best decided,
where the man who is a coward and the brave man show themselves clearly:
the skin of the coward changes color one way and another,
and the *thumos* in his *phrenes* has no control to make him sit steady,
but he shifts his weight from one foot to another, then settles firmly
on both feet, and the *kradiē* inside his chest pounds violent
as he thinks of death spirits, and his teeth chatter together:
but the brave man's skin will not change color, nor is he too much
frightened, once he has taken his place in the hidden position,
but his prayer is to close as soon as may be in bitter division:
and there no man could make light of your *menos* or your hand's work.

Idomeneus's hypothetical scenario is realized elsewhere in the *Iliad*.[125] Ajax's lauded courage, for example, materializes in his reaction to a dangerous situation. It takes Zeus to drive him to flight, and he draws back slowly and reluctantly (11.546–47), his reluctance confirming the character apparent in his *eidos*. Ajax's response suggests that if a warrior has an innate dispensation of *aretē*, he is able to resist, at least to a degree, the daemonic pressure to flee; in some cases, this resistance might secure a space to consider the consequences of fighting or fleeing.[126] The coward, conversely, is defined by the reflexivity of his response: the skin pales, the limbs tremble, the teeth chatter, the *thumos* becomes erratic.[127]

It is worth noting that fear is realized equally in both the felt and the seen domains. That is, fear is defined both by the feeling of terror and by the tremor that seizes the limbs. Neither of these experiences takes priority: there is no delay between the "internal" phenomenon and the "external" one; the latter is

---

[125] See also Pl. *R.* 3, 413d7–e5; *Leg.* 1, 647e–648e, where the city uses fear as a "test" of a warrior's courage.

[126] E.g., *Il.* 11.401–10. Deliberation will, in most cases, result in the hero holding his ground, but it may, in certain circumstances, permit retreat: see Loraux 1995.78; C. Gill 1996a.60–78.

[127] See, e.g., *Il.* 3.30–37, 7.215, 10.374–76, 14.506, 15.4, 280, 17.733, 20.44–45, 22.136–37, 24.358–59; *Od.* 22.68–69.

neither a sign nor an effect of the former.[128] What distinguishes them is the fact that visible changes attest heroic identity. Idomeneus's test at some level complicates the iconic truth of the seen, insofar as it assumes that character must be provoked into appearance by external stimuli: *aretē* is a dynamic state. At the same time, this dynamism reminds us that the boundaries of the self are not simply constituted by the relative unity of a conscious field or a static form but also affirmed in the face of external impacts.

Nevertheless, however much a daemonic force like fear reveals a warrior's *aretē*, it can always accommodate the abduction of a god's intentions: Zeus, for example, is often said to stun entire armies.[129] These intentions, as we have seen, intertwine with the self in complex ways. The touch of a god can be more or less forceful. It thus leaves more or less room for responses that are salient to heroic identity, such as deliberation or the expression of *aretē*.

The less room a hero has to respond to the god's force, the more the poet seems to stress blindness and the asymmetries between mortal and immortal knowledge. Narrating Patroclus's *aristeia*, he observes,

> ἀλλ' αἰεί τε Διὸς κρείσσων νόος ἠέ περ ἀνδρῶν·
> ὅς τε καὶ ἄλκιμον ἄνδρα φοβεῖ καὶ ἀφείλετο νίκην
> ῥηϊδίως, ὅτε δ' αὐτὸς ἐποτρύνῃσι μάχεσθαι·
> ὅς οἱ καὶ τότε θυμὸν ἐνὶ στήθεσσιν ἀνῆκεν.
>
> (*Il.* 16.688–91)

> But always the mind of Zeus is a stronger thing than a man's mind.
> He terrifies even the warlike man, he takes away victory
> lightly, when he himself has driven a man into battle
> as now he drove on the fury in the heart of Patroclus.

By emphasizing the uneven distribution of power between the two minds, the poet flags the impending harm to Patroclus, harm that will eventually appear in the form of Apollo the aggressor. In describing that encounter, we can recall, the poet draws on the asymmetrical relationships of seeing that are familiar from the battlefield. But we have not yet adequately addressed the question of *why* these relationships come into play. That is, if the poet can just say that the mind of Zeus is stronger than a man's mind, what need is there to endow agents like Apollo and Poseidon with human form? If gods act so easily in the world,

---

[128] Onians quotes William James observing "that the bodily changes follow directly the perception of the exciting fact and that our feeling of the same changes as they occur *is* the emotion" (1954.53, emphasis in original). See also Larock 1930.385; Harrison 1960.66; Loraux 1995.75–87, although Larock and Harrison appeal to the weakness of primitive thought to explain Homer's failure to distinguish between the inner condition of cowardice and its symptoms. (Cf. Böhme 1929.10–11, defending Homer's awareness of "das innere Erlebnis.")

[129] Individual fear and collective panic on the battlefield are often distinguished in the ancient sources. On the latter, later associated closely with Pan, see Borgeaud 1988.98–102.

why saddle them with bodies that occupy space and time?[130] Why, even when the gods' actions seem to disregard the boundaries of seen bodies, do the traces of the human form, like an afterimage, remain in representations of mortal-immortal contact?

How Gods Act

How, exactly, does a god affect a human? One strategy for answering this question is to claim that the how question is irrelevant.[131] In criticizing Frazer's theory of sympathetic magic, Gell writes:

> Frazer's mistake was, so to speak, to imagine that magicians had some non-standard physical theory, whereas the truth is that "magic" is what you have when you *do without* a physical theory on the grounds of the redundancy, relying on the idea, which is perfectly practicable, that the explanation of any given event (especially if socially salient) is that it is caused intentionally.[132]

Magic, Gell concludes, "registers and publicizes the strength of desire."[133] The agency of the gods, too, "registers and publicizes the strength of desire." Zeus, we have just seen, effortlessly "drives on" Patroclus's *thumos* (*Il.* 16.691); he sends terror against armies without ever descending to the battlefield. Indeed, only once do we see Zeus come into contact with the mortal hero when, in book 15, he pushes Hector from behind "with his great hand" (χειρὶ . . . μεγάλῃ, 695). Commentators have worried that the image verges on the grotesque.[134] It may appear less disturbing if we shift away from the norms of our realism to think about the expressive potential of the hand and other such figures.

Homer adopts the image of the great hand to mediate the relationship between Zeus and Hector. Why is the image useful? It is true that, because of the uncommon efficacy of the gods' intentions, force circulates freely between gods and humans in the register of the felt. In conceptualizing those exchanges, however, the poet appropriates the very instruments that mediate agency in the visible world. The hand, in other words, not only enables action but also symbolizes

---

[130] On the idea that gods act easily (ῥεῖα), see West 1978.139–40.

[131] Boyer 2001.138–40, 196–98, arguing that indifference to the "how" of daemonic interaction is cross-cultural, emphasizes that interest in such interaction is usually pragmatic (why?): the cultural tradition provides conventional guidelines for imagining how gods act. Cf. Samuelsen 2004.100–103 on the absence of body-to-body contact in the transmission of disease by sorcerers and spirits among the Bissa of Burkina Faso. See also Pelliccia 1995.80–83 on magical causality in Homer.

[132] Gell 1998.101 (emphasis in original).

[133] Gell 1998.101.

[134] Janko 1992.304. Janko thus prefers the vulgate ὦρσεν (roused) in 694 to Aristarchus's ὦσεν (pushed), printed in the Oxford Classical Texts and Teubner editions. On the hand held over one as a form of protection, see, e.g., *Il.* 4.249, 5.433, 9.419–20, 24.374; *Od.* 14.184; and Groß 1970, citing Near Eastern parallels.

the capacity to act.[135] Elsewhere, Zeus pairs his *menos* with his invincible hands (μένος καὶ χεῖρες ἄαπτοι, *Il.* 8.450) in reminding Hera and Athena of his power, there understood as the unfettered capacity to cause harm.[136] Recall that when Poseidon transforms the Phaeacians' ship into a rock, he does so "with the flat of his hand" (χειρὶ καταπρηνεῖ, *Od.* 13.164). Hands also express constraints on agency. In *Iliad* 1, Thetis recalls when the other gods plotted to bind Zeus in order to block his sovereign power. She prevented them from doing so by calling on the hundred-handed Briareus, the very embodiment of the capacity to act and to protect, to sit beside Zeus (1.399–406).[137] Thinking back to the death of Patroclus, then, we can read Apollo's hand not simply as an instrument but as a sign of the god's power to act.

The figure of the hand may also be understood as the outcome of a process of objectifying a hidden thing or agent, a process catalyzed by symptoms or perceptions of otherness in the environment.[138] Scarry has argued that this process is particularly likely to be triggered by acute pain, in part because pain, unlike love or hunger or vision, does not move out toward an object in the world, while, at the same time, it resists expression in language.[139] The most common responses to pain, on her argument, exploit what she calls "the expressive potential of the sign of the weapon."[140] Surveying a broad field of literary and documentary evidence, she observes that people nearly always resort to the language of "as if" to express pain (as if a knife were turning in my stomach, as if a hammer were pounding down). In the Homeric poems, we can observe a close relationship between pain and the figure of the weapon, particularly the arrow. The arrow is said to be "freighted with dark pains"; *odunai*, "acute pains," are described with the same terms used to describe the arrow, such as *oxus*, "sharp," and *pikros*, "bitter."[141] Scarry's "as if" language continues to appear in Hippocratic and Galenic medical treatises—"something like a thorn seems to be in the inward parts"; "it bores like a trepan"—a phenomenon once chalked up to

---

[135] The hand continues to do this symbolic work in the classical period, e.g., in the expressions ἀπέχειν χέρας (e.g., A. *Eu.* 350; *Supp.* 756; Pl. *Smp.* 213d3–4), "to refrain from violence against someone," or ἐν χειρῶν νόμῳ (Aeschines 1.5; Hdt. 8.89; Plb. 1.34.5), "by violence."

[136] See also *Il.* 1.567, 7.309, 11.169, 13.49, 16.244, 20.503; *Od.* 11.502, 22.70, 248; Hes. *Th.* 649; *Op.* 148.

[137] See also *Il.* 5.385–91, 8.24–27, 15.19–20. On binding as the constraint on sovereignty, see Slatkin 1991.66–69. See also Faraone 1992.74–81; Dickie 1999 for binding in magic.

[138] See the discussion in Csordas 1990: the objectification of demons in Charismatic Christianity is the final stage of a process that begins through sensations of otherness that are then retrospectively (albeit "automatically") diagnosed as daemonic presence.

[139] Scarry 1985.5–23.

[140] Scarry 1985.17.

[141] See Mawet 1979.41–43; Holmes 2007.58–59. The goddesses of birth pangs, the Eileithuiae, appear in the *Iliad* armed with a sharp dart (βέλος ὀξύ, 11.269–70). For the association of Artemis, herself an archer, with the Eileithuiae, see D. S. 5.72.5; Plut. *Mor.* 658F. See also Farnell 1896–1909, 2:444, with 567–68 n.41.

the obstinacy of archaic thinking.[142] It is more likely that the tendency to objectify persists despite changing notions of cause. "The point here," Scarry writes, "is not just that pain can be apprehended in the image of the weapon (or wound) but that it almost cannot be apprehended without it."[143]

Both weapons and hands belong to a crucial point of convergence between the felt and the seen—namely, the point at which the felt gives rise to an *imagined*, potentially seen world. The image of the weapon calls up intuitive notions of causality (i.e., pain is caused through violence to the skin, particularly penetration). Yet, at the same time, like the hand, the weapon is nearly inseparable from the idea of the *intent* to cause harm. In the *Iliad*, spears desire to glut themselves on flesh; they are eager to pierce the chest.[144] Rather than chalk these expressions up to a vague animism, we can see these weapons not as initiating but as secondary agents, that is, as "objective embodiments of the *power or capacity to will their use*."[145] By assuming the force of desire, weapons extend agency beyond the embodied agent.[146] Of course, whether they hit their target depends on the good or ill will of the gods: just as Zeus trumps Teucer's desire to kill Hector, Poseidon strips a spear of *menos* (ἀμενήνωσεν, *Il.* 13.562) to spare the life of Antilochus.[147] Yet this dependence merely confirms that weapons and hands are instruments of intentions.

In the figure of the weapon desirous of flesh, we see conflated the vulnerability of the warrior's skin and his vulnerability to the malevolent intentions of others. The (unseen) weapons of the gods exaggerate the latter kind of vulnerability, while bypassing the skin altogether. Yet they convey no less than a visible weapon the power to harm. It is useless to distinguish between how early Greeks represented daemonic violence and how they thought it "actually" happened: the images of the weapon and the hand are neither poetic props nor "realistic" instruments, but, rather, responses, both naturally and culturally determined,

[142] *Morb.* II 72 (Li 7.108–10 = 211,15–16 Jouanna), δοκεῖ ἐν τοῖσι σπλάγχνοισιν εἶναι οἶον ἄκανθα καὶ κεντεῖν; Galen *Loc.Aff.* 2.5 (Kühn 8.81): ὡς τρυπάνῳ δοκεῖν διατιτρᾶσθαι. Louis Bourgey sees in these cases "une incapacité à dépasser le point de vue descriptif" (1953.152).

[143] Scarry 1985.16.

[144] λιλαιόμενα χροὸς ἆσαι: *Il.* 11.574 (cf. 15.317, 21.168); μαιμώωσα: *Il.* 15.542. Both are examples given by Aristotle in speaking of Homer's tendency to describe inanimate things as if they were animate (*Rh.* 1411b31–1412a8). Eustathius reports that cases where the spear is said to "desire" to glut itself on flesh were seen as the transference of feeling from the one who suffers to that which acts (ἀπὸ τοῦ πάσχοντος ἐπὶ τὸ ποιοῦν, *ad* Δ 126): the experience of pain makes one attribute sentience to the imagined cause.

[145] Gell 1998.21 (emphasis in original). See also Knappett 2006.240: "It is through contact with the body as a conduit of intentional action that objects come to be imbued with mindfulness." Boyer 2001.115–16 notes that recent cognitive research suggests that humans have a separate inferential system activated by the perception of tools and artifacts that relates them to human agents.

[146] By assuming desire, weapons become moral entities in a restricted sense: see E. *Supp.* 1205–7.

[147] See also *Il.* 4.127–33, 13.444, 15.521–22. Achilles' spear is unique in that it always reaches its mark (*Il.* 20.99).

to perceptions and sensations of otherness, particularly pain. Like Poseidon's staff when he bestows *menos* or the wand used by Hermes to put some men to sleep and wake others, these potentially seen instruments relate ruptures in the domain of the felt to other intentional agents.[148] It is through this process of objectification that unseen harm takes on meaning.

THE SEEN BODY AND SOCIAL AGENCY

In *Iliad* 14, Hupnos appears as an agent complicit in Hera's plan. His complicity is extracted on the basis of a sexual transaction (the nymph Pasithea in exchange for Hupnos's cooperation), as if it is because Hupnos himself is vulnerable to the pleasures promised by Aphrodite's erotic arsenal that he agrees to compound their effects on Zeus. If Zeus's susceptibility to *hupnos* is expressed in terms of the position he unwittingly assumes within Hupnos's field of vision, Hupnos is implicated in Hera's power play because he himself has desires subject to manipulation.[149]

Agamemnon's first error in the *Iliad* arises, in fact, because he miscalculates the strength of the gods' emotions. In dismissing the priest Chryses with the warning that his scepter will offer him scant protection should he linger among the Achaeans, the king fails to recognize that the priest's symbolic object represents a capacity for agency far in excess of that represented by his own scepter. This capacity is shortly realized through Chryses' appeal to Apollo, which testifies to the power of human speech and tears to exert pressure on sympathetic gods: Apollo the archer is set in motion (αὐτοῦ κινηθέντος) *because* he is first moved to anger (χωόμενος κῆρ) by a suppliant's prayer (*Il.* 1.44–47). The impetus of that prayer eventually translates into the flight of the plague-bearing arrows into the Achaean camps. The chain reaction with which we began this chapter is mobilized by a mortal's appeal.

Naturally, the suppliant's words do not *compel* the god to act in accordance with his or her wishes.[150] For where would the divine be, one Hippocratic author asks, "if the capacity of a god could be overpowered and enslaved by the thinking of a human being" (εἰ δὴ τοῦ θείου ἡ δύναμις ὑπ᾽ ἀνθρώπου γνώμης κρατεῖται καὶ δεδούλωται, *Morb. Sacr.* 1, Li 6.360 = 7,16–17 Jouanna)? Nevertheless, not only Homeric epic but also other literary sources such as lyric poetry and tragedy, as well as the material evidence available for archaic and classical cult practices, strongly suggest that reciprocity between gods and humans is a fundamental tenet of Greek religion.[151] Indeed, reciprocity is at the core of

---

[148] On Hermes' staff, see *Il.* 24.343–44. See also *Od.* 10.238 (Circe), 13.429 (Athena).

[149] Those desires, however, appear less ambitious than Hera's.

[150] See, e.g., *Il.* 2.419–20, 6.311, 16.249–52, all cases where the gods refuse to respond to a prayer.

[151] R. Parker 1998. See also G. Lloyd 1966.195–96. Reciprocity has been seen as disqualifying the gods as moral agents (e.g., Adkins 1960.133–35). But, under the influence of comparative anthropology, it is now widely seen as part of the social-ethical texture of archaic culture.

a set of assumptions familiar to any Hellenist: that the gods take an interest in human beings; that they enter into relationships with them governed by mutually intelligible desires (e.g., for *timē*, "honor"), emotions (love, hate, delight, envy), and expectations; that they can intensify the emotions and fulfill the desires of favored mortals. Attention, moreover, cuts both ways: "Wretched girl," Aphrodite admonishes Helen, "do not tease me lest in anger I forsake you and grow to hate you as much as now I terribly love you" (μή μ' ἔρεθε, σχετλίη, μὴ χωσαμένη σε μεθείω, / τὼς δέ σ' ἀπεχθήρω ὡς νῦν ἔκπαγλα φίλησα, *Il.* 3.414–15).

Relationships of reciprocity are mediated, first, by speech.[152] After rousing the Aiantes with his staff, Poseidon incites the rest of the Achaeans to battle with winged words (*Il.* 13.94). Heroes, too, stir one another and their armies to action through language: when Agamemnon, speaking in the assembly, urges the Achaean army to abandon the war, he drives the *thumos* in the chests of his troops, and this, in turn, results in the whole assembly being moved (κινήθη) like a great wave on the sea (*Il.* 2.142–46). Speech accomplishes what force alone cannot, which is why the hero is not only a doer of deeds but also a speaker of words: "Power among humans is not simply the physical force with which one material body may move another; it is the force to distract, detour, maneuver, and command."[153] Such power is magnified when a god speaks: "No word will be fruitless, if [Zeus] speaks it" (*Il.* 24.92).

Reciprocity between mortals and immortals is further enabled by the gods' human-like form insofar as this form enables them to participate in the nonverbal behaviors crucial to intersubjective exchanges that Marcel Mauss called "*techniques du corps*."[154] In Homer, "the description of bodily reactions and relevant artifacts," as Donald Lateiner writes, "makes vivid the lively web and texture of human interrelations and interactions."[155] What Mauss calls "*techniques du corps*" combine with the visible signs of character and *aretē* that we saw earlier to embed embodied actors in an economy of power as social and ethical agents above and beyond their physical capacities.[156] Through anthropomorphism, the gods, too, are located in this economy. Thetis supplicates Zeus with the same techniques—embracing his knees, grasping his chin with her right hand (*Il.* 1.500–501)—used by humans; Zeus assents to her request by nodding his head, a gesture whose local efficacy in the human world resonates on a cosmic scale when performed by Zeus (1.528–30). The gods' anthropomorphism allows the divine world to be imagined as a potentially seen mimesis of the

---

[152] Human speech (αὐδή) and human form (δέμας) are often paired in descriptions of the gods moving through the mortal world: see Clay 1974.

[153] Lingis 2000.18.

[154] Mauss 1979.

[155] Lateiner 1995.6; see also Adkins 1960.21: "The only system which is forced upon the notice of Homeric man is the social system." Lateiner's rich analysis supports the claim that gods cannot participate in the social world of epic without bodies; see also Worman 2002.

[156] See above, pp. 70–72.

human world. Such a world can be unveiled to show gods feasting on food that is not food, holding assemblies, comforting and abusing one another.[157] The mirroring of the two worlds is like the language of *kharis*, which "sustains, indeed creates, the fiction that the relation between human and god can be assimilated to that between human beings and so brought within a comprehensible pattern."[158]

The weapon or the hand, we have seen, both symbolizes and concretizes the capacity of an intentional agent to act. Anthropomorphism, in turn, seems to ground that agency in the panoply of human motivations: anger, sorrow, envy, love, and the desire for recognition, among others. If, then, gods are imagined to act as potentially seen, embodied agents, it is because their actions are embedded in a social and emotional web. In other words, even if it is the nature of daemonic agency to *bypass* the "seen," spatialized boundaries of the person, thereby acting directly on the felt, the gods need visible forms to participate in the very economy of desires and intentions that motivate their interaction with persons. Thus, the "seen" dimension of the person in Homer involves more than a physical object's "realistic" occupation of space. That dimension *clarifies* the crucial elements in Patroclus's encounter with Apollo: the visual-epistemic asymmetry between assailant and victim and the unforeseeable arrival of the symptom; the origins of the attack in an agent whose intent to harm is embedded in a complex network of emotions (e.g., anger) and shadowy directives from Zeus and fate; the efficacious translation of that agent's intentions into action, through the blow; and the resulting damage that, though due to an invisible weapon (i.e., the hand), is nevertheless very real. In short, in Homer's accounts of daemonic attack, "metaphysics" and physics converge on a (potentially) visible human form.

The seen person, bound by skin, is not the only way of imagining boundaries. The descriptions of daemonic contact in Homer and other archaic and classical sources also present the agent in terms of a conscious field sensitive to perceptions of difference. Gods and divinized forces penetrate this domain as easily as breath enters the person or as violently as a spear breaks through the skin. Nevertheless, despite the fact that the circulation of daemonic force largely bypasses the visible, spatial boundaries of the person, the embodied agent remains crucial to how mortal-immortal interaction is conceptualized. By imagining discontinuities in experience in terms of potentially seen embodied agents, early Greeks embed suffering in a complex set of relationships with the gods, relationships that are orchestrated by social values, expectations, and emotions. Harming becomes an intentional act, open to social meaning. It comes as no surprise, then, that this mortal-immortal web is central to practices of healing in the archaic and classical worlds.

[157] See G. Lloyd 1966.193–200.
[158] R. Parker 1998.120.

Interpreting Disease and Practices of Healing

In the final moments before his death, Patroclus assumes the position of a seer. He recognizes Apollo as his assailant, as well as the roles played by Zeus and "harmful destiny" in his death (*Il.* 16.844–50). His insight succeeds in making sense of the eruption of daemonic power through him, just as Calchas's skills reveal Apollo's motives in the first book of the poem. In both cases, the requisite knowledge is guaranteed by a heightened relationship to the divine: Patroclus, on the threshold of death, achieves more-than-mortal knowledge; those upon whom Achilles calls when plague strikes are the seer, the holy man, and the interpreter of dreams (*Il.* 1.62–63).

Absent from Achilles' list is the *iatros*, the "healer."[159] In the *Iliad*, the *iatroi*, the two most famous of whom are Asclepius's sons Machaon and Podalirius, are concerned primarily with the treatment of flesh wounds through the application of *pharmaka*, "drugs," and the skilled use of the knife: in a famous passage, the *iatros* is worth many men for his ability "to remove arrows and apply soothing medicaments" (ἰούς τ' ἐκτάμνειν ἐπί τ' ἤπια φάρμακα πάσσειν, *Il.* 11.515; cf. 4.218).[160] Together with the recitation of a charm, which occurs once, in the *Odyssey*, and is not attributed to an *iatros*, these skills create a troika of faculties that Émile Benveniste christens the medical doctrine of the Indo-Europeans.[161] Although we are told in the *Odyssey* that, in Egypt, "everyone is an *iatros*, surpassing all men in their knowledge" (ἰητρὸς δὲ ἕκαστος ἐπιστάμενος περὶ πάντων / ἀνθρώπων, *Od.* 4.231–32), the kind of knowledge we actually see healers commanding, at least in the *Iliad*, concerns not the motivations of the gods but the extraction of weapons and *pharmaka*. Such knowledge is also the province of certain heroes, like Achilles and Patroclus.[162] Admittedly, it is the pains of the wound that dominate the *Iliad*. It is true, too, that we gain a slightly different picture of healing professionals in the *Odyssey*, where a "healer of evils" (ἰητὴρ κακῶν) is included, with seers and singers, in a list of itinerant craftsmen (*Od.* 17.382–85).[163] It is possible that the expertise of the *iatros* off the

---

[159] The healer's absence is noted already in ancient histories of medicine: see Cels. *De med.* procem. 4 (17,15–16 Marx), hypothesizing that healers are absent because disease is attributed to the anger of the gods.

[160] Pharmacological treatment: *Il.* 4.190–91, 218–29, 11.830, 844–48; see also 5.401, 900–901, in the context of wounded gods.

[161] On the charm, see *Od.* 19.457, with Renehan 1992. Benveniste 1945 finds the tripartite "doctrine médicale des Indo-Européens" conserved at Pi. *P.* 3.40–54. See also S. *Aj.* 581–82. A loose tripartite division into surgery, pharmacology, and dietetics can be discerned in the Hippocratic writings (esp. *Aph.* VII.87, Li 4.608 = 216 Jones) and becomes standard in later texts: see Cels. *De med.* procem. 9 (18,17–20 Marx), with von Staden 1999b.257–58; Thivel 2000.35–37; van der Eijk 2005b.110–14.

[162] Salazar 2000.136–40. Heroes with healing capabilities are connected to the centaur Chiron (*Il.* 4.217–19, 11.828–32): see Laser 1983.96; Mackie 1997; 2001; Edelstein and Edelstein 1998, 2: 4–5.

[163] On itinerant craftsmen, see esp. Burkert 1983; 1992.41–46.

battlefield extends beyond the treatment of wounds to include internal ailments.[164] Nevertheless, in the most explicit evidence we have from Homer, the knowledge of the *iatros* is worth little against Apollo's weapons.

The roles of the healer and the seer, the *mantis*, can, however, be conflated in myth and the early historical period in the mysterious figure of the *iatromantis*, of whom Calchas is sometimes seen to be a representative.[165] The term *iatromantis* itself does not appear until Aeschylus, where it is used of Apollo (*Eu.* 62) and his son Apis (*Supp.* 263); but healing capabilities are attributed to a number of seers in myth, such as Abaris, Bacis, Branchus, Melampus, and Thaletas, as well as to historical figures like Epimenides and Empedocles.[166] The bond between healing and divination, not only in the case of epidemic diseases like plagues but also in individual cases, is well attested throughout antiquity in both literary and epigraphic evidence.[167] In the later fifth century, the cult of Asclepius, the hero-son of Apollo who eventually becomes a god, begins to spread throughout the Greek world, flourishing in the Hellenistic period and

---

[164] There is a long-standing debate about whether archaic *iatroi* treated internal ailments, by either magical or pharmacological means. The κακά mentioned at *Od.* 17.384 imply a wide range of expertise. But a division of labor between healers is familiar in other cultures, as with the *āšipu* and the *asû* in Babylonian medicine: these figures are traditionally seen as a magician-exorcist and a physician (Ritter 1965). But see Scurlock 1999, arguing that the former would have dealt with all diseases requiring a diagnosis (with no differentiation between "natural" and "supernatural" causality), whereas the latter, like the Homeric *iatros*, would have been knowledgeable about drugs and capable of bandaging and setting bones; a third expert, the *bārû*, the diviner, could have supplied prognoses. On internal medicine in Homer, see Daremberg 1865.84–93; Cordes 1991; Hoessly 2001.86–90; Dean-Jones 2003.99–100.

[165] See R. Parker 1983.209. Cf. Hoessly 2001.95–96 (insisting on the importance of purification, in which Calchas does not engage directly, to the role of the *iatromantis*).

[166] The methods of healing that these figures use vary. Abaris is said to both foretell and ward off plague from the Spartans (Iamb. *Vit. pyth.* 91–92); he is mentioned as a Thracian who heals with *epōdai* at Pl. *Chrm.* 158b5–c1. Thaletas is sent by the Pythia to cure the Spartans of plague through music (Pratinas fr. 713 iii [*PMG*] = Plut. *Mor.* 1146B–C). Bacis cleanses the Spartan women of madness (Theopompus Hist. *FGrHist* 115 fr. 77). The Apollonian priest Branchus cures the Milesians of plague with laurel (Callim. fr. 194.28–31 Pfeiffer). Melampus cures the maddened daughters of Proetus, perhaps through *pharmaka* or homeopathic Dionysiac rites: see, e.g., Apollod. 2.2.2; Hdt. 9.34; Hes. frr. 37, 129–33 (M-W); Paus. 2.7.8, 2.18.4, 5.5.10, 8.18.7–8; [Plut.] *Fluv.* 21.4; Str. 8.3.19, with Vian 1965; Hoessly 2001.149–63. On Epimenides, who diagnoses the cause of plague in Athens, see Arist. *Ath. Pol.* 1; D. L. 1.110; Plut. *Sol.* 12 (where he deals with pollution already identified), with Burkert 1972.150–52. On the evidence for Empedocles as a healer, see below, chapter 5, n.38. On these healers, the figure of the *iatromantis*, and further discussion of his healing capacities, see Rohde 1925.294–97; Kudlien 1968.305–10; R. Parker 1983.208–12; Vegetti 1996; Hoessly 2001.173–81; Gorrini 2005.135–38.

[167] Although, Parker sees a splintering of the empire of the seer in the archaic and classical periods (1983.210). For literary evidence of the role of oracles and seers in healing, see Conon *FGrHist* 26 fr. 1.18; Hdt. 1.19–22, 4.155; Paus. 1.3.4, 3.19.11–13, 5.4.6, 9.8.2, 10.11.5; S. *OT* 149–50; Theopompus Hist. *FGrHist* 115 fr. 392; Th. 2.54. For epigraphic evidence, see Parke 1967.267–68, nos. 12–15 (Dodona) on individual consultations; and Graf 1992 on an oracle responding to plague from second-century CE Asia Minor. See also Faraone 1992.36–37.

under the Roman Empire.[168] Suppliants to the shrines of Asclepius and those of more minor healing gods and heroes typically gained access to the god's healing powers by sleeping in the temple precinct (incubation), then interpreting their dreams with the help of resident priests.[169] But unlike Calchas, who communicates Apollo's motives, or the magico-religious healers described in *On the Sacred Disease*, who correlate symptoms with the agency of specific gods, Asclepius seems to primarily provide therapeutic instructions (or at times enacted treatment in the dream), rather than identifying culpable agents and reconstructing causal narratives.

The emphasis in the Asclepius cult on healing, rather than diagnosis, reminds us of the wide range of responses to symptoms that would have been possible in the ancient Greek world. Some of these responses would have been pharmacological or surgical, others divinatory or purificatory. Yet, despite the heterogeneity of these responses, they cannot be separated from the magico-religious sphere, insofar as healers must have taken for granted the power of the gods to affect their therapies.[170] In many cases, they would have assumed that a person's exposure to the daemonic is unlike his exposure to mortal weapons: if a warrior's armor reflects an understanding of how to protect the innards from a spear, protecting oneself from the anger of a god or a *daimōn* involves a different

---

[168] On the evidence for the Asclepius cult, see Edelstein and Edelstein 1998; Nutton 2004.103–14; Wickkiser 2008. For the evidence from Epidaurus, see also LiDonnici 1995. It has been often observed that while the medical writers do attack their magico-religious rivals, as in *On the Sacred Disease*, they do not engage in polemics against Asclepius, suggesting a level of symbiosis with the cult. R. Parker 1983.249–50 suggests, in fact, that the Asclepius cult is shaped by the exaggerated expectations created but not fulfilled by the medical *tekhnē*; see also Chaniotis 1995.331; Gorrini 2005.146–47; and esp. Wickkiser 2008.39–61. Moreover, Gorrini 2005.143–45 cites epigraphic evidence showing the presence of physicians at Asclepieia and other healing shrines, and there is increasing overlap between contemporary medical therapeutics and the kinds of remedies recommended by Asclepius in the Hellenistic and imperial periods: Boudon 1994.165–68; Chaniotis 1995.334–35; LiDonnici 1995.48; Horstmanshoff 2004.

[169] On incubation, see Edelstein and Edelstein 1998, 2:145–58. Our evidence suggests that healing functions can be attributed to any hero or god. See, on Heracles, for example, von Staden 1992d.131 n.2; Kingsley 1995.275 n.88; Faraone 2001.6–7 with n.16; Salowey 2002; on Demeter, Richardson 1974.229; on Podalirius, Lyc. *Alex.* 1047–55 (Edelstein T158) and Str. 6.3.9 (Edelstein T205); on Machaon, Lyc. *Alex.* 2048 (Edelstein T205), Paus. 3.26.9 (Edelstein T186), and Paus. 2.11.6, 2.23.4, 2.38.6, 4.3.2, 4.30.3 (= Edelstein T187–91) on his sons. The author of *On Regimen* recommends praying to the heroes, along with the Earth and a host of other gods, to avert disease (*Vict.* IV 89, Li 6.652 = 224,25–28 Joly-Byl). See, in general, Rohde 1925.132–33, with nn.92–103; Brelich 1958.113–18; and the recent review of the evidence in Wickkiser 2008.50–53.

[170] The pharmacological knowledge of ancient healers, for example, may appear to lie outside the webbed social world that I have described, but the charm sung at *Od.* 19.457 reminds us that the efficacy of *pharmaka* could be bound to the gods' good and ill will. Their use, moreover, appears to have been governed in part by symbolic frameworks of meaning that persisted in the medical treatises (von Staden 1992a; 1992b), even as overt explanations of efficacy were aligned with the texts' causal principles (Scarborough 1983; A. Hanson 1991). See also the remarks of Hoessly 2001.93–95 on the impossibility of isolating sanitary cleansing from magico-religious cleansing.

apotropaic logic.[171] Ancient Greek cities, for example, set statues of a bow-bearing Apollo with his back to their gates, compelling or persuading him to aim the other way.[172] And because the gods' proximity to the self is not necessarily realized in physical space, healers can deal with the causes of suffering independently of the person afflicted. When Chryses, appeased, asks Apollo to give up his anger, he is working at some distance from the persons whose lives are at stake.[173]

In these examples, healer-seers succeed because they have a privileged relationship with an unseen divine-daemonic world. In the first fragment of the lost epic *The Sack of Troy* (attributed to the seventh-century Lesbian poet Arctinus), we encounter healing expertise that depends on a different understanding of the unseen. The fragment describes the onset of madness in Telamonian Ajax as it is first perceived by Podalirius, the less visible of Asclepius's two sons in the *Iliad*:[174]

αὐτὸς γάρ σφιν ἔδωκε πατὴρ †γέρας† Ἐννοσίγαιος
ἀμφοτέροις· ἕτερον δ' ἑτέρου κυδίον' ἔθηκεν·
τῷ μὲν κουφοτέρας χεῖρας πόρεν ἔκ τε βέλεμνα
σαρκὸς ἑλεῖν τμῆξαί τε καὶ ἕλκεα πάντ' ἀκέσασθαι,
τῷ δ' ἄρ' ἀκριβέα πάντα ἐνὶ στήθεσσιν ἔθηκεν
ἄσκοπά τε γνῶναι καὶ ἀναλθέα ἰήσασθαι·
ὅς ῥα καὶ Αἴαντος πρῶτος μάθε χωομένοιο
ὄμματά τ' ἀστράπτοντα βαρυνόμενόν τε νόημα.

(Fr. 2 West = Edelstein T 141 & 142)

For their father the Earth-Shaker himself gave them both the healing gift; but he made one higher in prestige than the other.[175] To the one he gave defter hands, to

---

[171] Although the shields in *Seven Against Thebes* or the Gorgons that protect the warriors' knees (places of life-force) do not defend only the "anatomical" self (Deonna 1939).

[172] On the statues of Apollo, see Faraone 1992.57–64. On the social agency of Greek statues, see Collins 2003.37–44. On sympathetic magic as persuasive, ritual enactment, see Taussig 1993, esp. 12–18, 100–43; 2003.288–95; see also Gell 1998.99–104.

[173] Compare the analysis of proximity and boundary violation in illness concepts in terms of physical bodies and social bodies in Samuelsen 2004. But the purification that the Achaeans undertake at *Il.* 1.312–16 (presumably on the advice of Calchas) treats the disease in more concrete terms; see also, e.g., *Morb. Sacr.* 1 (Li 6.362 = 9,3–7 Jouanna).

[174] For Podalirius, see *Il.* 2.729–33, 11.833. The scholiasts make Podalirius the root cutter (ῥιζοτόμος) in order to account for his relative absence in Homer (e.g., Eust. *ad* N 830 = Edelstein T197), while Machaon is said to practice the treatment of wounds and be more "warlike," given his name (Eust. *ad* Δ 202 = Edelstein T139). The scholia also link Podalirius to dietetics, noting that, in cases of injury, only Machaon is summoned (e.g., Eust. *ad* Λ 514 = Edelstein T142). This *argumentum ex silentio* neatly accounts for the double absence in Homer of the second Asclepiad and the branch of medicine that will become so important in later centuries.

[175] *The Sack of Troy* is the only instance where Poseidon is named as the father of Machaon and Podalirius or associated with healing, save at *Od.* 9.412 and 9.520–21, where he is summoned as Polyphemus's father.

remove missiles from flesh and cut and heal all wounds, but in the other's heart he placed exact knowledge, to diagnose what is hidden and to cure what does not get better. He it was who first recognized how the eyes were flashing and how the thought was growing distressed in raging Ajax. (trans. West, slightly modified)

Dealing with what is hidden or irreparable damage, as we have seen, does not appear to be part of the epic healer's *métier*. Podalirius's epistemic advantage thus appears to encroach on the seer's expertise. Yet he neither diagnoses the cause of madness nor predicts it. Instead, he alone recognizes how Ajax's eyes are flashing and how his thought is growing distressed through phenomena that, if not unseen, are in some way puzzling. Podalirius is thus endowed with a special capacity to see and comprehend obscure or confusing changes that a person experiences.

In representing Podalirius's knowledge and Ajax's madness, the poet of *The Sack of Troy* suggests that strange disruptions to the integrity of the person, that is, symptoms, are objects of expert vision and potentially useful to the treatment of difficult diseases. Such a suggestion anticipates the semantically rich body of the medical writers. In fact, though our evidence about the expertise of archaic healers is fragmentary and limited, the passage from *The Sack of Troy* might reflect a post-Homeric interpretation of the place of the healer on the roster of skilled workers and the rise of a medicine focused on symptoms as the key to the interpretation and treatment of illness.[176] What is clearer is that the fragment grants the healer expertise in perceiving what others do not. The representation of the expertise of the *iatros* in terms of his negotiation of the relationship between the seen and the unseen worlds becomes standard in the classical period. This shift in the understanding of the healer's epistemic advantage accompanies a reconceptualization of the unseen world onto which symptoms open. Understanding the nature of this world requires first examining the inquiry into nature.

---

[176] Ancient sources put the floruit of Arctinus around 775 BCE, but cf. Davies 1989.3, 5–6, 11 n.6 for arguments in favor of a later date. The post-Homeric forms in our fragments from the epic cycle suggest they were written after the *Iliad* and the *Odyssey* and may have been subject to some form of rationalization: see Davies 1989.65. Davies finds the above fragment "deeply unHomeric," in part because of the portrayal of the healer (1989.77). The term ἀκρίβεια first appears here, eventually becoming an important idea in medical epistemology: see, e.g., *Epid.* III 16 (Li 3.102 = 238,11 Kühlewein; cf. *Dieb. iudic.* 1 [Li 9.298]); *VM* 9 (Li 1.588–90 = 128,9–15 Jouanna), with Schiefsky 2005a.13–18. Mattes sees Ajax's madness, with the suffering of Bellerophon in the *Iliad*, as "die ersten Zeugnisse für eine natürliche Erklärung des Wahnsinns" (1970.66). Nevertheless, we must be cautious about speaking of a naturalizing explanation without clear verbal cues that the speaker sees his explanation in these terms.

CHAPTER TWO

The Inquiry into Nature and the Physical Imagination

There is always the violence of a sign that forces us into the
search, that robs us of peace. The truth is not to be found by
affinity, nor by goodwill, but is *betrayed* by involuntary signs.

Gilles Deleuze

IN MANY OF OUR archaic and classical sources, when the perceptible world is
suddenly and mysteriously disrupted, people look to the gods. By the fifth century, such disruptions may call to mind another web of power. In his biography
of Pericles, Plutarch reports a story that, while probably apocryphal, illustrates
how signs can draw different worldviews into competition in the classical period. Someone brings a one-horned ram for inspection to Pericles; he, in turn,
solicits two interpretations of the prodigy. One of the experts consulted, the
seer Lampon, taking into account Pericles' position as the head of one of two
factions struggling for control of Athens, announces that the leader on whose
estate the ram appeared will soon secure power. Lampon thus treats the ram as
a conduit of divine knowledge about the future of the *polis*. Given the opportunity to offer his own interpretation, his rival, the physicist Anaxagoras, cuts
open the animal's head in order to demonstrate that the single horn has been
caused by a defect in the brain. Instead of filling out its proper position, the
brain "had all slipped together to a point, like an egg, at that particular spot
from which the root of the horn begins" (*Per.* 6.2). Anaxagoras thus identifies
the cause of the irregularity by probing beneath the surface of the skin. The by-
standers are duly impressed, at least until Pericles does, indeed, assume power.
At this point, Plutarch tells us, everyone decides that Lampon has been right all
along. Anaxagoras's story is forgotten, and the ram's single horn is reconciled
with a political community.

Anaxagoras may not, on Plutarch's account, succeed with the crowd. Nevertheless, his assumptions can serve as a working introduction to the biological
fragments and medical writings extant from the fifth and fourth centuries BCE.
First, Plutarch's Anaxagoras acts as though we see in the absence of obstacles to
vision, rather than in the light of the gods' favor. In this case, nothing bars him
from removing what stands in his way—the skin. In making his cut, he upholds a fundamental principle in the inquiry into nature: phenomena can be

understood by looking below the surface to their hidden causes.[1] So, whereas Lampon takes the appearance of the ram as mimetic of future power relations in the *polis*, thereby displacing the meaning of the sign from its bearer,[2] Anaxagoras refers appearance to biological growth and a potentially seen subcutaneous world. When this world is revealed, he sees, in one sense, what an Iliadic warrior sees when flesh is cut away. Yet, in another sense, he sees something else entirely, insofar as his looking is conditioned by new ideas about the *phusis* of a complex organism.[3] Seen in this way, the world beneath the skin supports a framework of explanation robust enough to compete with one based on a divine-daemonic web of sympathies and antipathies.

Plutarch's vignette also shows, however, how difficult it can be to make sense, quite literally, of the world beneath the skin. For Anaxagoras ends up *denying* meaning to the mystery of the ram's single horn by referring it to a world buried below the threshold of our perception, indifferent to our interpretations, our needs, our politics. If the gods embody human values and excellence, this buried world is ill suited to the narratives that give our lives meaning. No less a biologist than Aristotle observes that "it is not possible to look at parts that constitute the human race [ἐξ ὧν συνέστηκε τὸ τῶν ἀνθρώπων γένος], such as blood, flesh, bones, vessels, and other such parts, without considerable distaste" (*PA* 645a28–30). A physical reality that we want nothing to do with and has nothing to say to us lies at the core of Anaxagoras's account. Once he shows why the horn formed as it did, his story is over and done with.[4] And yet, in the end, Anaxagoras's story cannot compete with that of Lampon, who relates the anomalous event to the people in whose midst it occurs. Lampon's success should remind us of how difficult it is to speak of objects without considering subjects. This will prove especially true when the objects are also subjects.

In this chapter, I step back from symptoms in order to sketch the larger conceptual context of the physical body's emergence. I focus on the gradual formation in the sixth and fifth centuries BCE of a community of objects joined together by their participation in what I have called physicality, rather than by a web of social relationships. I begin by following the shift from personal agents

---

[1] On the inquiry into nature, see above, introduction, n.5.

[2] Cf. the sneeze at *Od.* 17.539–47, with Pease 1911.431–32: the sign has little bearing on Telemachus himself, but confirms that Penelope's prediction of the suitors' death will come true. On somatic divinatory signs more generally, see Halliday 1913.174–83; Langholf 1990.248–49.

[3] Gregory Vlastos, describing *phusis* as it is used by Herodotus, gives a definition with broader applicability: "The *physis* of any given thing is that cluster of stable characteristics by which we can recognize that thing and can anticipate the limits within which it can act upon other things or be acted upon by them" (1975.19). See also Heidel 1910; Curd 1998.43–47; Andò 1999; and esp. Naddaf 2005.11–35, stressing the importance of origins and development to the concept of *phusis*. Gallego Pérez 1996.419–21 nn.1–11 offers a full bibliography on *phusis*.

[4] Democritus may have been the first to articulate the principle that there is no use looking for a reason for what is necessary in nature (DK68 A65 = Arist. *Phys.* 252a32–b1). Anaxagoras does have a principle of cosmic Mind, but it is unclear how it affects his interpretation of the horn.

to impersonal causes in the inquiry into nature. This is, of course, a well-known story. Nevertheless, I would like to revisit it in light of the discussion of social agents and symptoms in chapter 1. Early Greek poetry is deeply attuned to the behavior of fluids and winds, forces that are, nevertheless, pliable in the hands of gods and *daimones*. By uncoupling these forces from intentions, the physicists shift the weight of explanation to the interaction of contingent forces and natures. The *sōma* emerges through this process as a major site of becoming, through which human nature and other natures are necessarily implicated in newly elaborated webs of power. Reading *sōma* in this way may shed light on a famously puzzling fragment of the Eleatic philosopher Melissus, where what exists is said not to have (a) *sōma*.

In the latter part of the chapter, I take a closer look at how physicists and medical writers conceptualize a community of composite physical objects and begin to consider the place of human beings in this community. I show first how, through the use of analogy, these thinkers establish continuities between bodies in physical, rather than social, terms. I also explore their interest in interactions at the level of potentially seen stuffs in their accounts of perception, pain, and pleasure. By developing the idea of physical change that can be understood without being experienced, the physicists lay the groundwork for the conceptualization of a plane of events inside the *sōma* that escapes awareness, as well as a reappraisal of the felt in terms of the mechanisms of its production.

My focus in this chapter, then, is on two aspects of physicality that I suggest are particularly important to the emergence of the physical body: first, the transfer of power from unseen social agents to impersonal forces that drive ongoing, albeit often imperceptible, transformations in composite objects; and, second, the conceptualization of all such objects in terms of an objective nature rather than subjective experience. In the following two chapters, I examine in more detail the emergence of the physical *human* body, primarily in medical writing, and begin to explore the problems that this body poses to the idea of the person.

In putting so much emphasis on the physical world, I may seem to be adopting a rather outmoded way of approaching early Greek philosophy. In recent years, scholars have been less concerned—though not unconcerned—with whether early philosophers have an empirical understanding of the natural world and whether their methods deserve the label "scientific"; they have challenged the labeling of the Presocratics as "naturalists" and pointed to modern misunderstandings of Greek *phusis*.[5] Moreover, if we turn these thinkers into materialists, some have argued, we overlook how important the divine or Mind is to their work.[6] And, in fact, this very term, "materialism," which presumes a

---

[5] For the difficulties with the label "Presocratics," which was popularized by Diels's *Die Fragmente der Vorsokratiker* (1903), see Laks 2002.17–25. See also, introduction, n.5.

[6] On the importance of the divine, see Jaeger 1947, with the criticisms of Vlastos 1952; see also Kingsley 1995; Collins 2003.21–23.

concept of matter, raises all kinds of problems. By addressing some of these problems very briefly at the outset, I hope to clarify my aims in this chapter.

In a well-known passage from the beginning of his *Metaphysics*, Aristotle tells us that the earliest philosophers conceived of the "first principles of all things solely as a form of matter [ἐν ὕλης εἴδει]," principles he describes elsewhere as "corporeal" (σωματικαί).[7] Each thinker, on this account, posits a single stuff (or group of stuffs) that persists through any modification. One difficulty with this description is that *hulē*, Aristotle's technical term for "matter," designates a concept specific to his own ontology, where it is defined through its relationship to philosophical problems articulated in an Aristotelian manner, as well as to other concepts like form or composite body.[8] Aristotle, of course, never claims to be giving a disinterested history of philosophy. His discussion of his predecessors, rather, is openly "driven by the need to introduce, in addition to matter, the further explanatory kinds of principles, and to get clearer about the nature of these explanatory factors."[9] His account, then, can be read as a survey of how close prior thinkers come to his own doctrine of four causes and his metaphysics more generally. In light of Aristotle's method, it is not surprising that when he evaluates "a kind of matter" in earlier thinkers, that "matter" tends to satisfy one condition of *hulē* while violating another. To take an example: insofar as Aristotle sees the "material principles" of figures like Thales and Anaximenes as unchanging substrates,[10] he must exclude these principles from world formation on the grounds that *hulē*, on his own account, is inert.[11] Thus,

---

[7] Arist. *Metaph.* 983b7; see also 984a5–7, 987a4; *Phys.* 194a18–19. On the expression ἐν ὕλης εἴδει, see Ross 1958, 1:128–29, translating "of the nature of matter."

[8] Graham 1984 argues that we can pinpoint the "discovery" of matter within Aristotle's corpus, a claim reiterated at Graham 2006.64. On the function of Aristotle's matter concept, see Graham 1984; 1987. The difficulty involved in knowing matter empirically—at *Metaph.* 994b25–26, we are told "matter must be known through the thing that changes (ἐν κινουμένῳ)"; see also *Phys.* 191a7–12, where the substrate can be known only on analogy with phenomenal types of matter, like bronze— underlines that it is mostly a metaphysical concept.

[9] M. Frede 2004.14. For the classic negative assessment of Aristotle as a historian, see Cherniss 1935, esp. 218–88 on the concepts of cause and matter. Cf. Guthrie 1957. More recent studies tend toward the proverbial middle way: see Collobert 2002; M. Frede 2004; Leszl 2006; see also Baltussen 2000.28–29, emphasizing the shift toward a reception-based approach that sees Aristotle's historical overviews as critical in a constructive way. But there is still a healthy distrust of Aristotle's representation of prior philosophers (e.g., Kingsley 1995, esp. 384–91; Most 1999.332–33; Laks 2006.55–56), though few would argue that we should ignore his historical account altogether.

[10] Most scholars believe that, insofar as he represents Thales' water as an unchanging substrate, Aristotle is extending what was probably a cosmogonic principle beyond its intended function: see Kirk, Raven, and Schofield 1983.89–95. Mansfeld 1985.118–19 and Algra 1999.50–51 emphasize Aristotle's reticence about the role of water in Thales' philosophy. See also Graham 2006, esp. 48–112, who claims that Aristotle misapplies the substrate model ("Material Monism") to all the Milesians and argues that the *arkhē* for these thinkers is a generating substance that undergoes real change after the cosmogonic event.

[11] See, e.g., *Metaph.* 984a21–25: "It is surely not the substrate itself that makes itself change [οὐ γὰρ δὴ τό γε ὑποκείμενον αὐτὸ ποιεῖ μεταβάλλειν ἑαυτό] . . . wood does not make a bed, nor bronze a statue, but something else is the cause of the change." Similarly, although Aristotle considers principles like

although problems addressed by Aristotle under the rubric of *hulē* appear in earlier thinkers, *hulē* does not easily align with its purported predecessors, nor is there an obvious unifying term that it replaces. "Matter" is something of a moving target before Aristotle. Can we say, then, that the Presocratics deal with the notion of matter "without being able to refer to it abstractly?"[12]

This question is difficult to answer. It is not that Aristotle's formulation of the problem of matter is irrelevant, given that, in some sense, it grows out of his predecessors' work. Nevertheless, it is of limited use for understanding earlier thinkers. In this chapter, then, I do not approach matter as the philosophical problem articulated by Aristotle. That is to say, I am interested neither in categorically denying a respectable concept of matter to pre-Aristotelian thinkers nor in narrating the struggle to discover such a concept. Rather, I begin here to sketch a messier set of problems around the idea of physicality, a word that keeps *phusis* in the foreground while deflecting the assumptions associated with the term "materialism" and, indeed, the presumed coherence of any -ism. Consistent with my approach to the physical body, I treat physicality in terms of neither philosophical discovery nor an empirical grasp of the natural world but in terms of a provocative shift of explanatory emphasis. Thus, although physicality encompasses a number of ideas we would call philosophical or scientific, I am interested in pursuing conceptual consequences that have tended to escape histories of philosophy and science oriented toward the development of ideas deemed (philosophically or scientifically) viable.

At the same time, it bears repeating that there is an undeniable conceptual shift in the sixth and fifth centuries. Aristotle may or may not be giving us an adequate or accurate account in the *Metaphysics* when he describes how the Ionians rejected theogony in favor of identifying first principles.[13] Nevertheless, although it will always be possible to identify continuities from the eighth to the fifth century BCE, it is clear that by the late fifth century there are new paradigms of the natural world and divine power circulating in the Greek world, paradigms that provoke reconsideration of existing assumptions and anxiety.[14]

Empedocles' Love and Strife as possible precursors of the Unmoved Mover, they are ultimately disqualified on the grounds that they occupy space: see *Metaph.* 1075b2–6 (cf. Emp. [DK31] B17.19–20); see also *Metaph.* 988a33–34; *GC* 314a16–17, with Inwood 2001.51; Graham 2006.233–35. Cf. G. Lloyd 1966.251–52 and M. R. Wright 1995.32–34, arguing that because Love and Strife are inherent in the roots (Lloyd) or manifest in their balance and movement (Wright), they do not occupy space. Curd 2007.200 n.14 argues against the materiality of both Love and Strife and Anaxagoras's *Nous*. For the Presocratic "failure" to grasp the relationship between matter and spatial extension, see Renehan 1980; Kirk, Raven, and Schofield 1983.364, and the discussion of Melissus below.

[12] Graham 1999.172.

[13] For a negative view of this break, see Pl. *Leg.* 10, 886b10–e2. At the same time, Aristotle is, at times, willing to see continuities between myth and philosophy. Moreover, ancient historians of philosophy did not take Aristotle's story of the birth of philosophy for granted, as Mansfeld 1985 shows.

[14] In surveying the disruptive effects of these paradigms, modern scholars tend to emphasize different aspects: (a) the intent of the thinker in question; (b) the historical effects of the ideas; (c) the implications of those ideas as the original audience perceived them. See, e.g., Bett 2002.236 n.4, who focuses on (a), with some attention to (c). Cf. Graham 2006.194–95, in a discussion of

If Plutarch, who lived in an age when it was possible to accept both the (physical) *aitia*, "cause," and the (divine) *telos*, "reason," of a given event, finds little threat in Anaxagoras's elimination of politics from the interpretation of signs, we cannot assume that fifth-century Greeks were so easily reconciled to physicalizing explanation. Elsewhere, Plutarch registers the discomfort created by Anaxagoras's claim that lunar eclipses occur, not in response to the gods' will, but when a planetary body screens the moon. He observes:[15]

οὐ γὰρ ἠνείχοντο τοὺς φυσικοὺς καὶ μετεωρολέσχας τότε καλουμένους, ὡς εἰς αἰτίας ἀλόγους καὶ δυνάμεις ἀπρονοήτους καὶ κατηναγκασμένα πάθη διατρίβοντας τὸ θεῖον. (*Nic.* 23.4)

For people could not tolerate the physicists and the stargazers, as they were then called, on the grounds that they whittled the divine down to irrational causes and powers lacking intention and necessary incidents.

Is there contemporary support for Plutarch's picture of public unease with the inquiry into nature? Plato's *Apology* makes it clear that the claim that the planetary bodies are just rocks was a particularly incendiary assertion in the late fifth century (26d4–5), and the "Socrates" who appears in Aristophanes' *Clouds* as a natural philosopher is represented as a threat to the city and its youth.[16] Even those who have been skeptical about the reports of later writers like Plutarch about intolerance in classical Athens have seen as likely "a suspicion of intellectual or religious speculation" in the late fifth century.[17] In Euripides' *Electra*, the Chorus recalls how Zeus reacted in horror to Thyestes' crime by changing the path of the sun, before admitting that:

λέγεται [τάδε], τὰν δὲ πί-
στιν σμικρὰν παρ᾽ ἔμοιγ᾽ ἔχει,
στρέψαι θερμὰν ἀέλιον
χρυσωπὸν ἕδραν ἀλλά-
ξαντα δυστυχίᾳ βροτεί-
ῳ θνατᾶς ἕνεκεν δίκας.
φοβεροὶ δὲ βροτοῖσι μῦθ-
οι κέρδος πρὸς θεῶν θεραπεί-
ας.

(E. *El.* 737–45)

Parmenides, privileging (b). I find it hard to see how those active in debates about nature could not have foreseen the world-shaking ramifications of at least some of their ideas—their ambition is part of the point—but I am primarily interested in (b) and (c).

[15] See Anaxag. (DK59) A42 (= Hippol. *Ref.* 1.8.9).

[16] On the scandalous claim that the sun is a rock, which was associated with Anaxagoras, see Guthrie 1962–69, 2:307–8; Willink 1983. Euripides, in the [lost] *Phaethon*, calls the sun a "golden rock"; see also *Or.* 4–10, where theodicy seems to target the meteorosophist with a vengeance (Scodel 1984; Willink 1986.79–80).

[17] Wallace 1994.135; see also 138. Wallace otherwise largely upholds the skepticism about the persecution of intellectuals in Athens expressed in Dover 1976. Cf. Janko 2001.6, 11–15, strongly defending the view of an "anti-intellectual climate" in the last decades of the fifth century in Athens (14).

This is what is said, but the trust it gains from me is slight, that the golden-faced sun would turn and change its hot position for the purpose of mortal misfortune, because of a human dispute. Such fear-inducing stories are a boon to mortals, furthering the worship of the gods.

By using multiple adjectives for "mortal"/"human" (βρότειος, θνατός), the Chorus draws attention to the human world. Yet they do so only to suggest its isolation: behind the collective fictions, there may be only cosmic indifference to human misfortune and human crimes.[18] The possibility of such indifference is the danger posed by the physicists to a culture lacking sacred texts. In book 10 of Plato's *Laws*, for example, the Athenian castigates the physicists for claiming that things up above "are simply earth and stone, being incapable of taking heed of human things [ὄντα αὐτὰ καὶ οὐδὲν τῶν ἀνθρωπείων πραγμάτων φροντίζειν δυνάμενα]" (886d8–e1).[19]

Naturalizing explanation never decisively edges out the agency of the gods in classical antiquity; in some quarters its challenge was never felt. Nevertheless, by extending the forces of nature, contingency, and necessity into the domain of the god's hand, the physicists encourage those around them to see behind phenomena not embodied social agents but disembodied fragments of nonhuman power.

Depersonalizing Causes

In the *Sophist*, Plato declares that the materialists, that is, those who drag everything from the heavens down to earth, "actually getting hold of rocks and trees with their hands" (ταῖς χερσὶν ἀτεχνῶς πέτρας καὶ δρῦς περιλαμβάνοντες,

---

[18] The clearest evidence for the idea the gods may simply be a human creation is at DK88 B25, usually attributed to the sophist Critias, although sometimes assigned to Euripides; the fragment is thought to be from a satyr play, perhaps *Sisyphus*. In the fragment, the gods are invented by a clever man as a deterrent to crime. The *Electra* passage is more opaque, but it at least implies the otherness of the physical world and doubt about the gods' involvement in human affairs. See also the doubts about theodicy at E. fr. 506K (= *Melanippe* fr. 6 J.-V.L.). In a recent discussion of the Critias fragment, Bett 2002.251–54 reaffirms its atheistic nature while stressing the author's interest in an ordered society, thereby downplaying its radical implications. But the word ἄθεος was inflammatory in the fifth century. It could designate not only those who denied that the gods exist but anyone who departed from conventional views of them (Obbink 1996.1–2; Janko 2001.11–15). Lists of "atheists" were probably already circulating in the late fourth century: see Philodemus's *On Piety* Part I, col. 19.523–41 (Obbink), evidence for such a list in Epicurus's *On Nature*, with Obbink 1996.349–60. See further Janko 2001.7–8 (on Diagoras); Henrichs 1975; 1976 (on Prodicus and Democritus).

[19] See also X. *Mem.* 1.4.1–18. Even Epicurus, a philosopher who was deeply committed to physical explanation, takes his predecessors to task for "blaming everything on necessity and automatism" (ε[ἰ]ς τὸ [ε[ἰ]ς τὸ Sedley: ἔν· τὸ Gigante] τ[ὴ]ν ἀνάγκην καὶ ταὐτόματ[ο]ν πάντα α[ἰτι]ᾶσθαι, *Nat.*, liber incertus, 34.30 = Long-Sedley 20C.50–51).

246a8–9), claim that only what can be touched is real. Hostile critic or not, Plato points to a relatively uncontroversial fact about those working in the inquiry into nature—namely, that they invest meaning in the everyday details of the physical world. Their basic stuffs are things like air, water, fire, and earth. When Aristotle says that Thales posited water as his material principle, he makes it clear that water here is, at least in some sense, just what we think it is, something we can see or feel.[20]

At the same time, though, by delving into the physical world, the physicists seek to go beyond familiar acquaintance: "*Phusis*," as Heraclitus writes, "is wont to hide" (φύσις . . . κρύπτεσθαι φιλεῖ, DK22 B123). They build universalizing accounts of physical reality around natural processes like rarefaction, condensation, mixture, and separation, processes that lay bare the ephemeral nature of bounded solids and dispel the mirage of their unity. Their cosmogonies expose the present world's debt to an unseen source and prefigure, if not its demise, at least radical transformation.[21] The sun is created anew each day as a collection of little bits of fire.[22] Things that appear solid are unraveling at another level of reality. Gold, stone, and "everything else that seems to be strong" turn out to be born of water; iron is invisibly worn away; whatever we think has a form and a strength of its own relentlessly becomes other to itself.[23] The tenuous grasp these physical objects have on form recalls the *sōma* in Homeric epic, caught between the image of the person and the flesh that disappears into an economy of interincorporation.

Those seeking to describe and understand these changes in the natural world typically draw on some combination of the causes that Plato ascribes to the materialists in the *Laws*: *tukhē*, "chance"; *anankē*, "necessity"; and *phusis*.[24] Take, for example, an account, ascribed to Anaximander, of how wind, if, by chance, it is subjected to the right conditions, naturally and necessarily produces thunder and lightning. According to later sources, Anaximander claims that wind arises when the finest vapors are separated off from the air under the heat of the

[20] Aristotle speculates that Thales' claims are built on the empirical observation that all things are nurtured by the moist (*Metaph.* 983b22–23 = DK11 A12). Theophrastus conjectures that Thales privileges water as the principle of life after noticing that corpses dry up (Simp. *In ph.* 23.21–29 = DK11 A13), but he is probably thinking of Hippon's argument that the soul-seed of all things is moist (see Arist. *De an.* 405b1–3), as Kirk, Raven, and Schofield 1983.91–92 argue.

[21] "Il serait . . . plus exact de parler de 'cosmo-gono-phthories,' que de simples cosmogonies" (Laks 2006.10).

[22] Xenoph. (DK21) A40 (= Aët. 2.20.3); cf. A33 (= Hippol. *Ref.* 1.14.3). See also Heraclit. (DK22) B6; Emp. (DK31) B41. Aggregate creation can be expressed in genealogical-biological terms, e.g., Xenoph. (DK21) B30, where sea is named both a source and a begetter of winds and clouds. On biological language in early cosmology, see G. Lloyd 1966.232–72.

[23] Melissus (DK30) B8.

[24] *Leg.* 10, 889b1–c6; cf. *Phlb.* 28d5–9; *Sph.* 265c1–10. For the conjunction *phusis-anankē*, see further below, nn.57–58. In the *Timaeus*, Plato finds a place for the physicists' causes within his own cosmology (*Ti.* 46c7–e6), creating an uneasy alliance between *nous* and *anankē* (47e5–48a7); on this alliance, see Strange 1985.

sun and set in motion by being gathered together.[25] When the wind, "becoming trapped in a thick cloud, breaks out under force, because of its fineness and lightness," it causes thunder and lightning: "The bursting makes a noise while the rift against the blackness of the cloud produces the flash" (DK12 A23 = Aët. 3.3.1). The account resembles other early meteorological explanations in our sources.[26] It also bears a remarkable similarity to an extended parody of such explanations in Aristophanes' *Clouds*.[27] In that play, the character "Socrates," having declared that Zeus does not exist, argues that rain and thunder are caused by the rolling and crashing of the clouds: having happened to fill with water, these clouds are forced (κἀναγκασθῶσι, 376) to drift along, weighted down, necessarily (δι' ἀνάγκην, 377; cf. 405, ὑπ' ἀνάγκης), with water, until they finally burst, thundering on account of their density (διὰ τὴν πυκνότητα, 384; cf. 406).[28]

Aristophanes is clearly seeking maximum comic effect in this scene. Yet, in dramatizing how a physicist might have presented his theory to a skeptical audience, he is also showing us what might happen when new models of explanation encroach on domains traditionally under the aegis of Zeus. When Strepsiades, a wealthy but unsophisticated Athenian hoping to have his son educated at Socrates' Thinkery, is told that Zeus is not responsible for thunder and lightning, his first reaction is to ask *how* (τῷ τρόπῳ, 375) these phenomena arise.[29] Socrates, in turn, describes a series of events (the saturation of the clouds, their movement, the outcome of their collisions) that he explains in terms of both necessity and the nature of wind and clouds (denseness, fineness, lightness). This series allows him to fill in the space typically spanned by symbols of divine agency. Strepsiades, however, is reluctant to give up Zeus's agency: even after he has heard Socrates' account, he wants to know *who* forces the clouds to move (ὁ δ' ἀναγκάζων ἐστὶ τίς αὐτάς ... ὥστε φέρεσθαι, 379), triggering the chain of meteorological events. But Socrates heads him off here, too, by making "cosmic whirl" the initiating cause.[30] Like Anaximander, then, the Aristophanic Socrates sees thunder and lightning not in terms of Zeus's intentions or his technologies of action (the thunderbolt), but as the result of a mechanical process mobilized

---

[25] Anaximander (DK12) A11 (= Hippol. *Ref.* 1.6.7); see also A24 (= Aët. 3.7.1) and Kahn 1960.100–102.

[26] Compare, e.g., the testimonia at Anaxag. (DK59) A84.

[27] Although the *Clouds* was first performed in the latter part of the fifth century, more than a century after Anaximander, it reflects the popularity of these kinds of explanations in this period.

[28] Socrates' later explanation of the lightning bolt—a dry wind rises, gets trapped in the clouds, and bursts out, making a terrible noise because of its density and burning up because of friction and speed (*Nu.* 404–7)—is particularly close to the Anaximander testimonium: see Kahn 1960.108–9.

[29] Aristophanes makes the application of the how question to Zeus's own actions into a joke: "Indeed," says Strepsiades, "previously I thought that rain was Zeus pissing through a sieve" (καίτοι πρότερον τὸν Δί' ἀληθῶς ᾤμην διὰ κοσκίνου οὐρεῖν, 373).

[30] For the cosmic whirl see, e.g., Emp. (DK31) B35.4 (δίνη) and Democr. (DK68) B167 (δῖνος). The atomists, in particular, were known for their refusal to name any principle of directed motion: see DK68 A69 (= Arist. *Phys.* 196a24–35).

by a principle of random motion. Thunder and lightning make the force aggregated through this process blindingly visible: the cloud-hole left by the wind, writ large in the sky, lights up a world that runs on chance, nature, and necessity, a world independent not only of the gods' agency but also of the social framework of its realization (Socrates makes a point of disabusing Strepsiades of the idea that Zeus uses lightning to punish perjurers, 398–402).

It has become common, though not uncontroversial, to see the kinds of explanations parodied by Aristophanes, together with the larger physical world they assume, as supporting a "notion of self-regulating cosmological relationships, i.e., an idea of cosmological *order*."[31] Scholars defending this position typically point to the only Anaximander fragment we have: "For they pay penalty and recompense to one another for their injustice according to the assessment of time" (διδόναι γὰρ αὐτὰ δίκην καὶ τίσιν ἀλλήλοις τῆς ἀδικίας κατὰ τὴν τοῦ χρόνου τάξιν, DK12 B1).[32] The use that Anaximander makes of the legal language of exchange and retribution has led scholars to identify a "rule of law" in his physical theory that seems to render the gods' agency superfluous.[33]

But terms like "cosmological order" or "natural law" are loaded; behind them the risk of anachronism always lingers.[34] While it can hardly be denied that thinkers like Anaximander and Anaximenes are pioneering new ideas about how power works in the world, we need to be cautious about pinpointing what is new in these ideas. It is not sufficient, for example, to say that the gods disappear. If Socrates is trying to get Strepsiades to see thunder and lightning differently so that he will stop interacting with the traditional gods—sacrificing to them, offering them incense, pouring libations—it is because he wants him to honor three new ones: Chaos, the Tongue, and the Clouds themselves, the play's Chorus. Rethinking divinity was one of the hallmarks of the Ionian tradition. Aristotle tells us that Anaximander equates his first principle, *to apeiron*, "the unlimited," with the divine because it is deathless and imperishable, and he indicates that other physicists make their main principles divine.[35] Heraclitus

---

[31] G. Lloyd 1966.213 (emphasis in original); see also Vlastos 1952.114–15.

[32] The subjects of Anaximander's fragment are not specified, although they are usually seen as the opposites or the elements that come to be from and perish into their opposites: see Vlastos 1947.169; Kahn 1960.178–96; Graham 2006.34–38. On the ontological status of the opposites here and in other physicists, see G. Lloyd 1964.

[33] Vlastos 1947.168–73 offered an influential "democratic" reading of the fragment. Cf. Graham 2006.36–38, arguing that Anaximander's justice is monarchical or even anarchic; Engmann 1991; Gagarin 2002.

[34] See esp. Finkelberg 1998, arguing that *kosmos* in the sixth and fifth centuries does not mean "world order" or (primarily) "world" but "arrangement." On natural law in the Anaximander fragment, see G. Lloyd 1966.212–32 and 1979.33 on legal terms in the Presocratics more generally. Cf. Broadie 1999, arguing that a "truly naturalized natural world" is not found until Leucippus and Democritus (221); Guthrie 1962–69, 2:114; Graham 2006.276.

[35] Anaximander (DK12) A15 (= *Phys.* 203b10–15). See also Aët. 1.7.12 at A17 and examples in Vlastos 1952.97–100, Broadie 1999.205–6, and Collins 2003.22–23. On the unlimited, see Kahn 1960.231–39; Kirk, Raven, and Schofield 1983.109–11; Naddaf 2005.68–70; Graham 2006.28–34.

declares god to be "day night, winter summer, war peace, satiety hunger … becom[ing] other in the way that fire,[36] whenever it is mixed with spices, is named according to the pleasure [or flavor, scent: ἡδονή] of each" (DK22 B67). God for Heraclitus thus appears to be immanent in the ceaseless mutability of the phenomenal world. At the same time, the divine continues to be associated in early Greek philosophy with hegemony and efficacious intelligence. Aristotle says, for example, that Anaximander's *to apeiron* "steers and controls all things" (*Phys.* 203b11–13 = DK12 A15), and adds that others—presumably Anaxagoras and Empedocles—ascribe a similar power to *Nous* and Love, respectively; Xenophanes' god "without toil shakes all things by the thought of his mind" (ἀπάνευθε πόνοιο νόου φρενὶ πάντα κραδαίνει, DK21 B25).[37]

In Xenophanes' case, the relationship between a new concept of the divine and the human becomes particularly complex. He does not deny mind to his god. But he does call into question other dominant anthropomorphizing projections. In a famous series of fragments, he faults Homer and Hesiod for ascribing what is shameful among men—theft, adultery, deceit—to the gods (B11) and challenges those who believe that the gods are born and that they have their own clothes, a voice, and a *demas*, a "bodily structure" (B14). He declares that if horses and cattle and lions had the means to draw, they, too, would represent gods in their own image, presumably just as the Egyptians and the Thracians make gods in their own likeness (B15–B16). Xenophanes is not alone in questioning conventional representations of the gods. Heraclitus claims that those who pray to statues might as well be chatting with houses, "not recognizing who gods and heroes are" (DK22 B5). Empedocles' Sphere, which precedes every cosmic cycle and is called god, has no human head on limbs (ἀνδρομέη κεφαλῇ κατὰ γυῖα), no "twin branches" sprung from its back, no feet, no nimble knees, no fertile parts (DK31 B134; see also B29).[38] Xenophanes' god appears to lack neither a *demas* nor the capacity for thought, but he is different from mortals in both these respects (οὔτι δέμας θνητοῖσιν ὁμοίιος οὐδὲ νόημα, B23).[39] He sees, thinks, and hears with his whole being (οὖλος, B24); he shakes all things with thought (B25); he has no need of locomotion, which requires one to take up a position relative to others at different points in time and space (ἄλλοτε ἄλλῃ, B26). Xenophanes may be deliberately decoupling the god's

---

[36] πῦρ. suppl. Diels.

[37] Compare A. *Supp.* 96–103, where Zeus is capable of hurling mortals down, not with violence or toil, but with thought (φρόνημα) alone. See, too, Anaxag. (DK59) B12 on hegemonic Nous; Emp. (DK31) B134, where god is equated with φρὴν ἱερή; Diog. Apoll. (DK64) B5 on the divine Air that steers and controls all things.

[38] See also DK31 B31, where the γυῖα θεοῖο refer, on M. R. Wright's reading (1995.192), to "the totality of spatial parts," rather than anthropomorphic limbs. But note that, in addition to the cosmic deity, Empedocles recognizes "long-lived" (but not immortal) gods (B21.12) and counts himself among them (B112.4).

[39] For the limitations of *human* thought, see DK21 B34, with the summary of interpretations of the fragment at Lesher 1992.161–66. See also Hussey 1990.17–24; Lesher 1992.182–86.

efficacious intelligence from the human form, whose blind spots, we have seen, express gaps of knowledge in Homer.

At the same time, that very decoupling challenges our intuitive sense of agency, that is, doing this instead of doing that. Although in theory nothing escapes the mind of Zeus, in practice what he sees or hears at a given moment shapes how and where he acts in the world:[40] as the painter Agnes Martin once wrote, "one who has become all eyes does not see."[41] If gods see and know more than humans, humans are harmed or helped by this epistemic excess because they can, wittingly or unwittingly, *attract* it. The double sense of the verb *eukhomai*, "to pray" and "to boast," for example, casts prayer as the act of getting the gods' attention. Religious festivals and ritual activities are "an invitation for the attention of the superhuman."[42] But because Xenophanes' god sees everything and acts everywhere, it is difficult to embed his actions in a mortal-immortal community: as Vernant asks, "how could humankind institute regular exchange with the gods in which homages and benefits balance out, unless the Immortals appear in this world in a visible and specific form, in a particular place and at a particular time?"[43] Given Xenophanes' emphasis on his god's intelligence, it is not easy to see divine agency as immanent in the physical changes he describes elsewhere.[44] Nevertheless, by attending to those changes, he and other physicists begin to sketch a web of power relations capable of taking the place of the invisible web of mortal-immortal reciprocity assumed in poetry and ritual practice. On what terms do humans participate in this world?

NATURAL JUSTICE

In the first book of the *Iliad*, before swearing an oath to avenge his anger against Agamemnon, Achilles takes hold of the scepter that "the sons of the Achaeans carry ... in their hands in state when they administer the decrees of Zeus" (1.237–39). By appropriating the scepter, he implicates not just the entire Achaean community but Zeus himself in the insult to his honor and his demand for reparation.[45] The scepter makes Zeus's power to act concrete. Stripped

---

[40] See Hussey 1990.12, with n.5.

[41] Agnes Martin 1992.18.

[42] Athina Kavoulaki, cited at Nightingale 2004.45.

[43] Vernant 1991b.47. Although Xenophanes could eliminate traditional gods (e.g., DK21 B32), see the testimonia gathered at A13, which suggest that he would have accepted sacrifice to the gods; see also B1.13–16, approving hymns and libations, with Lesher 1992.115–16.

[44] It is difficult to reconcile Xenophanes' physical theories with his theology, a difficulty already recognized by Aristotle (*Metaph.* 986b21): see Lesher 1992.100–102 for modern approaches to the problem. Concerns about the tension between intelligence and mechanism were also often raised with respect to Anaxagoras's Mind, again already in antiquity: see Arist. *Metaph.* 985a18–21; Pl. *Phd.* 97b8–98c2.

[45] "The sceptre serves as a demonstrable sign of a wrong, as a silent, but certain, manifestation of injustice" (Lynn-George 1993.201–2). See Vernant 1991e.156–58 on the relationship between the scepter and other sacred objects.

of bark and denied the possibility of leafing out again, it ceases to participate in the life of the forest and becomes a means of harnessing the gods and the order they represent to the protection of human justice.[46] After all, there is no *dikē*, "justice," for fish and fowl, no oaths between lambs and wolves nor between men and lions.[47] The scepter stands as a powerful instrument of collective, mortal-immortal social and ethical agency.

The concept of *dikē* continues to do considerable work in the inquiry into nature, as the Anaximander fragment, with its reference to cosmic forces paying penalties to one another, suggests. Parmenides writes that the gates of Night and Day are controlled by "avenging *dikē*" (DK28 B1.14), which, by holding the fetters of what-is, keeps it from coming to be or perishing (B8.13–15). Heraclitus claims that should the sun overstep its boundaries, the Erinyes, ministers of cosmic *dikē*, would find him out (DK22 B94; cf. B28). Empedocles claims that Strife periodically succeeds Love to claim its right to dominance in the cosmos in accordance with a "broad oath" (DK31 B30).[48]

Many scholars have understood these fragments, with their strong commitment to the binding force of law, in terms of the changing political landscape of the sixth-century Greek world, a period when power was moving from aristocratic hierarchies into the more open channels identified with the *polis* and its legal innovations.[49] But, as Gregory Vlastos recognizes in an early and elegant exposition of this argument, even if the physicists, under the sway of nascent democratic or *polis* ideology, are assuming that the physical world obeys a kind of natural justice—and this claim remains subject to challenge—that assumption has "a strictly physical sense . . . accepted not as a political dogma but as a theorem in physical inquiry."[50] In other words, the physicists are not simply refashioning Olympian politics in more egalitarian terms, but are reworking what it means to speak of power on a macrocosmic scale by broadly eliminating the gods' social agency. In so doing, they complicate the very task of reconciling the macrocosm with the microcosm.

The challenge of reconciliation becomes evident when contemporary scholars try to explain the rapport between new physical macrocosms and the sociopolitical microcosm: "In the final analysis," one historian of philosophy writes,

---

[46] The idea that the gods uphold justice, however, is not monolithic in archaic poetry, through which runs a strong streak of pessimism: see Lloyd-Jones 1983.36–53.

[47] *Il.* 22.262–63; Hes. *Op.* 278 (cf. Arist. *EN* 1161b1–3). In Homer, *dikē* can also denote what is customary (e.g., *Od.* 4.691, 11.218, 14.59, 24.255), although these norms treat gods and especially humans in terms of social position (the king, the mortal man, the slave, the old man).

[48] For the continuity of these ideas with concepts of nature and order in Hesiod, see Slatkin 2004.

[49] Vernant 1983.197–211. See also Vlastos 1947.174–78; 1953a; G. Lloyd 1966.210–32; Naddaf 2005; and above, introduction n.76, on the sociopolitical context of early Greek science. Gagarin 2002 contests the historical argument, claiming that from Homer onward justice looks very much like the justice that Vernant equates with the *polis*; Seaford 2004.177–80 offers a similar critique.

[50] Vlastos 1947.175. Vlastos goes on to underscore the robustness of the "democratic idea." See also Vlastos 1952.114–15, where the stress is on the distance between cosmic and human justice; G. Lloyd 1966.227–28; and Laks 2006.98. Cf. Lloyd-Jones 1983.80–84.

"what we have is *a sort of* reciprocal relation between the microcosm of the city and the macrocosm of the universe."[51] Our ancient evidence is not much clearer. In one fragment, Heraclitus says:

ξὺν νόῳ λέγοντας ἰσχυρίζεσθαι χρὴ τῷ ξυνῷ πάντων, ὅκωσπερ νόμῳ πόλις καὶ πολὺ ἰσχυροτέρως· τρέφονται γὰρ πάντες οἱ ἀνθρώπειοι νόμοι ὑπὸ ἑνὸς τοῦ θείου· κρατεῖ γὰρ τοσοῦτον ὁκόσον ἐθέλει καὶ ἐξαρκεῖ πᾶσι καὶ περιγίνεται. (DK22 B114)

Those who speak with sense must put firm trust in what is common to all, like a city must rely on its law, and even more firmly. For all human laws are nourished by one [law], the divine one. For it has as much power as it wishes and is sufficient for all, with more left over.

Heraclitus is here focusing on the universality of the divine law. Yet against this universality stands the small word "like" (ὅκωσπερ), which establishes that the city's laws and the divine law have different scopes and operate on different scales (the divine law dwarfing that of the city). Heraclitus does not specify how the universal law, elsewhere expressed as "all things come to be through strife and necessity" (B80), nourishes the city. Nor does he clarify how, if "to god all things are beautiful and good and just, but men have supposed that some things are just, others unjust" (B102), divine justice dovetails with human justice. Some scholars have argued that these how questions are not Heraclitus's concern.[52] They may be right. Yet there is evidence that the question of how to relate a physical macrocosm to human communities has become urgent and open to discussion by the late fifth century.

Consider, for example, the debate about political power at the heart of Euripides' *Phoenissae*. Jocasta, in an attempt to avert civil war between her sons and reestablish rotating rule in the city, speaks first in praise of Isotēs, "Equality," hymning it as a necessary component of political alliances and friendships before casting it as a principle that transcends the city yet, nevertheless, finds its true meaning in the exempla it offers to human lives: "For it is Isotēs that has set up for man measures and divisions of weights, and has determined number" (541–42). She then shifts to the cosmos as a whole, where "night's lightless eye and the radiant sun walk an equal portion of the yearly course, and neither of them, defeated, is resentful" (543–45).[53] Yet Equality, like Jocasta herself, cannot compel anyone to imitate the order of nature. Indeed, the tragedy unfolds from the failure of Jocasta's plea.[54] In his rejoinder to his mother, Eteocles demonstrates his

---

[51] Naddaf 2005.7, emphasis added. Naddaf argues that the genre of prose treatises that begins with Anaximander would have included politogony, in addition to cosmogony and anthropogony, though there is very little evidence to support this claim. See also Laks 2006.11 n.1, suggesting that politogony became a later element of *Peri phuseōs*-type works.

[52] Schofield 1991.20. See also Vlastos 1952.115 n.84; Striker 1987.91 n.8.

[53] See also E. fr. 910K on the ethical benefits of observing order in nature.

[54] On the function of Euripides' "optimistic rationalists," see Mastronarde 1986; on Jocasta, see also Mastronarde 1994.297–98. Empedocles' call to his fellow citizens to pursue Love instead of Strife resembles Jocasta's plea (DK31 B136; B145) and admits the same possibility of failure. Slatkin

affinities with the young elites in Plato's *Laws* who are led by men of science to believe that justice is not about yielding but about succeeding by force.[55] The idea that it is naturally just for the stronger to triumph shows up elsewhere, as in Thucydides' Melian Dialogue. It was also possible to argue that laws go against human nature altogether, as the sophist Antiphon does in the fragments of *On Truth*.[56] These debates indicate that the question of how the "is" described by the inquiry into nature intersects with the "ought" of the sociopolitical realm is wide open in this period.

In their attempts to relate the sociopolitical order analogously or mimetically to the laws of nature or to oppose it to these laws altogether, fifth-century thinkers end up conferring on it a measure of autonomy. For physical laws take effect in the political sphere primarily by being enacted by social and ethical agents whose implication in these laws is at least to some degree dependent on how they interpret them.[57] Euripides suggests in the *Phoenissae* that how someone translates models drawn from nature into action depends on how he understands their prescriptive force and whether he chooses to accept it.[58] Eteocles stands with his mother's counsel on one side and ideas about natural domination on the other and chooses.[59] It is not that this decision—and its consequences—cannot in some way be explained in terms of physical forces. But anyone who wants to give such an explanation needs to develop a model of how human beings are embedded in a world that has largely been drained of social and ethical agency.

2004.30, 47–49 rightly observes that in archaic poetry, too, figuring out how the natural world is prescriptive of human "due measure" takes work—the task of poetry.

[55] Pl. *Leg.* 10, 890a2–9.

[56] Antiphon Soph. fr. 44 (Pendrick). On *nomos* as a constraint on human nature, see also, e.g., Hippias at *Prt.* 337d1–e2; Thrasymachus at Pl. *R.* 1, 343d1–344c8. On difficulties with the concepts of natural law and natural justice (in the human sphere), see Striker 1987; Woodruff 2002. For general overviews of the *phusis-nomos* question, see Beardslee 1918.68–81 (73–81 on late nineteenth- and early twentieth-century discussions of the question); Heinimann 1945, esp. 110–69; Guthrie 1962–69, 3:55–134; Kerferd 1981.111–30; Thomas 2000.102–34 (on Herodotus); Bett 2002.254–61. Darwinism opened up a similarly uncertain space of translation between the natural and social worlds, and Darwin himself could neither define nor control the implications of his theory for people and societies (Beer 2000.51–53, 92–96).

[57] The idea of a norm (νόμος) of nature (Pl. *Grg.* 483e3, perhaps the first instance) seems to imply an "ought," rather than a "must" (Kerferd 1981.112; see also Bett 2002.246). The idea of the necessity (ἀνάγκη) of nature is more complex in relationship to persons. The phrase is difficult to interpret at E. *Tro.* 886, where it may imply nature as a whole or human nature. Elsewhere, it implies sexual desire (Ar. *Nu.* 1075), a "will to power" (Th. 5.105), or death (Isoc. 4 [*Panegyricus*] 84).

[58] At Antiphon Soph. fr. 44 (a), col. I.25–27 (Pendrick), even if things in nature are necessary (τὰ δὲ [τῆς] φύσεως ἀ[ναγ]καῖα), whereas laws are imposed, it is up to us whether we pursue what is naturally advantageous. But note that the harm incurred by transgressing nature is "in reality," rather than in the eyes of men (col. II.21–23). In this last respect, Antiphon's approach is close to that of the medical writers: see Heinimann 1945.129, 138–39; Pendrick 2002.319–20.

[59] The relationship of this decision to figures of necessity is another question altogether, which I take up in chapters 5 and 6.

In fact, alongside fifth-century debates about the prescriptive force of the natural world, a rich discourse had been developing about precisely how we participate in that world not *qua* ethical subjects but *qua* physical compounds. For those writing in this tradition, the microcosm of the human being mirrors the larger world rather differently.[60] The author of the Hippocratic treatise *On Regimen*, for example, declares that all living beings are composed of fire and water, which master and are mastered, in turn, within a dynamic mixture, just as in the external world (*Vict.* I 10, Li 6.486 = 134,13–20 Joly-Byl). Alcmaeon, a physicist active in the early fifth century who was perhaps also a physician,[61] is reputed to have described health as an *isonomia*, "equal relationship," of forces such as the wet and the dry or the bitter and the sweet: disease is the *monarkhia*, "single rule," of one of these powers.[62] He thus recasts the struggle between various basic powers or stuffs in the world as a whole, a struggle common to many sixth- and fifth-century physical theories, as a struggle inside the microcosm. The author of *On Ancient Medicine* writes in the same vein when he emphatically declares that the different powers that he identifies in foods (the sweet, the bitter, and so on) are "both inside a human being and outside a human being" (καὶ ἐν τῷ ἀνθρώπῳ καὶ ἔξω τοῦ ἀνθρώπου, *VM* 15, Li 1.606 = 139,1 Jouanna).[63]

Because many of the things inside the body also exist outside it, the relationship between the macrocosm and microcosm is more than an analogy. Just as in early Greek poetry, in which the gods not only have a society like that of humans but also actively intervene in human society, the physical world not only is a mirror of the human microcosm but directly affects the balance of power within it.[64] Alcmaeon is reported to have thought that disease is caused either by an excess of heat or cold, created by a surfeit or deficiency of nourishment—nourishment being one of the primary means through which what is outside

---

[60] On the microcosm-macrocosm analogy in medicine and biology, see Joly 1960.37–52; Magdelaine 1997; Le Blay 2005. The first reference to the person as a *mikros kosmos* is at Democr. (DK68) B34, although Finkelberg 1998.120–22 challenges the fragment's authenticity. Cosmological and biological phenomena could independently support general claims without participating in an explicit analogy: see Kirk, Raven, and Schofield 1983.91.

[61] Diogenes Laertius reports that Alcmaeon wrote primarily on medical things (DK24 A1 = D. L. 8.83), but he is not mentioned in the Anonymous Londinensis papyrus, nor does he appear in Galen's list of Italian physicians (*MM* 1.1 = Kühn 10.6). Testimony from Chalcidius (*In Plat. Tim.* 246 [256,16–257,15 Waszinck], printed from 256,22 at A10) does imply that he practiced dissection: for discussion, see G. Lloyd 1975a; Mansfeld 1975. For Alcmaeon's influence on the medical writers, see Wellmann 1930, who called him "der Stammvater dieser ganzen Säftetheorie" (302); Thivel 1981.338–57.

[62] Alcmaeon (DK24) B4. Much has been made about the term *isonomia* as evidence of democratic influence on Alcmaeon: see esp. Vlastos 1947.156–58; 1953a.361–65; Schubert 1996.125–28. Yet the word is suspect: see the remarks of Heinrich von Staden and Jacques Jouanna at Schubert 1996.148–49, arguing that the fragment should not be classed among the *ipsissima verba* of Alcmaeon; see also the reservations of MacKinney 1964.

[63] Note, however, that an author can also stress the particularity of the things in the human body (e.g., the humors). W. Smith 1992 contrasts medical and philosophical theories of mixture.

[64] Le Blay 2005.253–54.

affects what is inside—or through more immediate external causes (κἀκ τῶν ἔξωθεν αἰτιῶν, B4), an etiology whose different elements resurface in later medical writing.[65] Thus, traversed by the same powers and composed of the same stuff(s), macrocosm and microcosm are engaged in continual exchanges governed by necessity and the nature of these forces and stuffs.

Alcmaeon's understanding of the person as constituted out of different kinds of basic stuffs bears a similarity to ideas about all composite objects in many of the major fifth-century writers on nature, including Anaxagoras, Empedocles, and the atomists Leucippus and Democritus. Whereas most sixth-century thinkers seem to have seen the origin of perceptible reality as a single basic stuff, these thinkers rely on a plurality of basic stuffs that neither come to be nor pass away.[66] In Empedocles, we find four *rhizōmata*, "roots" (air, water, earth, fire); in Anaxagoras, a plurality of *khrēmata*, "things," bits of everything that are present in everything (except Mind); and in Leucippus and Democritus, atoms, indivisible micro-bodies. In each case, imperceptibly small basic stuffs combine to create perceptible compound objects. For Empedocles, for example, all "mortal things," people and plants, bones and blood, are mixtures:[67]

φύσις οὐδενός ἐστιν ἁπάντων
θνητῶν, οὐδέ τις οὐλομένου θανάτοιο τελευτή,
ἀλλὰ μόνον μίξις τε διάλλαξίς τε μιγέντων
ἐστί, φύσις δ᾽ ἐπὶ τοῖς ὀνομάζεται ἀνθρώποισιν.

(DK31 B8)

> Of all mortal things no one has birth, or any end in pernicious death, but there is only mixing, and separating off of what has been mixed, and to these men give the name "birth." (trans. M. R. Wright)

Similar sentiments are attributed to Anaxagoras: "For no thing comes into being or perishes but is rather compounded or dissolved from the things that really exist" (οὐδὲν γὰρ χρῆμα γίνεται οὐδὲ ἀπόλλυται, ἀλλ᾽ ἀπὸ ἐόντων χρημάτων συμμίσγεταί τε καὶ διακρίνεται, DK59 B17). Compound objects for Democritus are aggregates of atoms.

---

[65] See also the system attributed to Philistion at Anon. Lond. 20.32–50 (36–37 Diels) and *Morb.* I 2 (Li 6.142 = 6,5–12 Wittern), where the causes of disease are divided into τῶν μὲν ἐν τῷ σώματι ἐνεόντων, here bile and phlegm, and τῶν δ᾽ ἔξωθεν, that is, exertions, wounds, and excessive heat and cold; see also 11 (Li 6.158 = 28,3–5 Wittern).

[66] For the view that the pluralists are, by denying substantial change to their basic stuffs, responding to Parmenides, see Curd 1998; 2002, esp. 143–45; Graham 2006.186–276 (esp. 186–95).

[67] For bones, blood, and flesh: DK31 B96; B98, with Solmsen 1950.435–45. Empedoclean mixtures must be assemblages of a sort, not true fusions. Mourelatos 1986.168–78 argues that each of the four elements has characteristic *poroi*, through which it interlaces with others. The result is not fusion but an interlocking that explains the qualities of the created object and its stability. See also M. R. Wright 1995.34–40 (on B23); Curd 1998.160–71; 2002.147–53 (arguing that the roots are "semi-particulate"); Ierodiakonou 2005.5–8.

In developing these physical theories, the so-called pluralists help to foster a new understanding of reciprocity between people and the larger world. For they embed people in this world not as social and ethical beings but as composite objects engaged in an ongoing process of becoming: "And these things," Empedocles says of the roots, "never cease from constantly interchanging [καὶ ταῦτ' ἀλλάσσοντα διαμπερὲς οὐδαμὰ λήγει], now through Love all coming together into one, now again each carried apart by the hatred of Strife . . . and they have no stable life [οὔ σφισιν ἔμπεδος αἰών]" (DK31 B17.6–8, 11).[68] If this is justice, it is not a justice that one chooses (with all the tragic weight of that word) to uphold or reject but, rather, a system into which every compound object is automatically inscribed. The site of these processes of becoming could by the fifth century be identified as *sōma*. Recognizing this may shed light on our first known attempt to deny the existence of *sōma*.

MELISSUS AND THE DENIAL OF BODY

Melissus of Samos (fl. ca. 440 BCE), long known as a follower of Parmenides of Elea, has, in recent years, been seen as a thinker in his own right.[69] In a long hexameter poem dated to the early part of the fifth century, Parmenides outlines a series of stringent logical conditions for what can exist: *to eon*, "what-is," must be ungenerated and imperishable, a homogeneous whole, unmoving, and complete (DK28 B8.1–4). In his elaboration of these conditions, Melissus adds that what-is must be spatially unlimited, specifies ways in which it does not change, and denies that it has (a) *sōma*.[70]

The last claim, that what-is lacks (a) *sōma* (DK30 B9), has been vexing for many modern scholars.[71] The trouble is that in other fragments Melissus argues that what-is is unlimited with respect to *megethos*, usually translated "spatial extension" (B3), and full, by which he presumably means "without interstitial void" (B7).[72] It has seemed virtually inconceivable, not only to modern thinkers but also to Simplicius, our sixth-century CE source for the fragment,

---

[68] Kirk, Raven, and Schofield note that these lines apply to the birth and death of the universe and to the lifecycle of compound bodies (1983.288). See also Curd 2002.140: mixture and separation also explain qualitative change in those compounds.

[69] See esp. Palmer 2004.41–48.

[70] For Melissus's contributions to Parmenides' theory, see Palmer 2004.22–41. If, as Curd 1998 argues, Parmenides is defending predicational monism, rather than numerical monism, Melissus is further distinguished by his clear commitment to numerical monism; see also Curd 1993; Graham 2006.148–85.

[71] Although the authenticity of B9 has been periodically challenged, Melissus's denial of *sōma* to what-is, stated twice by Simplicius (*In ph.* 85.6, 109.34–110.2), is generally accepted: see Palmer 2003.6 for a defense of this part of the fragment.

[72] The limited-unlimited distinction was seen already in antiquity as the major difference between Parmenides, who saw what-is as a perfect sphere bounded by the chains of necessity, and Melissus (Arist. *Phys.* 207a15–17).

that what-is can be spatially extended and "full" while lacking a *sōma*.[73] We cannot assume, however, that these three concepts—fullness, *megethos*, and *sōma*—are inextricably bound together in the fifth century. Our grasp of their respective semantic fields in this period is tenuous at best. Nevertheless, let us review what little we know about *sōma* before trying to understand what Melissus is denying in B9.

In the introduction, I sketched the unusually narrow semantic field of *sōma* in the Homeric epics, as well as the broader range of meanings evident in other archaic and classical texts.[74] These meanings all concern animate bodies. In the fifth century, we find several examples where *sōma* is used of inanimate objects in ways that anticipate the word's usage in the later philosophical tradition. In a fragment attributed to the fifth-century Pythagorean Philolaus, earth, fire, water, and air are referred to as *sōmata*; though the fragment is probably not genuine, we find the idea of constituent stuffs as *sōmata* from Plato onward.[75] In the late fifth century, Diogenes calls Air "an eternal and immortal *sōma*" (ἀΐδιον καὶ ἀθάνατον σῶμα, DK64 B7), whereas everything else comes into being and passes away. A second meaning of *sōma* is seen in Gorgias's *Encomium to Helen*, where he endows *logos* with a very tiny, invisible body, with which it accomplishes the most godlike things (σμικροτάτῳ σώματι καὶ ἀφανεστάτῳ θειότατα ἔργα ἀποτελεῖ, 8). The idea that *sōma* confers the power to act will be integral to Stoic ideas of corporeality. In yet another context, Gorgias's *On Nature, or What Is Not*, as it is transmitted by Sextus Empiricus, Gorgias differentiates between *megethos* and *sōma* in the course of outlining four possible ways to establish the unity of what-is.[76] Although the passage makes it easier to accept that Melissus accords *megethos* to what-is while denying it *sōma*, Gorgias, unlike Melissus, thinks that every kind of unity, including *megethos*, can be divided. In the case of *sōma*, he bases its divisibility on its tripartite nature: it has length, breadth, and depth—yet another definition that becomes significant in the later philosophical tradition.[77]

The spatial definition of *sōma* has dominated the concerns of those puzzled by Melissus's denial of *sōma* to a what-is that is full and in possession of *megethos*. It is favored in part because the equation of body with space is almost taken for granted in philosophical circles. But the spatial definition also

---

[73] Palmer 2003.1–6, noting that the problem has long been "notorious," revisits the various strategies designed to combat it; see also the comprehensive review of earlier literature in Reale 1970.193–220.

[74] See above, pp. 32–36.

[75] Philol. (DK44) B12. Huffman 1993.392–95 thinks the fragment is a post-Aristotelian forgery. For Plato, see *Ti.* 53c4–5.

[76] S. E. *M.* 7.73 (Gorg. fr. 3 Buchheim). Cf. [Arist.] *MXG* 979b36–980a2. Although the text is too corrupt to rescue, Buchheim's translation in his edition of Gorgias represents incorporeality as the absence of extension. But there is no internal reason to assume this reading.

[77] On Aristotle's conceptualization of *sōma* as "a magnitude divisible in three directions," see Falcon 2005.31–35. Bodies have depth (βάθος) at *Ti.* 53c5–6, although Plato does not speak of divisibility.

accounts for Melissus's statement in B9 that *sōma* threatens the unity of what-is because it has parts. Yet divisibility need not entail dimensions. It seems clear, moreover, on the basis of our limited evidence, that the semantic field of *sōma* is quite broad in the fifth century: in different contexts, it can entail not only three-dimensionality but also the capacity to act; it can describe constituent or basic stuffs, or objects constituted from these stuffs.[78]

If we assume that Melissus is not thinking of spatial extension when he denies that what-is has (a) *sōma*, we are left with two viable strategies for determining what is being denied in B9. In Simplicius, the claim that *sōma* has parts involves the intermediary step of endowing it with *pakhos*, "thickness" or "coarseness" (εἰ δὲ ἔχοι πάχος, ἔχοι ἂν μόρια). We can, then, try to understand *sōma* by inquiring into its relationship to *pakhos* and asking how *pakhos* relates to having parts. One of the more persuasive attempts to do this is G.E.L. Owen's hypothesis that Melissus has in mind an "ordinary" view of a physical solid, according to which it is "divisible in the sense that parts can be identified and distinguished in it, either by finding or making gaps between them or by characterizing them as having more or less of something (hardness, say, or heat) than their neighbor."[79] Owen's claim gains support from the fact that the adjective *pakhus* can describe not only thickness but also graininess or cloudiness, qualities that suggest heterogeneity within a stuff.[80] An understanding of *pakhos* in this sense offers the most workable solution to B9, at least if we accept that Melissus makes *pakhos* integral to his definition of *sōma*.

But no doubt things would be easier if we consider *sōma* independently of *pakhos* altogether, as John Palmer has recently proposed. Palmer argues that the final sentence of B9 (εἰ δὲ ἔχοι πάχος, ἔχοι ἂν μόρια) should be rejected as Simplicius's own gloss on Melissus's proposed incorporeality. He attributes to Melissus only the claim that what-is does not have (a) *sōma*.[81] He argues that, by denying *sōma* to what-is, Melissus, like Xenophanes in his denial of a human-like *demas* to god, is repudiating anthropomorphism.[82]

---

[78] For modern views of *sōma* in the fifth century, see H. Gomperz 1932, arguing that it was defined by visibility, tangibility, and spatial containment; see also Guthrie 1962–69, 2:111; Reale 1970.215–18, 225. Furley 1967.61 argues that *sōma* primarily denotes solidity or bulk; see also Curd 1993.16–18 (*sōma* denotes solidity in the sense of indivisibility). It seems best to allow for a wide semantic field. There is no single definition of *sōma* in the later philosophical tradition either. Rather, the local and conceptual context continues to determine which aspects are salient: see, e.g., Falcon 2005.37–38, on different meanings of *sōma* in Aristotle.

[79] Owen 1960.101. See also Untersteiner 1953.603–6, arguing that the denial of *sōma* in B9 is a denial of quantitative and qualitative difference ("ἰ ἀνόμοιον").

[80] See *Acut. Sp.* 19 (Li 2.434, ch. 8 = 77,19 Joly): cloudy urine; *Aer.* 8 (Li 2.32 = 204,16 Jouanna): briny water. See also *Il.* 23.697: thick blood.

[81] Palmer 2003.6–9.

[82] Palmer 2003.4, treating *sōma* as a virtual synonym of *demas*. See, too, Sedley 1999.129–30. Responding to Palmer, Ferrari 2005.93 sees a need to reconcile this anti-anthropomorphism with the remarks on pain and suffering in B7. Reading *sōma* as composite body smoothes over the tension identified by Ferrari.

Palmer's argument, careful in its attention to the often-uncertain line between fragment and testimonium, is attractive insofar as it allows us to focus our attention on *sōma* alone. Nevertheless, despite adopting a strategy very different from that of Owen, Palmer follows him in one respect. Both scholars circumvent the perceived conflict between B9 and the other fragments by declining to treat *sōma* as an abstract notion of space. They assume, rather, that, before the conceptual changes that make it possible to think of body *qua* space, *sōma* should be understood in a strictly "ordinary" sense, whether that means, as for Owen, a physical solid or, as for Palmer, a human body.

Yet we need not be restricted to imagining, on the one hand, a philosophically sophisticated idea of body or matter and, on the other, an unreflective, ordinary one. Melissus may have been using *sōma* to describe a composite object formed from more durable stuffs and dynamically embedded within reconceived networks of power. This usage is confirmed by other fifth- and fourth-century evidence. For example, the author of *On Regimen* (ca. 400 BCE), a text deeply indebted to the inquiry into nature, defines *sōma* as that which is never the same by nature or by necessity, on the grounds that it dissolves into all things and mixes with all things.[83] Empedocles speaks of the various limbs "allotted to a *sōma*" joining in love and being torn apart by strife.[84] In *On the Sacred Disease*, the author categorically rejects the idea that the *sōma* is defiled by a god, "what is most perishable [τὸ ἐπικηρότατον] by what is most pure [ὑπὸ τοῦ ἁγνοτάτου]" (1, Li 6.362 = 9,8–10 Jouanna). The *sōma* here epitomizes corruptibility, recalling the semantic field of the word in the Homeric epics. By the time Plato wrote the *Philebus*, he assumed that anyone would agree that, when the various basic stuffs are joined together, the resulting compound is called *sōma*.[85]

Plato's dialogues also offer us the first secure instances, five in total, of the adjective *asōmatos*, "incorporeal."[86] These examples lend credence to the idea that what is problematic about *sōma* for Melissus is precisely its relationship to

[83] σῶμα δὲ οὐδέποτε τωὐτὸ οὐδενὸς οὔτε κατὰ φύσιν οὔτε ὑπ᾽ ἀνάγκης, τὸ μὲν γὰρ διακρίνεται ἐς πάντα, τὸ δὲ συμμίσγεται πρὸς ἅπαντα (*Vict.* I 28, Li 6.502 = 144,18–20 Joly-Byl). The contrast is with *psukhē*, which is "the same" (ὁμοίη) in living creatures.

[84] DK31 B20: ἄλλοτε μὲν φιλότητι συνερχόμεν᾽ εἰς ἓν ἅπαντα / γυῖα, τὰ σῶμα λέλογχε, βίου θαλέθοντος ἐν ἀκμῇ· / ἄλλοτε δ᾽ αὖτε κακῇσι διατμηθέντ᾽ ἐρίδεσσι / πλάζεται ἄνδιχ᾽ ἕκαστα περὶ ῥηγμῖνι βίοιο (at one time, in the maturity of a vigorous life, all the limbs that are the body's portion come into one under love; at another time again, torn asunder by evil strifes, they wander, each apart, on the shore of life; trans. M. R. Wright). See, too, P. Strasb. gr. Inv. 1665–66 a(ii) 23 (Martin and Primavesi), where the likely conjecture σώμ[ατι seems to refer to the composite bodies of animals, persons, and plants (see further Alain Martin and Primavesi 1998.227–28).

[85] See *Phlb.* 29d7–8: πάντα γὰρ ἡμεῖς ταῦτα τὰ νυνδὴ λεχθέντα ἆρ᾽ οὐκ εἰς ἓν συγκείμενα ἰδόντες ἐπωνομάσαμεν σῶμα; (for when we see all these things just now mentioned by us gathered up into a unity, do we not name that "body"?). On the idea of *sōma* as a collective unity in contexts where the meaning of person is predominant, see Hirzel 1914.17–18.

[86] Pl. *Phd.* 86a2–3; *Phlb.* 64b6–8; *Plt.* 286a5; *Sph.* 246b8, 247d1.

becoming. Moreover, they evince little interest in spatial extension.[87] Simmias, describing the soul in the *Phaedo*, contrasts the harmony of a lyre, which is not only *asōmatos* but also invisible, divine, and beautiful, with its strings, which are "bodies and body-like and composite and earthy and kindred with what is mortal" (σώματά τε καὶ σωματοειδῆ καὶ σύνθετα καὶ γεώδη . . . καὶ τοῦ θνητοῦ συγγενῆ, 86a2–3).[88] In the *Philebus*, Socrates declares that, by banishing the false pleasures of becoming, he has imposed a kind of incorporeal order (κόσμος τις ἀσώματος) on an ensouled *sōma* prone to limit-defying pleasures and pains (64b6–8), destabilizing movements that preclude health and virtue.[89] Plato often treats the *sōma* as the point of our entanglement in a dynamic, impersonal world subject to *tukhē*, *anankē*, and *phusis* and resistant to *logos* and *noos*, a world that, unmoored from the Good, endangers our true nature.

It is probable, then, that *sōma* in B9 cues the volatile world of mixture and dissolution described by the fifth-century pluralists.[90] This hypothesis is strengthened by the presence of that world as a foil to what-is in another fragment where Melissus denies that what-is perishes, grows larger, is reordered, or suffers pain or anguish, all examples of suffering and becoming other. He puts particular emphasis on the claim that what-is suffers neither pain nor anguish:[91]

οὐδὲ ἀλγεῖ· οὐ γὰρ ἂν πᾶν εἴη ἀλγέον· οὐ γὰρ ἂν δύναιτο ἀεὶ εἶναι χρῆμα ἀλγέον· οὐδὲ ἔχει ἴσην δύναμιν τῷ ὑγιεῖ· οὐδ᾽ ἂν ὁμοῖον εἴη, εἰ ἀλγέοι· ἀπογινομένου γάρ τευ ἂν ἀλγέοι ἢ προσγινομένου, κοὐκ ἂν ἔτι ὁμοῖον εἴη. οὐδ᾽ ἂν τὸ ὑγιὲς ἀλγῆσαι δύναιτο· ἀπὸ γὰρ ἂν ὄλοιτο τὸ ὑγιὲς καὶ τὸ ἐόν, τὸ δὲ οὐκ ἐὸν γένοιτο. καὶ περὶ τοῦ ἀνιᾶσθαι ὡυτὸς λόγος τῷ ἀλγέοντι. (DK30 B7)

---

[87] Plato's lack of interest in extension has been noted by other scholars. David Sedley, speaking of the *Timaeus*, sees the soul as distinguished "not by necessarily being altogether non-spatial, but by lacking essential characteristics of body, such as visibility and tangibility" (2000.800); see also Johansen 2000.91–93. Cf. Renehan 1980, crediting Plato with establishing the relationship between corporeality and spatial extension.

[88] The word σωματοειδής first appears in Plato and primarily describes what is sensible, corruptible, and without order: see *Phd.* 81b5, 81e1, 83d5; *Plt.* 273b4; *R.* 7, 532d1; *Ti.* 31b4, 36d9. See also *Sph.* 246a10-b2, where the Friends of the Forms are contrasted with those who make everything into *sōma*; at *Smp.* 208b3–4, the *sōma* represents mortal things.

[89] Corporeal and incorporeal also correspond to epistemological categories: see *Sph.* 246b7–8, 247c9–d1 on antimaterialists who argue that true reality consists only of intelligible and incorporeal forms. At *Plt.* 285e4–286a7, knowledge of sensible things is contrasted to knowledge of incorporeal reality.

[90] Sedley 1999.131 sees Melissus taking up Parmenides' project with "a physicist's appeal to the principles of current scientific thinking"; see also Palmer 2004.22–41. More specifically, Graham 1999.172–76 argues that Melissus is debating the pluralists (Empedocles, Anaxagoras, Democritus) about the implications of Parmenides' arguments for physical inquiry; see also Ferrari 2005.91–92.

[91] The arguments against pain recur in the pseudo-Aristotelian account of the doctrines of Melissus, Xenophanes, and Gorgias (DK30 A5 = [Arist.] *MXG* 974a18–21), where anguish and disease are also mentioned: τοιοῦτον δὲ ὂν τὸ ἓν ἀνώδυνόν τε καὶ ἀνάλητον ὑγιές τε καὶ ἄνοσον εἶναι οὔτε μετακοσμούμενον θέσει οὔτε ἑτεροιούμενον εἴδει οὔτε μιγνύμενον ἄλλῳ.

Nor does what-is suffer pain. For it would not be whole if it were in pain, for a thing that suffers pain could not exist forever. Nor does it have a power equal to what is healthy. Nor could it be homogeneous, if it suffered pain. For it would suffer pain by the subtraction or the addition of something, and it would not still be homogeneous. Nor could what is healthy suffer pain. For what is healthy and what-is would be destroyed, and what-is-not would come into being. And the argument about suffering anguish is the same as for pain.

Like Melissus's denial of *sōma*, these lines have generated bewilderment among commentators. "The interesting thing is that Melissus should think the point worth mentioning at all," observes Guthrie.[92] Far from just mentioning the point, however, Melissus represents the thing-in-pain as the very antithesis of what-is: it is neither whole, nor eternal, nor homogeneous (for pain occurs when something is added or taken away). The internal difference that produces pain eventually leads to death: "If what-is were to become different [ἑτεροῖον] by a single hair in ten thousand years, it would all perish in the whole of time" (B7).

Although they resonate powerfully with late fifth-century intellectual concerns, Melissus's references to pain and *sōma* also recall an old anxiety, powerfully expressed in Priam's vision of the postmortem transition from person to *sōma*: "When an old man is dead and down, and the dogs mutilate the gray head and the gray beard and the parts that are secret, this, for all sad mortality, is a sight most pitiful" (*Il.* 22.74–76). In the inquiry into nature, the dogs are always at work: even what looks solid is imperceptibly crumbling below the surface, undermining the coherence of form. Modern commentators tend to be confused about why Melissus is dealing with something as banal as pain in a rarefied pursuit like metaphysics.[93] Yet, as Melissus tries to find something to hold on to in a world where everything familiar has come under threat from the unseen dynamics of flux, it would seem that bodies and pain, as well as other natural processes like growth, transposition, and decay, best capture the world of becoming that he wishes to deny.

For Melissus, suffering pain and anguish is a counterfactual condition. If sensory evidence were allowed, however, to be in pain would be a sign of membership in a community of composite objects gaining and losing parts and eventually falling to pieces.[94] In fact, it is precisely such a sign that is marshaled in the Hippocratic text *On the Nature of a Human Being*, whose author turns out to have a strategic familiarity with Melissus's philosophy. The treatise begins with

---

[92] Guthrie 1962–69, 2:113. See also Kirk, Raven, and Schofield 1983.397; Palmer 2004.24. Longrigg 1985.113 n.44 speculates that Melissus has Empedocles in mind here.

[93] They also tend to assume that Melissus is talking about the *feeling* of pain. Sentience, however, need not be implied, as I argue further below, pp. 111–14.

[94] As Curd says of Parmenides, "Any purported claim about what-is that fails the tests enumerated in the signs of B8.2–4 is really a claim about what-is-not" (1998.51).

an attack on contemporary material monists.[95] The author argues that, because the basic stuff of the physical world is not *phaneron*, "manifest"—presumably because the phenomenal world is so diverse—these monists have no empirical means of adjudicating between their competing primary stuffs and must resort to *marturia te kai tekmēria*, "evidence and proofs": "But in my view such men overthrow themselves through the terms of their own arguments because of misunderstanding, but they set the argument of Melissus upright" (ἀλλ᾽ ἔμοιγε δοκέουσιν οἱ τοιοῦτοι ἄνθρωποι αὐτοὶ ἑωυτοὺς καταβάλλειν ἐν τοῖσιν ὀνόμασι τῶν λόγων [τῶν] ἑωυτῶν ὑπὸ ἀσυνεσίης, τὸν δὲ Μελίσσου λόγον ὀρθοῦν, *Nat. Hom.* 1, Li 6.34 = 166,9–11 Jouanna). It is clear that the author is faulting his colleagues' failure to move beyond words to the more important criterion of truth, namely phenomenal evidence.[96] Less clear, however, is the reference to Melissus. The author may be co-opting the Eleatic's arguments that what really exists is not a part of the physical world, in order to block the application of material monism to human nature.[97] In any event, he certainly knows who Melissus is.

Even more striking evidence of the author's awareness of Melissus emerges in his attack on a subset of the material monists, the physician-monists. Here he is confronting opponents who, like him, verify their truth claims with evidence provided by the *sōma*. He begins his line of attack by rejecting monism *tout court*: "I say that if a human being were one, he would never be in pain. For certainly there would be nothing from which he, being one, could suffer pain" (ἐγὼ δέ φημι, εἰ ἓν ἦν ὤνθρωπος, οὐδέποτ᾽ ἂν ἤλγει· οὐδὲ γὰρ ἂν ἦν ὑπ᾽ ὅτευ ἀλγήσειεν ἓν ἐόν, 2, Li 6.34 = 168,4–5 Jouanna).[98] The medical writer thus repurposes the counterfactual argument used by Melissus to prove the impossibility of what-is suffering pain in order to show that human nature is not uniform but, on his account, made up of four basic stuffs (phlegm, blood, yellow bile, black bile) found inside the *sōma*. What had been initially advanced as disembodied, metaphysical truth becomes embodied truth: human nature is composite and, hence, internally divided. Beneath our sense of well-being—a sense, that is, of being an integrated whole—different constituent stuffs are in constant flux.

[95] We hear of various material monists active in the late fifth century (Jouanna 2002.226–29), though Diogenes of Apollonia is the most familiar to us. On the basis of a stylistic analysis of Diogenes' fragments, Jouanna 1965 argues that he is the author's target, but cf. Ducatillon 1977.131–32; Thivel 1981.249 n.281, responding that this is too narrow an interpretation. See also Wesoly 1987: Gorgias is the target of attack.

[96] The author of *On Ancient Medicine* similarly denounces cosmological speculation divorced from empirical evidence (*VM* 1, Li 1.572 = 119,7–11 Jouanna).

[97] Cf. Jouanna 1965; 2002.41–43, 238–39, arguing that the author means the speakers, despite their disagreement, end up supporting Melissus's claim that only one thing exists.

[98] See also *Nat. Hom.* 3 (Li 6.36–38 = 170,8–172,12 Jouanna): generation and corruption prove that bodies comprise multiple elements. The fact that the dichotomy presented by our author is "being in pain" and "being healthy" (ἀλγεῖ καὶ ὑγιαίνει 4, Li 6.40 = 172,15 Jouanna) also suggests a direct engagement with (and appropriation of) Melissus's arguments. See Jouanna 1965 for additional textual clues of this engagement.

The model advanced in *On the Nature of a Human Being* assimilates human nature to other natures being described in the fifth century. The pluralist line, as we have seen, is that the world is populated with compounds always undergoing change. These changes, however, are often imperceptible, with the result that we often fail to recognize the true composition of physical reality. Democritus famously declares: "We know nothing in reality; for truth is in the depths" (ἐτεῇ δὲ οὐδὲν ἴδμεν· ἐν βυθῷ γὰρ ἡ ἀλήθεια, DK68 B117).[99] Sextus Empiricus, in the context of transmitting the dictum "the phenomena are a sight of unseen things," reports that Anaxagoras proposes an experiment—take two colors, black and white, and pour one into the other drop by drop—to demonstrate that sight, because of its "weakness," cannot register the incremental changes underlying perceptible reality and, hence, the truth (*M. 7.90 = DK59 B21*). In *On the Nature of a Human Being*, as well, the reason the author marshals proof in defense of his account is we do not have an intuitive grasp of our own nature.

There are important philosophical consequences for the view that we fail to grasp what is going on below the threshold of the visible world outside us. The consequences of the idea that we are unaware of what is happening inside us are equally significant. In the previous chapter, I argued that the boundaries of the felt coincide with the boundaries of the person in early poetry and that the unfelt, unseen space from which symptoms erupt is understood as daemonic and external. Our evidence is too scanty to prove this point decisively. Nevertheless, I believe we can conclude that the idea of an *unseen* and *unfelt* space inside the person, that is, a space concealed by the skin and located mostly below the threshold of sensation, is crucial to the emergence of the physical (human) body and, more specifically, to the emergence of that body as an object of expert care. To consider how the basic idea of objective, unfelt space comes about, we can first examine how composite bodies are assimilated to one another through analogical arguments and then look briefly at some accounts of perception, pleasure, and pain that depend on potentially seen but not necessarily felt changes to those bodies. In the process, we can begin to get a sense, too, of the strategies being developed to see into the hidden physical world.

A COMMUNITY OF OBJECTS

One of the distinguishing features of sixth- and fifth-century physical and medical theories is that all compounds participate in the same economy of impersonal force. As the author of *On the Sacred Disease* observes, the south wind

---

[99] See also Democr. (DK68) B6–B10. B117 does not license pure skepticism. Elsewhere, the senses, by giving rise to inference, grant entry to the nature of atomic reality (e.g., B9 [cf. B125]; A135 = Thphr. *De sens.* 65, where sweetness, for example, is caused by larger, rounder atoms): see Bailey 1928.177–85; von Fritz 1946.24–30; Guthrie 1962–69, 2:438–40; C. Taylor 1967.19–24; 1999a.216–22; Farrar 1988.197–215; Curd 2001; Salem 2007.135–36.

acts in the same way (τὸ δ' αὐτὸ τοῦτο . . . ἐργάζεται) on the earth, the sea, rivers, springs, and wells, and, indeed, on every growing thing that has moisture, which is to say, everything, because everything has moisture (13, Li 6.384 = 24,5–8 Jouanna).[100] On the grounds that everything is subjected to the power of the south wind, the author thinks we can pursue knowledge about hidden things— in this instance, things inside the *sōma* like the brain and the vessels—by looking at analogues that are easier to observe. He accordingly introduces two such ana- logues: earthenware jars that change their shape in response to the wind; and the sun, moon, and stars, whose visibility is dimmed by the wind's force. If wind can master such great and powerful things, he points out, it can easily affect things inside the body. He concludes that, under the south wind's moist influence, the brain *necessarily* relaxes and the vessels in the body widen.[101]

It is clear from this passage that analogy, once dismissed by modern scholars as a merely ornamental device, plays a crucial methodological role in early Greek speculation about the natural world.[102] Physical analogies bear some clear similarities to similes in archaic poetry. Archaic similes often travel across the luminous surfaces of the world, gathering together the radiance of persons, stars, and flowers and thus giving the sense that the vital forces coursing through rivers and plants also animate people. These forces are imbued with newfound explanatory potential by the physicists. By advancing theories about the world's basic stuff(s) and qualitative change, they make analogy an increasingly useful means of explaining how one thing works by invoking another *qua* model. Such functional analogies identify similarities guaranteed by physical necessity. The analogue becomes an observable instance of a general principle while illumi- nating the specific process or effect in question, thereby shedding light on the unseen.

It is admittedly questionable whether the earliest Milesian analogies, which tend to focus on meteorological phenomena, are truly functional. When Thales answers the question of what keeps the earth from falling by observing that wood floats in water, he seems to be assuming that the image itself (an object stabilized by water) is a sufficient explanation of something that cannot be seen (the earth resting on water).[103] By the fifth century, however, physicists and medical writers are more explicitly invoking principles of regularity in their

---

[100] See also *Morb. Sacr.* 13 (Li 6.384 = 23,14–17 Jouanna), where the north wind, too, acts on all things in the same way (κατὰ δὲ τὸν αὐτὸν τρόπον) by separating "the moist" and "the dull" from everything, and from human beings, too (ἐξ αὐτῶν τῶν ἀνθρώπων).

[101] *Morb. Sacr.* 13 (Li 6.384–86 = 24,5–25,8 Jouanna).

[102] On the use of analogy, see esp. Regenbogen 1930; G. Lloyd 1966.172–420. See also Lonie 1981.77–86, on the evidential use of analogy in *On Generation/On the Nature of the Child* and *On Diseases* IV; G. Manetti 1993.43–47; Humphreys 1996.20–21; Vegetti 1996.72–74; Hankinson 1998a.21–23. Snell 1953.191–226 privileges the difference between the Homeric simile and physi- cal analogies in his telling of the *muthos* to *logos* story; see also Vernant 1983.378, with 490 n.22.

[103] See Arist. *Cael.* 294a28–33, at DK11 A14, with G. Lloyd 1966.306–9, 319–20. The illustrative function of analogy can block further examination, as Lonie 1981.86 observes.

analogies, as we saw in *On the Sacred Disease*. The author of *On Generation/On the Nature of the Child*, for example, claims that embryos grow to a size and shape that is equal to their enclosure. He notes that the principle can be observed directly by placing a jar over a young cucumber as it grows, before extending it universally: "For it is generally true that all things behave in this way [τὰ φυόμενα οὕτω πάντα ἔχει], however one compels them to" (9, Li 7.482 = 51,9–10 Joly).[104] Or consider the detailed explanation attributed by Aristotle to Empedocles of how breathing occurs through the alternating pressure of blood inside the body and air outside it: the process is both illustrated and verified by the alternation of water and air in the clepsydra, a vessel used for the transfer of liquids.[105] Analogy is "predictive metaphor."[106] By describing one object's behavior, the writer tells a vivid story about invisible changes to another.

In the majority of analogies cited thus far, the unseen domain in question is the inside of a body where brains grow damp, embryos take shape, and respiration occurs. By assimilating bodily structures and processes to plants, planetary bodies, and artifacts, these fifth-century thinkers are encouraging their audience to conceptualize things and events inside the *sōma* as potentially seen and to imagine the *sōma* itself as an object under the power of nature and necessity. It is true that in Homeric epic the innards are potentially seen; they are perceived as concrete. Yet, of equal importance is a primarily felt domain within the person that does not seem to be imagined as visible space: if the *ētor* rises or the heart beats faster, it is a subjective experience, communicable to others through the language of feeling. Conversely, when Empedocles uses the clepsydra to model breathing, he assumes that physical processes are not transparent to us because we experience them; they are, however, reproducible in a common field of vision. Whereas, in archaic poetry, animals primarily model characters, behaviors, and feelings, often "sharpen[ing] the portrayal of pathos," the animals used as analogues in physiological and biological contexts function primarily as structural models.[107]

---

[104] The treatise begins with the maxim "law governs all" (νόμος μὲν πάντα κρατύνει, 1, Li 7.470 = 44,1 Joly). See also *Genit./Nat. Puer.* 1 (Li 7.470 = 44,13 Joly), 29 (Li 7.530 = 78,3–4 Joly).

[105] Emp. (DK31) B100. See G. Lloyd 1966.328–33 and M. R. Wright 1995.245–46 for discussion of the main problems of interpretation. See also B84, a detailed analogy between the lantern and the eye; *VM* 22 (Li 1.626–30 = 149,4–151,7 Jouanna), where the author compares the organs of the body to cupping instruments, an analogy that Mario Vegetti makes critical to "la preistoria dei raffinati intrecci fra anatomia e tecnologia" (1996.73–74); see also Schiefsky 2005a.320–27, 333–34; 2005b.80–82, contrasting the analogy to Empedocles' analogies. Lonie 1981.367–70 presents similar experiments in *Morb.* IV 51 (Li 7.588 = 110,21–28 Joly) and 57 (Li 7.612 = 123,12–16 Joly).

[106] Beer 2000.74.

[107] Lonsdale 1990.7. Lonsdale later reaffirms this: "From a linguistic point of view animal similes [sc. in the *Iliad*] share more in common with the narrative than other groups, and the point of contact lies in vocabulary commenting on emotions" (1990.15, with appendix B, 133–35). For animals in archaic similes, see also G. Lloyd 1966.184–85. On the use of animals as analogues in biological and physiological contexts, see *Artic.* 8 (Li 4.94–98 = 121,12–123,10 Kühlewein); *Carn.* 8 (Li 8.594 = 193,20–22 Joly); *Epid.* VI 4.6 (Li 5.308 = 86,3–5 Manetti-Roselli); *Genit./Nat. Puer.* 18 (Li 7.502 =

Georges Canguilhem once observed that "a model only becomes fertile by its own impoverishment. It must lose some of its own specific singularity to enter with the corresponding object into a new generalization."[108] The models in early Greek science and medicine are, indeed, strategically limited representations of objects.[109] Yet these models, in turn, impoverish the object under observation. The subjective experience of being embodied gives way to the state of an object body. The emotionally rich nexus of social relations among gods and persons and animals fades before an emergent community governed by winds and humidity, the hot and the cold.

The mapping of objective space in the fifth century is encouraged by the extension of *aisthēsis*, "sensing" or "perceiving," to *all* compound bodies to describe how they respond to external forces.[110] The author of *On the Sacred Disease*, for example, expresses the impact of the powerful south wind by declaring that all things (cosmological bodies, earthenware vessels, and so on) *aisthanetai*, "sense," it; he goes on to assert that the wind forces the *sōma* "to sense," *aisthanesthai*, and "to change," *metaballein*.[111] In *On Generation/On the Nature of the Child*, we are told that a woman's body, being especially moist, *aisthanetai*, "senses," temperature fluctuations during the month: sensing results in the agitation of the blood, rather than subjective awareness of these changes (15, Li 7.494 = 57,18–22 Joly). Sensing in these instances does not coincide with sentience but describes, rather, physical interaction with the environment.[112] Thus, when these writers claim that vessels or bodies sense winds or changes in temperature, we should see this not as animism but as a kind of anti-anthropomorphism

---

62,6 Joly); *Haem.* 4 (Li 6.440 = 148,14–16 Joly); *Int.* 23 (Li 7.224 = 148 Potter); *Mul.* I 6 (Li 8.30 = 100,10–11 Grensemann); *Mul.* II 113 (Li 8.242); and the Hellenistic *Cord.* 2 (Li 9.80–82 = 190,14–191,10 Duminil). See also Annoni and Barras 1993.192–94; Ayache 1997.

[108] Canguilhem 1963.515.

[109] See Lonie 1981.296–97 on *Morb.* IV 39 (Li 7.556–60 = 92,12–94,9 Joly): "The model is not an exact replica of the anatomical conditions." Annoni and Barras 1993.202 note that, until Aristotle, the use of animal dissection is limited to the extent that it is deployed to prove a single point, rather than to establish "une conception 'organisée' du corps."

[110] Aristotle may have been the first thinker to limit αἴσθησις to animals (Solmsen 1955.152–53).

[111] For αἰσθάνομαι with parts of the body, see also *Morb. Sacr.* 17 (Li 6.392–94 = 31,6–7 Jouanna), with Ioannidi 1992. At *VM* 15 (Li 1.606 = 138,11–14 Jouanna), objects in leather, wood, and other materials are "less sensitive" (ἀναισθητότερα) than people. See also the "objective" account of sensing at *Vict.* I 35 (Li 6.512–22 = 150,29–156,18 Joly-Byl), where the αἰσθήσιες are not encounters between a mixture and incoming particles or forces but the particles themselves (before striking the soul): see Jouanna 2007a.19–26, 35–38 on similarities between the Hippocratic text and the discussion of αἰσθήσεις at Pl. *Ti.* 43b–44a. In both *On Regimen* and the *Timaeus*, while the meeting of the αἰσθήσεις/αἰσθήσιες with the soul implies sentience, the αἰσθήσεις/ αἰσθήσιες exist before conscious apprehension.

[112] See also Pl. *Tht.* 167b7–c2, where "Protagoras," ventriloquized by Socrates, says that gardeners, like physicians treating human bodies, instill beneficial and healthy sensations (χρηστὰς καὶ ὑγιεινὰς αἰσθήσεις) in plants. Earlier, he had spoken of sensations produced by a healthy body as felt (e.g., foods taste bitter), but this need not imply that the plants are sentient: the gardener is probably monitoring their reactions to their environment.

different from that found in Xenophanes, an anti-anthropomorphism that rede-scribes felt, socially embedded experience in terms of physical change.

Those writing on nature more generally appear to have adopted a similarly objective approach toward perception, pain, and pleasure. We owe most of our evidence for their ideas to Theophrastus's *De sensibus*. In keeping with the prin-ciples of Peripatetic "critical endoxography," Theophrastus adopts a highly combative stance toward previous theories of perception, one informed by his own sense of the explanatory burden of such a theory. While the degree to which his account distorts the theories in question cannot be gauged, it is, at the very least, an account shaped by its author's own terms and expectations.[113] Nevertheless, it is quite clear from Theophrastus's reports that many fifth-century physicists conceptualized perception, pain, and pleasure in objective, rather than subjective, terms. Empedocles states in one fragment that every-thing that has been "fitted together," presumably from the roots, not only feels pleasure and pain but also thinks.[114] More specifically, Theophrastus reports that Empedocles holds that "feeling pleasure is through things similar in their parts and in their mixture" (ἥδεσθαι δὲ τοῖς ὁμοίοις κατά τε [τὰ] μόρια καὶ τὴν κρᾶσιν), whereas being in pain, inverting this principle, occurs by things that are opposite (λυπεῖσθαι δὲ τοῖς ἐναντίοις).[115] Empedocles, then, may have seen

---

[113] On Theophrastus's method, see Baltussen 2000 (esp. 140–94 on the Presocratics), who argues that he is a relatively objective source, who must be read in light of what we know about Peripatetic dialectical method (for the term "critical endoxography," see 41–42). See also Sedley 1992.29–31; J. Warren 2007b.37–39.

[114] ἐκ τούτων [γὰρ] πάντα πεπήγασιν ἁρμοσθέντα / καὶ τούτοις φρονέουσι καὶ ἥδοντ᾽ ἠδ᾽ ἀνιῶνται (DK31 B107, transmitted at *De sens.* 10). If, with M. R. Wright (1995.123–24 = frr. 77 and 78; see also 233–34; Guthrie 1962–69, 2:229 n.3; Sedley 1992.27–28), we read B109 as beginning the quota-tion, both ἐκ τούτων and τούτοις refer to the four roots and Love and Strife. Empedocles would then be saying that thinking, feeling pleasure, and feeling pain are due to the roots and the principles of Love and Strife, just as all things are fitted together and constructed from them. Inwood 2001.285, following Barnes, argues that "ἐκ τούτων" are Theophrastus's words; but given that they would refer to the roots, the sense is basically the same. Long (1966.267), Andriopolous (1972.36–37), and M. R. Wright (1995.234–35) understand "thinking," "being in pain," and "feeling pleasure" in the broadest, nonanimistic sense possible here, although their focus is on thought, rather than pleasure and pain. For the claim that all things possess "wisdom and a share of thought" (φρόνησιν . . . καὶ νώματος αἶσαν), see B110.10, with S. E. *M.* 8.286 (our source for the fragment); A70 (= [Arist.] *De plantis* 815b16–17: see below, n.116, on this text).

[115] Thphr. *De sens.* 9; see also 16 (DK31 A86). On the principle of like-to-like, which Aristotle sees as central to Empedocles' program (*EN* 1155b6–8), see, e.g., B62.6; B109; B110.9. Perception is also defined by a like-to-like principle. An object is sensed only if its parts (or in the case of, e.g., seeing, the ἀπορροαί, "effluences": see DK31 B89; A92 [= Pl. *Men.* 76c4–d5]) are fitted to the channels of the perceiving organ: see Thphr. *De sens.* 7 (DK31 A86). Theophrastus protests that if every percep-tion occurs through like-to-like, every perception should be pleasurable (*De sens.* 16–17), but he may be unfairly conflating two different applications of the like-to-like principle. If "fitting-together" is a necessary condition for one object to affect another, it remains possible that, of the objects compatible with the channels, some may "fit" the mixture (of the body part or the whole body) and some may not (see B22.6–9, where things can differ from one another in birth, mixture, and the molding of their forms, γέννῃ τε κρήσει τε καὶ εἴδεσιν ἐκμάκτοισι). Perceptions may thus

pain as the antagonistic relationship between compounds that, while capable of interaction, are immiscible; pleasure would name the harmonious interpenetration of two compounds, which presumably results in a beneficial mixture in the incorporating object.

If pain, pleasure, and perception encompass a range of phenomena, Empedocles may have thought that different compounds "sense" differently, much as clay vessels and brains sense the south wind differently in *On the Sacred Disease*. But it is hard to know whether he, or indeed other pluralists, see all these compounds as sentient. In *On Plants*, a later Peripatetic text based on works by Aristotle and Theophrastus that survives only in translations of varying quality,[116] Empedocles is reported to have said that plants are moved by desire, perceive, and feel joy and sadness (*tristari delectarique*).[117] The same position is attributed to Anaxagoras, who is also alleged to have written that plants are living things that feel joy and sadness (*laetarique et tristari*), drawing this conclusion from their changing leaves.[118] It is difficult to make sense here of what these thinkers mean by joy and sadness (if, indeed, the text transmits their views correctly). Perhaps Anaxagoras infers that the plants *feel* pain or pleasure when their mixtures change, just as humans feel pain in disease or joy in health. Or perhaps he sees changing leaves as signs of an "objective" sorrow and joy.[119] But even if Empedocles or Anaxagoras does attribute sentience to plants, what would be the implications? Does plant sentience mean the same thing as the human experience of pain and pleasure? Stories of wounded plants (usually trees) from Greco-Roman literature, probably preserving cultic and folk traditions,

---

designate all bodily responses to an external stimulus, while pain and pleasure characterize the quality of that response. See also Aët. 4.9.15, 5.28 (DK31 A95): pain and pleasure are determined by whether the affecting object is "suited" (reading Diels's conjecture, ἐξ [οἰκείου], at Aët. 5.28 [*DG* 440, *ad* 19]; I thank David Wolfsdorf for bringing the conjecture to my attention) to the affected part or mixture. On this account, pleasure is the restoration of balance within a mixture: see further Gosling and Taylor 1982.20–22.

[116] The original Greek text is attributed to Nicolaus Damascenus, a Peripatetic active in the Augustan period who is thought to have compiled and commented on extracts from a lost Περὶ φυτῶν by Aristotle and Theophrastus's botanical works. The compilation passed through a Syriac translation, which survives only in a few fragments, into Arabic, then into Hebrew and Latin; from the Latin translation, dated to the twelfth to thirteenth century, a Greek retroversion was created. For an overview of the text's history, see Drossaart Lulofs and Poortman 1989.1–16.

[117] [Arist.] *De plantis* 815a15–18 (= DK31 A70): *Anaxagoras autem et Abrucalis desiderio eas* [sc. *plantas*] *moveri dicunt, sentire quoque et tristari delectarique asserunt.* Cf. Plut. *Mor.* 688A (= A70), reporting that [Empedocles says] plants preserve their nature unconsciously (ἀναισθήτως) by drawing up appropriate nutrition from the environment, though it is not clear whether Empedocles specifies ἀναισθήτως.

[118] [Arist.] *De plantis* 815a19–20 (= DK59 A117): *Anaxagoras animalia esse has* [sc. *plantas*], *laetarique et tristari dixit fluxum foliorum argumentum assumens.* See also Thphr. *De sens.* 44 (Diog. Apoll. [DK64] A19), claiming that Diogenes of Apollonia believed plants to have some kind of capacity for thought. For ancient philosophical opinions on plants as living things (ζῷα), see Aët. 5.26 (*DG* 438).

[119] That is, the process is just "a description of the disruption and restoration of the plants' natural, leafy state" (J. Warren 2007b.40).

grant them recognizable signs of pain (blood, crying out) that locate hurt within an emotional web of reciprocity and revenge.[120] Yet it is unlikely, though not impossible—especially for Empedocles—that this web is relevant to the physicists' descriptions of pain and pleasure.[121] Our evidence, though fragmentary and minimal, suggests that these thinkers understand pain, pleasure, and perception primarily in terms of mixtures and passages.

By taking such an approach, physicists and medical writers shift attention away from intentional, socially embedded harming. They also downplay the question of whether and how animate and inanimate bodies differ. The *lack* of difference is clearly a concern for Theophrastus, who faults Empedocles for not distinguishing between animate and inanimate compounds in his theory of perception, observing rightly that "parts are fitted into the passages of lifeless things too" (ἐναρμόττει γὰρ καὶ τοῖς τῶν ἀψύχων πόροις, *De sens.* 12).[122] Modern scholars, too, have been troubled by the blurred line between the objective and the subjective in Presocratic accounts of pleasure and pain.

Perhaps, however, the physicists are not so much blurring these categories as simply subordinating the latter to the former. Rather than privileging the subjective experience of, say, pain, they turn it into a subspecies of the category of physical change: "suffering harm." But this does not mean that they fail to recognize commonsense notions of sentience, at least in humans. Analogies identify not only sameness but also difference: on the one side stands the proliferation of likeness; on the other, the comfort of a dividing line (we are speaking not of x but of something only *analogous* to x). In the realm of sensing, compound bodies may be differentiated by whether they are aware of their own sensing.

Consider what we know, again largely from Theophrastus, about Anaxagoras's theories of perception and pain. Whereas Empedocles defines perception in terms of like-to-like, Anaxagoras seems to understand it in terms of difference, arguing that like is unaffected by like.[123] That is, if you experience something as hot, the hotness is registered because of the difference between the cold in you—recall that, according to Anaxagoras, a bit of everything is in everything—and the hot coming from outside. Anaxagoras also holds that every contact with what is unlike causes distress.[124] From these two premises, he

---

[120] E.g., Call. *Cer.* 39–41; Ov. *Met.* 8.757–64; V. *Aen.* 3.23–34, with Henrichs 1979, discussing both Greco-Roman and cross-cultural evidence of tree spirits. Henrichs argues that the Callimachean evidence attests an older concept of animate trees and tree nymphs in the Mediterranean (92).

[121] The case of Empedocles is complicated by his commitment to metempsychosis: he claims, for example, to have been a bush in another life (DK31 B117). The taboo against slaughtering animals rests on the claim that it is tantamount to human murder (B136; B137), which suggests that souls retain some qualities of other incarnations. For further evidence of ancient Greco-Roman beliefs in plant reincarnations, see D. L. 8.4; Porph. *Abst.* 1.6; Burkert 1972.133 n.74.

[122] See also Thphr. *De sens.* 23, 36; cf. 25, where Alcmaeon is credited with establishing the specificity of human perception. On the importance of the animate-inanimate contrast in both Aristotle and Theophrastus, see Baltussen 2000.74–75, 156–57, 181 (with n.146).

[123] Thphr. *De sens.* 27 (DK59 A92): τὸ γὰρ ὅμοιον ἀπαθὲς ὑπὸ τοῦ ὁμοίου.

[124] Thphr. *De sens.* 29 (DK59 A92).

arrives at a paradoxical idea—namely, that all perception is painful.[125] Theophrastus raises an obvious objection: because many perceptions are not painful at all, the claim that all perception is painful is manifestly untrue. But he also reports that Anaxagoras had empirical evidence to support his claim: bright colors and excessively loud noises often cause intolerable pain. In these cases, the degree of unlikeness is presumably strong enough to make us *feel* pain, that is, become aware of the state of conflict in our sensory organs.[126] But by pointing out that we feel pain only under these circumstances, Anaxagoras implies that the clash of opposites in perception—that is, pain—more commonly occurs below the threshold of consciousness. In other words, we feel pain only if the clash of opposites crosses a level of intensity.[127]

The very idea of a threshold of perceptibility in Anaxagoras implies someone *to whom* physical changes become manifest.[128] It recalls the claim in *On the Nature of a Human Being* that we perceive our composite nature only if difference within the mixture escalates into (felt) pain. The notion of a threshold reappears in another medical treatise, *On Ancient Medicine* (using λυπέω to refer to felt pain):[129]

ταῦτα μὲν μεμιγμένα καὶ κεκρημένα ἀλλήλοισιν οὔτε φανερά ἐστιν οὔτε λυπεῖ τὸν ἄνθρωπον, ὅταν δέ τι τούτων ἀποκριθῇ καὶ αὐτὸ ἐφ᾽ ἑωυτοῦ γένηται, τότε καὶ φανερόν ἐστι καὶ λυπεῖ τὸν ἄνθρωπον. (*VM* 14, Li 1.602 = 136,12–16 Jouanna)

These things [sc. constituent stuffs inside the body], when mixed and compounded with one another, are neither apparent nor do they hurt a person; but when one of them is separated off, and stands alone, then it is apparent and hurts a person.

---

[125] See esp. Thphr. *De sens.* 29 (DK59 A92), who uses the phrase μετὰ λύπης. See also Arist. *EN* 1154b7–8, where Anaxagoras is implied, and Asp. *In EN* 156.14–22 (Thphr. fr. 555 FHSG).

[126] Compare Elaine Scarry's comments on perception and pain: "The more a habitual form of perception is experienced as itself rather than its external object, the closer it lies to pain.... While forms of perception, like touch and vision, can be differentiated from one another by the relative degree of emphasis within them on the feeling state or instead on the object, any one of them in isolation contains the potential for being experienced either as state or as object, and thus has within it the fluidity of moving now toward the vicinity of hurting, now toward the vicinity of imagining. Although vision and hearing ordinarily reside close to objectification, if one experiences one's eyes or ears themselves—if the woman working looks up at the sun too suddenly and her eyes fill with blinding light—then vision falls back to the neighborhood of pain" (1985.165).

[127] The concept of "unfelt pains" is difficult for contemporary philosophers: see J. Warren 2007b.45–52, esp. 47 n.42.

[128] Though Anaxagoras assumes some kind of threshold, it is difficult to say what determines it. In most cases (e.g., with the pain of perception or the mixture of black and white), perceptibility appears to be correlated with basic human perception, which differs from that of other animals on account of the different mixture of humans. (*Nous* knows the nature of all the things that are in the mixture, DK59 B12.) At the same time, the idea of a nature implies that, although everything is in everything, there are basic stuffs or "ingredients" at the elemental level that determine the nature of a mixture, which is independent of subjective perceptions: in support of this view, developed by Strang, see Curd 2007.189–91, 196–205.

[129] On the vocabulary of pain in the corpus, see H. King 1988.58–60; Byl 1992; Rey 1995.17–23; Horden 1999; Marzullo 1999; Villard 2006.

Here, too, we are not hurt by the stuffs inside the body, as long as they are mixed together, which is to say, they are not *phaneron*, "apparent."[130] In each of these examples, the inside of the physical body is a space largely beyond the reach of consciousness. By splitting conscious subject from physical object, these thinkers help embed the line between seen and unseen in the inquiry into nature inside the human being.

BODIES, PERSONS, KNOWLEDGE

On the basis of what we have seen thus far, conscious sensing looks rather impoverished compared to bodily sensing. Bodies, strangely enough, would seem to be "more sensitive" than persons to the world around them. We can, however, adopt another perspective on the sensitivities of bodies and persons. After all, the encounter between persons and the external world is not limited to the body's reflexive sensing of temperature changes or even our conscious awareness of harmony or disharmony between our mixture and that of an object with which we come into contact. In the case of the most conventional modes of sensing (i.e., the five senses) and mental sensing, being affected by something focuses attention as much on its nature as on the quality (painful, pleasurable) of the changes it brings about. That is to say, the encounter produces some kind of knowledge of the external world (its basic stuffs, its underlying relationships), rather than simply knowledge of one's own experience.[131] Indeed, when earlier I described the physical body as the primary point of our implication in the natural world, I may have appeared to be overlooking the significance vested by many physicists in *observing* and *thinking* as privileged relationships with that world. Thus, Heraclitus, Empedocles, and Parmenides all state or suggest that thinking the right kinds of thoughts positively transforms our relationship to our environment.[132] If thoughts are the right kind, it is presumably because they build on the particular receptivity of human nature to true knowledge about the nature of things, knowledge that, in turn, brings the person into

---

[130] At *Morb.* I 20 (Li 6.178 = 54,16 Wittern), the adjectives ἄδηλον and ἀνώδυνον are used in a similarly tautological way.

[131] The degree to which the encounter can be said to produce objective knowledge will depend on a given thinker's perspective on the value of empirical evidence and the relative "interference" of the subjective state of the percipient (on which, see esp. Democr. [DK68] B7; B9; B125, and Diog. Apoll. [DK64] B5). Nevertheless, a working difference between knowledge (or opinion) about the object itself and the sensing of its effect on one's mixture is generally assumed.

[132] See Emp. (DK31) B17.21–24; Heraclit. (DK22) B1; Parm. (DK28) B6.4–7. In Empedocles, the moral order of the physical world is particularly important, most likely on account of the Orphic-Pythagorean context of his philosophy, on which see Kingsley 1995. Thus, thought and action connect the physical order to the social or the political: to achieve a high state of thinking through a perfect mixture informed by love precipitates action in the world that brings about order, rather than disorder; love, rather than strife.

greater harmony with the world around him. Thought is thus a uniquely trans-formative encounter with reality.

At the same time, virtually all of those working in the inquiry into nature conceptualize thought as a physical encounter.[133] As a result, they often make the capacity to know dependent on the state of the perceiving mixture.[134] In Empedocles, thinking requires that our own mixture be harmonious—he holds that thinking occurs through blood around the heart (DK31 B105)—so that acts of cognition are "acts of love."[135] Heraclitus declares that "a dry *psukhē* is wisest and best" (DK22 B118). If the *psukhē* gets too wet, for example, from ex-cessive drinking, one stumbles along, led by a slave. For Parmenides, the mix-ture of the "limbs" appears to affect the quality of thought (DK28 B16).[136] Dem-ocritus is reported to have held that thoughts change in accordance with the physical state of the soul.[137] And in the *Clouds*, Strepsiades first finds Socrates investigating meteorological matters by hanging in a basket where he can min-gle his thinking with fine and subtle air (229–30), probably a parody of Dio-genes of Apollonia. These thinkers thus establish a situation where we are igno-rant not because the gods see and know more but because our thinking can become muddled by the forces that govern other kinds of physical change.

This evidence ought to make us hesitate before treating the significance of thought in the inquiry into nature in terms of mind-body dualism. Rather, what we have begun to see is a more complicated situation. On the one hand, many

---

[133] Aristotle famously attacks his predecessors for conflating sensation-perception and thought (*De an.* 427a21–29; *Metaph.* 1009b12–31). Laks 1999.255–58 notes that the very opposition be-tween the senses and inferential or contemplative knowledge in the Presocratics disproves that they believe that perceiving and thinking are equivalent. But Aristotle appears concerned with something more precise. As Lesher 1994.11–12 notes, Aristotle says his predecessors see thinking and perceiving as the same, insofar as they see each as ἀλλοίωσις, "(physical) alteration." And it is true that the *act* of thinking is conceptualized by the Presocratics in terms of physical stuffs and change.

[134] The physicists tend to privilege substance over organs or sites; the latter become important in later discussions of mind, which are increasingly influenced by anatomy (Singer 1992.138). See esp. Pl. *Phd.* 96b3–8, where Socrates lists air, blood, and fire as possible mediums of thought, before of-fering the brain as another explanatory mechanism. For air, see Diog. Apoll. (DK64) A19 (Thphr. *De sens.* 44–45); B4–5. For blood, see Emp. (DK31) A86 (Thphr. *De sens.* 23); A97 (= Aët. 4.5.8); B105; cf. *Flat.* 14 (Li 6.110 = 121,9–11 Jouanna); *Morb.* I 30 (Li 6.200 = 86,19–88,6 Wittern). For fire, see Heraclit. (DK22) B36; B77; see also *Vict.* I 7 (Li 6.480 = 130,18–20 Joly-Byl), implying that thought involves fire and water. Alcmaeon is the clearest proponent of locating the perceptual and cognitive faculties in the brain (DK24 A5 [Thphr. *De sens.* 26]).

[135] Laks 1999.267; see also Long 1966.270; M. R. Wright 1995.57–69. Wright claims that, because *daimōn* is both bloodless and intelligent, Empedocles must have imagined "thinking at a higher and a lower level" (1995.71–74); see also 1990.218–25.

[136] See Hussey 2006, defending a materialist reading. Dilcher 2006 takes up the opposite position, arguing that *nous* is not determined by the composition of the mixture.

[137] Aristotle (*De an.* 404a27–31 = DK68 A101) says that Democritus reinterpreted the Homeric verb ἀλλοφρονέω (*Il.* 23.698; *Od.* 10.374) in this way; at *Metaph.* 1009b26–31, he ascribes the same in-terpretation to Anaxagoras. On Democritus's views on thinking, see also Thphr. *De sens.* 58 (DK68 A135) and below, p. 216.

of these thinkers seem to be working with the idea of a continuum of sensing, understood broadly as responsiveness to external forces, that extends through all physical bodies and body parts, whether they are human beings, plants, or earthen vessels. In this context, there is neither body nor mind. There are simply different kinds of mixtures. On the other hand, by recognizing a threshold of consciousness within the person, thinkers like Anaxagoras or the author of *On Ancient Medicine* demarcate two distinct domains. Conscious sensing, moreover, admits of a further division between registering the pain or pleasure created by incorporating or engaging a given mixture and achieving true knowledge of that mixture and reality more broadly. These thresholds—between the nonconscious and the conscious, between perception and knowledge—are thus not only points on a continuum but also opportunities to establish the categories of the body, the senses, and the mind.

The fifth- and fourth-century physicians, I argue, have an important role to play in demarcating these categories. Physicians offer, on the one hand, robust accounts of human nature—perhaps, as Jacques Jouanna has said, the first "*science de l'homme*"—that are grounded in the study of the *sōma* as an object.[138] It is precisely because these accounts rely so heavily on the physical body, as I suggest further in chapter 5, that they encourage others to develop accounts of human nature focused on the mind or the soul.

On the other hand, the medical writers tacitly but consistently acknowledge the difference between the person and the body, as well as the difference between sensing and knowledge. These differences are grounded in the physician-patient relationship. For in this relationship, the physician assumes an essentially disembodied position of knowledge about the physical body. By "disembodied," I do not mean that the physician does not use his senses; the senses, in fact, are indispensable to his acquisition of knowledge.[139] Rather, I mean the physician stands outside the body looking in. The basic dynamics of medical knowledge, then, including knowledge of human nature, split the person into the knower, who strives to understand and manipulate the body, and the body itself.

Located uncomfortably between the knowing physician and the body is the patient, the one who suffers.[140] The patient's presence points to another schism, this time between the person and his own body, which, *qua* physical object, is alien to him. The strangeness of the physical body means that if the person is to

---

[138] Jouanna 1992.92.

[139] See, e.g., *Epid.* VI 8.17 (Li 5.350 = 180,3–4 Manetti-Roselli); *Off. Med.* 1 (Li 3.272 = 30,2–7 Kühlewein). In these cases, however, the five senses are joined by a sixth, *gnōmē* or *logismos*, which turns the physician's sensory apparatus into an instrument of rational investigation.

[140] The relationship is expressed in the Hippocratic triangle. See *Epid.* I 11 (Li 2.636, ch. 5 = 190,3–6 Kühlewein): ἡ τέχνη διὰ τριῶν, τὸ νόσημα καὶ ὁ νοσέων καὶ ὁ ἰητρός· ὁ ἰητρὸς ὑπηρέτης τῆς τέχνης· ὑπεναντιοῦσθαι τῷ νοσήματι τὸν νοσέοντα μετὰ τοῦ ἰητροῦ (The *tekhnē* has three parts: the disease, the sick person, and the physician. The physician is the servant of the *tekhnē*; the sick person fights the disease with the help of the physician). The third limb here belongs to the disease, but the disease is internal to the body.

know anything about it and, hence, take care of it, he must *adopt the position of a physician*. Consider how the author of *On the Nature of a Human Being* uses phenomenological pain to prove that a human being is not one. Pain itself does not create the proposition "we are not one." Rather, it merely confirms the assumed principle that there is nothing from which the one could feel pain. Pain does not allow us to see the stuffs inside.[141] The clarity it provides relies on existing assumptions about how things work.

If the meaning of pain, and, indeed, any bodily phenomenon, depends on beliefs about cause, this is because symptoms stimulate worldviews that are conjectured, conceptualized, and imagined by people. Sign inference is common in the ancient Greek world, as it has been throughout human history. We have seen, for example, that someone who suffers a sudden and mysterious pain is likely to attribute it to a powerful unseen social agent. In fragments from Alcmaeon and Xenophanes, we begin to find a more self-conscious interest in the inference from signs as the basis for human knowledge about the invisible.[142] But it is the medical writers who demonstrate the most obvious commitment to making inferences from empirical data, which they use, in a complex circular process, both to underwrite and to build on claims about the nature of the body and human nature.[143] Taken together, the texts of the Hippocratic Corpus, despite the diversity of ideas and styles, undeniably attest a new self-consciousness about how knowledge about what is unseen is created.

---

[141] The relationship between pain and other forms of perception, especially seeing, remains a controversial issue in modern philosophy: see Aydede 2005, esp. 11–14. Scarry, for example, has argued that pain is a perception that lacks an object (1985.161–62). Others claim that pain does represent information about bodily damage to the mind: M. Evans 2007 argues that Plato holds this position in the *Philebus*. In the medical treatises, pain can reveal the location of the disease *qua* peccant stuff, especially in the nosological and gynecological treatises. See, e.g., *Aff.* 29 (Li 6.240–42 = 52 Potter): wherever the diseased blood settles in the leg, pain becomes manifest. Patients can also indicate where it hurts: see, e.g., *Epid.* V 91 (Li 5.254 = 41,6–8 Jouanna; cf. *Epid.* VII 100 [Li 5.454 = 108,6–8 Jouanna]). At *Art.* 10 (Li 6.18 = 237,1–3 Jouanna) and *Morb. Sacr.* 3 (Li 6.366 = 11,9–13 Jouanna), pain is used to prove the presence of some structure in the body (the bicameral brain and "cells" around the joints, respectively). Yet what is important in the medical texts is that the experience of the body does not represent the facts most relevant to its suffering, namely the causes.

[142] See Xenoph. (DK21) B18, with Lesher 1991; 1992.150–55; Alcmaeon (DK24) B1. Mario Vegetti has argued that it is Alcmaeon who initiates the break away from the tradition of analogy in favor of inferential reasoning based on empirical evidence (1976.31–34); see also Snell 1953.146–47; G. Manetti 1993.44; and cf. Dettori 1990–93, rethinking the "epistemological" reading of the fragment. At the same time, Presocratic examples of *sēmeia* and *sēmata* are rare and usually concern proofs involving logical deduction: Melissus (DK30) B8.1–2; Parm. (DK28) B8.2–4. See also Diog. Apoll. (DK64) B4.1. See further G. Lloyd 1979.69–71.

[143] G. Lloyd 1979.146–55. On sign reasoning in the medical writers, see Lonie 1981.72–86; di Benedetto 1986.97–125; Perilli 1991; G. Manetti 1993.36–52; Vegetti 1996.74–81; 1999; Langholf 1997–2004; Thomas 2000.168–212, who draws connections with Herodotus. Besides semiotic inference, the medical writers adopt other kinds of argumentation, such as modus tollens arguments (if A, then B; but not B, therefore not A): see, e.g., *Aer.* 22 (Li 2.76–80 = 238,12–241,5 Jouanna); *Morb. Sacr.* 1 (Li 6.356–58 = 5,13–17 Jouanna), with G. Lloyd 1979.71–78; Fausti 2002.241–42; Laskaris 2002.108–10.

I think we can better understand this self-consciousness by seeing it as part of a collective effort in the fifth and fourth centuries, primarily among physicians, to build a robust account of the physical body and the web of forces in which it is caught, an account competitive with existing strategies of interpreting symptoms. Neither the active forces in medicine—things inside the *sōma*, for example, or the impersonal powers of foodstuffs—nor daemonic agents are evident. Blaming symptoms on agents is a social practice too common to need proof, though experts may, of course, be consulted about *which* agents are responsible and how to appease or combat them. If physicians wanted to break the habit of inferring agents, they had to do the conceptual, imaginative, and rhetorical work to persuade their audience to "see" what neither pain nor health nor habit shows, that is, to see into the *sōma* with the sight of the mind. I turn now to consider both *how* and *what* physicians see when they use symptoms, and corporeal phenomena more generally, to look inside the *sōma*, beginning with their perception of a new daemonic space.

CHAPTER THREE

Incorporating the Daemonic

MEDICINE IN THE CLASSICAL period is distinguished from previous healing traditions by its representation of disease, *nousos* or *nosēma*, as a natural process that happens inside the *sōma*. It comes as no surprise, then, that the opacity of the *sōma* is a concern for physicians. Nowhere is this concern clearer than in *On the Tekhnē*, a short, rhetorically agile text most likely intended for oral performance before a lay audience in the late fifth century and thus valuable evidence of how physicians, medically informed rhetoricians, and medical writers were shaping the physical body as an object of the public imagination in this period.[1] The author introduces the *stegnotēs*, the "density," of the *sōma*, "in which diseases live not in plain view" (ἐν ᾗ οὐκ ἐν εὐόπτῳ οἰκέουσιν αἱ νοῦσοι, 11, Li 6.20 = 238,17–18 Jouanna), as a problem about halfway through the treatise, when he divides diseases into two kinds: those easily visible (ἐν εὐδήλῳ) and those in harder to see places (ἐν δυσόπτῳ); hidden diseases are in the majority.[2] The text goes on to initiate us, as it would have initiated the original listeners, into the topography of the *sōma*'s shadowy depths.

The medical writers, particularly in the surgical treatises, demonstrate some anatomical knowledge, much of which was probably handed down from earlier generations. But such knowledge has little bearing on how the inside of the body is described in *On the Tekhnē*.[3] The *sōma*, the author tells us, has not one cavity, but many. Yet, after specifying only two, he trails off.[4] Henceforth, his description is determined less by fidelity to detail, anatomical or otherwise, than by the leitmotif of hollows, voids, and interstices (νηδύς, κοῖλος, κενόν, διάφυσις,

---

[1] For arguments in favor of a late fifth-century date, see Jouanna 1988b.190–91; Jori 1996.43–54. On the epideictic function of the speech, see Jouanna 1988b.167–74. For a discussion of the epideictic milieu and other texts probably destined for oral performance, see Jouanna 1984; Thomas 1993; Wittern 1998.32–34; Laskaris 2002.73–124, esp. 73–75.

[2] *Art.* 9 (Li 6.16 = 234,13–15 Jouanna). See also *Flat.* 1 (Li 6.90 = 103,10–12 Jouanna). At Hdt. 2.84, one category of Egyptian specialists is called "those [specialists] in unseen diseases" (οἱ τῶν ἀφανέων νούσων), a phrase that Thomas 2000.41 finds "unmistakably Hippocratic" (see also 2000.204–5). Geller 2004.33–38 points out a similar distinction in a roughly contemporary Akkadian text. It is impossible to know, however, whether the taxonomies developed independently or, if not, the lines of influence.

[3] Given the lack of systematic dissection, it is not surprising that the medical writers' understanding of the cavity was less detailed than their knowledge of joints, bones, tendons, and other phenomena that they dealt with more directly: see Gundert 1992.453–54. On the influence of cultural and theoretical expectations on what physicians see inside the body, see G. Lloyd 1979.126–60.

[4] *Art.* 10 (Li 6.16 = 235,12–15 Jouanna).

ἀγγεῖον, θαλάμη).[5] Like a fifth-century physicist thinking about the cracks in apparently solid objects, the author imagines a space underneath the skin full of gaps—"all things have little chambers around them"—and trafficked by air and fluids.[6] He uses the word *nēdus* to describe these cavities, as if the mysterious inner space of the female body were fragmenting into hundreds of smaller hollows, each capable of concealing and nourishing disease in a kind of "demonic pregnancy."[7]

The lungs, for example, can contain many things, "some of which harm the possessor, some of which benefit him."[8] These cavities allow diseases to evade detection as they gather momentum and thus gain an advantage over the physician. The physician is not to blame, then, if hidden diseases overwhelm patients, but, rather, the nature of bodies (ἡ φύσις αἰτίη ἡ τῶν σωμάτων).[9] By describing this nature, the author turns the blind spot in the Homeric warrior's field of vision into a blind spot within the self.

The author of *On the Tekhnē* is interested, however, not only in darkness but also in light. If hidden diseases do not derive their power from an excess of knowledge and vision, as in the magico-religious model, but from the fact they develop out of sight, the physician needs a way of bringing them into the light. Given that he cannot open up the body, he uses symptoms, either yielded "willingly" by nature or forced by the physician to appear.[10] His description of symptoms is worth quoting at length.

ἰητρικὴ δέ, τοῦτο μὲν τῶν ἐμπύων, τοῦτο δὲ τῶν τὸ ἧπαρ ἢ τοὺς νεφρούς, τοῦτο δὲ τῶν συμπάντων τῶν ἐν τῇ νηδύι νοσεύντων ἀπεστερημένη τι ἰδεῖν ὄψει ἢ τὰ πάντα πάντες ἱκανώτατος ὁρῶσιν, ὅμως ἄλλας εὐπορίας συνεργοὺς εὗρε· φωνῆς τε γὰρ λαμπρότητι καὶ τρηχύτητι καὶ πνεύματος ταχυτῆτι καὶ βραδυτῆτι, καὶ ῥευμάτων, ἃ διαρρεῖν εἴωθεν ἑκάστοισι δι' ὧν ἔξοδοι δέδονται [ὧν] τὰ μὲν ὀδμῇσι τὰ δὲ χροιῇσι τὰ δὲ λεπτότητι καὶ παχύτητι διασταθμωμένη τεκμαίρεται ὧν τε σημεῖα ταῦτα ἅ τε πεπονθότων ἅ τε παθεῖν δυναμένων. ὅταν δὲ ταῦτα τὰ μηνύοντα μηδ' αὐτὴ ἡ φύσις ἑκοῦσα ἀφιῇ, ἀνάγκας εὕρηκεν ᾗσιν ἡ φύσις ἀζήμιος βιασθεῖσα μεθίησιν· ἀνεθεῖσα

[5] *Art.* 10 (Li 6.16–18 = 235,15–237,3 Jouanna).

[6] *Art.* 10 (Li 6.18 = 236,17–237,1 Jouanna): καί τούτων οὐδὲν ὅ τι οὐχ ὕπαφρόν [ὕπαφρόν A M Ermerins Jouanna: ὕποφρόν Erot. Heiberg: ὑπόφορόν Zwing^mg edd.: ὑποφρύ Reinhold] ἐστι καὶ ἔχον περὶ αὐτὸ θαλάμας (and none of these things does not contain foam, but each has around it little chambers). The rare term ὕπαφρος was glossed by Heraclides of Tarentum (cited by Erotian) as κρυφαῖος. Modern editors (Littré, Gomperz, Jones) have tended to prefer ὑπόφορος, "porous." Jouanna prints ὕπαφρος, "containing foam inside," writing that "l'écume contenue en dessous est le signe que les parties sont creuses" (1988b.261). Cf. *Loc.* 7 (Li 6.290 = 46,17–27 Craik).

[7] "Demonic pregnancy" appears in Susan Sontag's compendium of oncological metaphors (1978.14).

[8] *Art.* 10 (Li 6.18 = 236,12–13 Jouanna).

[9] *Art.* 11 (Li 6.20 = 238,7–9 Jouanna). More specifically, in this passage, the author is blaming the body for the slowness of the physician's response to disease. Jori 1996.238–39 sees the emphasis on the body's opacity as part of a strategy to exculpate physicians.

[10] See Jori 1996.93–94 n.17; von Staden 2007b.28–32.

δὲ δηλοῖ τοῖσι τὰ τῆς τέχνης εἰδόσιν ἃ ποιητέα. βιάζεται δὲ τοῦτο μὲν πύου[11] τὸ σύντροφον φλέγμα διαχεῖν σιτίων δριμύτητι καὶ πωμάτων ὅπως τεκμαρεῖταί τι ὀφθὲν περὶ ἐκείνων ὧν αὐτῇ ἐν ἀμηχάνῳ τὸ ὀφθῆναι ἦν· τό τ' αὖ πνεῦμα, ὧν κατήγορον, ὁδοῖσί τε προσάντεσι καὶ δρόμοισιν ἐκβιᾶται κατηγορεῖν· ἱδρῶτάς τε τούτοισιν τοῖσι προειρημένοισιν ἄγουσα [καὶ] ὑδάτων θερμῶν ἀποπνοίῃσι, τεκμαίρεται. ἔστι δὲ ἃ καὶ διὰ τῆς κύστιος διελθόντα ἱκανώτερα δηλῶσαι τὴν νοῦσόν ἐστιν ἢ διὰ τῆς σαρκὸς ἐξιόντα . . . ἕτερα μὲν οὖν πρὸς ἑτέρων καὶ ἄλλα δι' ἄλλων ἐστὶ τά τε διιόντα τά τ' ἐξαγγέλλοντα, ὥστε οὐ θαυμάσιον αὐτῶν τάς τε πίστιας[12] χρονιωτέρας γίνεσθαι τάς τ' ἐγχειρήσιας βραχυτέρας, οὕτω δι' ἀλλοτρίων ἑρμηνειῶν πρὸς τὴν θεραπεύουσαν σύνεσιν ἑρμηνευομένων. (12, Li 6.22–26 = 240,1–241,4; 241,7–11 Jouanna)

Now despite the fact that in cases of suppuration, or with diseases of the liver or the kidneys, or with all those diseases of the cavity, the medical *tekhnē* is deprived of seeing anything by means of the sight through which everyone sees everything perfectly adequately, it has nevertheless discovered resources to assist it. Having taken into account the clearness or the hoarseness of the voice, and the quickness or shortness of the breath, and, of the discharges that habitually flow out through each of the paths that are given to egress, sometimes the odors, sometimes the colors, and sometimes the fineness or thickness, the physician conjectures of which body parts these are the signs, what they have suffered, and what they are capable of suffering. But whenever nature itself does not willingly yield these informants, the *tekhnē* has discovered the means of compulsion by which nature, without being harmed, is forced to give them up. Once released, nature makes clear to those who know the matters of the *tekhnē* what must be done. The *tekhnē* forces the innate phlegm to flow from the pus by means of the acridity of foods and drinks so that on the basis of what is seen it can make inferences about those things that before it was without means to see. Then again it forces the breath, through uphill runnings, to accuse those [diseases] of which it is the accuser. Inducing sweats, too, by the aforementioned means and by evaporations of hot water, it makes conjectures. There are also things that pass through the bladder that are more suited to revealing the disease than what exits through the flesh. . . . Thus, those things that pass out of the body and

---

[11] πυοῦ A Jouanna (πύου): ποιοῦσα A²⁻³: πῦρ M. The reading of M, printed by Littré ("la médecine force la chaleur innée à dissiper au dehors l'humeur phlegmatique . . ."), has been followed by Gomperz, Heiberg, and Jori. Jouanna prints the reading of A ("l'art contraint d'abord le phlegme, humeur innée, à verser du pus . . ."). It is difficult to decide between the two readings. Nevertheless, πύου is better suited to the context, as Jouanna observes (1988b.266–67), and while the innate heat becomes particularly important in post-Hippocratic medicine, it tends to be visible more in its actions than in name in the early medical writings (see below, chapter 4, n.51). Jones omits the phrase as a gloss, supplying φύσις as the implied object of βιάζεται.

[12] τε πίστιας A M^corr (π in ras. M²) I² Corn. (Bas.): ἀπιστίας I: τ' ἀπιστίας Ald. Jouanna prints τε πίστιας and translates "les diagnostics sûrs exigent plus de temps," arguing that "dans chaque cas, la conviction (πίστιας) est longue à se faire" (1988b.268). This reading is preferable to the one given by Jones ("disbelief in this information is prolonged," printing ἀπιστίας), given the discussion at *Art.* 11 (Li 6.20 = 238,7–9 Jouanna).

communicate information are drawn out one by one means, another by another, and pass one by one way, another by another, so that it is not surprising that trustworthy judgments are long in coming, and that therapeutic actions are given less time, since it is foreign interpreters who interpret on behalf of therapeutic intelligence.

Symptoms mediate between the inside and the outside of the *sōma*, as the prefixed verbs (διαρρεῖν, διιόντα, ἐξιόντα, διελθόντα) make clear. They thus have a dual identity. They can be allies of the physician, providing evidence in a mock trial to determine both cause and therapy and thus helping the physician master the disease.[13] But they can also be strange messengers from a strange land, messengers whose communications initiate a lengthy process of interpretation.[14] That strange land is the physical body.

The strangeness of this body, specifically those characteristics which allow it to perform some of the work previously ascribed to gods and *daimones*, is the primary focus of this chapter: not only its unseen and often unfelt cavities but also its potentially treacherous constituent stuffs, the volatile economies of physical force in which it participates, and its uncanny automatism. I begin, however, by giving a bit more attention to how medical interpretations of the symptom facilitate the emergence of this body, showing how, by locating symptoms at the crossroads of the language of cause and the language of visibility, the medical writers establish them as springboards to hidden truths about the physical world. That world is sometimes extended beyond the *sōma* to include diet or environmental factors. Nevertheless, because symptoms are produced by things inside the *sōma*, the world they reveal is primarily that which lies between external catalysts and visible effects, what I have been referring to as the cavity.

One of the hardest things to "see" in medicine is the disease itself. We can best understand it as a cluster of effects to be referred to a specific *phusis* that is endowed with a specific *dunamis*, that is, a capacity to act and to suffer in a predictable way.[15] Through a close reading of a passage from *On Diseases* I, I demonstrate how one medical writer uses symptoms to represent the disease not so much as a thing—though it takes on thinglike qualities—but as a process. As the disease unfolds, we come to see, too, not only the troubling instability of the physical body and its complicity in its own destruction but also the challenge this instability poses to the physician's desire for epistemic and pragmatic mastery of the cavity.

---

[13] The chapter is peppered with legal language. Nature is forced, like a slave, to provide evidence: see comparanda and bibliography at von Staden 2007b.46 n.39. On the "deceitful" body, see H. King 1998.40–53.

[14] Despite medicine's advances, "[sc. these diseases] require more labor and more time than if they were seen by the eyes to be known" (μετὰ πλείονος μὲν γὰρ πόνου καὶ οὐ μετ᾽ ἐλάσσονος χρόνου ἢ εἰ τοῖσιν ὀφθαλμοῖσιν ἑωρᾶτο, γινώσκεται, 11, Li 6.20 = 237,9–11 Jouanna).

[15] On the *phusis* of the disease, see *Aff.* 25 (Li 6.236 = 46 Potter); *Epid.* I 23 (Li 2.668–70, ch. 10 = 199,9–200,2 Kühlewein); *Prog.* 1 (Li 2.112 = 194,3–5 Alex). On the character of the disease, see also *Epid.* III 16 (Li 3.100–102 = 232,7–19 Kühlewein; cf. *Dieb. iudic.* 1 [Li 9.298]); *Epid.* VI 8.14 (Li 5.348 = 178,4–8 Manetti-Roselli), 8.24 (Li 5.352 = 186,1–2 Manetti-Roselli); *Mul.* I 17 (Li 8.56). On *dunamis*, see below, pp. 134–35.

What a symptom refers to depends largely on the question posed to it. That is, symptoms enable physicians to see a range of obscure things depending on whether they are interested in what is happening inside a given body at a given moment; in the probable outcome of the disease; or in securing evidence for a general claim—diagnosis, prognosis, and proof, respectively.[16] Most treatises are organized around one class of questions more than another. In what I refer to loosely as "nosological" treatises, symptoms are used primarily to identify a disease and its treatment, whereas, in "prognostic" treatises, symptoms tend to be used to determine the outcome of the disease; other texts routinely exploit the symptom to prove claims about the nature of the human body and its diseases.[17] At the same time, symptoms often function in different and complementary ways in the same text.[18]

I stress the symptom's polyvalence in part as a reminder that fifth- and fourth-century medical writing exhibits considerable heterogeneity. At the same time, though, that polyvalence attests the complexity of what I take to be the common object of these writings—the physical body.[19] That is, the different questions posed to the symptom reflect the different angles these writers take

[16] It was for many years a scholarly commonplace that the medical writers, or at least the genuinely "Hippocratic" ones, were interested primarily in prognosis, attaching little or no importance to diagnosis. Littré decisively shaped the idea in modern criticism: see Lonie 1978.77–92. For its fate since Littré: Thivel 1981.39–67; Langholf 1990.12–36. The tenacity of the opposition between prognosis and diagnosis can be credited to the fact that it dovetails with ideas about rival schools at Cos and Cnidos: the Coans, who privilege "dynamic" disease concepts, ostensibly prefer prognosis, while the (inferior) Cnidians, committed to "ontological" disease concepts, favor diagnosis. On "ontological" and "physiological" concepts of disease, see Temkin 1963, who cautions against polarizing the two approaches. The gradual disappearance of the Cos-Cnidos binary has made it possible to see how much diagnosis and prognosis involve one another, a point stressed by Grmek 1989.292–94; see also Lichtenthaeler 1963.48; Thivel 1981.55–56. Nevertheless, interpretations of the symptom *do* depend on context, with the result that the division between prognostic and diagnostic functions remains useful; see also di Benedetto 1986.97–100; Langholf 1997–2004.

[17] While I do not discuss the surgical treatises in detail, complications are understood there on the basis of a humoral logic shared with other treatises. The nosological treatises are best represented by *On Diseases* I–IV [note: these texts do not constitute a series, but are by different authors, as is the case with other numbered titles], *Internal Affections, On Affections, Diseases of Women* I–III, and *On Places in a Human Being*; see also *On the Nature of a Human Being, Regimen in Acute Diseases*, with *Appendix*. The prognostic function is best seen in the seven *Epidemics, Prognostic, Prorrhetic* I and II, *Coan Prognoses*, and *Aphorisms*. On points of contact between *Prognostic* and the *Epidemics*, see Li 2.588–89; Vust-Mussard 1970; Robert 1975; Langholf 1983; 1990.159–64, 222–31; Jouanna 2000.lxiv–lxviii. There is a relatively high number of proofs in *On Diseases* IV and *On Generation/On the Nature of the Child, On the Sacred Disease, On Breaths*, and *On Ancient Medicine*—all texts that were probably intended for epideictic performance.

[18] Symptoms can, for example, indicate imminent death or recovery in the nosological treatises, though this function is not systematic there: e.g., *Int.* 39 (Li 7.262 = 200 Potter); *Morb.* II 16 (Li 7.30 = 150,16–151,1 Jouanna); *Morb.* III 2 (Li 7.120 = 70,22–23 Potter), with Langholf 1990.61–68. Conversely, one finds diagnostic uses of the symptom in primarily prognostic contexts: e.g., *Epid.* I 25 (Li 2.676 = 200,22–201,17 Kühlewein); *Prog.* 8 (Li 2.130–32 = 203,8–204,8 Alex); *Prorrh.* II 17 (Li 9.42–44 = 258 Potter).

[19] In the next two chapters, I assume that the extant medical texts share a set of basic ideas about the body and the disease process. I indicate variation where it is salient to my argument.

on that body. Emerging through a cluster of phenomena and ideas, the physical body is at once a hidden space of bones, sinews, and joints, hollows and channels; a mixture of stuffs with different capacities to act and suffer; dense but labile flesh; and a principle of growth and flourishing. It is precisely because it is so complex that it fosters so many divergent narratives within its broader intellectual and cultural milieu, narratives that transform the conditions under which human nature can be imagined.

Symptoms at the Threshold of Seen and Unseen

If a symptom is to indicate what is wrong inside the *sōma*, those interpreting it need some ideas about how the things inside the *sōma* work.[20] Take, for example, a chapter from *On Affections*: the head starts to hurt because a lot of phlegm, having become agitated, has accumulated there.[21] Regardless of how, when, and where these concepts (the presence of a stuff called "phlegm" in the *sōma*; its accumulation in the head when agitated; its capacity to produce pain) first appear, such a world is taken for granted from the first lines of the treatise, where the author declares that anyone with any sense must know that "all human diseases come to be because of bile and phlegm" (1, Li 6.208 = 6 Potter).[22] Bile and phlegm are always present in the body, but they produce disease only under specific conditions:

ἡ δὲ χολὴ καὶ τὸ φλέγμα τὰς νούσους παρέχει ὅταν ἐν τῷ σώματι ὑπερυγραίνηται ἢ ὑπερξηραίνηται ἢ ὑπερθερμαίνηται ἢ ὑπερψύχηται· πάσχει δὲ ταῦτα τὸ φλέγμα καὶ ἡ χολὴ καὶ ἀπὸ σίτων καὶ ποτῶν, καὶ ἀπὸ πόνων καὶ τρωμάτων, καὶ ἀπὸ ὀσμῆς

---

[20] Scholarship on the relationship of etiology to symptoms and treatment has been entangled in the Cos-Cnidus debate. Lonie 1965a argues that the "Cnidian" treatises (for him, *On Affections*, *Diseases* I–III, *Internal Affections*) share an etiological system derived from the lost *Cnidian Sayings*. Cf. Jouanna 1974, arguing for a gradual homogenization of causal factors within the Cnidian treatises (Lonie's "Cnidian" works plus the gynecological writings). Jouanna does not eliminate etiology from what he argues is the earliest strand (= *Diseases* II 12–75) but argues that humoral explanation is fully present only in the later texts. Grensemann 1975 independently identifies *Diseases* II 12–75 as the most archaic layer of texts, together with chapters from the gynecological treatises ("Schicht A"), and also argues for etiological development (1975.55–56). Note, however, that even in the archaic layer, treatment is still directed toward factors inside the body (blood, water), and Mansfeld 1980.381–88 rightly argues that stronger theoretical presuppositions are suggested by the treatment in *Diseases* II 12–75 than Jouanna and others, such as Bourgey 1953, allow. On these presuppositions, see also Joly 1966; Thivel 1981.67–90; Langholf 1990.52–72.

[21] *Aff.* 2 (Li 6.210 = 8 Potter).

[22] On φλέγμα, "phlegm," perhaps derived from φλέγω (to inflame), see Jouanna 1974.92–108; Mansfeld 1980.388–90; Lonie 1981.277–79; Thivel 1981.306–7; Thomas 2000.36. References to χολή, "bile," are found as early as the seventh century: [Archil.] fr. 234 (W²); Hipponax fr. 73.3 (W²). See also Guardasole 2000.118–30, reviewing the evidence from tragedy. On the relationship between χόλος (anger) and χολή, see W. Smith 1966.555–56; Langholf 1990.37–40. On the concept of κίνησις, "agitation": Lonie 1965a.27–28; Jouanna 1974.143–48, 238, 350.

καὶ ἀκοῆς καὶ ὄψιος καὶ λαγνείης, καὶ ἀπὸ τοῦ θερμοῦ τε καὶ ψυχροῦ· πάσχει δέ, ὅταν τούτων ἕκαστα τῶν εἰρημένων ἢ μὴ ἐν τῷ δέοντι προσφέρηται τῷ σώματι, ἢ μὴ τὰ εἰωθότα, ἢ πλείω τε καὶ ἰσχυρότερα, ἢ ἐλάσσω τε καὶ ἀσθενέστερα. (*Aff.* 1, Li 6.208 = 6 Potter)

Bile and phlegm produce diseases when, inside the body, one of them becomes too moist, too dry, too hot, or too cold; phlegm and bile undergo these changes because of foods and drinks, exertions and wounds, smell, sound, sight, and sexual inter-course, and because of heat and cold; they suffer when any of the things described are administered to the body at the wrong time, contrary to what is habitual, in too great an amount and too strong, or in insufficient amount and too weak.

It is with this etiological schema in mind that we read the explanation of the patient's head pain.[23]

Not all the medical writers make the causal relationships in a disease explicit (although these relationships are often implied). Yet whenever etiology is fore-grounded, it is, as one would expect, attracted to the symptom. So pervasive are expressions such as "y (= phenomenal event or condition) happens when x (= hidden event, condition) happens," "if x happens, y happens," "y happens on account of x," "y arises from x," "x produces y," and combinations thereof in ex-tant medical writing that they often escape notice.[24] In such cases, etiology cre-ates an implicit rationale for recommended treatment.

On occasion, however, we find authors actively trying to secure their readers' assent to an explanation by offering what is identified as proof of the causal mechanisms that it posits.[25] In *Airs, Waters, Places*, for example, we are told that a bladder stone forms when the bladder grows feverish and heats (or "con-cocts") the urine within it: as a result, the heaviest part of the water taken in by the body remains in the bladder and masses together, while the lightest, clearest

---

[23] In *On Affections*, etiology follows therapy so that the symptom ("if pains befall the head") is aligned with therapeutic action expressed as an imperative ("warm his head by washing it with copi-ous hot water") before its specific origins are explained. But texts vary in how these components—etiology, treatment, and symptoms—are arranged. Moreover, although symptomatology is the only constant, the organization of symptoms varies: see Lonie 1965a.3; Wittern 1987.74–82; Langholf 1990.55–72; Potter 1990, esp. 240–42; Roselli 1990.

[24] On the phrase "y happens when [ὅταν, ἐπειδάν, ὁπόταν, or genitive absolute] x happens": see, e.g., *Aff.* 23 (Li 6.234 = 42 Potter); *Loc.* 9 (Li 6.290–92 = 46,30–31 Craik), 12 (Li 6.296 = 52,1–2 Craik); *Morb.* II 9 (Li 7.16 = 140,7–9 Jouanna). "If [ἤν] x happens, y happens": see, e.g., *Glan.* 7 (Li 8.562 = 117,16–18 Joly). On "y happens on account of [διά] x": see, e.g., *VM* 11 (Li 1.594 = 131,11 Jouanna). On "y arises from [ἀπό] x": see, e.g., *Morb.* I 14 (Li 6.164 = 36,2 Wittern); with ὑπό: e.g., *Loc.* 14 (Li 6.304 = 56,19 Craik); with ἐκ: e.g., *Int.* 28 (Li 7.240 = 170 Potter). On "x produces [παρέχει] y": see, e.g., *Vict.* III 81 (Li 6.628 = 212,25–26 Joly-Byl). Causal language often accumulates: e.g., *Aff.* 10 (Li 6.218 = 20 Potter): ἡ δὲ νοῦσος γίνεται ὑπὸ χολῆς, ὅταν κινηθεῖσα πρὸς τὰ σπλάγχνα καὶ τὰς φρένας προσίζῃ (the disease arises from bile, when being set in motion it falls against the innards and the diaphragm).

[25] In Herodotus, too, the language of proof signals that he is self-consciously making a claim (Thomas 2000.193, 195–98 on the medical writers). On the vocabulary of proof in the classical pe-riod, see G. Lloyd 1966.425–26; 1979.59–125; G. Manetti 1994.

part exits as urine.[26] The proof (τεκμήριον)? People suffering from stones have very clear urine. Here the role of the symptom shifts. For the author is not simply making sense of the phenomenon by referring it to causal mechanisms (here a mechanism by which water separates into light and heavy parts when heated). He is also using the symptom to make his listeners believe in the bodily process behind it. Putting the symptom in the service of proof, he appropriates its visibility for events hidden inside the *sōma*.[27]

If attention is shifted back to the symptoms of a particular patient, however, this mechanism (i.e., separation of water in the bladder and the massing together of the heaviest part) is once again taken for granted.[28] Under these circumstances, the symptom indicates that a known mechanism is active in a particular patient. That is, if the physician accepts the account of bladder stones in *Airs, Waters, Places*, he can diagnose stones on the basis of a patient's clear urine. We thus return to the scenario "y happens when x happens," but with a twist: now the phenomenon "y" is not simply explained by "x" but can reveal its presence. This "diagnostic" function of the symptom is common in classical medical writing: spontaneous discharge of blood or urine signifies that the small vessels in the kidney are broken; if sperm exits the woman's body with a lot of moisture, it is clear that the womb is too wet; if the patient is neither nauseous nor heavy-headed and the fever is mild, the disease is "settled," allowing the lower cavity to be purged.[29] The surgical treatises, too, are full of signs indicating the nature of the dislocation.[30]

In such contexts, the medical writers often use a transitive verb such as *sēmainō*, "to signify." The verb lays stress on the phenomenon's power to indicate something hidden. At the same time, it quietly marks the symptom as a threshold that cannot, in the end, be crossed: because the body cannot be opened and because cause cannot be seen, we can access the unseen only indirectly, through a conceptual leap from signs to hidden truths.

---

[26] *Aer.* 9 (Li 2.38–40 = 209,11–210,13 Jouanna); cf. *Nat. Hom.* 12 (Li 6.62–64 = 198,18–200,4 Jouanna). See Diller 1932.17–19 for an analysis of a similar argument in ch. 8 of *Airs*.

[27] For other proofs, see *Aer.* 20 (Li 2.72–74 = 235,8–236,7 Jouanna); *Carn.* 4 (Li 8.588–90 = 191,7–12 Joly), 8 (Li 8.594 = 193,20–23 Joly); *Flat.* 12 (Li 6.108–10 = 119,11–120,10 Jouanna); *Genit./Nat. Puer.* 8 (Li 7.480–82 = 50,12–14 Joly), 18 (Li 7.502–4 = 62,19–63,1 Joly), 29 (Li 7.530 = 77,19–78, 9 Joly); *Glan.* 4 (Li 8.558 = 115,18 Joly), 17 (Li 8.574 = 122,11–18 Joly); *Int.* 51 (Li 7.292 = 242 Potter); *Morb.* IV 56 (Li 7.606–8 = 120,3–121,22 Joly); *Morb. Sacr.* 4 (Li 6.368 = 12,17–20 Jouanna); *Mul.* I 71 (Li 8.150); *Nat. Hom.* 7 (Li 6.46–50 = 182,4–186,12 Jouanna); *Steril.* 233 (Li 8.446); *VM* 17 (Li 1.612 = 141,15–142,5 Jouanna).

[28] On the circularity involved here (the assumed cause explains the phenomenon, the phenomenon proves the cause), see Vegetti 1976.48–51; Lonie 1981.85; Langholf 1990.221–22; Perilli 1991.163; G. Manetti 1993.46–47.

[29] *Aph.* IV.78 (Li 4.530 = 156 Jones); *Mul.* I 12 (Li 8.48); *Epid.* V 64 (Li 5.242 = 29,7–10 Jouanna; cf. *Epid.* VII 60 [Li 5.426 = 87,14–17 Jouanna]).

[30] E.g., *Artic.* 19 (Li 4.132 = 142,20–143,1 Kühlewein; cf. *Mochl.* 9 [Li 4.354 = 252,15–17 Kühlewein]), 20 (Li 4.134 = 143,4–5 Kühlewein; cf. *Mochl.* 10 [Li 4.354 = 252,20–21 Kühlewein]); *Fract.* 42 (Li 3.552 = 105,9–12 Kühlewein).

At other times, however, the medical writers use the very perceptibility of the symptom to turn inference into emergence. Symptoms (together with similar phenomena such as the menses) are often enmeshed not only in the language of causality but also in the language of appearance, particularly compounds of the verb *phainomai—prophainomai, epiphainomai, emphainomai*.[31] The visibility of the symptom is thus appropriated for what lies below the threshold of perception. Consider an example from *Internal Affections*, where the author is describing a jaundice caused when the subcutaneous moisture congeals with blood. He introduces the symptoms, which here both confirm the alleged cause and identify the disease in a particular patient, with the phrase "as is clear from the following" (τοῖσδε δὲ ἀποδηλοῖ ὡς οὕτως ἔχει, 36, Li 7.256 = 192 Potter). By shifting the symptoms into the instrumental dative, he establishes them as merely auxiliary to insight while exploiting their connection to the clarity of phenomenal reality. He thus allows an unseen condition to become the subject of an intransitive verb of appearing, as if it were coming to light directly. In a common variant of this expression, writers shift symptoms into the dative in order to make a hidden physical condition the direct object of verbs of knowing: "You will know x by y."[32] By instrumentalizing the phenomenon in this way, they lend credence to medicine's claim to offer "second sight": knowledge of the unseen is not mediated by a logical operation but is evident, given, *real*.[33]

Despite inflecting it differently in different contexts, then, the medical writers consistently use the symptom to connect the visible and invisible dimensions of

[31] For φαίνομαι, e.g., *Acut. Sp.* 23 (Li 2.440, ch. 9 = 79,9 Joly); *Epid.* II 3.17 (Li 5.118 = 64 Smith); *Epid.* VII 83 (Li 5.438 = 98,1 Jouanna); *Prog.* 2 (Li 2.116 = 196,3 Alex), 25 (Li 2.190 = 231,3 Alex); *Mul.* I 4 (Li 8.26 = 96,28–98,1 Grensemann); *Mul.* II 118 (Li 8.254), 128 (Li 8.274); *Nat. Mul.* 74 (Li 7.404 = 75,2 Bourbon); *Prorrh.* II 26 (Li 9.58 = 274 Potter), 35 (Li 9.66 = 282 Potter); *Superf.* 18 (Li 8.486 = 80,9 Lindau). For προφαίνομαι: *Aer.* 8 (Li 2.34 = 205,8 Jouanna); *Iudic.* 4 (Li 9.276), 35 (Li 9.286); *Mul.* II 129 (Li 8.276); *Nat. Mul.* 36 (Li 7.378 = 52,14 Bourbon), 40 (Li 7.384 = 57,7 Bourbon); *Prorrh.* II 21(Li 9.50 = 264 Potter). For ἐπιφαίνομαι: *Aph.* I.12 (Li 4.464 = 104 Jones), IV.72 (Li 4.528 = 154 Jones); *Coac.* 340 (Li 5.656), 524 (Li 5.704); *Epid.* I 16 (Li 2.648, ch. 8 = 193,14 Kühlewein); *Epid.* II 1.6 (Li 5.74 = 20 Smith), 3.1 (Li 5.100 = 46 Smith), 3.17 (Li 5.116 = 62 Smith); *Epid.* IV 56 (Li 5.196 = 148 Smith); *Hum.* 4 (Li 5.482 = 70 Jones); *Mul.* I 28 (Li 8.72); *Mul.* II 61 (Li 8.124); *Prorrh.* II 14 (Li 9.38 = 254 Potter); *Steril.* 217 (Li 8.418), 245 (Li 8.458); *Superf.* 1 (Li 8.476 = 72,11 Lindau), 29 (Li 8.494 = 86,8 Lindau). For ἐμφαίνομαι: *Nat. Mul.* 53 (Li 7.394 = 66,13 Bourbon). For the language of visibility in the Babylonian medical texts, see Stol 1993.12, with nn.63–64. Symptoms can also be paired with neutral verbs or presented through parataxis, compositional features that are consonant with the catalog structure and brachylogy of many medical texts, on which, see Lonie 1983; W. Smith 1983; G. Miller 1990; Humphreys 1996.8–9; van der Eijk 1997.102–6.

[32] See, e.g., *Int.* 9 (Li 7.188 = 100 Potter): τούτῳ δὲ γνώσῃ; *Loc.* 10 (Li 6.294 = 48,33–50,2 Craik): τῷδ᾽ ἐστὶ γιγνώσκειν; *Morb.* II 61 (Li 7.94 = 200,12–13 Jouanna): τούτῳ ἂν γνοίης; *Morb. Sacr.* 15 (Li 6.388 = 27,6–7 Jouanna): γνώσει δὲ ἑκάτερα ὧδε; *Mul.* I 22 (Li 8.62): γνώσῃ δὲ τῷδε. These expressions are discussed at di Benedetto 1986.101–2. They are particularly common in the gynecological treatises: *Mul.* I 58 (Li 8.116), 59 (Li 8.118); *Mul.* II 150 (Li 8.326); *Nat. Mul.* 21 (Li 7.340 = 24,2 Bourbon), 22 (Li 7.340 = 24,9 Bourbon), 49 (Li 7.392 = 64,16 Bourbon); *Steril.* 215 (Li 8.416), 230 (Li 8.438). Such expressions can be combined with semiotic language, e.g., *Artic.* 10 (Li 4.102 = 126,1–2 Kühlewein): γινώσκειν δὲ εἰ ἐκπέπτωκεν ὁ βραχίων τοισίδε χρὴ τοῖσι σημείοισι.

[33] See von Fritz 1943.87 on the absence of inferential reasoning in archaic uses of the verb νοεῖν.

the physical body, implicating suffering in a world of somatic stuffs and forces that can be neither easily observed nor intuitively known, while, at the same time, bringing that world to light.

THE INTERVAL

By granting causal significance to the physical body, the medical writers, of course, do not exclude the role of external catalysts.[34] In fact, when an author wishes to draw attention to these factors, he will often downplay the role of the cavity. In one chapter from *On Affections*, the author interprets symptoms by bypassing causes inside the body altogether:

> καὶ τῶν σιτίων, ἃ δύναμιν ἕκαστα ἔχει, τεκμαίρεσθαι χρὴ ἀπὸ τῶν φανερὴν τὴν δύναμιν ἐχόντων, ὅσα ἢ φῦσαν ἢ δῆξιν ἢ πλησμονὴν ἢ ἐρευγμὸν παρέχει ἢ στρόφον, ἢ διαχωρέει ἢ μὴ διαχωρέει, καὶ φανερά ἐστιν ὅτι ταῦτα ἐργάζεται. ἀπὸ τούτων χρὴ τὰ ἄλλα σκοπεῖν· ἔχει γὰρ τὰ ἕκαστα τῶν ἐδεσμάτων, διότι ὠφελέει καὶ βλάπτει· ἀλλὰ τὰ μὲν φανερώτερά ἐστιν ἐργαζόμενα ἃ ἐργάζεται, τὰ δὲ ἀμυδρότερα. (*Aff.* 47, Li 6.254–56 = 70 Potter)

> About foods, each of which has its own *dunamis*, one must conjecture on the basis of those which have a visible *dunamis*, those which produce gas or pangs or satiety or belching or colic, or pass off below or do not pass off, being visible in effecting these things. On the basis of these things you must investigate the others. For each of these foodstuffs has something because of which it helps and harms; but some are very perceptible in producing the effects they do, while others are more obscure.

Here, the author is inquiring into the general powers of foodstuffs. The Hippocratic physician might also be interested in environmental factors. The major objects of the physician's knowledge in *Airs, Waters, Places*, for example, are what effects each season is capable of producing (ὅ τι δύναται ἀπεργάζεσθαι) in human nature, as well as the *dunameis* of winds and waters.[35] Physicians also engage in this kind of testing in specific scenarios. The physician-author of *On the Use of Liquids*, instructing the reader on the therapeutic uses of water, recommends pursuing a course of action with the patient until some obvious benefit or harm allows its correctness to be gauged.[36]

Inquiries into the effects of external forces are slightly complicated in *On Diseases* IV. The author first establishes that, like roses, garlic, and all other organic things, the *sōma* attracts the *ikmas*, "juice," that is most like it from food

---

[34] The external catalyst is sometimes called the *prophasis*, as opposed to the primary or necessary cause, e.g., *Morb. Sacr.* 3 (Li 6.366 = 11,6–9 Jouanna). Rawlings 1975 argued that the *prophasis* (from φαίνω) is always the visible, external cause; but cf. G. Lloyd 1979.54 n.231, cautioning against seeing the medical lexicon as too precise; see also Jouanna 2002.291–92.

[35] *Aer.* 1 (Li 2.12 = 186,2–187,4 Jouanna).

[36] *Liq.* 1 (Li 6.118–20 = 164,19–24 Joly). See also, e.g., *Loc.* 34 (Li 6.326 = 72,20–22 Craik).

and drink.[37] He then claims that, if a food contains too much of a given juice, the *sōma* grows sick from the excess, offering the following proof. If we eat or drink something particularly bitter, the bile in the liver, its natural home, will increase. The liver is immediately pained, and "we take note of this occurring, and it is clear to us that this occurs because of the food and drink" (τοῦτο ἐσείδομεν γινόμενον καὶ ἐμφανὲς ἡμῖν ἐστιν ὅτι ἀπὸ τοῦ βρώματος ἢ τοῦ ποτοῦ ἐγίνετο, *Morb.* IV 36, Li 7.550 = 89,7–8 Joly).[38] If, however, the amount of incoming bile is small enough, the body, "since it is very big" (ἄτε μέγα τὸ σῶμα ἐόν), absorbs it, and we feel nothing.[39] We can note, first, that, although the author singles out bile in the food as a catalyst, harm is actually produced through the (increased) bile in the liver. The role of the internal bile reminds us of one of naturalizing medicine's core precepts—namely, that it is the things inside the body that hurt a person, or, to quote Plato's appropriation of this principle, "external badness induces the natural badness (of the body)."[40] Second, the fact that food or drink can have an impact on the constituent stuffs without a perceptible effect reminds us that much of what happens inside the *sōma* is not consciously felt, as we saw in the previous chapter.

In the introduction, I suggested that we can speak of the space between cause and effect as what Dupréel calls an interval or "une réalité intercalaire," by which he means a space of possible interference within the production of an effect. The cavity realizes such an intercalated space, hidden and volatile. For every reaction to an external force is a delayed reaction, complicated by its passage through the mysterious interval. In *On Diseases* IV, for example, the effect of the food always depends on the "old bile" already present. That bile might immediately

---

[37] *Morb.* IV 34 (Li 7.544–48 = 85,25–87,18 Joly). On ἰκμάς, see Thomas 2000.49–52.

[38] Given that the liver is the subject of the verb ἀλγέω, the author seems to make a point of noting when the person registers the damage to the liver.

[39] *Morb.* IV 36 (Li 7.552 = 89,21–23 Joly). See also *Morb.* IV 35 (Li 7.550 = 88,19–22 Joly); 45 (Li 7.568 = 99,13–17 Joly).

[40] See *R.* 10, 609e1–610a3: ἐννόει γάρ, ἦν δ᾽ ἐγώ, ὦ Γλαύκων, ὅτι οὐδ᾽ ὑπὸ τῆς τῶν σιτίων πονηρίας, ἥ ἂν ᾖ αὐτῶν ἐκείνων, εἴτε παλαιότης εἴτε σαπρότης εἴτε ἡτισοῦν οὖσα, οὐκ οἰόμεθα δεῖν σῶμα ἀπόλλυσθαι· ἀλλ᾽ ἐὰν μὲν ἐμποιῇ ἡ αὐτῶν πονηρία τῶν σιτίων τῷ σώματι σώματος μοχθηρίαν, φήσομεν αὐτὸ δι᾽ ἐκεῖνα ὑπὸ τῆς αὐτοῦ κακίας νόσου οὔσης ἀπολωλέναι· ὑπὸ δὲ σιτίων πονηρίας ἄλλων ὄντων ἄλλο ὂν τὸ σῶμα, ὑπ᾽ ἀλλοτρίου κακοῦ μὴ ἐμποιήσαντος τὸ ἔμφυτον κακόν, οὐδέποτε ἀξιώσομεν διαφθείρεσθαι ("For consider, Glaucon," I said, "that we do not even believe that a body would be destroyed by the deficiency belonging to foods, whether it is staleness, rottenness, or anything else. But if the foods' own deficiency induces bodily deterioration, we will say the body was destroyed through them by its own badness, which is disease. But we will never admit that the body is destroyed by the deficiency belonging to foods—since they and the body are different things—except when external badness induces the natural badness"; trans. Reeve). Plato, however, is working with a slightly different notion of what in food induces disease (staleness, rottenness), which can be explained by the fact that the body's badness is introduced as an analogy to that of the soul. Whereas, in the medical writers, the *dunamis* of the food is not good or bad absolutely but only relative to the strength of the body, Plato needs a more obvious "badness" in order to make the analogy with vice (= always bad) work. For the body-soul analogy, see chapter 5 and, on Plato, Holmes, forthcoming (b).

increase enough to be felt. But, having absorbed the new bile, it can also become the unperceived seed of a disease that will take root only later.

At the same time, the author asserts the role of internal bile in order to control the interval represented by the cavity by identifying an intervening causal mechanism between the visible, external catalyst and the phenomenon. In so doing, he, like many other medical writers, is trying to eliminate unpredictability. But he is also helping to establish mechanisms through which disease unfolds inside the body, mechanisms that make the daemonic world from which symptoms arise intelligible. A similar process is at work in *On the Sacred Disease*, where the author, trying to persuade his listeners that phlegm, not a god, is responsible for epileptic symptoms, goes inside the cavity, as it were, in order to describe each mechanism triggered when phlegm invades the network of channels that circulate air.[41] He continues to assume a hairbreadth of time between the catalyst and the symptoms. Nevertheless, by charting how phlegm produces each individual symptom, he dilates that moment to accommodate the complex, concealed workings of the physical body.

The interval can, however, also expand in time more literally. Such an expansion is often marked by the escalation of symptoms. Discussing a lung disease, the author of *On Diseases* III observes, "as time passes, the disease reveals itself more clearly" (προϊόντος δὲ τοῦ χρόνου μᾶλλον καὶ ἡ νοῦσος σαφὴς δηλοῦται, 16, Li 7.150 = 92,31–32 Potter).[42] He goes on to note that if the physician fails to expel the pus from the patient's lung, it breaks into the chest. On the surface, the patient "seems to be healthy" (δοκέει ὑγιὴς εἶναι). In truth, the chest is silently filling with pus until, through coughing, fevers, and other complications, "the disease shows through" (καὶ ἡ νοῦσος διαδηλοῦται, Li 7.152 = 94,8 Potter). The longer that emergence takes or the more complex the symptoms, the more potential there is for the cavity to appear daemonic.[43] Let us consider now what it means to refer symptoms not to specific events, conditions, or external forces (e.g., the dampness of the womb, a bilious food), but to the more prolonged phenomenon of disease.

---

[41] *Morb. Sacr.* 7 (Li 6.372–74 = 14,21–16,23 Jouanna).

[42] See also *Morb.* I 22 (Li 6.186 = 66,12 Wittern): ὅταν δ᾽ ἡ νοῦσος ἐμφανὴς γένηται; *Mul.* I 4 (Li 8.28 = 98,10 Grensemann): ἐπιφαίνεται τὰ νοσήματα; *Mul.* II 113 (Li 8.242): ἢν δὲ μηκύνῃ, ταῦτα πάντα ἐπὶ μᾶλλον ἀνθέει, καὶ δῆλος ἡ νοῦσος. See further *Aph.* VI.41 (Li 4.572 = 188 Jones); *Artic.* 41 (Li 4.180 = 166,10–11 Kühlewein); *Coac.* 275 (Li 5.644); *Epid.* V 7 (Li 5.208 = 5,9–11 Jouanna); *Loc.* 14 (Li 6.306 = 58,23 Craik); *Morb.* IV 44 (Li 7.566 = 97,24–98,4 Joly); *Vict.* I 2 (Li 6.472 = 126,1 Joly-Byl).

[43] See *Nat. Hom.* 13 (Li 6.64 = 200,13–14 Jouanna): ὅσα τῶν νοσημάτων ἐξ ὀλίγου γίνεται, καὶ ὅσων αἱ προφάσιες εὔγνωστοι, ταῦτα δὲ ἀσφαλέστατά ἐστιν προ[σ]αγορεύεσθαι (Diseases that develop right away and whose exciting causes are well known are the easiest to give an advance account of). Jouanna 2002.290–91 gives good reasons for translating ἐξ ὀλίγου in a quantitative sense ("d'un petit dérangement"), but the temporal sense is idiomatic enough to seem natural here; it may give the sense that diseases that "spring" right away are easier to understand than those that develop over time in the cavity.

Explaining Disease

Hippocratic disease lacks "any clear objective correlative which could serve as an *unambiguous* referent."[44] The classical medical writers virtually ignore the concept of contagion, perhaps because it reminds them too much of the magico-religious idea of *miasma*.[45] Even in the nosological and gynecological treatises, which were long seen as the bastion of archaic, ontological disease concepts and in which disease is endowed with a strong spatial identity—it becomes fixed in places, seizes parts of the body, travels as a flux—the identity of a disease depends mostly on the kind of trouble it causes.[46] The disease that slowly reveals itself in *On Diseases* III 16, for example, in the passage just cited, does so through the patient's dry cough, fever, shivering, rapid breathing, deepened voice, and flushed face. The form, *eidos* or *ideē*, of a disease is not something visible, let alone an anthropo- or zoomorphic figure, but, rather, a constellation of symptoms—a syndrome, in modern parlance—organized by the mind into an object of thought.[47]

Disease does, at times, glint at the edge of the seen. The skin might fall away, exposing the pus below.[48] Nevertheless, the pus is but a relic of the once dynamic interaction between the disease and the body: once seen, it becomes another symptom. In *On the Sacred Disease*, the reader is invited to cut open the head of an epileptic goat in order to confirm for himself the author's account of the disease's causes. Yet seeing the goat's phlegm-corroded brain is not tantamount to

---

[44] Lonie 1983.152 (emphasis in original), arguing that, with the rise of literacy, written catalogs objectify the disease. See also G. Miller 1990, esp. 35–36. Cf. the reservations about a relationship between literacy and ancient science at von Staden 1992c.589–90; van der Eijk 1997.93–99 (specifically addressing the hypotheses of Lonie and Miller). On the slipperiness of disease concepts, see also Edelstein 1967b.65–66; di Benedetto 1986.11–34; and the essays in Potter, Maloney, and Desautels 1990.

[45] R. Parker 1983.220; Hankinson 1995a. But see *Flat.* 6 (Li 6.98 = 110,7 Jouanna) on *miasmata* transmitted by winds, with Jouanna 2001.14–19. See also Hoessly 2001.274–78, emphasizing continuities between medical and magico-religious ideas of *miasma*. By the time we reach Galen, the resistance to an idea of contagion is pronounced (Nutton 1983.14–16; Jouanna 2001.20–27, esp. n.22). On the more clearly delineated adversaries of modern medicine, see Sontag 1978.62–66; Horstmanshoff and Rosen 2003.96.

[46] Ontological disease concepts in the "Cnidian" texts: Lonie 1965b.59–60 n.3; Boncompagni 1972; Byl 1992.205. Cf. the criticisms of the ontological label in di Benedetto 1986.106–10. Langholf 1990.151–52, 162–63 speaks rather of "disease units" in the nosological treatises. On the movement of the disease through the inner body, see above, n.22, on κίνησις.

[47] On *eidos/ideē*, see, e.g., *Aer.* 11 (Li 2.52 = 219,8 Jouanna); *Int.* 20 (Li 7.214 = 136 Potter); *Morb.* IV 57 (Li 7.612 = 124,2–3 Joly); *Nat. Hom.* 2 (Li 6.36 = 168,8–9 Jouanna), with Gillespie 1912.183–90. But cf. *Flat.* 2 (Li 6.92 = 105,9 Jouanna), where ἰδέη is allied with the commonalities of diseases (objects of mental vision) and contrasted to symptomatic variation (see Jouanna 1988b.132–33). *Eidos* can still refer to the visible body of the patient, as at *Oss.* 11 (Li 9.182 = 149,12 Duminil), or other seen forms, like a bruise (*VC* 5, Li 3.200–202 = 68,12–13 Hanson), as well as to a patient's constitution (*Hum.* 1, Li 5.476 = 64 Jones; *Nat. Hom.* 9, Li 6.52 = 188,8 Jouanna).

[48] πύον ὑποφαίνεται: *Epid.* V 97 (Li 5.256 = 43,9–10 Jouanna; cf. *Epid.* VII 35 [Li 5.402 = 73,5 Jouanna], with ὑπεμένετο).

seeing the disease. Rather, the author assumes that by confronting rotted flesh, the reader will be persuaded to trade a story about agency for a story about physical causality: "And you will know clearly by this that it is not a god but the disease that violates the body" (καὶ ἐν τούτῳ δηλόνοτι γνώσῃ ὅτι οὐχ ὁ θεὸς τὸ σῶμα λυμαίνεται, ἀλλ᾽ ἡ νοῦσος, 11, Li 6.382 = 22,2–4 Jouanna).[49] But even as the author borrows the sights and smells of the physical body to endow his claims about the disease with clarity, the disease itself remains elusive. In *Epidemics* V, it is noted that when the swollen skin is cut away from a patient with broken ribs, the purulence is shown to extend deep into the body.[50] Following this, "it was recognized that the nature of the disease was farther off than below the skin" (ἐγνώσθη τὸ εἶναι πορρωτέρω τὴν φύσιν τοῦ νοσήματος ἢ ὑπὸ τὸ δέρμα, 26, Li 5.226 = 16,17–18 Jouanna). This clipped observation makes a nice aphorism: although disease is often rooted in some *materia peccans* whose elimination may produce health, it is, in truth, always out of reach, known only by the damage it creates.[51]

The fact the disease is so elusive reminds us that the medical writers are working with two kinds of "imperceptibility": what is potentially seen and what is seen with the mind. The former can be correlated with the embodied daemonic agent, the latter with his intentions. Rather than openly acknowledging these two classes of imperceptibles, however, the medical writers usually conflate them. By doing so, they allow their claims about the nature of the body or the disease to masquerade as concrete objects of perception, as we saw in relation to the language surrounding symptoms. The pus or the corroded brain is not the disease, but, rather, further inducement to inference, perceptible traces that allow events to be reconstructed through the knowledge of causes. That is to say, they allow an investigation into those things that before the art was at a loss to see altogether.[52] Among the things that the art needs to see are the *phusis* and the *dunamis* of the disease.

As we have begun to see, the capacity to act and suffer is of particular importance to the visibility, as well as the identity, of the disease.[53] In Homer, *dunamis*

---

[49] See G. Lloyd 1979.23–24: postmortem examinations were not standard procedure.

[50] *Epid.* V 26 (Li 5.224 = 16,5–7 Jouanna): ἀνατμηθὲν τὸ δέρμα ὅπη [ὅπη Jouanna: ὅπη M V] ἐφάνη, ἐς τὸ δέρτρον ἐπὶ θάτερα ἀφήκουσα καὶ πρὸς τὸν νεφρὸν καὶ πρὸς τὰ ὀστέα ἐπῆλθε σαπρίη. See Jouanna 2000.138–39 on this passage. Other editors print ὀπὴ ἐφάνη ... : Smith translates "an opening into the peritoneum appeared which led in both directions: a rotten channel ran to the kidney and to the bones," which, as Jouanna notes, improbably suggests an autopsy.

[51] Parker has likened the *kakon* eliminated from the body to the polluted matter targeted by purifiers (1983.213–16). See also Hoessly 2001.247–313 and esp. von Staden 2007a.36–38, stressing the specificity of medical *katharsis*. Niebyl 1969.28–56 discusses the difference between a corrupted substance that causes pain and a foreign body.

[52] ὅπως τεκμαρεῖταί τι ὀφθὲν περὶ ἐκείνων ὧν αὐτῇ ἐν ἀμηχάνῳ τὸ ὀφθῆναι ἦν (*Art.* 12, Li 6.24 = 240,15–17 Jouanna), cited above, p. 123. Touch, too, although it allows for direct perception of unseen things—the mouth of the womb, for example, can be felt for wetness or smoothness (*Mul.* I 21, Li 8.60 = 118,18–20 Grensemann)—produces evidence that must be interpreted. On the vocabulary of touch in the corpus, see Boehm 2003.

[53] On *dunamis* in the medical writers, see H. Miller 1952; 1959; Plamböck 1964; von Staden 1998. On the "verbal" nature of the disease, see also Preiser 1976.60–71; von Staden 1990.99–102.

describes the power of an agent to act, whether to fight or to protect, to punish or to heal.[54] In the previous chapter, we saw this kind of intentional agency being replaced by physical causes in the sixth and fifth centuries (e.g., in the physicists' explanations of meteorological events). Yet our limited evidence suggests that it is not the physicists but the physicians who are primarily responsible for transferring the term *dunamis* to physical stuffs. This impression may be due to an accident of textual transmission. Nevertheless, it is telling that, in the *Phaedrus*, Plato defines the "Hippocratic" approach to nature in part as an inquiry into *dunameis* (270c10–d7).[55] If we turn to the medical writers themselves, we see that many of them attribute a *dunamis* to virtually everything—foods, drinks, drugs, and therapies, as well as the constituent stuffs of the body, body parts such as the brain or the nostrils, and the whole body.[56] In so doing, they extend and reframe the power of things around them, stuffs like honey, oil, and bran,[57] as well as the seasons and the winds. In *On Breaths*, for example, wind—"invisible to sight, visible to reasoning" (τῇ μὲν ὄψει ἀφανής, τῷ δὲ λογισμῷ φανερός)—is a *megistos dunastēs*, a "most powerful master," capable of not only bending trees and upsetting ships but also piercing human flesh "like an arrow" (ὥσπερ τόξευμα) and producing the whole spectrum of human diseases.[58]

The "like" (ὥσπερ) in this last simile cues an important difference between the "expressive potential of the weapon" that we saw in chapter 1 and the function of the medical writer's arrow. Apollo's (unseen) arrows, for example, are the immediate cause of the plague, but only insofar as they fill in the "how" space between the god's fully efficacious intention to harm and the Achaeans. The arrow in *On Breaths*, however, is only analogous to the wind. That is, the wound it creates *illustrates* the violence that the author imagines is being inflicted by breaths inside the body. The mechanics of that violence still have to be explained by the wind itself—its nature and its *dunamis*. At the same time, because there is no god behind the wind to assume responsibility for the damage, it is all the more important to know how exactly wind and breaths, absent a god's efficacious agency, cause harm. The author of *On Breaths* seems well aware that his account, clearly adapted to an epideictic context (and, hence, a lay

---

[54] See *Il.* 8.294, 13.786–87, 22.20; *Od.* 2.62, 10.69, 23.128. See also *Od.* 20.237 and 21.202, where *dunamis* is paired with the hands (γνοίης χ' οἵη ἐμὴ δύναμις καὶ χεῖρες ἕπονται). On the hand as a symbol of agency, see above, pp. 73–74.

[55] The idea of *dunamis* in Plato, moreover, resembles that found in medicine (Souilhé 1919; von Staden 1998). On the Presocratic evidence, see von Staden 1998.265, with n.16.

[56] *Dunameis* of food and drink: *Aff.* 47 (Li 6.254 = 70 Potter); *Vict.* II 39 (Li 6.534 = 162,9 Joly-Byl). *Pharmaka: Aff.* 18 (Li 6.228 = 32 Potter). Therapies: *Vict.* II 66 (Li 6.586 = 190,24 Joly-Byl). Body parts: *Morb. Sacr.* 16 (Li 6.390 = 29,4–5 Jouanna). Bodies: *Prog.* 1 (Li 2.112 = 194,4 Alex). I have drawn these examples from the more extensive list at von Staden 1998.274–75 nn.6–13.

[57] In this respect, naturalizing medicine in Greece anticipates what Michael Pollan has called "nutritionism" in contemporary Western culture (Pollan 2008). Think, for example, of an apple, with its familiar shape and familiar taste. Now think of being told about its antioxidant properties. The different relationship to the apple created by the "expert" information approximates what may have happened with the rise of naturalizing medicine in Greece.

[58] *Flat.* 3 (Li 6.94 = 106,2–10 Jouanna), 9 (Li 6.104 = 116,2–3 Jouanna).

audience), must respond to this question.[59] Indeed, at one point, he introduces a skeptical listener to ask just this: "So how [πῶς] do breaths cause fluxes? In what way [τίνα τρόπον] does wind cause hemorrhages in the chest?" (10, Li 6.104 = 116,10–12 Jouanna).

Answering these kinds of questions is no easy task. Part of the problem is that they require the author to provide an explanation not simply of a uniform power, for example, the capacity to cut. They require him to explain how breaths produce a series of events that collectively replace the sudden blow of a god's anger. We can see this process of replacement at work in a chapter from *On Regimen in Acute Diseases*, in which the author polemically advances his own explanation of those whom "the ancients" thought to be *blētoi*, "stricken," "just because the flanks of those who have died are found to be livid, *as if* a blow had been received [ἴκελόν τι πληγῇ]" (17, Li 2.260–62, ch. 5 = 43,4–6 Joly).[60] While the simile allows the author to acknowledge that the symptom is sudden and bruise-like, it also blocks the abduction of agency.[61] Having signaled his distance from daemonic blows, he offers his own *aition*, "account," of the symptom, focusing on the dangers of feeding a patient without first ensuring that the pain in his side has been "loosened."[62] It is this massed pain that becomes responsible for the livid mark on the body. That mark is thus appropriated by the medical writer to signal not unappeased anger but concealed pain below the skin. But what *is* pain here? And what happens to anger? Is it simply absorbed by the strangely concrete pain that the physician fails to relieve? One clue to the changes in the traditional story is the author's use of the passive voice when discussing harm: damage happens (βεβλάψεται, 16, Li 2.256, ch. 5 = 42,9 Joly), rather than being inflicted by an agent. This is true even though it is the physician who, by feeding the patient, commits the initial error. That error is not so much an act as a catalyst for a series of bad outcomes inside the *sōma* that "feed off one another" (ἀλλήλοισι συντιμωρεῖ) until finally "it"—whatever it is—is strong enough to cause death in most cases (καὶ ὅταν ἐς τοῦτο ἔλθῃ, θανατῶδες ὡς ἐπὶ τὸ πολύ ἐστι, 17, Li 2.262, ch. 5 = 43,12–13, 15–16 Joly).[63] Once the author eliminates the daemonic agent, then, anger and intention fragment into a series of events through which the power of "bad things" gains momentum. The bruise brings this power to light while cuing the unseen process of its accumulation.

The idea that trouble can grow from a small catalyst has deep roots in archaic

---

[59] On the epideictic nature of the treatise, see Jouanna 1988b.10–24.

[60] On the *blētoi*, cf. *Coac.* 394 (Li 5.672); *Morb.* II 8 (Li 7.16 = 139,1–140,6 Jouanna), 25 (Li 7.38–40 = 158,10–159,8 Jouanna); *Morb.* III 3 (Li 7.120–22 = 72,10–19 Potter). The conditions from which these patients suffer vary, however: for discussion of the differences, see Mansfeld 1980.374–78; Duminil 1992.

[61] See also, e.g., *Epid.* VII 11 (Li 5.384 = 60,2 Jouanna): a patient leaps up "*as if* from a blow" (ὥσπερ ἂν ἐκ πληγῆς).

[62] On these concepts—loosening (λύσις), coction (πεπασμός), and expulsion (ἔκκρισις) of the damaging humor—see further below, pp. 153–54.

[63] On the expression ὡς ἐπὶ τὸ πολύ, see von Staden 2002.

ideas about suffering. Solon, for example, writes in the sixth century BCE—in the context of disease—that, "from a small pain a great pain often arises" (πολλάκι δ' ἐξ ὀλίγης ὀδύνης μέγα γίγνεται ἄλγος, fr. 13.59 W²).[64] Yet the medical writers turn this maxim into a major conceptual tool capable of crowding out agent-based explanation: serious diseases tend to arise "from small catalysts" (ἀπὸ σμικρῶν προφασίων); they grow "bit by bit" (κατὰ [σ]μικρόν).[65] By depersonalizing cause and distributing power over a series of micro-events, these writers rewrite the drama behind the symptom in terms of physical processes.

I say "drama" because, despite elevating processes over agents, the medical writers do not give up the language of conflict and attack.[66] The hostility they describe, however, is transformed by the fact that power in their explanations is so fluid, untethered to the discrete aims of other minds. On the one hand, the *sōma* has a fundamentally agonal relationship to the world around it: every encounter is a high-stakes struggle for power. If, for example, the liver cannot resist the power of the wind, it cannot *not* suffer harm or escape pains.[67] In digestion, the cavity must conquer, through heat, whatever enters it.[68] If it fails to do so, normal processes of growth and life are reversed:

ἐπὴν δὲ μάσσον προσενέγκηται, ἢ ἀλλοίως μεταλλάξαν κρατῆται, κρατέουσι καὶ τὰ σιτία· καὶ ὁπόταν κρατῆται τὸ σῶμα ὑπὸ τῶν προσοισμάτων, [ἃ] θάλλειν ποιεῖ ταῦτα καὶ κρατέει ἅμα τοῦ σώματος τά τε ὑπεναντία ποιέουσιν. (*Loc.* 43, Li 6.336 = 80,15–18 Craik)

But when too much is administered, or being changed in some other way the body is mastered, then the foods, in fact, take control; and when the body is mastered by the things administered to it, the same things [that] make it thrive prevail over the body and produce the opposite effect.

Yet, on the other hand, as this passage makes clear, the hostility of the incoming foods is conditional. That is to say, the foods become hostile only at the moment they overpower the cavity. That which the cavity conquers and assimilates becomes nourishment.[69]

---

[64] On this passage, see Noussia 1999, who sees the influence of early naturalizing medicine.

[65] *Aff.* 33 (Li 6.244 = 56 Potter); *Morb.* IV 50 (Li 7.580 = 106,12 Joly); *Vict.* I 2 (Li 6.472 = 124,28–126,1 Joly-Byl).

[66] On the body as battlefield: Cambiano 1983.448–51; Vegetti 1983.463–65; von Staden 1999a; 2007a.22–24. On therapies in the battle against disease, see, e.g., *Acut. Sp.* 4 (Li 2.400, ch. 3 = 70,4–5 Joly); *Aff.* 20 (Li 6.230 = 36 Potter). On the physician or his tools as the adversaries of the disease, see von Staden 1990.87–89, 97–99.

[67] *VM* 22 (Li 1.632 = 152,1–11 Jouanna).

[68] See *Aff.* 47 (Li 6.256 = 70 Potter); *Salubr.* 7 (Li 6.82 = 216,12–17 Jouanna, as *Nat. Hom.* 22); *Vict.* III 75 (Li 6.616 = 206,32–34 Joly-Byl), 79 (Li 6.624 = 210,25–27 Joly-Byl); Anon. Lond. 5.39–6.4 (8 Diels). See also *Vict.* I 10 (Li 6.484 = 134,7–8 Joly-Byl): the cavity is the "nurse of all creatures suited to it, destroyer of those not suited" (ζῴων συμφόρων τροφόν, ἀσυμφόρων δὲ φθόρον).

[69] See also *Morb.* IV 36 (Li 7.552 = 89,26–90,4 Joly). There are some foods, however, such as cheese, at *VM* 20 (Li 1.622 = 147,1–4 Jouanna), that are always hostile to a specific stuff in the body.

The *sōma* has a similarly ambiguous relationship to its constituent stuffs. For when it fails to conquer things coming from outside, the power to harm is transferred to the things inside. Like a foodstuff, a humor is both beneficial and threatening. The pathogenic humor "innately belongs to the affected organism, but is functionally alien to it."[70] In medical writing, the capitulation of something in the body seems to make an enemy out of it, a process that continues until the whole body has turned (or been turned) against life: "The body, having changed and being ineffective and conquered by everything, begins to fester" (τὸ γὰρ σῶμα μετατρεπόμενον καὶ ὀλιγοεργὲς ἐὸν καὶ ὑπὸ παντὸς νικώμενον τὰς παλιγκοτίας παρέχει, *Loc.* 43, Li 6.338 = 80,25–26 Craik). Here is the paradox of corporeal change: it is precisely when the *sōma* has been conquered that it acquires the power to hurt itself. Culpability, diffuse and mobile, is attracted not only to things outside the *sōma* but also to the *sōma* itself.

Scholars of ancient medicine are familiar with the idea that the antagonism between inside and outside is always latent within the physical body, making that body highly fragile. By defamiliarizing the cliché of precarious balance, however, we can shed light on the physical body's emergence and, more specifically, on the way in which the conceptualization of that body allows it to appropriate the signs of the unseen world of daemonic agents. Crucial to this appropriation, as we have seen, is the idea of a cavity, an opaque inner space below the threshold of sensing that conceals fundamentally untrustworthy physical stuffs. I would like to examine this untrustworthiness by looking at one writer's account of how disease unfolds in the cavity. The text in question allows us to see how the symptom could be used to support not simply claims about cause but new narratives of suffering, narratives in which the physical body takes on blame even as culpability is fractured.

THE DYNAMICS OF THE CAVITY

Thus far we have been focusing primarily on clusters of symptoms with a diagnostic function, symptoms that enable the identification and, hence, the treatment of a disease. Symptoms, however, can also be used to track disease as a dynamic process. The dynamism of disease lies, on the one hand, in the fluxes it causes within the cavity and, on the other, in its identity as an incremental process that, barring successful treatment, often leads to death. Both these characteristics take on an exaggerated clarity in medical accounts of suppuration, a disease that causes putrefaction of the flesh and the humors, and dropsy,

---

[70] Bratescu 1990.275, my translation. The Anonymous Londinensis papyrus suggests that some thinkers did not see bile and phlegm as part of the healthy body: Thrasymachus of Sardis, for example, understood pus, bile, and phlegm as forms of blood corrupted by heat or cold (Anon. Lond. 11.42–12.8 = 17–18 Diels). The "Hippocrates" who appears in the text believes that "residues" of food left undigested in the cavity turn into pathogenic vapors (5.35–6.43 = 10 Diels).

which turns flesh to water; both conditions often supervene on other diseases.[71] The corruption of stuffs inside the body dominates Plato's vivid account of disease in the *Timaeus*, which is often seen as deeply informed by contemporary medical writing.[72] Equally vivid is the account of suppuration in *On Diseases* I, which tracks the outcome of a small tear in the inner tissue.[73]

The author of the treatise begins by reconstructing the tear's early history, before any symptoms appear. The flesh is torn through overexertion, but the tear is not signaled by the expectoration of blood. As it attracts moisture, the tear becomes slightly livid. Still, however, the patient either feels nothing because of his good health (μὴ αἰσθάνηται παθὼν ὑπὸ ῥώμης καὶ εὐεξίης) or, if he does sense something, deems it of no account (ἢν δὲ καὶ αἴσθηται, μηδὲν πρῆγμα ἡγήσηται, *Morb.* I 15, Li 6.166 = 38,9–10 Wittern).[74] The author thus tacitly registers a lag before symptoms appear. In so doing, he introduces at the outset a misalignment between the story of the seen and the story of the unseen, with the latter clearly privileged as the primary, more complete account.

The tear's presence becomes perceptible only when some exciting cause—a fever, perhaps, or sexual indulgence—dries and warms the injured tissue, forcing it to attract moisture from surrounding fleshes and vessels.[75] The process soon gets out of hand; one bad thing leads to another. Eventually the attracted moisture putrefies, and the flesh ulcerates and begins to melt away. Henceforth, the disease's victory is assured: "The harmful things flowing toward the pus overpower what flows off, and the fleshes are more wasted by the disease than nourished by the things coming in [αἱ δὲ σάρκες τηκόμεναι μᾶλλον ὑπὸ τῶν

---

[71] In *On Diseases* I, suppuration is dealt with at such length (esp. 11–22) that Ermerins identifies the treatise as the text περὶ ἐμπύων promised at *Aff.* 33 (Li 6.244 = 56 Potter). On dropsy, which is often fatal, see Skoda 1994.256–57, 263 and the description at *Aff.* 22 (Li 6.232–34 = 38–40 Potter): ὕδερος δὲ γίνεται τὰ μὲν πλεῖστα, ὅταν τις ἐκ νούσου μακρῆς ἀκάθαρτος διαφέρηται πολὺν χρόνον· φθείρονται γὰρ αἱ σάρκες καί τήκονται καὶ γίνονται ὕδωρ . . . τὸ δὲ ὕδωρ γίνεται οὕτως· ἐπειδὰν αἱ σάρκες ὑπὸ φλέγματος καὶ χρόνου καὶ νόσου καὶ ἀκαθαρσίης καὶ κακοθεραπείης καὶ πυρετῶν διαφθαρῶσι, τήκονται καὶ γίνονται ὕδωρ (Dropsy comes about, in most cases, when someone goes on for a long time after a lengthy illness in an unclean state; for the fleshes become corrupted, melt, and turn to water. . . . The water in dropsy arises as follows: when the fleshes become corrupted as the result of phlegm, the passage of time, disease, lack of cleanliness and bad treatment, and fevers, they melt and turn to water).

[72] See *Ti.* 81e6–86a8, esp. 82e2–83a5.

[73] *Morb.* I 15 (Li 6.166–68 = 38,5–40,17 Wittern). This author is particularly interested in integrating symptoms into a story of what is happening inside the body: "Il n'y a plus deux niveaux. Tout se fond chez lui dans un même langage: l'évidence des processus invisibles n'est pas moins forte pour lui que celle des phénomènes visibles" (Jouanna 1974.339). In other treatises, such as *On Affections* and *Internal Affections*, the symptom, while *implicated* in the etiological account, does not participate as systematically in a story about the disease. Note, too, that the account is written on the assumption that the patient is neglected (ἢν ἀμεληθῇ, 15, Li 6.166 = 36,19–20 Wittern; cf. 12, Li 6.160 = 28,10 Wittern; 14, Li 6.162 = 34,4 Wittern).

[74] On the patient's lack of awareness, see also *Morb.* I 13 (Li 6.160 = 28,20–30,3 Wittern); 22 (Li 6.184 = 64,11–12 Wittern).

[75] The attraction of fluids is a common mechanism in Hippocratic pathology: see Lonie 1981.266–68; Gundert 1992.460–62.

κακῶν ἢ τρεφόμεναι ὑπὸ τῶν ἐσιόντων]" (15, Li 6.168 = 42,4–7 Wittern). Yet, at the very moment the disease is acting most decisively, its power to act is most elusive. What commands the verb "to overpower" is not the disease or the tear but, rather, "harmful things that flow toward the pus" (πρὸς μὲν τὸ πύον τὰ ἐπιρρέοντα κακά).[76] The antagonist in this story, then, refuses to crystallize, even as verbal agency persists. In one scenario, in fact, the enemy is the cavity itself: though initially the subject of passive verbs—"to be heated," "to be melted," "to be disordered"—it eventually turns on the patient and kills (ἔφθειρε) him (15, Li 6.168 = 40,10 Wittern).[77]

What begins as a slight tear, then, becomes the locus of a growing and ultimately fatal force. It is important to remember, however, that the author's description of this transformation is largely speculative, conditioned by expectations about the humors, rather than confirmed by autopsy. In developing it, he counters the body's initial silence, making sense of its slow destruction by extending its deterioration into the concealed space-time of the cavity. From the beginning, his language, peppered with the prefix *hupo-*, fosters the sense of incremental deterioration. The tear initially attracts a little moisture and grows a little livid (ὑποπέλιος). Catalyzed by a further misstep on the part of the patient, it heats and dries a bit (ὑποξηραίνεται, ὑποθερμαίνεται). Symptoms begin to corroborate this gradualism: the pain is, at first, light, the cough intermittent. As the disease develops, the adjectives assigned to the symptoms intensify: the pain is stronger, the cough more frequent (ἰσχυροτέρην,[78] πυκνοτέρην). But the situation remains embryonic, as is shown by the transfer of the prefix *hupo-* to the track of the symptom: what is coughed up is a little purulent (ὑπόπυον), a little livid (ὑποπέλιον), a little bloody (ὕφαιμον). Nevertheless, the more time passes, the more moisture the tear draws to itself (ὅσῳ δ᾽ ἂν ὁ χρόνος προίῃ, ἕλκει τε μᾶλλον ἐς ἑωυτήν). When the tissue finally ulcerates, the symptoms become decisive: severe (ἰσχυρή) pain and frequent, violent (πυκνή, πολλή) coughing that produces unadulterated (εἰλικρινές) pus. Through all of this, the concealed events *inside* the *sōma* remain in the foreground, driving the narrative. Symptoms serve primarily as echoes of that story, rather than as sites of inference. Crucially, "the person" disappears from the scene after his failure to sense the lesion and reappears only as the object of the verb "to kill."

The idea of wasting diseases exercises a powerful hold on the Greek imagination. The process of disarticulation painstakingly described here calls to mind

---

[76] Such periphrases are common: see, e.g., *Loc.* 12 (Li 6.298 = 52,16 Craik): "the stuff flowing to the ears" (τοῦ ἐς τὰ ὦτα ῥέοντος) becomes pathogenic; 30 (Li 6.322 = 70,13 Craik): τὸ τὴν νοῦσον παρέχον. At *Epid.* II 1.7 (Li 5.78 = 24 Smith), the stuff that fixes is not the disease but something "from a strong disease" (ἐκ νούσου ἰσχυρῆς).

[77] Elsewhere, too, the κοιλίη is dangerous and lively: at *Int.* 6 (Li 7.180 = 90 Potter), it roars, turns, and rumbles (βρέμει . . . καὶ στρέφει καὶ βορβορύζει). On instances where the cavity is the subject of verbs of killing or maiming, see von Staden 1990.101–2.

[78] The reading of M, printed by Potter and Wittern. Θ gives ἰσχυρὴν.

the *dolikhē nousos*, "long disease," that Odysseus suspects as a cause of his mother's death in the *Odyssey* (11.172); in her response, Anticleia speaks of a disease that destroys life with "hateful wasting" (τηκεδόνι στυγερῇ, 201). Love's effects, too, are *takera*, "liquefying," in archaic poetry: like sleep, grief, and death itself, *erōs* undoes the articulation of the body.[79] In the Hippocratic account, however, dissolution is envisioned as a potentially seen physical process. The reader is invited to imagine the heating and the melting of the fleshy inner parts through a well-paced, detailed story in which verbal agency is artfully shunted from the wound to stuffs and tissues to the cavity itself, effectively shutting out the daemonic agent.[80] I am not denying that there are obvious continuities between the Hippocratic author's assumptions about wasting and those of an archaic poet. Nevertheless, by transferring the bulk of causal responsibility to unseen stuffs inside the cavity and specifying the mechanisms by which those stuffs cause harm, the medical author helps to transform the meaning of disease.

Such an explanatory shift needed to be defended. "In the face of entrenched beliefs," writes another medical author, "it is necessary to offer many proofs if you intend to persuade, by means of your account, a listener to turn away from the judgment he already holds" (ἀνάγκη ἐστὶ πρὸς τὰ ἰσχυρῶς δοκέοντα τὰ πολλὰ ἱστόρια ἐπάγεσθαι, εἴ τις μέλλει τὸν ἀκούοντα[81] ἐκ τῆς πρὶν γνώμης μεταστρέψαι τοῖσιν ἑωυτοῦ λόγοισι πείσειν, *Morb.* IV 56, Li 7.608 = 121,19–22 Joly). The same author also stresses the importance of offering what he calls an *alēthēs logos*, a "true story," designed, we can assume, to compete not only with the accounts of rival physicians but also with magico-religious stories about daemonic violence, stories animated by social agents and underwritten by an intuitive physics.[82] For, those who were minimizing or eliminating the role of daemonic agents in the classical period had to come up with a persuasive answer to the how question posed by listeners accustomed to the efficacy of divinized intention, as we have already seen with Socrates and Strepsiades in the *Clouds*, for example, or with the author of *On Breaths* and his hypothetical interlocutor. The author of *On Diseases* I, too, who in the prologue of the text imagines his reader engaged in a debate about healing with bedside rivals, is developing a narrative that uses symptoms to make a different kind of sense of

---

[79] For τακερός: Anacr. fr. 459 (*PMG*); *AP* 7.420; Ibyc. fr. 287 (*PMG*); Luc. *Am.* 14. For λυσιμελής, see Archil. fr. 196 (W²); Hes. *Th.* 121; Sappho fr. 130 (L-P), with Vermeule 1979.154–62.

[80] For the wasting demon, see *Od.* 5.394–97, with Laser 1983.63–64.

[81] ἀκούοντα M Erm. Joly: ἀκόντα [*sic*] Littré recc.

[82] On the "true story," see Lonie 1981.72–74. *On Diseases* IV may have been epideictic: see D. Manetti 1973.430. By the late fifth century, physical explanations of many diseases may have acquired credibility, at least in some (urban, elite) circles: see esp. *Morb. Sacr.* 1 (Li 6.352–54 = 3,1–4 Jouanna), where the author says that there are many diseases that no one considers sacred. But even in their arguments with rival physicians, those advancing physical explanations help to establish the *sōma* as the reality behind the symptom.

suffering and death. Much has been written about the importance of rhetoric to the physician.[83] What I would like to emphasize is that this rhetoric, together with the battery of techniques for seeing the unseen developed by physicians, not only transforms the meaning of disease but also facilitates the crystallization of the physical body *qua* conceptual object.

That the things inside the body turn so easily on a patient and that this turning is precipitated by nothing more than a misstep or an unfortunate encounter with an impersonal world are ideas deeply rooted in medicine's conceptualization of the physical body. Health is fragile. Of a recovering patient, one author writes, "Let him, having recently regained health, not run against the wind nor ride a horse nor [ride] in a wagon, and have him avoid shouting and excitement; for there is a risk of relapse, and it is necessary to take care [φυλάσσεσθαι χρὴ] with regard to all these things" (*Int.* 1, Li 7.170 = 76 Potter). The imperative to take care becomes something of a mantra, as we will see in chapter 4, issued to counteract the dangerous passivity of patients like those in *On Diseases* I 15, whose only actions are nonactions (*not* to perceive the trouble inside, *not* to recognize the meaning of whatever he does feel).

Both the persuasiveness of the physician's story and the power to take care rely on the disease's conformity to a kind of plot; plot minimizes the role of the cavity as a mysterious interval between catalysts and symptoms. Yet things inside the cavity often remain volatile and unpredictable, part of a dynamic whose laws appear beyond the physician's grasp. They thus retain something of the strange and threatening nature of the daemonic. I close this chapter by considering this aspect of the cavity before turning, in the next chapter, to those vital forces in the body that support health and life.

The Automatic Body

In *On Diseases* I 15, variations in the disease are so many routes to death. In other contexts, however, the treatise's author is unusually skeptical about the viability of prognosis.[84] Describing erysipelas, a localized inflammation of the skin, he gives the patient two to four days for the fluids that have accumulated in the lung to disperse—for *to endon*, "what is within," to move *exō*, "outward"—

---

[83] See esp. Edelstein 1967b; G. Lloyd 1979.86–98; 1987.56–70; Jouanna 1984; Humphreys 1996.12–13; van der Eijk 1997; Thomas 2000, esp. 249–54.

[84] See esp. *Morb.* I 16 (Li 6.168–70 = 42,8–44,3 Wittern), expressing skepticism about predictions of the number of days within which a patient will recover or die, with Edelstein 1967b.73–74 and Thivel 1981.232–33; see also the local skepticism of *Morb.* III 1 (Li 7.118 = 70,10–11 Potter). The uncertainty in *On Diseases* I appears to be related to the author's acute awareness of variability: it is not only bodies that differ from one another (διαφέρει . . . σῶμα σώματος), e.g., according to age (*Morb.* I 22, Li 6.182–88 = 62,14–70,3 Wittern), but also the affections, the seasons, and the patient's level of endurance (16, Li 6.170–72 = 42,8–44,3 Wittern). Nevertheless, he does not disavow completely the system of critical days and prognosis: see, e.g., 26 (Li 6.194 = 78,5–6 Wittern).

lest they putrefy and become dangerous. If this does not happen, the patient dies.[85] What causes this dispersal?

One answer appears in the methodological reflections at the beginning of the treatise. There we learn that foremost among the factors that complicate prognosis are *tukhē* and *to automaton*, "the spontaneous." In acknowledging contingency, however, the author is also seeking to contain it. He first identifies those diseases in which bad things, including death, necessarily follow, and then distinguishes these from diseases whose outcomes are uncertain.[86] For these latter cases, he goes on to designate two classes of events that encourage or thwart the disease: things that happen to patients *apo tou automatou*, "spontaneously," and those achieved by therapy through good or bad fortune, of which the turning inward or outward of epysipelas is an example.[87] The sense of necessity that drives his account of suppuration thus expands to admit apparent indeterminacy. Whereas the Hippocratic triangle traditionally joins the disease and the physician to the patient, here the third point is occupied by *to automaton* or *tukhē*. Insofar as this third actor may harm or help, it acts as a wild card, disrupting the story's regularity and collapsing distinctions between protagonist and antagonist.

By including *tukhē* and *to automaton* within the scope of *tekhnē*, the author would seem to be defending a delicate position.[88] Indeed, placed alongside other medical texts, *On Diseases* I looks strikingly heterodox. It is true that the author of *On the Tekhnē*, for example, accepts that some patients might chance upon the same treatments a physician would have prescribed.[89] Yet, to the extent the physician grasps the effect of each therapy in advance—although the author is willing to concede there are things medicine does not yet know, he is confident that everything about the body *can* be known—he has no need for *tukhē*.[90] Even greater optimism is on display in *On Places in a Human Being*:

ἰητρικὴ δή μοι δοκεῖ ἤδη ἀνευρῆσθαι ὅλη, ἥτις οὕτως ἔχει, ἥτις διδάσκει ἕκαστα καὶ τὰ ἤθεα καὶ τοὺς καιρούς. ὃς γὰρ οὕτως ἰητρικὴν ἐπίσταται, ἐλάχιστα τὴν τύχην ἐπιμένει, ἀλλὰ καὶ ἄνευ τύχης καὶ σὺν τύχῃ εὖ ποιηθείη ἄν. βέβηκε γὰρ ἰητρικὴ πᾶσα, καὶ φαίνεται τῶν σοφισμάτων τὰ κάλλιστα ἐν αὐτῇ συγκείμενα ἐλάχιστα τύχης δεῖσθαι· ἡ γὰρ τύχη αὐτοκρατὴς καὶ οὐκ ἄρχεται, οὐδ᾽ ἐπ᾽ εὐχῇ ἐστιν αὐτὴν

---

[85] *Morb.* I 18 (Li 6.172 = 46,18–20 Wittern). See also *Aph.* VI.25 (Li 4.568 = 184 Jones); *Coac.* 360 (Li 5.660).

[86] *Morb.* I 3 (Li 6.142–46 = 6,13–10,12 Wittern).

[87] *Morb.* I 8 (Li 6.154 = 20,19–20, 22,10 Wittern). See also Democr. (DK68) B275 on ἐπιτυχίη/ ἀτυχίη.

[88] Jori 2002.208 argues that the recognition of contingency so compromises the conditions of "correctness" and "incorrectness" in medicine as to strip those terms, and the very idea of a *tekhnē*, of meaning. I discuss this objection further below. On the opposition *tukhē-tekhnē*, see Schiefsky 2005a.5–13, with further bibliography.

[89] *Art.* 5 (Li 6.6–8 = 228,6–230,2 Jouanna); see also *Aff.* 45 (Li 6.254 = 68 Potter).

[90] See also *VM* 1 (Li 1.570–72 = 118,10–119,4 Jouanna).

ἐλθεῖν· ἡ δ᾽ ἐπιστήμη ἄρχεταί τε καὶ εὐτυχής ἐστιν, ὁπόταν βούληται ὁ ἐπιστάμενος χρῆσθαι. ἔπειτα τί καὶ δεῖται ἰητρικὴ τύχης; (*Loc.* 46, Li 6.342 = 84,17–25 Craik)

> Medicine in its present state, it seems to me, has now been fully discovered insofar as it teaches the details and the constitutions and the correct measures. For if someone knows medicine in this way, he waits the least for luck, but, with or without luck, everything is properly accomplished. For all medicine has been founded, and the finest of its accepted methods seem to be in little need of luck. For chance takes its power from itself and cannot be ruled, and does not come at one's wish. But knowledge can be commanded and successful, whenever the person who knows wishes to make use of his knowledge. Why, then, does medicine have any need of luck?

Knowledge, in short, enables control not only over the depths of the body, as we saw early in this chapter, but over the factor of arbitrariness that so often thwarts or unexpectedly rewards mortal ambitions. Whereas *tukhē* is self-ruled, refusing any and all masters, including prayer, knowledge is available whenever the knower wishes to use it. For this writer, then, *tukhē* simply names ignorance about when and how to act on the body.

What about *to automaton*? The author of *On the Tekhnē*, in addition to his remarks on *tukhē*, has a categorical observation to make on this subject, too:

ὅπου οὖν οὐδὲν οὔτ᾽ ἐν τοῖσιν ἀγαθοῖσι τῶν ἰητρῶν οὔτ᾽ ἐν τῇ ἰητρικῇ αὐτῇ ἀχρεῖόν ἐστιν, ἀλλ᾽ ἐν τοῖσι πλείστοισι τῶν τε φυομένων καὶ τῶν ποιευμένων ἔνεστιν τὰ εἴδεα τῶν θεραπειῶν καὶ τῶν φαρμάκων, οὐκ ἔστιν ἔτι οὐδενὶ τῶν ἄνευ ἰητροῦ ὑγιαζομένων τὸ αὐτόματον αἰτιήσασθαι ὀρθῷ λόγῳ· τὸ μὲν γὰρ αὐτόματον οὐδὲν φαίνεται ἐὸν ἐλεγχόμενον· πᾶν γὰρ τὸ γινόμενον διά τι εὑρίσκοιτ᾽ ἂν γινόμενον, καὶ ἐν τῷ διά τι τὸ αὐτόματον οὐ φαίνεται οὐσίην ἔχον οὐδεμίαν ἀλλ᾽ ἢ ὄνομα. (*Art.* 6, Li 6.10 = 230,9–18 Jouanna)

> Seeing that there is nothing that is without a use for good physicians or for the art of medicine itself, but the greater part of things that grow or are made constitute the forms of treatments and drugs, it is not possible for anyone who recovers without a physician to credit the spontaneous with any justification. For the spontaneous turns out not to exist on examination. For everything that happens would be found to do so on account of something, and given this "on account of something," the spontaneous appears to have no other existence than as a name.

While this author can accept *tukhē* on the grounds that patients sometimes unwittingly help themselves, he cannot admit ignorance at the level of the body, where things necessarily happen *dia ti*, "because of something." But does the author of *On Diseases* I allow for spontaneity in this sense? That is, does he allow gaps and jumps in physical reality?[91]

---

[91] See Jori 2002.200, referring to *smagliature* and *salti*. Aristotle accuses the early atomists of the same error—admitting chance into a system supposedly governed by law and necessity (*Phys.*

If there is a gap at work in *On Diseases* I, it exists because the physician has a limited perspective on the causal series within the body. That is, in scenarios where *tukhē* and *to automaton* come into play, the inside of the physical body stands as the interval par excellence, that is, a space open to forms of unpredictable interference. Unpredictability appears to result not from the interference of something outside the causal laws accepted elsewhere in the treatise but, rather, from the nature of the *sōma* itself, and particularly the labile quality of the humors. Like a Homeric warrior, the author knows which wounds make death a foregone conclusion. He knows what kind of damage (e.g., head wounds, severed cords) necessarily produces certain effects.[92] At a certain point, though, the complex behaviors of things inside the body frustrate his understanding. By leaving room for *tukhē* and *to automaton*, this medical writer captures the symptom's inextricability from the daemonic, understood not as a divinized plane of reality but as a volatile economy of impersonal forces.

It is hardly sufficient, however, to equate the humors with contingency. After all, most medical speculation about disease relies on knowledge of how humors work. Moreover, despite his distrust (though not rejection) of prognosis, the author of *On Diseases* I is committed to considerable regularity in the disease process. So a bit more precision is needed.

We can first recognize that *tukhē* and *to automaton* are not quite the same things. The former characterizes the success or failure of the physician's actions. What happens "automatically," on the other hand, seems to be accomplished in (by?) the cavity without technical intervention.[93] When Herodotus reports that Egyptians shave their eyebrows if a household cat has died *apo tou automatou* (2.66), it is likely he is talking about what we would call the cat's natural death.[94] Something of this sense of mysteriousness in living things is perhaps present, too, when the medical authors contrast what happens because of the physician's drugs with what happens automatically. For example, the recovery process can be disrupted either by things administered or *apo tou automatou*; patients may recover *automatoi*, "on their own"; the belly may become disordered *automatē*, "by itself," without the physician administering a drug.[95] On one occasion, we

---

196a24–35 = Democr. [DK68] A69). But cf. DK68 A70 (Aët. 1.29.7), with C. Taylor 1999b.185–89, suggesting that Democritus calls *tukhē* what is beyond human understanding. I argue the same meaning is present in *On Diseases* I.

[92] *Morb.* I 3 (Li 6.142–44 = 6,13–8,2 Wittern), 4 (Li 6.146 = 10,13–12,3 Wittern).

[93] At *Morb.* I 7 (Li 6.154 = 20,16–17 Wittern), the expression ἀπὸ τοῦ αὐτομάτου καὶ ἀπὸ ἐπιτυχίης does refer to a series of events not involving the physician, but the author seems interested in drawing a contrast between everything that happens independently of the physician's knowledge and what he controls; he is adamant that *tukhē* lies outside the boundaries of knowledge and ignorance. In the following list of things blamed on *tukhē*, virtually every event is triggered by the administration of a drug.

[94] See also Pl. *Ap.* 38c5; Th. 2.77; X. *An.* 1.3.13. In Homer, αὐτόματος describes the gates of Olympus, which open by themselves, albeit in response to someone's intention (*Il.* 5.749).

[95] *VM* 21 (Li 1.624 = 148,6–7 Jouanna); *Morb.* II 71 (Li 7.108 = 210,15 Jouanna); *Nat. Hom.* 12 (Li 6.64 = 200,9–12 Jouanna). See also, e.g., *Acut.* 19 (Li 2.266, ch. 6 = 44,10–13 Joly); *Aph.* I.2

find a bodily change that happens automatically contrasted to one that happens because of a *prophasis*, which here probably means a "manifest" (rather than simply an "external") cause.[96] In many (but not all) of these cases, the "automatic" and, hence, hard-to-predict outcome involves the fluid dynamics of the humors, such as when and especially where a flux will occur or whether the cavity will be set in motion.[97] In contrast, authors seem more confident about specific causal mechanisms and the logic of deterioration, with its transubstantiation of stuffs (e.g., if blood flows into the upper cavity, it necessarily turns to pus).

Despite the many mechanisms that connect the catalyst and the symptom, then, the unstable identity of the foodstuff or the humor—beneficial or harmful—haunts the body as a complex system. Insofar as what happens spontaneously can either help or harm, the physical body and, more specifically, the cavity, is conceptualized as a terrain of unruly forces only contingently aligned with health. In fact, these forces can be seen as hard to control and potentially dangerous even when they are accomplishing something good:

φάρμακον δὲ μήτ᾽ ἰνηθμῷ μήτ᾽ ἐμετήριον [πιόντος add. Joly], χολὴ ἐπὴν αὐτομάτη ῥαγῇ ἢ κάτω ἢ ἄνω, χαλεπωτέρη παύειν· ἡ γὰρ αὐτομάτη ὑπὸ βίης γινομένης τῷ σώματι βιῆται· ἢν δ᾽ ὑπὸ φαρμάκου ῥέῃ, οὐχ ὑπὸ συγγενέος βιῆται. (*Loc.* 33, Li 6.326 = 72,12–15 Craik)

When bile breaks out spontaneously in either the upper or the lower part of a patient [who has taken] neither a laxative nor an emetic drug, it is harder to stop. For spontaneous (bile) is forced by a power with its origin in the body; whereas if it flows by the action of a drug, it is not forced by what is innate.

If the author is uneasy about the power of a *biē*, "force," with origins in the *sōma*, his concern appears due to the fact that, although this force mimics the action of the physician's purgatives, it threatens to subvert technical control. The spontaneous flux of bile does not "know" how or when to stop; the physician may or may not succeed in imposing measure on it. Left to its own devices, the *sōma* gets carried away by its predisposition to instability.

In the end, the remarks about *tukhē* in *On Diseases* I are not so anomalous. They seem strange only because they so openly acknowledge the volatile complexity of the physical body that is a quiet constant in many other texts. Even the author of *On Places in a Human Being*, so confident about *tekhnē*, turns out

---

(Li 4.458 = 98 Jones); *Artic.* 46 (Li 4.198 = 175,6–8 Kühlewein); *Genit./Nat. Puer.* 18 (Li 7.502 = 62,14–15 Joly); *Hum.* 5 (Li 5.482 = 70 Jones); *Int.* 21 (Li 7.218 = 140 Potter), 42 (Li 7.272 = 214 Potter); *Morb.* I 19 (Li 6.174 = 50,8–9 Wittern); *Morb.* II 30 (Li 7.48 = 165,14–16 Jouanna); *Mul.* I 7 (Li 8.34 = 102,14 Grensemann), 36 (Li 8.86 = 128,19–20 Grensemann), 40 (Li 8.98); *Superf.* 7 (Li 8.480 = 74,28–29 Lienau); *Ulc.* 8 (Li 6.406 = 56,15 Duminil). Less common is the verb αὐτοματίζω, e.g., *Acut. Sp.* 33 (Li 2.464, ch. 11 = 85,3 Joly). See also the expression at *Morb.* II 53 (Li 7.82 = 191,2–3 Jouanna): ἐπὴν αὐτὸς ἑωυτοῦ δοκῇ ἄριστα τοῦ σώματος ἔχειν.
[96] *Prorrh.* II 20 (Li 9.48 = 262 Potter).
[97] Initiating fluxes in the body is often dangerous: see von Staden 2007a.28–32.

to acknowledge not only the unruliness of innate forces but also good and bad luck in practice.[98] Moreover, *to automaton* does not keep the author of *On Diseases* I from making sense of disease. Rather, it introduces elements of uncertainty into that account. The degree of uncertainty leads him to restrict the predictive capacity of symptoms.

Elsewhere in the extant medical writings, however, symptoms refer precisely to specific outcomes (recovery, relapse, death). They thus support prognosis, rather than diagnosis or universalizing claims. This is not to say that humoral pathology ceases to matter. Yet the focus shifts to the battle between the *sōma* and the disease. One consequence of this shift, I argue, is that the nature of the *sōma* emerges with greater visibility in these contexts, not only as an opponent of the disease but also as the mysterious substratum of the person.

---

[98] See *Loc.* 24 (Li 6.316 = 64,29–30 Craik) on the most dangerous fluxes: ἐπιτυχὼν μὲν γὰρ ὑγιέα ποιήσεις, ἀτυχήσας δέ, ὅπερ καὶ ὡς ἔμελλε γίνεσθαι, τοῦτ᾽ ἔπαθε (for if you are lucky, you will create health, but if you fail, the patient suffers that which was likely to have happened anyway).

CHAPTER FOUR

Signs of Life and Techniques of Taking Care

The privilege of freedom carries the burden of need and
means precarious being. For the ultimate condition for the
privilege lies in the paradoxical fact that living substance, by
some original act of segregation, has taken itself out of the
general integration of things in the physical context, set itself
over against the world, and introduced the tension of "to be
or not to be" into the neutral assuredness of existence.

Hans Jonas

We master by means of *tekhnē* what we are conquered
by in nature.

Antiphon

WE HAVE BEEN WATCHING the medical writers interpret symptoms by making
imaginative leaps into the depths of the physical body. Their patients, however,
have remained largely at the margins. They take on sharper contours if we turn
to the case histories gathered in the seven *Epidemics*, a diverse group of treatises written by a number of different authors and dating from the late fifth and
early to mid-fourth centuries.[1] Here are the last days in the life of one Apellaeus, a wrestler who has been ill on and off for two years, as chronicled in
Epidemics V.

ἔχων δὲ τὸ σῶμα ἐπίχολον, παλαίσας πολλά, μάλα ἐρρίγωσε καὶ πυρετὸς ἐπέλαβε,
καὶ ἡ νοῦσος ἐς νύκτα. τῇ δ᾽ ὑστεραίη ἐδόκει ὑγιὴς εἶναι αὐτῷ, καὶ τῇ ἑτέρῃ. τῇ δ᾽
ἐπιούσῃ νυκτὶ ἡ νοῦσος ἐπέλαβε δεδειπνηκότα ἀπὸ πρώτου ὕπνου καὶ εἶχε τὴν

---

[1] Scholars typically divide the seven *Epidemics* into three groups: *Epidemics* I and III (dated on in-
scriptional evidence from Thasos to 410 BCE); *Epidemics* II, IV, and VI, dated by Deichgräber to the
early fourth century (though see the discussion of Deichgräber's dating at Grmek 1989.314–17,
317–19 on the grouping of II, IV, and VI); and *Epidemics* V and VII, dated to the mid-fourth century. On the *Epidemics*, see the general overview at Jouanna 2000.vii–xvii; see further the papers in
Baader and Winau 1989 and Langholf 1990.

νύκτα καὶ τὴν ἡμέρην μέχρι δορπηστοῦ· ἔθανε πρὶν ἐμφρονῆσαι . . . καὶ ὅτε δοκέοι διαναπεπαῦσθαι, κῶμα εἶχε καὶ ἔρρεγχε καὶ αὖτις ἐξεδέχετο ἡ νοῦσος. (*Epid.* V 22, Li 5.222 = 14,9–15, 17–18 Jouanna)

Given that he had a bilious body, after much wrestling, he had severe chills, fever seized him, and the illness seized him toward night. The next day he seemed well to himself, and on the next, too. The following night, after dinner, the sickness seized him after his first sleep, and so continued that night and the next day until dinner. He died before returning to his senses. . . . And whenever he seemed to get a moment of respite, coma held him, he would wheeze, and again the disease would usurp power.

Apellaeus, at first glance, does not seem so unlike the anonymous patient of *On Diseases* I 15. That patient, we can recall, appears briefly at the moment he failed to notice an internal lesion and reappears only when, after a series of escalating mishaps, it brings about his death. In a similar way, Apellaeus is given two important verbs: "to seem," which, in light of the eventual outcome, draws attention to his *illusion* of health, and "to die."[2] The disease, on the other hand, named three times, controls, with its symptoms, a series of verbs that call to mind daemonic violence:[3] *epilambanō*, "to seize"; *ekhō*, "to take hold"; and *ekdekhomai*, which usually means "to succeed in power," "to usurp."[4] Rather than explain this language in terms of latent archaism, we can read it in terms of the author's shift of focus vis-à-vis the texts examined in the previous chapter. Symptoms in this passage mark not so much a series of events inside the body as a struggle between two distinct forces, as the final verb, "to usurp," drives home. It is not exactly Apellaeus himself pitted against the disease. And yet his insistent presence makes it clear what is at stake in this fight: a human life. What does it mean to say this life belongs to Apellaeus?

In this chapter, I explore how an innate tendency toward life emerges in medicine's field of vision and how the nature of that life reshapes ideas about the person in medicine, as well as in a wider cultural context in the classical period. In considering the function of symptoms in prognosis, I argue that, by investing the symptom with value ("good" or "bad"), the physician enables it to refer not only to an implicit story unfolding in the cavity but also to the respective strengths of the agonists battling for control. One of these agonists, as the case of Apellaeus vividly illustrates, is the disease. The other is a force that, until now, has been blurry and elusive—namely, something in the *sōma* that safeguards not only basic functions but also those phenomena and behaviors most

---

[2] The verb δοκέω is sometimes used to distance the physician-writer from what the patient reports, e.g., *Epid.* II 2.24 (Li 5.96 = 42 Smith); *Epid.* V 43 (Li 5.232 = 21,12 Jouanna); *Epid.* VII 25 (Li 5.394 = 66,16–17 Jouanna). But it does not always imply a mismatch between appearance and reality. It can also mark how something feels to the physician or should feel to the patient, e.g., *Artic.* 50 (Li 4.224 = 188,14–17 Kühlewein); *Morb.* II 16 (Li 7.30 = 151,5–6 Jouanna).

[3] On "daemonic" verbs with the disease, see Jouanna 1988a; 1990a; 1999.335–36.

[4] E.g., Hdt. 1.16, 103.

essential to human nature, including the use of language, mental lucidity, and individual appearance. As this vital force emerges with greater clarity, we will see that the origins of the embodied subject in medicine are located in the same mysterious place from which symptoms arise.

In the latter part of the chapter, I demonstrate how physiological concepts of the human interact with the idea of technical agency, that is, strategies of manipulating the physical body informed by expert knowledge. I sketch out two positions of knowledge vis-à-vis the physical body, that of the patient and that of the physician, and explore how the technical agency identified with the physician informs the patient's relationship to his body. For if the patient's ignorance about the physical body makes him more vulnerable to its instability, medicine, with the knowledge it offers, enables him to exercise control over the flux in which he is riskily embedded. Indeed, in some quarters the care of the *sōma* has become an urgent task by the end of the fifth century, coloring the impersonal world of the cavity with ethical meaning. That urgency goes a long way toward explaining why medicine comes to the forefront of debates about how to define human nature, as well as how to protect it.

THE PROGNOSTIC SYMPTOM: FORCES OF LIFE AND DEATH

Symptoms, as we have seen, respond to different kinds of questions in medical writing. If we want to understand how they work in prognosis, we can begin by looking at a case from *Prognostic* that covers the same ground as *On Diseases* I 15.[5] Both treatises share the idea that bile and phlegm, if not evacuated from places where they have accumulated in excess, will putrefy. The technical terms that we find in *Prognostic*, such as *to empuēma*, *hē ekpuēsis*, and *hoi empuoi*, confirm, in fact, that concern about suppuration is common in naturalizing medicine and, indeed, by the fourth century, in the wider public exposed to it: the speaker in Demosthenes' *Against Conon*, for example, recounts being told by his physician that, absent a spontaneous hemorrhage of blood (κάθαρσις αἵματος αὐτομάτη), he would have died *empuos* (54.12).[6] Yet, unlike the author of *On Diseases* I, the author of *Prognostic* is not interested in describing the process of suppuration. Instead, he uses symptoms to predict whether the patient will live or die and when.[7] The prognosis begins pessimistically: if suppuration

---

[5] *Prog.* 15 (Li 2.146–50 = 212,1–214,2 Alex).

[6] The passage is even more interesting for showing physicians using the idea of *apostasis* (see below) to explain to patients what was happening to them.

[7] See *Prog.* 1 (Li 2.112 = 194,8–9 Alex): τοὺς ἀποθανουμένους τε καὶ σωθησομένους προγινώσκων τε καὶ προλέγων. For προλέγω, see also *Acut. Sp.* 24 (Li 2.442–44, ch. 10 = 80,4–6 Joly); *Prorrh.* II 2 (Li 9.10, ch. 1 = 222 Potter). The verb προλέγω has been interpreted as both "to predict" and "to speak publicly," and perhaps has both connotations: see Marzullo 1986–87.213–15. The public nature of prediction is stressed by Edelstein 1967b.69–70, influentially arguing that prognosis increased trust in the physician, improved his reputation, and established a consensus about treatment.

begins on the seventh day of the disease, while the patient is still coughing up bilious stuff, death will arrive on the fourteenth. Following this damning pronouncement, however, we find a conditional clause that opens up another outcome: the patient will die *unless* a good symptom supervenes. The opening up of temporally circumscribed possibilities, together with the promise of navigating them, brings us to the prognostic symptom.

One of the defining characteristics of prognosis in classical medical writing is that it designates specific zones of the body and classes of phenomena, such as the patient's urine, breathing, and posture, as particularly meaningful. The physician assigns meaning—and, more specifically, value—to these phenomena on the basis of what they communicate about a desired end, that is, recovery: white, smooth, homogeneous urine is a good sign; cold breath is a fatal one.[8] Typically, a single symptom is not sufficient to predict an outcome, unless that outcome is a single dramatic event like a hemorrhage or a spasm.[9] More often, symptoms are part of a group of signs realized in different bodily zones, not only synchronically, but also diachronically, at critical times over the course of days and weeks.[10] Therefore, if the physician wishes to make a prognosis, he needs to evaluate a specific set of signs vis-à-vis one another, taking into account both the good and the bad.[11]

See also Pagel 1939.388–89; Horstmanshoff 1990.181–82; von Staden 1990.110–11. But prognosis also risked eroding trust, as we see at *Prorrh.* II 2 (Li 9.10 = 222 Potter), and casting the physician as a showy diviner: see *Prorrh.* II 2 (Li 9.8 = 220 Potter): οὐ μαντεύσομαι. See also T. Barton 1994.140–43 on charges that Galen was a diviner. For the relationship of prognosis to divination, see further Marzullo 1986–87; Radici Colace 1992; Fausti 2002.

[8] *Prog.* 5 (Li 2.122 = 199,7–8 Alex), 12 (Li 2.138–40 = 208,4–5 Alex). Langholf 1983 and 1990.162–64 sees traces of a "questionnaire" in the symptoms reported in the *Epidemics* and *Prognostic*.

[9] σημεῖα αἱμορροώδεα, e.g., *Coac.* 306 (Li 5.650); [σημεῖα] σπασμώδεα, e.g., *Prorrh.* I 28 (Li 5.516 = 78,4 Polack), 104 (Li 5.542 = 89,1–2 Polack). These single symptoms are most common in compilations like *Coan Prenotations, Crises, Critical Days,* and *Prorrhetic* I.

[10] While sometimes it does not matter to their value when symptoms occur, e.g., *Acut. Sp.* 26 (Li 2.448, ch. 10 = 81,9–12 Joly), symptoms are often favorable at one point, less favorable at another, e.g., *Prog.* 14 (Li 2.146 = 211,10–13 Alex). If the disease disappears on a day that is *not* critical, it usually indicates death or relapse, e.g., *Prog.* 23 (Li 2.178 = 225,6–8 Alex); *Prorrh.* II 21 (Li 9.50 = 264 Potter). On critical days, see esp. *Epid.* I 26 (Li 2.680, ch. 12 = 202,5–8 Kühlewein). See also *Acut. Sp.* 21 (Li 2.436, ch. 9 = 78,7–9 Joly); *Carn.* 19 (Li 8.612–14 = 202,7–16 Joly); *Morb.* IV 46–47 (Li 7.572–76 = 100,23–103,16 Joly). On critical days and number theory, see Lichtenthaeler 1963.110–11; Thivel 1981.216–36; and esp. Langholf 1990.79–118. On critical signs (τὰ κρίσιμα [σημεῖα], τὰ κρίνοντα): *Epid.* IV 45 (Li 5.186 = 138 Smith), 46 (Li 5.188 = 142 Smith); *Epid.* VI 3.21 (Li 5.302 = 72,6–8 Manetti-Roselli); *Hum.* 5 (Li 5.482–84 = 70 Jones), 6 (Li 5.484–86 = 72 Jones). All these treatises are traditionally dated to the early fourth century, suggesting that the formalization of critical signs may be a slightly later phenomenon than that of critical days. The *krisis* doctrine itself is present but undeveloped in the nosological treatises, becoming significant in the *Epidemics* and related treatises: see Thivel 1981.174–89, 216–36; Langholf 1990.61–68, 119–35.

[11] *Prog.* 15 (Li 2.150 = 213,13–14 Alex). See also *Prog.* 12 (Li 2.142 = 209,6–7 Alex), 17 (Li 2.158 = 217,2–3 Alex), 19 (Li 2.164 = 219,8–12 Alex), 22 (Li 2.174 = 223,7–9 Alex), 24 (Li 2.188 = 230,1–3 Alex); *Prorrh.* II 15 (Li 9.40 = 256 Potter), 22 (Li 9.50 = 266 Potter). Lichtenthaeler 1963.125–27 goes so far as to treat signs as mathematical factors. But the common verbs suggest evaluation,

To make these kinds of evaluations, the physician may have relied on a text like *Prognostic*. One of the author's basic assumptions is that all acute diseases (i.e., diseases that come to a "decision" at specific times) unfold as predictable clusters of events.[12]

εὖ μέντοι χρὴ εἰδέναι περὶ τε τῶν τεκμηρίων καὶ τῶν ἄλλων σημείων καὶ μὴ λανθάνειν ὅτι ἐν παντὶ ἔτει καὶ πάσῃ χώρῃ[13] τά τε κακὰ κακόν τι σημαίνει καὶ τὰ χρηστὰ ἀγαθόν, ἐπεὶ καὶ ἐν Λιβύῃ καὶ ἐν Δήλῳ καὶ ἐν Σκύθῃσι φαίνεται τὰ προγεγραμμένα ἀληθεύοντα σημεῖα. εὖ οὖν χρὴ εἰδέναι ὅτι ἐν τοῖσι αὐτοῖσι χωρίοισιν οὐδὲν δεινὸν τὸ μὴ οὐχὶ τὰ πολλαπλάσια ἐπιτυγχάνειν, ἢν ἐκμαθών τις αὐτὰ κρίνειν τε καὶ ἐκλογίζεσθαι ὀρθῶς ἐπίστηται. ποθεῖν δὲ χρὴ οὐδενὸς νοσήματος τοὔνομα, ὅτι μὴ τυγχάνει ἐνθάδε γεγραμμένον. ἅπαντα γὰρ ὁκόσα ἐν τοῖσι χρόνοισι τοῖσι προειρημένοισι κρίνεται, γνώσῃ τοῖσιν αὐτοῖσι σημείοισι. (*Prog.* 25, Li 2.188–90 = 230,11–231,8 Alex)

Certainly it is necessary to know about the indices and the other signs and not overlook the fact that in every season and in every land bad signs signify something bad and beneficial ones something good, since the aforementioned signs prove to be true in Libya and in Delos and in Scythia. One must know, then, that there is nothing strange in the fact that someone hits upon the truth in the same regions in the majority of cases, if he, having learned them thoroughly, knows how to judge and calculate the signs correctly. And one ought not regret the absence of the name of any disease, because it is not written here. For you will know by the same signs all those diseases that come to a crisis at the times I have stated.

The expression "you will know x by y," familiar from chapter 3, here designates a startlingly vast field of knowledge to be targeted by a limited group of symptoms, namely, *all* acute diseases.[14] Of course, in practice, there is always the threat that symptoms will appear in a manner "entirely disordered, irregular, and uncritical" (πάνυ ἀτάκτως καὶ πεπλανημένως καὶ ἀκρίτως, *Epid.* I 8, Li 2.626 = 187,17–18 Kühlewein). Still, the alpha-privative adverbs in this passage, in capturing what is lost, recall what prognosis seeks: the organization of phenomena into a limited number of sequences with circumscribed outcomes.

Returning to the shifting mélange of phenomena at *Prognostic* 15, we can see how symptoms are weighed in practice. Recall that if empyema forms on the

---

rather than calculation, as di Benedetto 1966.322, 327–30 points out: ἀναλογίζομαι: *Prorrh.* II 7 (Li 9.26 = 240 Potter); σκέπτομαι: *Prorrh.* II 14 (Li 9.38 = 252 Potter); συμβάλλομαι: *Prog.* 20 (Li 2.172 = 222,7 Alex); τεκμαίρομαι: *Prog.* 17 (Li 2.158 = 217,3 Alex); ὑποσκέπτομαι: *Prog.* 18 (Li 2.158 [printing ἐπισκέπτομαι] = 217,6 Alex). The weighing of signs to achieve an overall impression recurs in the physiognomic tradition: Gleason 1995.33–37.

[12] Contrast *Epid.* III 16 (Li 3.100–102 = 232,7–19 Kühlewein), where prognosis requires knowing the constitution of the seasons and the patient.

[13] χώρῃ C' Jones: ὥρῃ other MSS Kühlewein Alex.

[14] The author's polemical rejection of disease names may be directed at the model used in nosological treatises. See also *Acut.* 3 (Li 2.226–28, ch. 1 = 37,4–10 Joly).

seventh day, death arrives on the fourteenth, unless something good (e.g., easy respiration, painlessness) happens. Having specified these good signs, the author predicts that, should all of these signs occur, the patient will survive; if only *some* of them occur, the patient will live another fourteen days, then die at some point after. He goes on to catalog the bad symptoms, a mirror image of the good ones: if one of them appears and the patient is still coughing up the wrong kind of stuff, he will die within fourteen days, on the ninth or eleventh day. Symptoms, then, can both confirm dangerous tendencies and mitigate, at least temporarily, signs of trouble.[15] In another case, trouble is averted only after part of the body has been sacrificed:

ἢν γὰρ εὐπετέως φέρων φαίνηται τὸ κακὸν ἢ καὶ ἄλλο τι τῶν περιεστικῶν σημείων πρὸς τούτοισιν ἐπιδεικνύῃ, τὸ νόσημα ἐς ἀπόστασιν τρέπεσθαι, ὥστε τὸν μὲν ἄνθρωπον περιγενέσθαι, τὰ δὲ μελανθέντα τοῦ σώματος ἀποπεσεῖν. (*Prog.* 9, Li 2.132–34 = 205,3–7 Alex)

For if the patient appears to be easily bearing the bad thing, or if another of those signs indicating recovery in addition to those just described should show itself, it is likely that the disease will turn to *apostasis*, with the result that the patient will survive, although he will lose whatever parts of the body were blackened.

Here, initial signs of defeat are called into question by conflicting signs that signal a twofold outcome: the patient survives; the affected part, the foot or the finger, does not.

Thus far, I have been vague about what is threatening the patient. In the passage just cited, the patient is bearing the "bad thing" (although, immediately after this, the author refers to the disease).[16] What is this bad thing? More specifically, does the author's understanding of the bad thing influence how he thinks about the connection between the prognostic symptom and the outcome it predicts? The question is important. For years, scholars have held up *Prognostic*, together with the *Epidemics*, as a model of clinical observation, that is, an accumulation of empirical data uninformed by theories of cause and, hence, unencumbered by fantastic ideas about the body.[17] The positivist characterization of prognosis, however, has been challenged in recent decades, particularly by Volker Langholf, who has demonstrated in detail how treatises oriented toward prognosis and case study incorporate and extend many of the theoretical presuppositions

---

[15] See also, e.g., *Prorrh.* II 40 (Li 9.70 = 286 Potter): καὶ γὰρ τοῦτο τὸ σημεῖον τούτοισιν ὁμολογέον ἐστίν (for this sign agrees with the others).

[16] τὸ κακὸν appears in M and V and is printed by Littré, Alexanderson, and Jones; C has νόσημα.

[17] On the correlation of sign and outcome, see Vegetti 1996.77: "La funzione predittiva del segno si basa invece sull'osservazione ripetuta (e presto affidata alla scrittura) di un nesso regolare tra fenomeni visibili, senza transito per la supposizione causale, e quindi garantita soltanto dalla costanza della reciproca associazione." See also Pigeaud 1990.28. This latter kind of empiricism does appear as a self-conscious methodological ideal in the Hellenistic period: see M. Frede 1988; Hankinson 1995b.

evident in the nosological treatises.[18] His conclusions suggest that ideas about how disease forms remain relevant to the meaning of prognostic symptoms, despite the importance of outcomes.

Consider the hope in *Prognostic* 9 that the disease will turn to *apostasis*. The texts we have do not provide a neat definition of *apostasis*, nor do they always communicate confidence about how it works: the author of *Epidemics* IV, having ventured some generalizing remarks, concludes, "but I do not really know" (25, Li 5.168 = 120 Smith). Nevertheless, physicians tend to recognize *apostasis*, essentially the isolation and expulsion of corrupted humors, when they "see" it, whether in symptoms such as varicose veins or nosebleeds, or through more complex calculations—for example, if a fever lasts more than twenty days in a patient showing signs of recovery, an *apostasis* is expected.[19] If *apostasis* is going to be beneficial, the peccant material needs to be cooked or "concocted," a condition particularly evident in the stuffs that exit the orifices—hence, the heightened attention to effluvia in the prognostic calculus.[20] Evidence of coction thus signifies a swift crisis and the recovery of health, whereas "raw" evacuations foretell a long illness, death, or relapse.[21]

Given how important coction and *apostasis* are to the meaning of the prognostic symptom, it seems fair to conclude that it does, indeed, refer to something happening inside the body.[22] Yet the prognostic sign goes beyond single events or localized trouble. Having cataloged the bad types of urine, the author of *Prognostic* concludes, "Do not be fooled if the bladder produces these kinds of urine when it is diseased, for this will be a sign not of the whole body [τοῦ ὅλου σώματος σημεῖον] but only of the bladder itself" (*Prog.* 12, Li 2.142 = 210,1–3 Alex).[23] If we think back to the explanation of bladder stones in *Airs*,

---

[18] Langholf 1990. See also G. Lloyd 1979.154–55; Grmek 1989.289–90; H. King 1998.54–74, esp. 55–58.

[19] *Prog.* 24 (Li 2.180 = 227,4–5 Alex). Langholf 1990.85–88 gathers incidental descriptions of *apostasis*. On the concept: Bourgey 1953.238–39; Thivel 1981.204–16; Langholf 1990.79–93.

[20] On *apostasis* and coction, see Langholf 1990.88–92. For coction and cooking, see also Schiefsky 2005a.280–83. On judging bodily effluvia, see, e.g., *Acut. Sp.* 19 (Li 2.434, ch. 8 = 77,18–23 Joly), 39 (Li 2.474, ch. 15 = 87,1–2 Joly); *Morb.* I 25 (Li 6.190 = 74,8–16 Wittern); *Morb.* IV 42 (Li 7.564 = 96,26–28 Joly); *Prog.* 12 (Li 2.138–42 = 208,4–210,3 Alex). It is also important that, if the peccant stuffs are isolated in a part of the body, that part can withstand their force: see, e.g., *Epid.* II 1.7 (Li 5.78 = 24 Smith) and, on the delicate role of the physician in such situations, *Epid.* II 3.8 (Li 5.112 = 56 Smith); *Epid.* VI 2.7 (Li 5.282 = 32,10–34,8 Manetti-Roselli), 2.14 (Li 5.284 = 38,1–5 Manetti-Roselli); *Hum.* 6 (Li 5.484 = 72–74 Jones).

[21] *Epid.* I 11 (Li 2.632–34, ch. 5 = 189,18–23 Kühlewein).

[22] Cases where a reason is given (with γάρ) for the goodness or badness of a symptom explicitly cue this referential field, e.g., *Aph.* IV.56 (Li 4.522 = 150 Jones; cf. *Iudic.* 29 [Li 9.286]), VII.49 (Li 4.590 = 204 Jones); *Prog.* 12 (Li 2.142 = 209,9 Alex).

[23] See Pigeaud 1988.322–23. Signs of the tongue (τὰ τῆς γλώσσης σημεῖα) are also signs of "the whole body," especially in *On Diseases* III, e.g., 6 (Li 7.124 = 74,18–21 Potter), 15 (Li 7.136 = 82,28–84,3 Potter), 16 (Li 7.146 = 88,29–30 Potter); see also *Epid.* VI 5.8 (Li 5.318 = 112,1–4 Manetti-Roselli), 5.10 (Li 5.318 = 114,1–3 Manetti-Roselli); *Hebd.* 42 (Li 8.660–61 = 64–65 Roscher). Diogenes of Apollonia reportedly held that because the tongue received all the vessels of the body, it

Waters, Places, it was precisely signs of the bladder that the author sought.[24] What, then, does it mean to seek a sign of the whole body?

One way to approach the question is to imagine that in prognosis the referential field of the symptom expands. By endowing symptoms with value (good or bad), the physician binds them both to forces operating inside the body and to the outcome of their struggle.

The physician engaged in prognosis, however, does not simply register the presence of the disease and its opponent as active forces. Rather, by interpreting symptoms in this way he participates in a process through which these forces are objectified within medicine's field of vision. Prognosis, in other words, turns forces of life and death into things that the physician can see. These forces become particularly vivid through their polarization: good signs are x, y, z; bad signs are "the opposites of these things" (τἀναντία τούτων).[25] Even when the symptomatic portrait is more complex, indicating a protracted illness or a mixed outcome, simply pitting good symptoms against bad strengthens the sense of a struggle between two hidden antagonists. In the prognostic context, then, disease is conceptualized less as an incremental process that fragments and redistributes verbal agency, as we saw in chapter 3, and more as a full-fledged actor capable of exerting a power over the patient that mimics a god's intention to harm. Perhaps even more important, prognosis creates the perception of a vital *dunamis* in the *sōma* that resists the disease. In fact, one of the most important things for physicians to know in *Prognostic* is how much a given disease exceeds the *dunamis* of bodies (ὀκόσον ὑπὲρ τὴν δύναμίν εἰσιν τῶν σωμάτων).[26] In the prognostic context, the *dunamis* of the body is closely associated with a specific end, namely the recovery of health. We could thus describe it as teleological (without assuming the Aristotelian baggage of that word).[27] By recognizing the teleological energy of the physical body, we expand our understanding of how it becomes visible. Although bodily health is often

---

could reflect the condition of the whole body, sick or well: see DK64 A19 (= Thphr. *De sens.* 43); A22 (= Aët. 4.18.2).

[24] *Aer.* 9 (Li 2.38–40 = 209,11–210,13 Jouanna), cited above, pp. 27–28.

[25] *Prog.* 15 (Li 2.150 = 213,3 Alex). See also *Aph.* I.25 (Li 4.470 = 108 Jones); *Coac.* 380 (Li 5.664), 387 (Li 5.668); *Epid.* II 1.6 (Li 5.76 = 22 Smith); *Epid.* VI 1.10 (Li 5.270 = 10,8–9 Manetti-Roselli), 4.22 (Li 5.314 = 100,4 Manetti-Roselli); *Hum.* 4 (Li 5.482 = 70 Jones); *Prog.* 17 (Li 2.156 = 216,9–14 Alex); *Prorrh.* II 6 (Li 9.22 = 236 Potter), 14 (Li 9.38 = 254 Potter). Patients, too, are located between two extremes, as at *Prog.* 20 (Li 2.170 = 222,2–7 Alex); *Prorrh.* II 11 (Li 9.30 = 246 Potter). On polar thinking in Greek thought, see G. Lloyd 1966.15–171. Note that polarization is evident, too, in the Akkadian medical prognostic texts (Heeßel 2004.105–8).

[26] See *Prog.* 1 (Li 2.112 = 194,3–5 Alex). On the *dunamis* of the *sōma* or the patient, see also *Morb.* III 16 (Li 7.148 = 90,24–26 Potter); *Mul.* II 133 (Li 8.296), 135 (Li 8.308); *Prorrh.* II 4 (Li 9.14 = 228 Potter); *VC* 20 (Li 3.256 = 90,6 Hanson); *VM* 3 (Li 1.578 = 122,15 Jouanna). See also Niebyl 1969.26–38.

[27] See Jaeger 1944.26–30 and Grmek 1991.16, both making *phusis* teleological, with the cautionary remarks at Jouanna 1999.346–47. The contrast that is often drawn by scholars between a quasi-democratic humoral balance and the pathological hegemony of a single stuff can obscure the dynamic striving (of the body or of nature) toward balance.

signified through the *absence* of pain, prognostic symptoms allow the tendency toward life and growth in that body to appear as an active force. By examining how this tendency registers perceptibly, we can better grasp how the dynamics of physicality are reshaping the terrain of the person in this period.

FRAGILE LIFE

The medical writers see the physical body's vital tendencies behind two different types of good signs. On the one hand, the physician looks for evidence, particularly in bodily effluvia, that the raw stuff of disease has been cooked and conquered. Such a defeat restages on a grand scale the little victory the cavity achieves each time it breaks down incoming food.[28] At the same time, whereas, in health, we infer victory from our feeling of well-being, in acute diseases, good signs are often specific to the disease context and, hence, intelligible to specialists alone: only a physician, for example, would know that a burst tumor, which signals an *apostasis*, is a good sign.[29]

On the other hand, symptoms are positive if they uphold the norms of health.[30] If disease exaggerates the natural heterogeneity of the physical body, the physician knows that internal differences have been tamed when he sees effluvia that are *homokhroa*, "uniform in color," and *homala*, "consistent."[31] He infers that the integrity of the body has been restored not only from the coction of physical stuffs but also from signs that belong to the public self, such as comportment, affect, and speech. These latter signs have been classified by some historians of medicine as "picturesque" observations, rather than what a modern physician would recognize as genuine clinical signs.[32] Yet, when a medical writer says that a patient holds his limbs *anōmalōs*, "askew," he is using the same vocabulary that he uses to talk about the humors, suggesting that he sees "picturesque" symptoms on a continuum with the more concretely physical ones.[33] In both cases, he is trying to determine the degree to which the patient resembles a healthy person. If a writer deems certain postures for the sick (reclining on the right or left side, with arms, neck, and legs slightly bent, and the whole body relaxed) best, it is because they are "most similar to those of the healthy"

[28] On the relationship between coction and digestion, see Langholf 1990.88–90.

[29] *Aph.* IV.82 (Li 4.532 = 156 Jones; cf. *Coac.* 463 [Li 5.688]).

[30] On the healthy body in prognosis, see Lichtenthaeler 1963.71–72; di Benedetto 1966.332–33. On ideas of health in medical writing, see the overview at Jouanna 1999.323–35, 344–47.

[31] See *Prog.* 7 (Li 2.130 = 203,5 Alex), 12 (Li 2.138 = 208,5 Alex), 17 (Li 2.156 = 216,8 Alex). For the vocabulary of ὁμαλός/ἀνώμαλος, see also *Acut. Sp.* 53 (Li 2.500, ch. 21 = 92,2 Joly); *Coac.* 273 (Li 5.642); *Epid.* II 3.11 (Li 5.112 = 56 Smith); *Epid.* VI 8.8 (Li 5.346 = 172,5 Manetti-Roselli); *Hum.* 13 (Li 5.494 = 86 Jones); *Prog.* 7 (Li 2.126 = 201,1 Alex), 15 (Li 2.150 = 213,5 Alex); *Prorrh.* II 7 (Li 9.24 = 238 Potter).

[32] "[Ces signes] nous apparaissent plutôt comme des notations pittoresques que comme de véritables signes de maladies" (Thivel 1981.43). See also Thivel 1985.487–88.

[33] Limbs askew: *Prog.* 3 (Li 2.120 = 197,13 Alex).

(αἱ ὁμοιόταται τῇσι τῶν ὑγιαινόντων, *Prog.* 3, Li 2.118 = 197,8 Alex).[34] It is a good sign if someone sleeps through the night and is awake during the day, "just as is habitual for us and in accordance with nature" (ὥσπερ καὶ κατὰ φύσιν ἡμῖν ξύνηθές ἐστιν, *Prog.* 10, Li 2.134 = 205,9 Alex).[35] The physician thus seeks normative signs of health beyond the effluvia, where coction is most evident.

In fact, some of the weightiest symptoms in prognosis are those that strike the major sites of the person *qua* social agent—delirium, aphonia, glossolalia, the loss of motor control. We can credit the significance of these symptoms in part to their immediate, intuitive intelligibility. The spectacle of a person "seized" by pain or biting his own tongue does not simply express his struggle with an amorphous, impersonal disease but powerfully dramatizes that struggle.[36] At the same time, the patient who cannot move or stop moving because of pain, or the patient who cannot stop weeping, or the patient deliriously beside himself is not simply enacting failed coction in the idioms of the volitional, the emotional, and the cognitive.[37] Rather, whether the patient has control over these faculties matters deeply to his survival. Delirious speech, for example, can be a fatal sign in *Prognostic*, perhaps because, as the verb *allophassō*—a Hippocratic *hapax legomenon* that Galen glosses as "speaking one thing at one time, another at another" (ἐκ τῶν ἄλλοτε φάσκειν ἄλλα)—suggests, it is incoherence of the highest order.[38] Indeed, the voice appears to be one of the most significant expressions of vital force. Its "release" can coincide with the triumph of the person's *phusis*, while the loss of articulation often signals further complications. Silvia Montiglio is only slightly exaggerating when she calls aphonia "the

---

[34] See also *Acut. Sp.* 23 (Li 2.440, ch. 9 = 79,7–9 Joly); *Epid.* VII 3 (Li 5.370 = 51,14 Jouanna); *Prog.* 11 (Li 2.134 = 206,4 Alex).

[35] On explanations of sleep in the Hippocratic Corpus, see Marelli 1983; Byl 1998.

[36] Tongue biting: *Epid.* V 53 (Li 5.238 = 24,14 Jouanna; cf. *Epid.* VII 74 [Li 5.432 = 93,7 Jouanna]). On the importance of narrative to case study in the *Epidemics*, see Pearcy 1992.

[37] Cannot stop moving from pain: *Epid.* I, case II (Li 2.686 = 204,1 Kühlewein), case VIII (Li 2.702 = 209,24 Kühlewein), case XII (Li 2.712 = 212,24 Kühlewein); *Epid.* V 61 (Li 5.242 = 28,2 Jouanna; cf. *Epid.* VII 33 [Li 5.402 = 72,4 Jouanna]); *Epid.* VII 10 (Li 5.382 = 58,12–14 Jouanna), 93 (Li 5.448 = 105,10–11 Jouanna); *Int.* 7 (Li 7.184 = 94 Potter); *Morb.* II 16 (Li 7.30 = 150,15–16 Jouanna); *Morb.* III 7 (Li 7.126 = 74,29–31 Potter), 13 (Li 7.132 = 80,19–20 Potter). Cannot move from pain: *Epid.* VII 3 (Li 5.370 = 51,16–18 Jouanna); *Int.* 1 (Li 7.168 = 72 Potter). Pigeaud 1987.16 nn.11–13 catalogs such cases in *Epidemics* I and III. See also Villard 2006.75–77 on the myriad effects of pain on the patient. Loss of control over voluntary functions: *Aph.* IV.52 (Li 4.522 = 148 Jones), VII.83 (Li 4.606 = 214 Jones); *Coac.* 485 (Li 5.694); *Epid.* III, case XII (Li 3.64 = 223,19–20 Kühlewein); *Epid.* IV 46 (Li 5.188 = 142 Smith); *Epid.* V 42 (Li 5.232 = 21,9–10 Jouanna); *Epid.* VI 1.13 (Li 5.272 = 14,9–10 Manetti-Roselli); *Epid.* VII 25 (Li 5.398 = 68,8 Jouanna); *Morb.* II 21 (Li 7.36 = 155,13–14 Jouanna); *Prog.* 11 (Li 2.138 = 207,8–10 Alex); *Prorrh.* I 29 (Li 5.516 = 78,5 Polack), 78 (Li 5.530 = 84,6–8 Polack). The Hippocratic writers have a rich vocabulary to express delirium: see Byl 2006.22–24. For patients "outside" themselves (ἐξ ἑωυτοῦ, ἔκτοσθεν): e.g., *Epid.* V 85 (Li 5.252 = 39,5 Jouanna; cf. *Epid.* VII 90 [Li 5.446 = 103,20 Jouanna]); *Epid.* VII 45 (Li 5.412 = 79,20 Jouanna), 85 (Li 5.444 = 101,3 Jouanna).

[38] *Prog.* 20 (Li 2.170 = 222,6 Alex); Galen *Hipp.Prog.* 3.8 (Kühn 18b.249). Galen offers two interpretations, "to be delirious" or "to toss about," but advocates the first on the basis of the gloss cited above. Others derive the word, he tells us, from the movement of the eyes.

defining symptom of the otherwise undefinable [*sic*] state of 'dying' " in medical writing.[39] Conversely, the voice is established at the most critical stage in child development in *Epidemics* II: once it appears, *ischus*, "strength," and the mastery of the hands follow, "nature being like speech" (ἡ γὰρ φύσις τῇ φθέγξει ὁμοίη, 6.4, Li 5.134 = 82 Smith).[40]

The face, too, which, "like a mirror, reveals what an individual is and what he stands for" in archaic poetry, is one of the richest semiotic zones in prognosis.[41] The significance of the face is particularly clear in the famous *facies Hippocratica*. The author of *Prognostic* exhorts the physician preparing to make an initial prognosis to examine the patient's face in order to determine "if it resembles those of healthy people" (εἰ ὅμοιόν ἐστι τοῖσι τῶν ὑγιαινόντων, 2, Li 2.112 = 194,11 Alex).[42] But the healthy face here is not only a generic phenomenon. The physician is also instructed to see to what degree the patient resembles his usual self: this resemblance is the best sign, while "the greatest divergence from it is the most fearsome" (τὸ δὲ ἐναντιώτατον τοῦ ὁμοίου δεινότατον, 2, Li 2.114 = 194,12–13 Alex), unless it can be blamed on insomnia or hunger.[43] For other prognostic signs, too, the physician must rely on more precise norms to determine what can be considered "paralogical," on the principle articulated in *Prorrhetic* II that both diseases and patients have specific *ēthea*, "characters," that have to be learned before prognosis.[44] For example, exposing a bit of the whites of the eyes when they are closed in sleep, or lying on one's belly, or grinding one's teeth are all bad signs *unless* these are habitual behaviors.[45] Likewise, an insolent reply from a usually well-mannered person portends ill.[46]

[39] Montiglio 2000.229; see also Ciani 1987; Boehm 2002.269. Already in Homer, the shades of the dead are marked by the qualities of their voices (*Il.* 23.101; *Od.* 24.5, 9).

[40] See also *Acut. Sp.* 6 (Li 2.402–4, ch. 4 = 70,16–21 Joly), 10 (Li 2.414, ch. 6 = 73,6–7 Joly); *Coac.* 91 (Li 5.532–34), 240–54 (Li 5.636–38); *Epid.* II 6.2 (Li 5.132 = 82 Smith); *Epid.* V 55 (Li 5.238 = 25,12 Jouanna; cf. *Epid.* VII 75 [Li 5.434 = 94,3 Jouanna]); *Epid.* VI 7.1 (Li 5.334 = 146,1–5 Manetti-Roselli); *Epid.* VII 41 (Li 5.408 = 77,6–7 Jouanna). On lack of articulation: *Epid.* V 74 (Li 5.246–48 = 34,6–8 Jouanna; cf. *Epid.* VII 36 [Li 5.404 = 74,11–12 Jouanna]); *Epid.* VI 7.1 (Li 5.334 = 148,8–9 Manetti-Roselli); *Epid.* VII 5 (Li 5.374 = 54,13–16 Jouanna), 8 (Li 5.378 = 56,21–25 Jouanna); *Morb.* III 13 (Li 7.132–34 = 80,21–22 Potter); *Prorrh.* I 54 (Li 5.524 = 81,7–8 Polack), 55 (Li 5.524 = 81,8–9 Polack; cf. *Coac.* 243 [Li 5.636]). See Gourevitch 1983 on the range of symptoms associated with the loss of the voice. Kuriyama 1999.136–37 relates the voice to corporeal articulation.

[41] Vernant 1991b.45.

[42] See Grmek 1987.132–35. For the impact of the face and eyes on prognosis, see *Epid.* II 2.8 (Li 5.88 = 32 Smith); *Epid.* VI 2.17 (Li 5.286 = 40,7–9 Manetti-Roselli), 4.22 (Li 5.312 = 98,4 Manetti-Roselli).

[43] See also *Morb.* III 2 (Li 7.120 = 72,6 Potter).

[44] *Prorrh.* II 3 (Li 9.12 = 226 Potter). On individual norms, see Temkin 1963.634–35, noting, too, the skepticism in later Greek medicine as to whether a science of the individual was possible; Gundert 2000.34–35; Giambalvo 2002.66–69.

[45] Eyes in sleep: *Prog.* 2 (Li 2.116–18 = 196,6–197,1 Alex). Lying on the belly: *Prog.* 3 (Li 2.120 = 198,1–3 Alex). Grinding teeth: *Prog.* 3 (Li 2.120 = 198,6–7 Alex); see also *Prorrh.* I 48 (Li 5.522 = 80,12–13 Polack).

[46] *Epid.* IV 15 (Li 5.152 = 104 Smith). See, too, *Prorrh.* I 44 (Li 5.522 = 80,8–9 Polack); *Epid.* III, case XI (Li 3.134 = 241,10 Kühlewein); *Epid.* VII 10 (Li 5.382 = 58,8–9 Jouanna), 11 (Li 5.384 = 60,15 Jouanna), 25 (Li 5.396 = 67,9–13 Jouanna).

Prognostic signs, then, are not limited to effluvia or other phenomena obviously associated with the physical body but are regularly located at the nodes of personal identity. Because treatises like *Prognostic* and the *Epidemics* invest these nodes with so much meaning, a number of scholars have praised them for recognizing the patient as an individual.[47] The individual may no longer pass muster as a transhistorical category. Nevertheless, it is evident that phenomena appropriated as good signs in prognosis are drawn from a group of behaviors and characteristics that together constitute the "social, regularized, embodied, and therefore visible phenomenon" of self-presentation in the archaic Greek world.[48] In early Greek poetry, as we saw in chapter 1, these phenomena often stand in, catachrestically, for something more fleeting, namely character. Theognis, for example, "often treats *ēthos* as something visible but ephemeral, a quality of mind that can be read by the attentive observer on the face and in the deportment of his fellow citizens."[49] By assigning semiotic weight to normative behaviors, particularly those through which identity was traditionally realized in public space, physicians appropriate these phenomena as expressions of a vital force working in the body, a force at the core of their physicalized model of both human nature and more individualized natures.

Still, like the disease, this vital force is half-disclosed, half-created by phenomena. As a result, it is hard to say what exactly it is.[50] Symptoms like paralysis or madness could be traced, like unconcocted effluvia, to the defeat of the body's innate heat, but this innate heat is only rarely mentioned.[51] Similarly, although the medical writers could see as well as anyone that breath is necessary to life, it is a principle of primary importance in only a handful of treatises.[52] And

---

[47] From very different perspectives: Pagel 1939; Vlastos 1946.55 n.11; Diller 1964.36; Hall 1974.285–90; Bourgey 1975; Pigeaud 1987.23–24; Wittern 1987.86–88; Schubert 1996; Andò 2002; Giambalvo 2002. Individualism was long associated with the Coan treatises, while Cnidian treatises were thought to be more focused on disease entities: see, e.g., Boncompagni 1972; Wittern 1987.71. For a corrective to this "anti-patient" view of the nosological treatises, see Langholf 1990.60–61. Nevertheless, as my own organization of the material suggests, different treatises adopt palpably different perspectives on the symptom.

[48] Worman 2002.5; 6–7, 17–40 on the importance of the visual field to the presentation of the self. See also C. Gill 1990b; Halliwell 1990.43–56; Winkler 1990b.64–67; Vernant 1991c.70; Bassi 1998; 2003; Holmes, forthcoming (a). On the semiotics of character in later antiquity, see Gleason 1995.

[49] Worman 2002.30.

[50] On the problem of what organizes the body, see also Grmek 1991.14–18.

[51] *Epid.* I 12 (Li 2.638 = 190,19 Kühlewein): τὸ θερμὸν κρατεῖται. On "vital," innate heat (τὸ σύμφυτον θερμόν, τὸ ἔμφυτον θερμόν, τὸ θερμόν): *Aph.* I.14 (Li 4.466 = 104 Jones), I.15 (Li 4.446 = 104–6 Jones); *Morb.* I 11 (Li 6.158 = 28,4–5 Wittern); *Vict.* II 62 (Li 6.576 = 184,23–24 Joly-Byl); *VM* 16 (Li 1.608 = 139,13 Jouanna). See also *Liq.* 2 (Li 6.122 = 165,23 Joly), referring to οἰκεῖον θάλπος. At *Carn.* 2 (Li 8.584 = 188,12–14 Joly), heat is immortal and endowed with omnisentience and omnipotence. In the *Timaeus*, fire and breath are necessary for life (76e7–77a2), although the *psukhē* organizes growth. Heat becomes a key concept in Aristotle's biology, where it is a precondition of the soul's functions (*GA* 739a9–12, b20–26; *PA* 652b7–17): see Solmsen 1957.

[52] At *Flat.* 4 (Li 6.96 = 107,10–12 Jouanna), air is both the cause of life (αἴτιος τοῦ βίου) in living things and the cause of disease, though intelligence is related to the blood (as for Empedocles).

while *psukhē* has been seen as one of the most important "life-force" words in the fifth century, it is rather rare in the medical writers, particularly with this connotation.[53] If we wish to give a name to the principle of flourishing that the medical writers see expressed through physical bodies—and it is worth stressing that not all of them feel the need to name this principle—*phusis* may be our best choice.[54] In *On Generation/On the Nature of the Child*, the principle that guides the creation of a human being, described on analogy with the development of plants, is called *phusis*.[55] *Phusis* can designate, too, the structure that stabilizes the organism and is sustained through maturity: to study the *phusis* of a human being in *On Regimen*, for example, is to examine not only what he is made of originally but also the constituent stuffs that are dominant in health.[56] One medical writer identifies the starting point of medicine with the *phusis* of the *sōma*.[57] *Phusis* can also name the force behind the body's automatism. In a passage from *Epidemics VI*, *phusis* is credited with the production of tears, ear wax, and saliva, as well as yawning, coughing, and sneezing: *phusis* is responsive to changes in the body, too, discovering how to adapt on its own, without thought (οὐκ ἐκ διανοίης).[58]

If we align the vital force of the body with *phusis*, however, the struggle staged by the prognostic calculus grows complicated. After all, if the physician uses individual norms to evaluate certain phenomena (e.g., emaciation, ruddiness) as deviant or not, he can also use them to determine how and, indeed, whether a given disease will unfold in a given person. In other words, individual natures not only oppose the disease but also inform its expression. The author of *On Regimen in Acute Diseases* chides his colleagues for failing to recognize how *phusis* and *hexis*, "habit," influence the form taken by a disease in a

---

At *Morb. Sacr.* 16 (Li 6.390 = 29,4–8 Jouanna), air is central to intelligence. For the relationship of both treatises to Diogenes of Apollonia (and Anaximenes), see Jouanna 1988b.26–29; 2003.lxv–lxx. The cause of the embryo's organic growth is πνεῦμα at *Genit./Nat. Puer.* 12 (Li 7.486–88 = 53,1–55,3 Joly), 17 (Li 7.496 = 59,9–12 Joly). Lonie 1981.148–56 compares the views of the Hippocratic author on this point to those of his Presocratic contemporaries.

[53] On life-force meanings, see Claus 1981, esp. 122–40. For the medical writers, see Gundert 2000.18 n.29. At *Nat. Hom.* 6 (Li 6.44 = 178,15–17 Jouanna), the author's opponents are said to consider blood flowing from a wound to be the *psukhē* in a person, but the author himself always talks about human *phusis*. See also *Vict.* I 28 (Li 6.502 = 144,17–22 Joly-Byl), discussed above, chapter 2, n.83.

[54] For the word's frequency, see the tables and lists in Gallego Pérez 1996.424 and Byl 2002.47. On *phusis* in the medical texts, see Beardslee 1918.31–42; Michler 1962; D. Manetti 1973; Ayache 1992; Andò 2002; Giambalvo 2002; von Staden 2007b. On *phusis* more generally, see above, chapter 2 n.3.

[55] *Genit./Nat. Puer.* 27 (Li 7.528 = 77,4–7 Joly). See D. Manetti 1973.436–37; Naddaf 2005.20–22.

[56] *Vict.* I 2 (Li 6.468 = 122,23–27 Joly-Byl).

[57] *Loc.* 2 (Li 6.278 = 38,4 Craik).

[58] *Epid.* VI 5.1 (Li 5.314 = 100,7–102,2 Manetti-Roselli). See also *Hum.* 9 (Li 5.490 = 80 Jones), with Pigeaud 2006.41–44; *Vict.* I 15 (Li 6.490 = 136,28–138,1 Joly-Byl): ἡ φύσις αὐτομάτη ταῦτα ἐπίσταται, with Ayache 1992; Andò 2002.116–20, pointing out that Hippocratic physicians tend to intervene, rather than letting nature run its course. See also *Alim.* 15 (Li 9.102 = 141,24 Joly), 39 (Li 9.112 = 145,12 Joly), probably from the Hellenistic period.

given patient.[59] But many of them do, indeed, note these factors. The authors of the *Epidemics*, in particular, often treat distinguishing features of the patient, such as age, sex, and physical characteristics, as relevant to the disease.[60] The author of *Airs, Waters, Places* systematically catalogs the relationships between bodily types, *eidea*, which he attributes to whole populations (e.g., Scythian, Phasian), environmental conditions, and recurrent diseases. And recall that the author of *Epidemics* V, in narrating the death of Apellaeus, made special mention of the patient's bilious body.

In this last case, one of the body's constituent stuffs has come to color its normal form, rather than emerging solely through disease. In this light, disease no longer appears to be alien to the person but, rather, an exaggeration of his nature. In *Epidemics* I and III, too, we find diseases habitually correlated with constitutions. One class of sufferers has a *phusis* that "tends toward the consumptive" (ἔρρεπεν ἡ φύσις ἐπὶ τὸ φθινῶδες, *Epid.* I 2, Li 2.604–6 = 181,17–18 Kühlewein).[61] Those with sanguine and melancholic constitutions are liable to fall prey to fevers, phrenitis, and dysenteries.[62] These tendencies are on occasion identified as hereditary, strengthening the notion that every *phusis* carries within it the seeds of its perversion.[63] Whether this perversion is expressed

[59] *Acut.* 43 (Li 2.316, ch. 11 = 54,22–23 Joly): ὅσα τε ἡμέων ἡ φύσις καὶ ἡ ἕξις ἑκάστοισιν ἐκτεκνοῖ πάθεα καὶ εἴδεα παντοῖα. The author's opponents are a matter of debate. His own practice is visible at *Acut.* 34 (Li 2.296, ch. 9 = 50,4–8 Joly), 53 (Li 2.336, ch. 15 = 59,8–11 Joly).

[60] On differences according to sex: see, e.g., *Acut.* 61 (Li 2.358, ch. 16 = 63,15–16 Joly); *Epid.* I 1 (Li 2.602 = 181,6 Kühlewein), 16 (Li 2.646 = 193,6–7 Kühlewein); *Epid.* II 3.16 (Li 5.116 = 60 Smith); *Epid.* V 89 (Li 5.254 = 40,12–14 Jouanna; cf. *Epid.* VII 95 [Li 5.450 = 106,10–12 Jouanna]); *Epid.* VI 7.1 (Li 5.334 = 146,11–148,1 Manetti-Roselli). On differences related to external appearance: e.g., *Epid.* I 19 (Li 2.656–58 = 195,15–196,13 Kühlewein); *Epid.* VI 3.10 (Li 5.296 = 62,1–3 Manetti-Roselli), 3.13 (Li 5.298 = 66,4–7 Manetti-Roselli); *Salubr.* 2 (Li 6.74 = 208,9–14 Jouanna, as *Nat. Hom.* 17), 7 (Li 6.84 = 216,18; 218,4–6 Jouanna, as *Nat. Hom.* 22). On differences according to age, e.g., *Epid.* I 10 (Li 2.630 = 188,23–189,1 Kühlewein), 12 (Li 2.638 = 190,16–20 Kühlewein); *Epid.* III 4 (Li 3.70–72 = 225,10–13 Kühlewein), 8 (Li 3.84 = 228,8–11 Kühlewein.); *Epid.* VII 105 (Li 5.456 = 110,3–4 Jouanna); *Loc.* 47 (Li 6.348 = 88,31–32 Craik); *Nat. Hom.* 15 (Li 6.68 = 204,15–21 Jouanna); *Salubr.* 2 (Li 6.74–76 = 208,14–20 Jouanna, as *Nat. Hom.* 17).

[61] See also *Hum.* 8 (Li 5.488 = 78 Jones) and Demont 2002 on ῥέπειν.

[62] *Epid.* III 14 (Li 3.96–98 = 231,12–18 Kühlewein). For types of constitution (phlegmatic, bilious, etc.), see also *Acut.* 62 (Li 2.358, ch. 17 = 63,25–64,1 Joly); *Epid.* II 3.15 (Li 5.116 = 60 Smith); *Epid.* IV 20f (Li 5.160 = 110 Smith); *Epid.* VI 4.19 (Li 5.312 = 96,4–7 Manetti-Roselli), 6.14 (Li 5.330 = 138,1–8 Manetti-Roselli), 7.6 (Li 5.340 = 156,7–158,4 Manetti-Roselli); *Morb.* III 16 (Li 7.146–48 = 90,15–22 Potter); *Nat. Hom.* 9 (Li 6.54 = 190,5–12 Jouanna); *Nat. Mul.* 33 (Li 7.370 = 45,17–46,7 Bourbon); *Steril.* 213 (Li 8.412 = 144,14–15 Grensemann); *Vict.* I 2 (Li 6.468 = 122,26 Joly-Byl). The role of the patient's constitution in disease is hotly debated in later medicine: see Hankinson 1998a.374–79 on the debate between Galen and Erasistratus on antecedent causes.

[63] E.g., *Epid.* III, case VI (Li 3.52 = 221,2 Kühlewein): ἦν δέ τι καὶ συγγενικὸν φθινῶδες. On the transmission of "sickly seed," see *Aer.* 14 (Li 2.60 = 224,17–225,4 Jouanna); *Genit./Nat. Puer.* 8 (Li 7.480 = 49,20–22 Joly); *Morb. Sacr.* 2 (Li 6.364 = 10,14–18 Jouanna); Democr. (DK68) A141 (= Aët. 5.3.6). On expressions used to denote hereditary and congenital causes, see von Staden 1990.94. On heredity in general: Grmek 1991.

depends on changing conditions in the *sōma*: the interaction of hot and cold, bile and phlegm, fire and water, and so on.

By explaining both symptoms *and* norms in terms of interaction between a nature and contingent conditions, the medical writers do more than trace daemonic transformations, such as the epileptic's rolling eyes or his sudden bolt from bed, to the uncanny workings of the physical body. They also infect the very idea of human nature with the unreliability of the humors, whose neutrality in the game of life and death is related to the labile nature of physical stuffs. What this means is that *phusis,* however much it is oriented toward life, emerges in medicine's field of vision as changeable and, hence, untrustworthy.

In the *Republic*, Plato has Socrates observe that it is not sufficient for a body to just be a body. Bodies "need something else" (προσδεῖταί τινος), and it is for this reason that the medical *tekhnē* was discovered (*R*. 1, 341e1–6). Although the medical writers differ from one another in many respects, the body that they see is, indeed, dependent on *tekhnē* for its well-being. We can see this dependence perhaps most clearly in the revisiting of medicine's discovery in the treatise *On Ancient Medicine*, where the difficulties created by an unstable body are compounded by the difficulty of knowing what it needs.

On Ancient Medicine and the Discovery of Human Nature

On Ancient Medicine is the most deliberate and ardent defense we have of medicine's stake in the question, What is a human being?[64] Of course, the need to advance such a defense presupposes rivals. The oblique appearance that these rivals make in the treatise provides invaluable evidence of the lively, fifth-century intellectual milieu that had sprung up around new kinds of "anthropological" inquiry.[65]

λέγουσι δέ τινες καὶ ἰητροὶ καὶ σοφισταὶ ὡς οὐκ εἴη δυνατὸν ἰητρικὴν εἰδέναι ὅστις μὴ οἶδεν ὅ τι ἐστὶν ἄνθρωπος, ἀλλὰ τοῦτο δεῖ καταμαθεῖν τὸν μέλλοντα ὀρθῶς θεραπεύσειν τοὺς ἀνθρώπους. τείνει τε αὐτοῖσιν ὁ λόγος ἐς φιλοσοφίην καθάπερ Ἐμπεδοκλέης ἢ ἄλλοι οἳ περὶ φύσιος γεγράφασιν ἐξ ἀρχῆς ὅ τι ἐστὶν ἄνθρωπος καὶ

---

[64] On medicine and debates about human nature, see also *Carn*. 1 (Li 8.584 = 188,6–11 Joly); *Nat. Hom*. 1 (Li 6.32 = 164,5–8 Jouanna); *Vict*. I 2 (Li 6.468 = 122,22–24 Joly-Byl); Pl. *Smp*. 189d5, where Aristophanes' declaration that he will speak on human nature (ἡ ἀνθρωπίνη φύσις) looks like part of his parody of Eryximachus's medical discourse. See also G. Lloyd 1979.92–97; Wesoly 1987; Jouanna 1992; 2002.223–24; Thomas 2000, esp. 153–61; Schiefsky 2005a.38–40. On lexical expressions for human nature in the medical writers, see Gallego Pérez 1996.426.

[65] The dating of this treatise has been controversial. Festugière (1948.60) argued that it should be placed as early as 440 BCE, while Diller claimed that the author is responding to Plato: see Jouanna 1990b.84–85, who places it around 420–410 BCE. For a late fifth-century date, see also H. Miller 1955.52, with n.7; G. Lloyd 1963; Vegetti 1998; Cooper 2004.6; Schiefsky 2005a.63–64. Hankinson 1992 leans toward a fourth-century date. I assume a date in the last quarter of the fifth century, given the reference to Empedocles and the popularity in this period of the *Kulturgeschichte* the author offers.

ὅπως ἐγένετο πρῶτον καὶ ὁπόθεν συνεπάγη. ἐγὼ δὲ τοῦτο μὲν ὅσα τινὶ εἴρηται ἢ
σοφιστῇ ἢ ἰητρῷ ἢ γέγραπται περὶ φύσιος ἧσσον νομίζω τῇ ἰητρικῇ τέχνῃ προσήκειν
ἢ τῇ γραφικῇ, νομίζω δὲ περὶ φύσιος γνῶναί τι σαφὲς οὐδαμόθεν ἄλλοθεν εἶναι ἢ
ἐξ ἰητρικῆς. τοῦτο δὲ οἷόν τε καταμαθεῖν ὅταν αὐτήν τις τὴν ἰητρικὴν ὀρθῶς πᾶσαν
περιλάβῃ—μέχρι δὲ τούτου πολλοῦ μοι δοκεῖ δεῖν—, λέγω δὲ ταύτην τὴν ἱστορίην,
εἰδέναι ἄνθρωπος τί ἐστι καὶ δι᾽ οἵας αἰτίας γίνεται καὶ τἆλλα ἀκριβέως. ἐπεὶ τοῦτό
γέ μοι δοκεῖ ἀναγκαῖον εἶναι ἰητρῷ περὶ φύσιος εἰδέναι καὶ πάνυ σπουδάσαι ὡς
εἴσεται, εἴπερ τι μέλλει τῶν δεόντων ποιήσειν, ὅ τι τέ ἐστιν ἄνθρωπος πρὸς τὰ
ἐσθιόμενά τε καὶ πινόμενα καὶ ὅ τι πρὸς τὰ ἄλλα ἐπιτηδεύματα καὶ ὅ τι ἀφ᾽ ἑκάστου
ἑκάστῳ συμβήσεται. (*VM* 20, Li 1.620–22 = 145,18–147,1 Jouanna)

But some physicians and sophists say that it is not possible to know the medical
tekhnē if someone does not know what a human being is—it is this that anyone
who is going to treat people correctly must learn completely. Their account concerns philosophy in the same way as Empedocles and others who have written on
nature[66] [have written] about what a human being is from the beginning, and how
he first came into being, and from what stuff he is put together.[67] But I believe, on

---

[66] I find attractive Langholf's suggestion that we transform the relative οἵ into the article οἱ to create
the expression "those [who have written] about nature" (see Jouanna 1990b.207). The verb
γεγράφασιν, which would be implied in the shorthand phrase οἱ περὶ φύσιος, could thus serve as
the main verb; otherwise, we need to read γεγράφασιν twice or supply a similar verb.

[67] Much in this phrase, and, indeed, in this passage as a whole, is ambiguous. On the term σοφιστής,
see Jouanna 1990b.206. I take φιλοσοφίη to refer to a form of inquiry that is primarily defined by
theoretical speculation, the exchange of arguments, and totalizing ambitions (see Laks 2006.67–81,
71–73 on this passage) and exemplified by those who write treatises "on nature," like Empedocles.
In these treatises, the physicists presumably would have extended their physical theories to encompass anthropogony, biology, and physiology (introduction, n.81). Indeed, it is what such treatises
say about "what a human being is" that interests both our author and those whom I take to be his
main targets: physicians and sophists who insist that the anthropological-anthropogonical aspects
of the inquiry into nature are indispensable to the practice of medicine. It is in part because the author is talking about what those who write on nature say about *human* nature that there is so much
confusion about what he means when he refers to φύσις. Matters are further complicated by the fact
that the author himself frequently uses φύσις in different senses—eighteen times in addition to the
four uses here (see also *VM* 2 [Li 1.572 = 119,18 Jouanna], where Jouanna prints φησί [φησί Lind.:
φύσι A: φύσει A³: φήσει M]). Of these twenty-two cases, thirteen refer to human nature (the other
uses pertain, e.g., to the φύσις of parts of the body), as indicated either by the context or, in six instances, by the genitive τοῦ ἀνθρώπου or the adjective ἀνθρωπίνη. Most commentators assume
that, in the passage cited above, every reference to φύσις means either "nature" in general (Cooper
2004.13–14 n.16, 38–39 n.47; see also Nestle 1938.23 n.1; Festugière 1948.18) or "human nature"
(Jouanna 1990b.208; Schiefsky 2005a.304–5, 311; 2005b). I think the author's position is more rhetorically complex than it has been portrayed. Two points are worth noting. First, elsewhere in the
treatise, he specifies "human" nature unless "human" is clear from the context. Second, the phrase
περὶ φύσιος, which occurs in the treatise only here, probably carries a quasi-technical meaning associated with the inquiry into nature. I interpret the first use of φύσις in terms of this meaning. In
the following cases, however, after the writer has specified the kinds of questions his opponents are
asking (e.g., what constitutes a human being?), περὶ φύσιος probably has the more narrow sense of
what of the inquiry into nature touches on human nature. Nevertheless, the phrase is sufficiently
ambiguous without the qualification of τοῦ ἀνθρώπου or ἀνθρωπίνης that the author feels the need

the one hand, that whatever has been said by someone, either a sophist or a physician, or written about nature has even less to do with the medical art than with painting; and, on the other hand, I think that nothing clear can be known about nature in any way, except through the art of medicine. This it is possible to learn when one has properly understood the medical *tekhnē* as a whole; until this point, it seems to me that much is lacking—I am referring to this kind of inquiry, that is, to know what a human being is and on account of what causes he comes to be and all the rest with precision. Since, indeed, it seems to me, what a physician must necessarily know about nature—and must be at great pains to know it—if he is going to do something of what he has to do, is this, namely, what a human being is in relation to what he eats and drinks and what he is in relation to other practices, and what will happen to each person because of each of these things.

Both the author and his rivals take for granted that the question of human nature will be answered by some kind of inquiry into nature.[68] Whereas philosophically inclined physicians and sophists advocate an inquiry into the origins and the composition of the human being,[69] our author insists we need to inquire into the *dynamics* of human nature, that is, what a human being is in relation to food, drink, and various practices, and what happens to him on account of these things. His conceptualization of human nature brings us back to the idea of the physical body as an interval between external causes and perceptible effects. At the same time, it foregrounds the problem of how we achieve knowledge about this hidden space, not only as disembodied experts but also as embodied subjects.

Epistemological concerns, in fact, dominate the first chapters. The author rejects at the outset the idea that what human nature suffers can be known through *hupotheseis*, "abstract postulates": examples include the hot and the

---

to restate his target area of concern, that is, what of the inquiry into nature touches on human nature, in the next sentence (λέγω δὲ ταύτην τὴν ἱστορίην . . .): see Schiefsky 2005a.310–11. In the last instance of περὶ φύσιος, the author may be confronting his opponents head-on by imbuing φύσις with the double sense of the object of his opponents' investigations (human nature as it falls within a larger inquiry into nature) and the object of his own (human nature more narrowly understood): the physician must know *this* (τοῦτο) about (human) nature, not what he gets out of treatises "on nature," but what a human being is πρὸς τὰ ἐσθιόμενά τε καὶ πινόμενα. By this point, the repeated specification of nature as "what a human being is . . ." makes it possible for the author to use φύσις twice more in the chapter to refer to human nature without a qualifying term. In short, I think the author has human nature foremost in his mind throughout the diatribe, as his specifications indicate. Yet he does not use τοῦ ἀνθρώπου or ἀνθρωπίνη to qualify φύσις in order to trade on the charge of the phrase περὶ φύσιος, a phrase that both easily identifies his opponents and sets them up to have their authority in matters of "what a human being is" appropriated by the author. By the end of the attack, he has succeeded in making the phrase περὶ φύσιος refer to his own views on human nature and, specifically, to "what a human being is in relation to what he eats and drinks."

[68] Stressed by Schiefsky 2005a.294–95; 2005b.72.

[69] See *Vict.* I 2 (Li 6.468 = 122,23–25 Joly-Byl), where constituent stuffs define human nature.

cold.[70] The problem with these postulates, he argues, is that the listener has no way of knowing clearly whether they have any relationship to the truth.[71] The author concedes that these kinds of postulates are necessary for explaining "invisible and doubtful things," such as what is up above or below the earth. But because medicine can make its claims empirically evident, he refuses to accept postulates as the basis of its inquiries.[72] His commitment to empirical knowledge has attracted the respect of modern scholars.[73] Yet the question of how knowledge, necessarily mediated by the symptom, is made manifest rewards further examination, as does the question of *to whom* knowledge becomes clear. For, in fact, there are different kinds of knowing in *On Ancient Medicine*.[74]

Central to the author's defense of medicine's expert knowledge is its *hodos*, "road" or "method." He retraces this road in the first chapters back to its origins in a half-mythic, precultural time when humans were struggling to survive in a world ill-suited to their natures. Whereas the natures of oxen, horses, and all other animals harmonized unthinkingly with the available nourishment, human nature stood apart, at odds with food in its raw, "bestial" state.[75] If humans were to live and grow, they needed to discover another diet.

> ὡς γὰρ ἔπασχον πολλά τε καὶ δεινὰ ὑπὸ ἰσχυρῆς τε καὶ θηριώδεος διαίτης ὠμά τε καὶ ἄκρητα καὶ μεγάλας δυνάμιας ἔχοντα ἐσφερόμενοι—οἷά περ ἂν καὶ νῦν ὑπ' αὐτῶν πάσχοιεν πόνοισί τε ἰσχυροῖσι καὶ νούσοισι περιπίπτοντες καὶ διὰ τάχεος θανάτοισιν ... διὰ δὴ ταύτην τὴν χρείην καὶ οὗτοί μοι δοκέουσι ζητῆσαι τροφὴν ἁρμόζουσαν τῇ φύσει καὶ εὑρεῖν ταύτην ἣ νῦν χρεώμεθα. (*VM* 3, Li 1.576 = 121,15–20, 122,6–8 Jouanna)

For as they suffered many terrible things on account of the strong and bestial nature of their diet, when they were taking in foods that were raw and unmixed and possessing great *dunameis*, such things as one would suffer now too, falling into violent pains and diseases and quickly death. . . . On account of this need, it seems to

---

[70] *VM* 1 (Li 1.572 = 119,4–5 Jouanna). On what is meant by *hupothesis*, see G. Lloyd 1963; Hankinson 1992; Cooper 2004.19–23; Schiefsky 2005a.120–26. For arguments against the hot and the cold as causal factors, see chapters 16–20.

[71] *VM* 1 (Li 1.572 = 119,7–10 Jouanna). Cf. 13 (Li 1.598–600 = 133,7–134,17 Jouanna) and *Nat. Hom.* 1 (Li 6.32–34 = 164,12–166,9 Jouanna). Cooper 2004.10–18 persuasively demonstrates that the opponents in chapters 2 and 13 are the same as those in chapter 20; see also Schiefsky 2005a.24; 2005b.74–75.

[72] *VM* 1 (Li 1.572 = 119,4–7 Jouanna). The idea of clarity recurs throughout the treatise: terms such as φανερόν and δῆλον often indicate both what is experientially clear and what is logically clear: e.g., 1 (Li 1.570 = 118,7 Jouanna), 2 (Li 1.572 = 120,2 Jouanna), 6, *tris* (Li 1.582 = 125,6,8,13 Jouanna), 18 (Li 1.612 = 142,6 Jouanna).

[73] See Hankinson 1998a.64–69; Cooper 2004; Schiefsky 2005a. The author has been accused of advancing hypotheses of his own: see G. Lloyd 1966.83; 1979.147.

[74] This point is usually overlooked. Scholars tend to align the knowing subject with the physician and equate perception with seeing. Pigeaud 1977 is a notable exception.

[75] *VM* 3 (Li 1.576 = 121,5–12 Jouanna).

me, they sought nourishment that harmonized with their nature and they discovered that which we use now.

Necessity, in other words, drives discovery.[76] While born of necessity, though, this discovery is not the same as necessary outcomes in the body, insofar as it involves a shift from the automatism of the physical world to conscious, rational inquiry.[77] The vital tendencies of human nature become the seeking of these first investigators; "cooking" in the cavity is anticipated by the deliberate modification of foods, as they "mold everything to suit human nature and its *dunamis*" (πλάσσοντες πάντα πρὸς τὴν τοῦ ἀνθρώπου φύσιν τε καὶ δύναμιν, 3, Li 1.578 = 122,14–15 Jouanna). Pain is no longer just pain, but what Jackie Pigeaud has felicitously called "la pédagogie de la douleur."[78]

Although in the beginning, all humans suffered from their diet, only a small group of insightful people, the forerunners of physicians, used their suffering to discover the *tekhnē*. In the present, however, "all are knowledgeable [ἐπιστήμονες] on account of necessity and use" (4, Li 1.578 = 123,10–11 Jouanna).[79] Dietetics is democratic not simply because everyone must eat, but because human nature, while defined collectively against the foil of the animal, comprises a range of individual natures, each with its own needs.[80] Some natures are too weak to tolerate the slightest deviation in dietary habits; others cannot handle specific foods, like cheese, that may well benefit someone else.[81] Because natures differ, the ancients' research must be restaged at the level of the individual, who learns his own nature by querying its capacities through painful trial and error.

Some kind of biofeedback also forms the bedrock of research in medicine. Indeed, medicine's origins mimic those of dietetics: just as pain once revealed the incompatibility of a raw diet with human nature, it has shown, too, that the same diets do not benefit the sick and the healthy. When patients who have

---

[76] *VM* 3 (Li 1.574–76 = 121,2–5 Jouanna). Compare Democr. (DK68) B144, although Schiefsky 2005a.50 is rightly skeptical about a direct Democritean influence. See also Dunn 2005.56–60, stressing the role of contingency in the Hippocratic author's account of progress. On the relationship of *On Ancient Medicine* to *Kulturgeschichte*, see H. Miller 1949.190–99; 1955; Dunn 2005; Schiefsky 2005a.157–60. On *Kulturgeschichte* more generally, see Cole 1990.

[77] On the automatism of nature versus intelligent and volitional human action, see also *Vict.* III 68 (Li 6.600 = 198,12–15 Joly-Byl), contrasting the unthinking adjustment of trees to seasonal change with the need for people to undertake preparations themselves, with Joly 1960.130–31; E. *Cyc.* 332–33 (ἡ γῆ δ᾽ ἀνάγκῃ, κἂν θέλῃ κἂν μὴ θέλῃ, / τίκτουσα ποίαν τἀμὰ πιαίνει βοτά, the earth out of necessity, willingly or unwillingly, producing grass feeds my flocks).

[78] Pigeaud 1977.207.

[79] Though dietetics keeps being refined for those with specialized needs, such as athletes (*VM* 4, Li 1.580 = 123,14–17 Jouanna).

[80] See *VM* 20 (Li 1.624 = 147,16–17 Jouanna): διαφέρουσιν … αἱ φύσιες. See also *Fract.* 35 (Li 3.536–38 = 99,22–100,1 Kühlewein); *Vict.* III 67 (Li 6.592 = 194,4–5 Joly-Byl); and above, chapter 3, n.84.

[81] Weak natures: *VM* 10 (Li 1.592–94 = 130,14, 131,9–10 Jouanna). Cheese: *VM* 20 (Li 1.622–24 = 147,1–148,2 Jouanna).

been given porridge suffer fever and pains, for example, they provide the physician with crystalline evidence that porridge is not always suitable in disease.[82]

Given the role played by pain in teaching the physician what he knows, medicine's claims to knowledge about human nature can appear like a reworking of the tragic axiom "knowledge through suffering," *pathei mathos*. At the same time, as we shift from dietetics to medicine, the person who suffers is no longer necessarily the same person who learns, or at least the primary learner.[83] Rather, the sufferer stands on one side, the physician-inquirer on the other, with the *sōma* in the middle. It is, in fact, the *sōma* on which the author, in a programmatic statement, makes all medical knowledge and therapy depend. It is necessary to shoot for some measure in treatment, he observes.[84] Yet "you will discover no measure, neither a number nor a weight, in relation to which someone could acquire precise knowledge, except the *aisthēsis* of the *sōma*" (μέτρον δὲ οὐδὲ ἀριθμὸν οὔτε σταθμὸν ἄλλον πρὸς ὃ ἀναφέρων εἴσῃ τὸ ἀκριβές, οὐκ ἂν εὕροις ἀλλ᾽ ἢ τοῦ σώματος τὴν αἴσθησιν, 9, Li 1.588–90 = 128,11–13 Jouanna).[85]

The phrase "the *aisthēsis* of the *sōma*" is obviously crucial to the author's point. But what does it mean? In particular, whether we read the genitive as subjective or objective determines how we understand the role of *aisthēsis* in medical epistemology, at least for this author. If we read an objective genitive, the author will be referring to the sensation the physician has of the patient's body. But, while it is true that the physician is a privileged subject of knowledge in the text, by translating *aisthēsis* in this way we neglect the crucial epistemic function of pain and privilege hands-on investigation over the kind of inferential prowess demonstrated by the physician elsewhere in the treatise.[86] If we read the genitive as subjective, sensing belongs to the patient's body. Sensing is often equated with "the sensation an individual has of their own body."[87] But given that, as we saw in chapter 2, *aisthēsis* can be extended to bodies and body parts independently of the sentient person, we should not assume this equation. Let us consider, then, to whom or to what *aisthēsis* belongs here.

---

[82] *VM* 6 (Li 1.582–84 = 125,5–126,2 Jouanna).

[83] Galen imagines a physician who has experienced every kind of pain himself as an impossible ideal (*Loc.Aff.* 2.6, Kühn 8.88–89). But cf. Pl. *R.* 3, 408d8–e5.

[84] On στοχάσασθαι, see Ingenkamp 1983 and Jouanna 1990b.172–73.

[85] See also *Vict.* I 2 (Li 6.470 = 124,17–24 Joly-Byl) on the difficulty of matching regimen "to the nature of each" (πρὸς ἑκάστου φύσιν).

[86] For a defense of the objective genitive, see Laín Entralgo 1975.305–10; Thivel 1981.331; Bratescu 1983. These scholars are hard-pressed to corroborate the claim with internal support (Bratescu offers no evidence, while all of Laín Entralgo's is from other treatises).

[87] Dean-Jones 1995.52; see also Jouanna 1990b.174. Schiefsky 2005a.191–92 distinguishes this position from the Protagorean doctrine "man is the measure of all things" as it is expressed in Plato's *Theaetetus*; Demont 2005.273–75 sees more overlap between the Hippocratic author and the Apology that Socrates assigns Protagoras. Deichgräber 1933 accepts the subjective genitive, but is so troubled by its implications for the authority of the physician that he proposes changing αἴσθησιν to διάθησιν (the patient's condition); Müri 1936 soundly rejects the emendation.

First, it is undeniable that, for this author, the experience patients have of their bodies is indispensable to medical knowledge. Concluding his methodological proem, he remarks:

μάλιστα δέ μοι δοκεῖ περὶ ταύτης δεῖν λέγοντα τῆς τέχνης γνωστὰ λέγειν τοῖσι δημότῃσιν· οὐ γὰρ περὶ ἄλλων τινῶν οὔτε ζητεῖν οὔτε λέγειν προσήκει ἢ περὶ τῶν παθημάτων ὧν αὐτοὶ οὗτοι νοσέουσί τε καὶ πονέουσιν. αὐτοὺς μὲν οὖν τὰ σφέων αὐτῶν παθήματα καταμαθεῖν, ὥς τε γίνεται καὶ παύεται καὶ δι᾿ οἵας προφάσιας αὔξεταί τε καὶ φθίνει, δημότας ἐόντας οὐ ῥηΐδιον, ὑπ᾿ ἄλλου δὲ εὑρημένα καὶ λεγόμενα εὐπετές· οὐδὲν γὰρ ἕτερον ἢ ἀναμιμνήσκεται ἕκαστος ἀκούων τῶν ἑωυτῷ συμβαινόντων. εἰ δέ τις τῆς τῶν ἰδιωτέων γνώμης ἀποτεύξεται καὶ μὴ διαθήσει τοὺς ἀκούοντας οὕτως, τοῦ ἐόντος ἀποτεύξεται. καὶ διὰ ταῦτα οὖν ταῦτα οὐδὲν δεῖ ὑποθέσιος. (*VM* 2, Li 1.572–74 = 120,3–15 Jouanna)

But most of all it seems to me that one must, when speaking about this *tekhnē*, speak of things known to average people. For it is a question of researching and describing nothing other than the affections that afflict these very people and on account of which they suffer. Certainly for them to figure out themselves their own affections—how they come about and cease, and on account of which causes they grow and subside—is not easy, because they are average people; but when their affections have been discovered and explained by someone else, it is simple. For this requires nothing more than for each one, listening, to remember what has happened to him. But if someone fails to connect with the understanding of average people and does not put his listeners in this condition, he will be out of touch with reality. And it is for the same reasons that medicine has no need of a postulate.

The "things known to ordinary people" would seem to be the affections that afflict them without encompassing everything there is to know about these affections. The particular knowledge of average people, we might infer, is what they sense of their own bodies, sensations that are particularly sharp and insistent when they are sick. The last sentence suggests that it is the patient's memory of what has happened to him (τῶν ἑωυτῷ συμβαινόντων), triggered by hearing the physician's account, that is the touchstone of medicine's truths about human nature, or, rather, in this case, simply "what is" (τοῦ ἐόντος). The patient's knowledge thus frees medicine from a dependence on *hupotheseis*.[88]

---

[88] On "reciprocal pedagogy," see Pigeaud 1977.200. Cf. *Art.* 7 (Li 6.10–12 = 231,11–17 Jouanna), where physician and patient are pitted against each other in a zero-sum contest to evade blame: οἱ μὲν γὰρ ὑγιαινούσῃ γνώμῃ μεθ᾿ ὑγιαίνοντος σώματος ἐγχειρέουσι, λογισάμενοι τά τε παρεόντα τῶν τε παροιχομένων τὰ ὁμοίως διατεθέντα τοῖσι παρεοῦσιν ὥστε ποτὲ θεραπευθέντα εἰπεῖν ὡς ἀπήλλαξαν, οἱ δ᾿ οὔτε ἃ κάμνουσιν οὔτε δι᾿ ἃ κάμνουσιν, οὐδ᾿ ὅ τι ἐκ τῶν παρεόντων ἔσται οὐδ᾿ ὅ τι ἐκ τῶν τούτοισιν ὁμοίων γίνεται εἰδότες ἐπιτάσσονται ([The physicians] take up their task with healthy judgment in a healthy body, having reasoned about the present case and past cases analogous to the present case in order to be able to say with what therapy other patients survived, but the others [i.e., patients] receive orders, knowing neither what they are suffering nor on account of what they are suffering, nor what will be the outcome of their present situation nor what usually happens in situations similar to this one).

In securing the patient as a subject of knowledge, though, we bring to light another complication. Recall that dietetics, that is, the art of harmonizing food with one's nature, is essentially a democratic practice supported, at least in part, by self-reflexively produced knowledge about one's own nature. In the passage just cited, however, this community of knowers breaks down, creating two different epistemic positions: that of the embodied sufferer and that of the physician.[89] We have seen that the experience of suffering is indispensable to learning the truth about disease. But if the physician, too, is needed to obtain that truth, then suffering alone must be insufficient for knowledge. Indeed, in this passage, the author emphasizes not only the clarity of embodied experience but also the nontransparent meaning of symptoms. Suffering reveals neither its origins nor its antidote; it does not indicate why it waxes and wanes. Pain becomes truly clear only once someone else has discovered and explained what has happened, that is, once pain is put in the context of hidden forces, stuffs, and structures, as we saw in *On the Nature of a Human Being* in chapter 2. Knowledge gained about one's own nature is never intuitively revelatory, but always depends on making connections between catalysts and symptoms.[90]

It is in the context of drawing such connections, and more specifically in a discussion of how to find a balance between overpowering the patient and depriving him of needed food, that the author introduces the *aisthēsis* of the *sōma* as the only guide available to the physician. The context suggests that we should read *aisthēsis* as the reaction of the *sōma* to incoming *dunameis*—that is, symptoms.[91] On this reading, while the patient has a more intimate acquaintance with the symptom—hence, his importance to medical knowledge—he is not necessarily the only one with empirical access to it: a fever, for example, can be felt by the physician, too.[92] Both the physician and the patient, then, can gather somatic data. At the same time, both of them can make inferences about cause on the basis of symptoms. Here, however, because the physician has a better understanding of causes, he has the advantage.

It was by tracing symptoms to causes that a small group of intelligent people first discovered techniques to survive. The author of the treatise assumes that these people undertook their experiments with winnowing, grinding, and

[89] The author routinely distinguishes the specialist (δημιουργός, χειροτέχνης, ἰητρός) from the layperson (δημότης, ἰδιώτης).

[90] The terms used of knowledge acquisition in the text pertain to reasoning, investigating, and searching, rather than "seeing": see, for example, ζητέω (*VM* 4, Li 1.580 = 123,16 Jouanna); λογισμός (12, Li 1.596 = 133,4 Jouanna); σκέπτομαι (11, Li 1.594 = 131,11 Jouanna); σκέψις (4, Li 1.580 = 123,13 Jouanna).

[91] For this reading, see Müri 1936.468–69. See also Festugière 1948.59–60; Pigeaud 1977.215–16. Schiefsky accepts *aisthēsis* as the body's reaction to a *dunamis*, but argues that, because the patient's body is not inanimate, the author means the body's reaction "*as it is perceived by the patient*" (2005a.199, emphasis in original). Yet the author indicates no such specification.

[92] Although, in the long list of symptoms (e.g., dizziness, troubled dreams, bitterness in the mouth, loss of pleasure in food) at *VM* 10 (Li 1.592–94 = 130,9–131,9 Jouanna), the patient is the primary observer—indeed, an unusual situation in the medical writings.

baking raw food because they had already "seen" that the causes of pain, disease, and death lie in foods that are too strong for human nature to master.[93] Later in the treatise, the author reports that the first investigators also saw the qualitative differences among these stuffs (the salty, the bitter, the acidic, and so on).[94] Their vision extends even beyond foods to things inside a human being:

> ταῦτα γὰρ ἑώρων καὶ ἐν τῷ ἀνθρώπῳ ἐνεόντα καὶ λυμαινόμενα τὸν ἄνθρωπον· . . . ταῦτα μὲν μεμιγμένα καὶ κεκρημένα ἀλλήλοισιν οὔτε φανερά ἐστιν οὔτε λυπεῖ τὸν ἄνθρωπον, ὅταν δέ τι τούτων ἀποκριθῇ καὶ αὐτὸ ἐφ᾽ ἑωυτοῦ γένηται, τότε καὶ φανερόν ἐστι καὶ λυπεῖ τὸν ἄνθρωπον. (VM 14, Li 1.602 = 136,8–9, 12–16 Jouanna)

> For they saw that these things [sc. constituent stuffs inside the body] are inside a human being and they hurt a human being. . . . These things, when mixed and compounded with one another are neither apparent nor do they hurt a person; but when one of them is separated off and stands alone, then it is apparent and hurts a person.

Having discovered that the powers outside a human being are also inside him, these early researchers arrive at a conclusion by now familiar from other medical writing: pain is most proximately caused by things inside the person. Their realization encourages those pursuing the study of human nature to inquire further into the stuffs and mechanisms that are directly responsible for suffering.[95]

The author positions himself as a direct heir to this method. He argues that physicians need to know not simply whether cheese, for example, is a bad food, but what kind of pain it produces, what causes it, and to what constituent stuff in a person it is unsuited (τίνα τε πόνον καὶ διὰ τί καὶ τίνι τῶν ἐν τῷ ἀνθρώπῳ ἐνεόντων ἀνεπιτήδειον, 20, Li 1.622 = 147,3–4 Jouanna).[96] Later he discusses the kinds of structures found inside the body and their role in the production of symptoms—he asks, for example, why we feel violent pain just below the diaphragm—as well as the ways in which different powers interact. In these last two cases, the route to knowledge bypasses the patient altogether: the physician can find structures analogous to those inside the body to examine; he can observe directly how different *dunameis* interact by mixing foods and liquids. Indeed, the author concludes by stating his preference for these disembodied

---

[93] VM 3 (Li 1.578 = 122,15–123,3 Jouanna). See also 14 (Li 1.600–602 = 135,14–136,5 Jouanna). This insight, though it has a basis in qualities (e.g., the salty, the bitter) that can be perceived in foods, is not obvious: others continue to (mistakenly) fault the hot and the cold for pain.

[94] The author's theory of powers has similarities with Alcmaeon's theories: see Wellmann 1930; cf. Schiefsky 2005a.48–49, with n.111, noting important differences. For a summary and discussion of the physiological theory in *On Ancient Medicine*, see Schiefsky 2005a.229–35, and 239, 246–48 on qualitative difference.

[95] Cited above, pp. 162–64. The author continues by remarking that the disruption caused by unblended foods is just like the disruption caused by a power that stands alone (VM 14, Li 1.602–4 = 136,16–21 Jouanna). The comparison supports Schiefsky's argument (2005a.234–35) that the model of the human body as a mixture is implicitly developed on analogy with the understanding of food as a mixture.

[96] See also VM 14 (Li 1.600 = 135,7–14 Jouanna).

methods of inquiry: "If someone in this way, conducting all his research outside the human body, were able to reach the truth, he would be able to always choose the best treatment" (οὕτως εἴ τις δύναιτο ζητέων ἔξωθεν ἐπιτυγχάνειν, καὶ δύναιτ᾽ ἂν πάντων ἐκλέγεσθαι αἰεὶ τὸ βέλτιστον, 24, Li 1.636 = 153,16–18 Jouanna). Presumably, because natures vary, treatment would continue to rely on bodily feedback. At the same time, the very desire to explore the causal factors at work inside the body by looking outside it makes clear that symptoms promise more clarity than they deliver.

The physician's skill in interpreting symptoms is particularly valuable in scenarios, such as a full-fledged disease, where the interval between catalyst and perceptible effect has grown complicated. In this context, the temporal proximity of a probable cause can become a red herring, and the patient, whose inferences tend to be based on that proximity, becomes a *negative* model of knowledge. The author lambastes those physicians who connect disturbances during recovery to whatever unusual thing the patient has done most recently for being as blind as patients.[97] Such imprecision should not affect the informed physician, who pairs an encyclopedic grasp of causes with a fine-grained analysis of symptoms in their specificity, specificity being that which enables him to move beyond simple temporal correlations of cause and effect:

> οὐδέποτε γὰρ ἡ αὐτὴ κακοπάθεια τούτων οὐδετέρου· οὐδέ γε ἀπὸ πληρώσιος οὐδ᾽ ἀπὸ βρώματος τοίου ἢ τοίου. ὅστις οὖν ταῦτα μὴ εἴσεται ὡς ἕκαστα ἔχει πρὸς τὸν ἄνθρωπον, οὔτε γινώσκειν τὰ γινόμενα ἀπ᾽ αὐτῶν δυνήσεται οὔτε χρῆσθαι ὀρθῶς.
> (*VM* 21, Li 1.626 = 148,15–19 Jouanna)

> For it is never the same bad feeling that arises from each of these two things, nor from surfeit, nor from one food or another. Whoever does not know how each of these particulars affects a person will be unable to know the things that arise from them, nor will he be able to use them correctly.

Knowledge is thus correlated with a system of translation between "bad feelings" and their causes.[98] Embodied experience may contribute to such knowledge, but it does not guarantee it. Even if it is the things inside us that hurt us, they—and, indeed, our very nature—remain alien without technical expertise.

Embodiment, Knowledge, and Technical Agency

Despite his avowed hostility toward physicists like Empedocles and his ilk, the author of *On Ancient Medicine* defines human nature through the dynamics of

---

[97] See also *Acut.* 1 (Li 2.224, ch. 1 = 36,2–10 Joly); *Vict.* III 70 (Li 6.606 = 202,11–12 Joly-Byl).

[98] For variation in the intensity of a "bad feeling," see also *VM* 10 (Li 1.592 = 130,9 Jouanna). In the imperial period, Archigenes, in the interest of improving the "translation" system, develops a more precise terminology for pain: see Pigeaud 1999.127–38. Criticizing this approach, Galen concludes that such precision is impossible: pain, being private, is unspeakable (ἄρρητος), so that pain suffered by another is ultimately *unknowable* (ἄγνωστος, *Loc.Aff.* 2.9 = 8.117 Kühn).

what I have called physicality. In so doing, he elaborates a concept of vulnerability markedly different from that assumed by magico-religious interpretations of symptoms. First and foremost, human nature, unlike every other animal nature, fails to harmonize automatically with the things growing in the earth.[99] But, moreover, it does not communicate its needs clearly to humans themselves. The belly, writes the author of On Regimen, is without understanding; although through it we become aware of hunger and thirst (ἀσύνετον γαστήρ· ταύτῃ συνίεμεν ὅτι διψῇ ἢ πεινῇ, I 12, Li 6.488 = 136,12–13 Joly-Byl), hunger, like pain, does not tell us what to eat or how to prepare our food. We need dietetics in order to secure the conditions under which our natures can master what enters from outside: the triad of growth, health, and life depends on interpreting symptoms and identifying causes.

The author of On Ancient Medicine does not simply stress that humans are different from other living beings because they do not harmonize unthinkingly with their environment. He also shows little interest in how human nature does balance itself automatically. He rejects the hot and the cold as pathogenic factors in part because they counteract each other's force apo tautomatou, "spontaneously": what is so deinon, "terrible" or "strange," about that, he asks.[100] If it is our nature to live so thoughtlessly, we might as well be animals, or barbarians—for barbarians, and even some Greeks, make no use of the medical tekhnē nor do they hold back from anything they might desire, even in illness, a life hapless enough to qualify as bestial.[101] Tekhnē, then, like dikē in Homer and Hesiod, draws a line between human and nonhuman. But whereas, in those poets, it is because animals lack dikē that they are excluded from the exchanges so critical to social concord, in On Ancient Medicine, animals lack tekhnē because they are already in harmony with the world. It is harmony of this kind, not among humans or between humans and gods but between different natures, that physicians aim to mimic by replacing the automatism of the physical body's interaction with the world with intelligent manipulation. Nevertheless, this is mimicry with a difference, insofar as harmony is achieved through reasoning. Human beings thus come to be defined not through the weakness of their natures but through their deliberate exercise of mastery over the physical world—both the world outside them and their own bodies. The care of human nature(s) is one of those "games of truth and error through which being is historically constituted as experience; that is, as something that can and must be thought."[102]

Herein, then, lies the gift of medicine: it enables reasoning agents to act on the dunameis in which they are necessarily and unseeingly implicated, rather

---

[99] VM 3 (Li 1.576 = 121,9 Jouanna): πᾶσιν ἐκτὸς ἀνθρώπου.

[100] VM 16 (Li 1.612 = 141,8–11 Jouanna). On "the spontaneous," see above, pp. 143–47.

[101] VM 5 (Li 1.580 = 124,7–9 Jouanna).

[102] Foucault 1985.6–7; see also Foucault 1997.223–51, 281–301. John Tambornino 2002.118–23 offers another angle on biofeedback and subject formation.

than merely suffering the reactions of the *sōma* to these forces. In *On Ancient Medicine*, the verb *dunamai*, "to be able," describes not only what human nature can do or withstand but also the ability of people, collectively expressed in *tekhnē*, to discover and, through reasoning, to use the forces that shape their experience in the service of health.[103] The author of *On the Tekhnē*, too, endows *tekhnē* with a *dunamis*, which translates the mere desire to know into efficacious inquiry and action. He argues that it is possible to investigate hidden diseases only if one has acquired the power to do so through education: just wanting to uncover them is not enough.[104] Knowledge, by making it possible to harness *dunameis*, thus creates a conduit between desire and its realization. Recall that, in *On Places in a Human Being*, knowledge is there whenever the knower wants to use it in contrast to *tukhē*, which is "self-ruled" (αὐτοκρατής).[105]

Most extant medical texts, unsurprisingly, vest the power to know and to act in the physician. Nevertheless, authors writing for a wider audience also recognize laypersons as subjects of medical, and not simply embodied, knowledge. Part of this recognition is implicit, embedded in the very structure of treatises addressed to nonspecialist audiences.[106] Yet it also explicit, insofar as many authors invite laypersons to adopt a specifically medical filter on their own embodied experiences, hoping to appropriate the often biting clarity of those experiences as "verification" of the explanations that they are offering. In making his case, the author of *On Ancient Medicine* regularly uses the first-person plural: *we* are disturbed, for example, when constituent stuffs separate out.[107] Or consider his use of the common cold, a condition in which we are all *empeiroi*, "experienced," and which he calls the "clearest of cases," as proof in his extended argument that it is not the hot and the cold but isolated humors that harm us.[108] If we find his extended account of a runny nose banal, it is worth remembering that this banality is tactical. Whereas the author of *On the Sacred Disease*, by tackling the causes of epilepsy, strives to create a new worldview behind the most spectacular symptoms, the author of *On Ancient Medicine* builds his

---

[103] For *phusis* with δύναμαι: *VM* 3, *bis* (Li 1.578 = 122,16, 123,2 Jouanna), 7 (Li 1.584 = 126,10 Jouanna), 14 (Li 1.602 = 136,4 Jouanna). The verb δύναμαι may also be used with people understood as virtually interchangeable with their natures (e.g., 5, Li 1.582 = 124,16 Jouanna). For δύναμαι used with knowing agents or the art, see 12 (Li 1.596 = 133,2–5 Jouanna), 14 (Li 1.600 = 135,7–10 Jouanna), 21 (Li 1.626 = 148,17–19 Jouanna).

[104] ἐξεύρηταί γε μὴν οὐ τοῖσι βουληθεῖσιν, ἀλλὰ τούτων τοῖσι δυνηθεῖσιν· δύνανται δὲ οἷσι τά τε τῆς παιδείης μὴ ἐκποδών, τά τε τῆς φύσιος μὴ ἀταλαίπωρα (*Art.* 9, Li 6.16 = 235,5–8 Jouanna). See also *Art.* 4 (Li 6.6 = 228, 2–5 Jouanna); Pl. *Phdr.* 268a9-b3.

[105] *Loc.* 46 (Li 6.342 = 84,17–24 Craik), cited in full above, pp. 143–44.

[106] On the relationship of the generic features of texts to their intended audiences, see van der Eijk 1997.86–89.

[107] *VM* 14 (Li 1.602–4 = 136,20–21 Jouanna): ταρασσόμεθα. See also 7 (Li 1.584 = 126,7 Jouanna), 15 (Li 1.604 = 137,19 Jouanna). The first-person plural is also extended to verbs of inquiry, for example, σκεψώμεθα at *VM* 5 (Li 1.580 = 123,18 Jouanna). On the appeal in medical writing to general human experience, see Diller 1932.40; van der Eijk 1997.116–17; Laskaris 2002.129–32.

[108] *VM* 18 (Li 1.612–16 = 142,6–143,6 Jouanna).

world-making case from everyday aches and pains. Both authors, however, are extending the indisputable reality of symptoms to a largely hidden, abstracted physical world.

The benefits of persuading listeners to see with the mind of a physician go beyond the epideictic arena to the bedside, where persuasion had more immediate and concrete consequences.[109] If bringing a patient to see things from the doctor's perspective encourages compliance, it is an obvious desideratum. In the Platonic dialogue named for him, Gorgias defends rhetoric's usefulness by boasting of having often convinced patients to submit to treatment after their physicians failed to do so (456b1–5). Even after a patient acquiesces, there is always a risk he will go astray in the physician's absence or mistake premature feelings of recovery for total recuperation.[110] In practice, then, physicians could hardly fail to see that the bodies in their care were attached to people, whose cooperation needed to be secured, albeit sometimes by proxy, for therapy to work.

If the patient unites with the physician against the disease, the Hippocratic triangle collapses into a battle between opposing forces. But what if the patient refuses to ally himself with the physician? Far from simply standing on the sidelines of the struggle between life and death, such patients are often tacitly understood to be complicit with the disease and sometimes openly so: in his eagerness to free physicians from blame, the author of *On the Tekhnē* declares outright that noncompliant patients are responsible for their own deaths.[111] When there is no physician to disobey, however, it is more difficult to figure out where the patient stands in relationship to his disease, as we can see in *On Ancient Medicine*. On the one hand, by making health dependent on the inferences and deliberate actions of an embodied agent, the author limns the possibility that a human being has control over his own nature. On the other hand, he recognizes that the requisite knowledge is difficult to acquire.[112] By acknowledging this difficulty, thereby circumscribing the control people have over their nature, he complicates the grounds for reproach. Even the author of *On the Tekhnē* accepts that the patient's agency is compromised, at least in disease.[113] But if the patient's own inclination toward health is as contingent and uncertain as the vital tendencies of his nature or the humors, can he ever be said to be *aitios* for his suffering? Let us stop and reconsider how medical etiology works.

[109] Langholf 1997–2004.920–21. In addition to the presiding physician, there would have been observing, and perhaps dissenting, physicians: see *Epid.* V 14 (Li 5.212 = 8,19–20 Jouanna), 95 (Li 5.254–56 = 42,3–14 Jouanna; cf. *Epid.* VII 121 [Li 5.466 = 116,17–117,9 Jouanna]), with Nutton 1995.16–17.

[110] *Prorrh.* II 3–4 (Li 9.12–20 = 224–34 Potter) outlines a series of signs for detecting disobedience. On premature feelings of recovery, see *Artic.* 9 (Li 4.100 = 124,7–11 Kühlewein).

[111] *Art.* 7 (Li 6.12 = 232,7–11 Jouanna).

[112] Of course, if the patient circumvents this difficulty by conversing with the physician, we return to a model where noncompliance is a possibility.

[113] *Art.* 7 (Li 6.10–12 = 231,11–232,3 Jouanna), cited in part above, n.88.

Extant medical writing affords us ample opportunity to see how, as responsibility migrates from social and ethical agents to impersonal stuffs and forces, the very idea of responsibility is adapted to natural causes. External forces, such as bilious foods or the south wind, still exercise considerable power over us; yet, as we saw in the previous chapter, their assault is stripped of intentions and emotions. With the disappearance of a desire to harm, the capacity to harm breaks down over a causal series, which unfolds largely inside the *sōma*. It is true that the earliest Greek poets believe both that things inside a person can hurt him and that individual identity can influence how daemonic force is realized. As the physical body emerges, however, this inner space is reconceived in terms of humors, structures, fleshes, the body's *dunamis*, and its *phusis*—things that can explain in relatively precise terms how an external catalyst is transformed into a symptom. Inner space comes to be defined as largely nonconscious, subject to necessity and physical automatism. Understood in these terms, the *sōma* both mitigates the power of blind fatalism in archaic explanations of disease and attracts responsibility for unseen harm from daemonic agents and, indeed, from the person himself insofar as, recklessly or inadvertently, he incurs daemonic anger.

But it may be precisely because the physical body is so estranged from the human, despite being closely allied with the idea of human nature, that the responsibility for suffering once vested with mortal and immortal social agents often seems to slide off it. Failing to absorb blame, the body sends it back into circulation. One natural candidate to receive it is the physician.[114] Another is the patient. Indeed, it is in the context of the causal shift just described, I suggest, that the person's relationship to his *sōma* assumes ethical potential, that is, the potential to be praised or blamed, beyond the narrow question of patient compliance.[115]

The patient has the capacity, through what he eats or does, to guard against the body's hair-trigger tendencies toward instability and formlessness. But that capacity is a double-edged sword. After all, by eating or acting he can just as easily upset the delicate economy of power in the cavity. The patient oblivious to the effects of his actions risks precipitating disaster or making a small problem worse. In *On Regimen*, for example, the author speaks at one point of people who "turn the disease into pneumonia through their use of baths and foods and bring themselves to the brink of ruin" (ἀλλὰ λουτροῖσί τε καὶ σίτοισι χρησάμενοι ἐς περιπλευμονίην κατέστησαν τὸ νόσημα, καὶ ἐς κίνδυνον τὸν ἔσχατον ἀφικνέονται, III 72, Li 6.610–12 = 204,14–15 Joly-Byl). In *On the*

---

[114] On the delicate question of the physician's blame, see von Staden 1990; see also Pigeaud 1990, arguing that the physician relieves the patient of responsibility; Horstmanshoff and Rosen 2003, on the honor at stake for the physician in tackling difficult diseases. Physicians may have been tried for incompetence, but they show up in our legal evidence more often as "expert witnesses" (Amundsen and Ferngren 1977).

[115] Hankinson 2006.44–50 discusses obligations to care for the body in the ancient world from the perspective of modern imperatives of body care.

Tekhnē, not only is the density of bodies to blame for disease but also the negligence of patients (διὰ τε τὴν τῶν καμνόντων ὀλιγωρίην, 11, Li 6.20–22 = 238,18 Jouanna). Yet, as we have seen, the person can manage his body, mysteriously located between what he does (taking baths, eating cheese, walking at noon) and what happens to him, only if he understands how it works. In the opening chapter of *On Affections*, before stating the causal role of bile and phlegm in disease, the author observes:

> ἄνδρα χρή, ὅστις ἐστὶ συνετός, λογισάμενον ὅτι τοῖσιν ἀνθρώποισι πλείστου ἄξιόν ἐστιν ἡ ὑγιείη, ἐπίστασθαι ἀπὸ τῆς ἑωυτοῦ γνώμης ἐν τῇσι νούσοισιν ὠφελέεσθαι· ἐπίστασθαι δὲ τὰ ὑπὸ τῶν ἰητρῶν καὶ λεγόμενα καὶ προσφερόμενα πρὸς τὸ σῶμα ἑαυτοῦ καὶ διαγινώσκειν· ἐπίστασθαι δὲ τούτων ἕκαστα ἐς ὅσον εἰκὸς ἰδιώτην. (*Aff.* 1, Li 6.208 = 6 Potter)[116]

> Any man of intelligence, having taken it into account that health is of the greatest value to human beings, ought to know by means of his own understanding how to help himself in diseases, and to know and to judge what is said by physicians and what they administer to his body, and to know each of these things to the extent that is fitting for a layperson.

In stressing the patient's own capacity for understanding (ἀπὸ τῆς <u>ἑωυτοῦ</u> γνώμης), the author anticipates the reflexive pronoun used with *sōma* several lines later (τὸ σῶμα <u>ἑαυτοῦ</u>). His repetition of the reflexive draws a line between the patient's ownership of the *sōma* and his responsibility to grasp it with his own mind. The author seems to suggest that only by exercising his ability to understand his body can the patient claim it as his own.

In the proem, the author of *On Affections* treats the patient as a subject of knowledge modeled on the physician. Shortly afterward, however, patients revert to their more typical role: marginal and passive. These possibilities represent the two positions that the medical writers imagine for a person in relation to his own body: either he takes up the perspective of the physician or he becomes the pawn of forces he neither understands nor controls—suffering without learning. The person is, in other words, either the first cause of what happens to him, intelligently determining his own experience, or the last effect of a chain of mechanically driven events, a symptom himself. Transformed by the incorporation of the daemonic energies that had cut through the Homeric hero, the person, quite *unlike* in Homer, threatens to dissolve into the impersonal force field from which he is created. Escaping this fate, at least for the medical writers, requires the knowledge that only they can supply. While dream interpreters may be well and good, the author of *On Regimen* observes, when it comes to health and disease, "they cannot instruct one how to take care" (οἱ δ'

---

[116] These lines are also found verbatim at *Salubr.* 9 (Li 6.86 = 220,8–10 Jouanna, as *Nat. Hom.* 24). The content of the treatise appears so technical that Paul Potter, the most recent editor, argues that the proem must be a frame, into which a specialist treatise has been set (1988a.4–5). Others, however, have seen the proem as further evidence of educated interest in medicine: see van der Eijk 1997.86–87; Schiefsky 2005a.41–42; see also Jouanna 1974.262–63.

οὖν οὐ διδάσκουσιν, ὡς χρὴ φυλάσσεσθαι). They simply recommend prayer—not a bad idea, but one ought to invoke the gods "while also helping oneself" (αὐτὸν συλλαμβάνοντα), a practice that requires an understanding of causes.[117] Indeed, "if people had knowledge," writes the author of *On the Tekhnē*, "they would never have fallen into their diseases" (εἰ γὰρ ἠπίσταντο, οὐκ ἂν περιέπιπτον αὐτοῖσι, 11, Li 6.20 = 238,1–2 Jouanna).[118]

Practices of care in Greek medicine and ethics have received a lot of attention in recent years. The assumptions behind these practices, however, have not been fully examined, in part because our own culture is so anxiously committed to the care of the physical body, making such care seem familiar, in part because the context in which these practices unfold has been insufficiently understood.[119] It is worth taking a closer look, then, at how the care of the *sōma* brings to light the ethical implications of its physicality.

TAKING CARE

More than any other extant medical text, *On Regimen* (ca. 400 BCE) attests the growing interest in the late fifth century in the care of the physical body.[120] In the opening chapter, the author notes that many before him have written on the subject of human *diaitē*, a term that encompasses not only diet but also exercise, sexual habits, and a range of other behaviors.[121] It is likely that he is referring to a recent—perhaps even within the past twenty years—spate of work. Most ancient writers, with the notable exception of the author of *On Ancient Medicine*, see regimen as a relatively late arrival to the medical tradition, and

---

[117] *Vict.* IV 87 (Li 6.642 = 218,20–22 Joly-Byl). On causes and care, see also *Vict.* I 2 (Li 6.468 = 122,27–124,4 Joly-Byl); *VM* 23 (Li 1.634 = 153,5–6 Jouanna): ἃ δεῖ πάντα εἰδέναι ᾗ διαφέρει, ὅπως τὰ αἴτια ἑκάστων εἰδὼς ὀρθῶς φυλάσσηται.

[118] The passage continues: τῆς γὰρ αὐτῆς συνέσιός ἐστιν ἥσπερ τὸ εἰδέναι τῶν νούσων τὰ αἴτια, καὶ τὸ θεραπεύειν αὐτὰς ἐπίστασθαι πάσῃσι τῇσι θεραπείῃσιν αἳ κωλύουσι τὰ νοσήματα μεγαλύνεσθαι (For it is the task of the same intelligence on which knowing the cause of diseases depends to know how to treat them with all the therapies that keep diseases from growing larger, Li 6.20 = 238,2–5 Jouanna); see also *Flat.* 1 (Li 6.92 = 104,1–4 Jouanna). On the idea that experience gives people some knowledge of their bodies, see, e.g., *Mul.* I 62 (Li 8.126 = 112,23–114,2 Grensemann), where, with time, women become experienced in their affections; on the experienced woman in Hippocratic gynecology, see further A. Hanson 1990.309–10. See also *Morb.* I 22 (Li 6.184 = 64,13–15 Wittern): older men "understand more and take better care of their affections" (ἐπαίουσι μᾶλλον καὶ ἐπιμέλονται μᾶλλον τῶν παθημάτων). On the patient's knowledge, see also above, p. 168.

[119] As I noted in the introduction, Foucault's work on the care of the self gives little sense of how this care takes shape. Most work by historians of ancient philosophy on the care of the self has not paid enough attention to medical writing.

[120] For the dating of the treatise, see Joly 1960.203–9.

[121] *Vict.* I 1 (Li 6.466 = 122,7 Joly-Byl). On *diaitē*, see Thivel 2000, esp. 30–35 on its use in medical texts. Wesley Smith sees *On Regimen* as "the culmination of the development of dietetic theory in the Classical Period" (1980.440). Dietetics does, however, continue to flourish in the fourth century: see esp. Diocles fr. 182 (van der Eijk); see also Mnesitheus fr. 18 (Bertier), on the diet of young children; frr. 22–40 (Bertier) on foodstuffs. For the importance of dietetics in the Hellenistic and imperial periods, see Scarborough 1970; W. Smith 1982; Foucault 1986.

modern scholars have generally concurred.[122] The later date fits well with what we see in *On Regimen*, which extends the causal theories and techniques of intervention familiar from other medical writings into the patient's daily life.[123] The author's approach is driven, above all, by the need to exercise foresight to head off the symptom before it erupts.[124] The treatise's orientation suggests a reciprocal strengthening of anxieties about the physical body and public confidence in the power of medicine to manage it.

The preemptive strategy of regimen targets potential triggers of disease. In the case of environmental factors, which lie outside his control, the physician aims to remake the person's nature to withstand their assault. He creates regimens capable of "warding off" seasonal changes as one might ward off the gods' anger.[125] If a cold and moist constitution is at risk in winter and spring, for example, regimen can supply warmth and dryness. Exercise molds the flesh so that the winds cannot.[126] The language of making and molding here is not trivial. In *On Regimen*, the author dwells at length on similarities between crafts like metallurgy and carpentry and the arts of fashioning the physical body, which include both medicine and gymnastic training.[127] By educating the layperson about the causes of disease, the physician also "remakes" him, preventing him from becoming another mindless force acting on his nature.

Crucial to the layperson's role in health is what the author calls pre-sufferings. In the introduction, we saw how Plutarch uses these pre-sufferings to counter Hesiod's "silent" diseases. In *On Regimen*, the author claims them as his own discovery:[128]

ἐμοὶ δὲ ταῦτα ἐξεύρηται, καὶ πρὸ τοῦ κάμνειν τὸν ἄνθρωπον ἀπὸ τῆς ὑπερβολῆς, ἐφ᾽ ὁπότερον ἂν γένηται, προδιάγνωσις. οὐ γὰρ εὐθέως αἱ νοῦσοι τοῖσιν ἀνθρώποισιν ἐπιγίνονται, ἀλλὰ κατὰ μικρὸν συλλεγόμεναι ἀθρόως ἐκφαίνονται. πρὶν οὖν

---

[122] At *Acut.* 3 (Li 2.226, ch. 1 = 37,2–4 Joly), "the ancients" are blamed for neglecting dietetics. See also Pl. *R.* 3, 407c8–408b6 (cf. 405d6–406a4); Galen *Thras.* 32–33 (Kühn 5.869–70), following Plato. On the history and prehistory of dietetics, see Temkin 1953.221–22; Edelstein 1967f; Lonie 1977; W. Smith 1980; 1992; Longrigg 1999.

[123] See esp. Edelstein 1967f on regimen's transformation of everyday life. See also Jaeger 1944.26–45; Temkin 1949.4–5; Kudlien 1973; Foucault 1985.97–108; 2005.75.

[124] χρὴ προμηθεῖσθαι: e.g., *Vict.* III 72 (Li 6.612 = 204,16 Joly-Byl), 73 (Li 6.612 = 204,33 Joly-Byl), 74 (Li 6.616 = 206,23 Joly-Byl). See also *Vict.* II 38 (Li 6.534 = 162,8 Joly-Byl): χρὴ ... παρεσκευάσθαι.

[125] *Salubr.* 1 (Li 6.74 = 206,15–16 Jouanna, as *Nat. Hom.* 16). On the vocabulary of "warding off" in medical and nonmedical sources, see Jouanna 1983a. On counterbalancing regimens, see, e.g., *Salubr.* 2 (Li 6.74–76 = 208,9–20 Jouanna, as *Nat. Hom.* 17); *Vict.* I 32 (Li 6.506–10 = 148,3–150,10 Joly-Byl), 35 (Li 6.512–22 = 150,29–156,18 Joly-Byl), III 68–69 (Li 6.594–606 = 194,17–202,4 Joly-Byl).

[126] *Vict.* I 2 (Li 6.470 = 124,8–14 Joly-Byl).

[127] *Vict.* I 13–22 (Li 6.488–94 = 136,15–140,16 Joly-Byl), discussed in Hawhee 2004.86–92.

[128] See also *Vict.* III 69 (Li 6.606 = 200,28–32 Joly-Byl). The practice of προδιάγνωσις may have become standard: see the possibly spurious Diocles fr. 183 (van der Eijk), with the largely inconclusive discussion of the arguments for and against its authenticity at van der Eijk 2000–2001, 2:353–58.

κρατεῖσθαι ἐν τῷ ἀνθρώπῳ τὸ ὑγιὲς ὑπὸ τοῦ νοσεροῦ, ἃ πάσχουσιν ἐξεύρηταί μοι, καὶ ὅπως χρὴ ταῦτα καθιστάναι ἐς τὴν ὑγιείην. (*Vict.* I 2, Li 6.472 = 124,28–126,3 Joly-Byl)

These things have been discovered by me, and also, before a person suffers from surfeit, a "pre-diagnosis" on the basis of what sort it is. For diseases do not come upon people all at once; rather, gathering themselves together gradually, they appear with a sudden spring. So I have discovered what a person suffers before what is healthy in him is mastered by what is diseased, and how one ought to restore these things to health.

In the third book of the treatise, the author provides ample documentation of this discovery, correlating various sensations with kinds of surfeit on the model of translation envisioned in *On Ancient Medicine*. Here, however, the embodied person is entrusted with interpreting corporeal signs, however faint. Like a physician, he looks past the surface of the body to its hidden troubles. His precaution turns every sensation into a potential symptom.

Such attention to the body calls to mind the portrait of the *deisidaimōn*, the "superstitious man," in Theophrastus's *Characters*, a text that dates from the latter part of the fourth century.[129] The *deisidaimōn* is plagued by an undue fear of the daemonic: he is terrified of the owl's hoot, the mouse in the grain sack, the weasel that crosses his path. His world abounds in signs requiring sacrifices and interpretation. Similar anxieties are scathingly ascribed to elite adherents of medicine in the third book of Plato's *Republic*,[130] with the important difference that the daemonic here comprises forces within the body. The threat these forces are seen to pose leads to what Socrates denounces as the "excessive care of the body" (ἡ περιττὴ αὕτη ἐπιμέλεια τοῦ σώματος).[131]

τὸ δὲ δὴ μέγιστον,[132] ὅτι καὶ πρὸς μαθήσεις ἁστινασοῦν καὶ ἐννοήσεις τε καὶ μελέτας πρὸς ἑαυτὸν χαλεπή, κεφαλῆς τινας ἀεὶ διατάσεις καὶ ἰλίγγους ὑποπτεύουσα καὶ αἰτιωμένη ἐκ φιλοσοφίας ἐγγίγνεσθαι, ὥστε, ὅπῃ ταύτῃ ἀρετὴ ἀσκεῖται καὶ δοκιμάζεται, πάντῃ ἐμπόδιος· κάμνειν γὰρ οἴεσθαι ποιεῖ ἀεὶ καὶ ὠδίνοντα μήποτε λήγειν περὶ τοῦ σώματος. (Pl. *R.* 3, 407b8–c6)

And most important of all, surely, is that [sc. this care] makes any sort of learning, thought, or private meditation difficult, by forever causing imaginary headaches or dizziness and accusing philosophy of causing them. Hence, wherever this sort of

---

[129] Thphr. *Char.* 16. This fear is presented by Theophrastus as unseemly: contrast, for example, the apparently legitimate concerns about the gods and the daemonic at Hes. *Op.* 706–829. Dale Martin argues that Theophrastus's judgment is based on class: "Superstitious beliefs are wrong because they cause people to act in ways that are socially inappropriate, embarrassing, and vulgar" (2004.34).

[130] On Plato's familiarity with contemporary medicine, see Craik 2001c; G. Lloyd 2003.152–57.

[131] Cf. X. *Mem.* 1.2.4, where Socrates is in favor of body care as long as it does not interfere with the care of the soul. At Pl. *Phd.* 66d2–7, it is the *sōma* itself that interferes with the pursuit of philosophy.

[132] Slings posits a lacuna here (and would supply something like ἦν δ' ἐγώ or ἔφην).

virtue is practiced and submitted to philosophical scrutiny, excessive care of the body hinders it. For it is constantly making you imagine that you are ill and never lets you stop agonizing about your body. (trans. Reeve)

Such vigilance is confirmed by the elaborate recommendations of *On Regimen*.

Given the labor involved in this "excessive" care of the body, we would expect that regimen was primarily an elite preoccupation. This is, indeed, what we are told by Plato, who contrasts the carpenter who, "if someone prescribes a lengthy regimen," promptly replies he does not have the leisure to be ill, with the wealthy man who can devote all his energy to pursuing the virtue of health (3, 406d2–407b2). Think of Phaedrus at the beginning of another Platonic dialogue, strolling outside the city walls on the advice of the doctor Acumenus.[133] The author of *On Regimen*, however, has higher hopes for the carpenter. He expressly designates two audiences for his text, of which the first comprises "the great majority of people who necessarily live haphazardly [ὅσοισιν ἐξ ἀνάγκης εἰκῇ τὸν βίον διατελεῖν ἐστι] and cannot take care of their health [τῆς ὑγιείης ἐπιμελεῖσθαι] by neglecting everything else" (III 69, Li 6.604 = 200,23–25 Joly-Byl).[134] The regimen he goes on to outline is so long that one begins to wonder about not only the carpenter's patience but also what more can be done. It turns out that the commitment required for optimal health is total, as befits an audience that is "well off, and convinced that there are no benefits of wealth or anything else without health" (III 69, Li 6.604–6 = 200,25–27 Joly-Byl). Even, then, if *On Regimen*'s intended double audience signals medicine's burgeoning ambitions, it also confirms that, despite the "democratization" of health theoretically supported by regimen, practices of care have the potential to resignify the relationship, conventionally guaranteed by the gods, between prosperity and well-being.[135] It is the wealthy, we are reminded in the *Republic*, who have time for virtue. In *On Regimen*, wealth translates into the freedom to learn about one's nature and manage its care.[136]

---

[133] Pl. *Phdr.* 227a2-b1.

[134] This audience is characterized as laborers at *Vict.* III 68 (Li 6.594 = 194,17–21 Joly-Byl). Ducatillon 1969.40 takes the passage as evidence of medicine's broad popular audience; see also Wilkins 2005.126–28. Cf. Joly 1960.134–36, who suggests that the ideal of two audiences may have been the author's response to earlier criticisms of regimen as too time-consuming for the average population.

[135] For the idea of "democratization," see Wohl 2002.30–72, who shows how the idealized elite self in Pericles' Funeral Oration is positioned as a goal for all classes. The idea that health can be bought from the gods is challenged at *Aer.* 22 (Li 2.76–82 = 238,6–241,20 Jouanna). The author, pointing to wealthy Scythians who suffer an effeminizing disease, argues that, if the disease is divine, it should attack the poor, who do not shower the gods with gifts. On his account, the disease is caused by horseback riding, a habit of the wealthy. On the pursuit of health as a mark of wealth and freedom, see also Edelstein 1967f.314–16.

[136] On medical learning among laypersons as part of *paideia* in the fifth and fourth centuries, see Jaeger 1944.3–45; Schiefsky 2005a.36–46. Nightingale argues that, at least in the fourth century, "The possession of a liberal or philosophical education . . . identified the elite by recourse to criteria other than wealth or power" (2004.15).

Plato views the elite status of medical knowledge in a more favorable light in the *Laws*. If, in *On Affections*, medical knowledge enables the person merely to assert control over his body in the face of diseases and physicians, in the *Laws*, this knowledge, born of an exchange of information not unlike the reciprocal pedagogy of *On Ancient Medicine*, defines the free patient against his slave counterpart:[137]

> ὁ δὲ ἐλεύθερος ὡς ἐπὶ τὸ πλεῖστον τὰ τῶν ἐλευθέρων νοσήματα θεραπεύει τε καὶ ἐπισκοπεῖ, καὶ ταῦτα ἐξετάζων ἀπ᾽ ἀρχῆς καὶ κατὰ φύσιν, τῷ κάμνοντι κοινούμενος αὐτῷ τε καὶ τοῖς φίλοις, ἅμα μὲν αὐτὸς μανθάνει τι παρὰ τῶν νοσούντων, ἅμα δὲ καὶ καθ᾽ ὅσον οἷός τέ ἐστιν, διδάσκει τὸν ἀσθενοῦντα αὐτόν, καὶ οὐ πρότερον ἐπέταξεν πρὶν ἄν πῃ συμπείσῃ, τότε δὲ μετὰ πειθοῦς ἡμερούμενον ἀεὶ παρασκευάζων τὸν κάμνοντα, εἰς τὴν ὑγίειαν ἄγων, ἀποτελεῖν πειρᾶται; (*Leg.* 4, 720d1–e2)

> But the freeborn doctor, for the most part, treats and examines the diseases of free men, and by investigating these diseases from their *arkhē* and in accordance with nature, by consulting with the patient himself and those close to him, he himself learns something from the sufferer and, to the extent that he is able to, he also teaches the patient himself, and he does not prescribe anything before persuading the patient, and, securing the patient's continued acquiescence with persuasion, he tries to complete the task of leading him back to health.

Given that Plato is making a point about how to educate citizens about the law, the relationship between physician and patient here is freighted with larger concerns about authority and obedience. Nevertheless, his remarks draw attention to the ways in which caring for the physical body had become relevant to larger questions of autonomy. By allying himself with the physician as a subject of medical knowledge—elsewhere, Plato tells us that the physician addresses the free man "almost like a philosopher, tracing the disorder to its *arkhē*, going over the whole nature of bodies" (ἐξ ἀρχῆς τε ἁπτόμενον τοῦ νοσήματος, περὶ φύσεως πάσης ἐπανιόντα τῆς τῶν σωμάτων, *Leg.* 9, 857d2–4)—the patient resists becoming the object of another's care. Indeed, by inquiring into his own nature, he may even escape physicians altogether. Xenophon reports that Socrates recommended his followers take their own notes on the effects of foods, drinks, and exercise on their bodies, on the grounds that "by such attention to yourselves you can discover better than any doctor what suits your constitution" (*Mem.* 4.7.9). What in Xenophon appears as a mild tension between the patient and the physician flares up in Plato's attack on medicine in *Republic* 3. Seeing the glut of doctors and lawcourts in Athens, his Socrates concludes that

---

[137] Slaves in classical Athens were distinguished by their lack of corporeal integrity (Winkler 1990b.47–49; duBois 1991; Hunter 1992), and there may be a sense that the slave patient, under the care of a "tyrant" healer, has given up ownership of his body; see also Nussbaum 1994.69–71, 74–75 on Aristotle's concerns about power in the physician-patient relationship. McKeown 2002 argues that the medical writers themselves do not distinguish between free and slave patients; see also Jouanna 1999.112–16.

free men, lacking their own resources, have had to start making use of a justice supplied by others, as if these men were their masters.[138]

Plato's fears about compromised autonomy in this last example do not simply concern the asymmetrical relationship between physicians and patients; they also target the free subject's very capacity to take care of himself. In Plato's view, as we will see further in chapter 5, this crisis can be traced to trouble in the *psukhē*. In medicine, however, virtually all threats to the person are traced back to a physical substratum most closely identified with the *sōma*. Although at times the medical writers seem to define human nature too narrowly to engage the self in its totality, as in *On Ancient Medicine*, at other times they address a fuller spectrum of faculties, including sensing, acting, speaking, judging, and thinking. I would like to close this chapter by returning to the topic with which it began, namely, the significance of physicality to the person, particularly the person *qua* ethical subject, by which I mean a subject capable of taking responsibility for the physical body, and thus of being praised or blamed for its care.

Shoring Up the Self

We have seen that prognosis incorporates and, indeed, heavily weights those phenomena through which personal identity is realized. By vesting these phenomena with significance, physicians tacitly present themselves as guardians of the self. In other contexts, the medical authors, often addressing a wider public, make the integrity of the self depend on medical expertise by relating cognitive and perceptual functions to physical stuffs. In *On the Sacred Disease*, for example, joys, sorrows, pains, and even judgments of value depend on the condition of the brain.[139] If the brain is overcome by moisture, madness and confusion arise:[140]

καὶ μαινόμεθα μὲν ὑπὸ ὑγρότητος· ὅταν γὰρ ὑγρότερος τῆς φύσιος ᾖ, ἀνάγκη κινεῖσθαι· κινευμένου δὲ μήτε τὴν ὄψιν ἀτρεμίζειν μήτε τὴν ἀκοήν, ἀλλὰ ἄλλοτε ἄλλα ὁρᾶν καὶ ἀκούειν, τήν τε γλῶσσαν τοιαῦτα διαλέγεσθαι οἷα ἂν βλέπῃ τε καὶ ἀκούῃ ἑκάστοτε· ὅσον δ' ἂν ἀτρεμίσῃ ὁ ἐγκέφαλος χρόνον, τοσοῦτον καὶ φρονεῖ ὥνθρωπος. (*Morb. Sacr.* 14, Li 6.388 = 26,13–27,4 Jouanna)

And we go mad because of moisture. For whenever [the brain] is wetter than it is naturally, it necessarily moves about, and if it moves, neither our vision nor our

---

[138] ἦ οὐκ αἰσχρὸν δοκεῖ καὶ ἀπαιδευσίας μέγα τεκμήριον τὸ ἐπακτῷ παρ' ἄλλων, ὡς δεσποτῶν τε καὶ κριτῶν, τῷ δικαίῳ ἀναγκάζεσθαι χρῆσθαι, καὶ ἀπορίᾳ οἰκείων (Pl. *R.* 3, 405b1–3).

[139] *Morb. Sacr.* 14 (Li 6.386–88 = 25,15–27,4 Jouanna).

[140] For other physical explanations of thinking and sensing in the medical writers, see chapter 2 n.134. For cases where physical changes affect mental states, see, e.g., *Int.* 48 (Li 7.284–86 = 232–34 Potter; cf. *Dieb. iudic.* 3 [Li 9.300–302]); *Morb.* II 72 (Li 7.108–10 = 211,15–212,10 Jouanna); *Virg.* 3 (Li 8.468 = 24,1–4 Lami). On explanations of mental and emotional functions in medical writing, see Pigeaud 1980; 1987.13–63; 2006.31–47, 71–112, 122–33; Claus 1981.150–55; di Benedetto 1986.35–69; Hankinson 1991.200–208; Singer 1992; Gundert 2000.20–31; Boehm 2002; van der Eijk 2005b.119–35.

hearing is steady, and we see and hear one thing at one time, another at another, and the tongue communicates the things that we see and hear at each point. But as long as the brain is stable, the person thinks rightly.

In *On Regimen*, too, moisture plays a critical role in intelligence and perception. This author, however, relates these faculties not to the brain but to the mixture of fire and water in the *psukhē* as it moves along a *periodos*, "circuit," in the body.[141] The relationship between intelligence and the *psukhē* is relatively rare in the late fifth century outside a handful of medical treatises and texts claiming Socratic influence.[142] Despite innovating in this respect, however—perhaps under the influence of Heraclitus or his fifth-century acolytes—the author folds his *psukhē* into a familiar model.[143] Like the *sōma*, the *psukhē* is shaped by exercise, diet, vomiting, bathing, and other such techniques, making it the object of medical care.[144] Similarly, the author of *On the Sacred Disease* uses the physicality of the brain to justify medicine's therapeutic authority: "Whoever knows how to create [ποιεῖν] the wet and the dry and the cold and the hot in human beings through regimen" can cure the "sacred" disease (*Morb. Sacr.* 18, Li 6.396 = 32,15–33,2 Jouanna). While these authors resemble physicists like Diogenes and Empedocles, who also offer physicalized models of cognition and affect, they are using these models to inform and to justify technical intervention aimed at securing not just bare survival but flourishing in the broadest sense of the term.

Yet, if physiological approaches to human nature guarantee not simply living but living well, the concepts of pathology and norm come under pressure. These concepts were in some sense always under pressure, insofar as the medical writers recognize that each nature is disposed toward particular affections and

---

[141] *Vict.* I 35 (Li 6.512–22 = 150,29–156,18 Joly-Byl). On how fire and water affect intelligence, see Jouanna 2007a.16–18.

[142] See *Hum.* 9 (Li 5.488–90 = 80 Jones), where the author identifies some behaviors (intemperance, endurance) as psychic. *Carn.* 1 (Li 8.584 = 188,8 Joly) promises to give an account of what the soul is (ὅ τι ψυχή ἐστι): chapters 15–18 on sensory perception may fulfill his earlier intention, as Gundert 2000.16 suggests. Claus 1981.150–51 draws attention to the *sōma-psukhē* contrast at *Aer.* 19 (Li 2.72 = 234,10 Jouanna), but rightly notes that it receives no special emphasis; the context, moreover, as at 24 (Li 2.88 = 246,1–4 Jouanna), suggests the *psukhē*'s traditional relationship to courage—on which, see Claus 1981.75–78—rather than a new psychological self. Elsewhere in the treatise, a sharp change to the *sōma* (μετάστασις ἰσχυρὴ τοῦ σώματος) can be paralleled by mental disturbances (ἐκπλήξιες τῆς γνώμης, 16, Li 2.62–64 = 228,3–4 Jouanna); body, soul, and intelligence, like character, are subject to the same environmental forces, although *nomoi*, too, are credited with formational power (16, Li 2.64 = 228,8–10 Jouanna): see Pigeaud 1983. On the text's environmental determinism, see Jouanna 1999.211–21; Isaac 2004.55–109; and esp. Calame 2005.

[143] For Heraclitus and the soul, see above, introduction, n.108. Jouanna 2007a.27–31 documents similarities between the Hippocratic author's account of intelligence and the account attributed by Theophrastus to Empedocles while also stressing the originality of *On Regimen*.

[144] Cambiano 1980 defends the author's physicalism against claims, based on *On Regimen* IV, that his *psukhē* is influenced by Orphic-Pythagorean doctrines. See also Jouanna 1998, on the unity of the treatise; 2007a.14–26 on the physicality of the *psukhē*.

expresses health in a particular way. Nevertheless, the more broadly health is understood, the more complicated the idea of pathology becomes. If, from one perspective, variation among natures is simply an empirical truth that explains why judgments in medicine are never rule-bound but always adaptive, from another perspective, variability creates a spectrum that restages the good-bad polarity of prognostic symptoms in terms not of survival but of different, and potentially ranked, classes of natures.[145] In one passage from the fourth-century *Epidemics* II, for example, bodily signs seem to support broad judgments about character: those with big heads, large, dark eyes, and a thick, blunt nose are *esthloi*, "good"; those with large heads and small eyes are *oxuthumoi*, "quick to anger," if they also stammer (6.1, Li 5.132 = 80 Smith).[146] The author of *On Regimen*, who believes that regimen can help or harm intelligence and character traits, also accepts that the mixture is not responsible for some attributes, including irascibility, craftiness, and benevolence. In these cases, "it is not possible

---

[145] Klibansky, Panofsky, and Saxl 1964.6 attribute the first "psychosomatic theory of character" to Empedocles. The watershed moment, however, is usually taken to be the famous pseudo-Aristotelian *Problem* 30.1 (953a–955a), where the melancholic constitution is related to both madness and extraordinary accomplishment in philosophy, politics, poetry, and the arts: see van der Eijk 2005b.155–60; Jouanna 2007b.29–37, who downplays the influence of the *Problem* on the later medical and ethical traditions. The search for earlier incarnations of the melancholic character type has had mixed results: it is difficult, first, to determine what qualifies as a sufficiently robust concept of character—most of what we see in the Hippocratic treatises seems to concern physiological tendencies; second, black bile is not widely seen in the Hippocratic texts as a constituent stuff in persons; and, finally, it is hard to know if terms like μελαγχολικός, μελαγχολώδης, and μελαγχολάω in classical nonmedical literature are "popular" or "physiological." Jouanna 2007b.11–22 distinguishes between the medical disease *melancholiē*, the humor black bile, and the melancholic temperament and demonstrates that they "n'apparaissent pas au même moment et ne se recoupent pas nécessairement" (21–22). It is nevertheless likely that the growing use of the term *phusis* in the classical period to describe character was influenced by contemporary physiological theories.

[146] See also *Epid*. II 5.1 (Li 5.128 = 74 Smith). The word φυσιογνωμονίη (*Epid*. II 5.1, Li 5.128; cf. 6.1, Li 5.132, φυσιογνωμονικόν; Smith omits these words, but Alessi retains them in his forthcoming Budé edition of *Epidemics* II) appears for the first time in *Epidemics* II. Galen, in fact, claims that Hippocrates invented physiognomy (*QAM*, Kühn 4.798; [Galen] *Prog.Dec.* 1, Kühn 19.530). The first extant treatise on physiognomy, probably of Peripatetic origin, dates from the late fourth or early third century BCE, but Antisthenes (mid-fifth to early fourth century) is reported to have written a treatise at least a century earlier (Ath. 14, 656f; D. L. 6.16). The lack of evidence makes it difficult to know how much weight to assign to the appearance of φυσιογνωμονίη in *Epidemics* II (which may have been added as a heading later). It is unclear as well to what extent the remarks in *Epidemics* II are, in fact, physiognomical, that is, observations about character, rather than observations where ἐσθλός and πονηρός are strictly physiological judgments: see Alessi 2008; see also Jouanna 2007b.14. For other discussions of physiognomy and character analysis in early Greek medicine, see Joly 1960.83–89; E. Evans 1969.19–20; Villari 2003.93–94. See also, more generally, Klibansky, Panofsky, and Saxl 1964.55–66; Marganne 1988; Gleason 1990; Sassi 2001.34–81; and esp. Boys-Stones 2007, who persuasively argues that physiognomy as a theoretical discipline rests on a given author's ideas about the relationship of the body to the soul or the person. It follows from Boys-Stone's argument that the idea of the physical body would transform what it means to infer character from someone's appearance, even if physicians were not actually practicing character diagnosis.

to remold unseen nature" (φύσιν γὰρ μεταπλάσαι ἀφανέα οὐχ οἶόν τε, I 36, Li 6.524 = 156,27–28 Joly-Byl): people with these traits are stuck in their ways. Insofar as craftiness, for example, or cowardice, is both fixed and negatively weighted, being alive does not entail living well.

The ambiguous relationship of bodily health to the health of the social, ethical subject, both inside and outside medical writing, is most powerfully illustrated by the sexed body. Female bodies have a natural norm.[147] Women can, and often do, get sick *qua* women—many of their diseases are tied to the womb and menstruation—and regain health. Yet the very characteristics that determine the normative expression of female nature can signify as pathological vis-à-vis a male norm. Bodily articulation, for example, what we call muscularity, is fundamental to Greek notions of beauty, strength, and overall flourishing.[148] It is also used by the medical writers as a significant criterion of difference between male and female bodies. Whereas the male fetus is articulated after thirty days, the female requires at least twelve more to achieve form because female seed is wet and moist.[149] Once outside the womb, the female body, with its porous and spongy flesh, never achieves the same level of articulation as the male body, and it degenerates more quickly.[150]

Although the medical writers often speak of the weakness of female nature in general terms, these differences are most plausibly caused by excessive moisture in the female body.[151] The dangers posed by wetness were well known.

---

[147] On female bodies in classical Greek medical writing, see Manuli 1980; 1983; Rousselle 1980; A. Hanson 1990; 1992b; 2007; Sissa 1990b; Dean-Jones 1991; 1994; H. King 1994; 1998; Bodiou 2004; 2006; Byl 2005; Bonnard 2007. On the female body more generally in Greek culture, see duBois 1988.37–166; Carson 1990; Sissa 1990a; Faranda 1993; Sassi 2001.82–139.

[148] The concept of muscles was slow to form in Greek medicine. Nevertheless, "before they became fascinated with special structures named muscles, the Greeks celebrated bodies that had a particular look—a special clarity of form, a distinct 'jointedness,' which they identified with the vital as opposed to the dying, the mature as opposed to the yet unformed, individuals as opposed to people who all resemble each other, the strong and brave as opposed to the weak and cowardly, Europeans as opposed to Asians, the male as opposed to the female" (Kuriyama 1999.143; see also 129–43). See Bolens 2000 on *le corps articulaire* in Homer. Stewart 1997.92–97 discusses the muscled ideal in classical Greek sculpture. In tragedy, for a man to be ἄναρθρος is a sign of disease, e.g., E. *Or.* 228; S. *Tr.* 1103. The word is also found, without context, at E. fr. 557K (= *Oedipus* fr. 22 J.-V.L.).

[149] *Genit./Nat. Puer.* 18 (Li 7.498–500 = 60,19–23 Joly; Li 7.502–6 = 62,19–64,7 Joly); *Oct.* 9 (Li 7.450 = 80,18–20 Grensemann), with A. Hanson 1992b. See also Emp. (DK31) A83 (= Orib. *inc.* 16 = 4:106,2–7 Raeder).

[150] Spongy, porous flesh: *Glan.* 16 (Li 8.572 = 121,20–122,7 Joly); *Mul.* I 1 (Li 8.12 = 88,24–90,4 Grensemann); see also Dean-Jones 1994.55–59. The female ages more quickly "on account of the weakness of her body and her regimen" (διὰ τὴν ἀσθενείην τε τῶν σωμάτων καὶ τὴν δίαιταν, *Oct.* 9, Li 7.450 = 80,23–24 Grensemann); see also E. fr. 24K (= *Aeolus* fr. 11 J.-V.L.) and Carson 1990.145–48. At *Vict.* I 32 (Li 6.508 = 148,23–25 Joly-Byl), wetter constitutions age more quickly.

[151] For the weakness of female nature: *Virg.* 1 (Li 8.466 = 22,8–9 Lami). On wetness, see *Aph.* III.11–14 (Li 4.490–92 = 124–26 Jones); *Steril.* 216 (Li 8.416); *Vict.* I 27 (Li 6.500 = 142,27–144,14 Joly-Byl), 34 (Li 6.512 = 150,23–28 Joly-Byl). See further Manuli 1980; A. Hanson 1990; 1992a.245–48; 1992b, esp. 48–56; Dean-Jones 1994.46. See also Carson 1990.137–45, 153, incorporating nonmedical material. There is less of a consensus on whether women are colder, e.g., Emp. (DK31) B65 and

For example, the author of *Airs, Waters, Places* takes for granted a correlation between too much wetness, in this case caused by environmental factors, and the improperly formed bodies of many foreign peoples. Scythians, for example, suffer from a monotonous, moist climate that produces a fleshy, unarticulated external form with a watery internal cavity.[152] The Phasians, too, live in a marshy, damp land that makes their bodies thick and formless; their fruit is stunted, feeble, and literally "feminized" (τεθηλυσμένοι), just as atrophied flesh, in *On Joints*, "becomes female" (θηλύνονται).[153] In these last two cases, the authors assume that flesh and fruit lose their shape only under pathological conditions. In using the verb "to become female" (θηλύνομαι) to describe these processes, however, these authors take wetness and weakness as defining female qualities. In fact, female bodies require wetness to survive. If a woman's body dries out, she may develop masculine traits—this is exactly what happens to two widows in *Epidemics* VI. Nevertheless, masculinity thus achieved is unsustainable: both widows quickly die.[154]

Despite their undesirable traits, female bodies are well equipped for survival. Indeed, sometimes they seem to be even better equipped than their male counterparts.[155] If the patient has a "naturally" diseased body or nature, he or she does not necessarily succumb more easily to disease, but may be able to take humoral disturbances in stride.[156] The same principle can explain why physicians often distrust the athlete's nature; it is unstable and "turns to the extremes; in these types of bodies, a good condition flourishes for only a short while" (καὶ τρέπεται ἐφ᾽ ἑκάτερα, καὶ ἀκμάζει ὀλίγον χρόνον ἡ εὐεξίη ἐν τοῖσι τοιουτοτρόποισι τῶν σωμάτων, *Salubr.* 7, Li 6.84 = 218,2–4 Jouanna, as *Nat. Hom.* 22).[157]

Nevertheless, even if naturally diseased bodies can stay alive, the conditions under which life is sustained preclude ideal human flourishing. Physicians certainly do not invent the idea that women are inferior to men. Yet in elaborating the idea of the physical body, they reconceptualize this inferiority by using the female body to exaggerate those aspects of the physical body that for men are

---

Vict. I 34 (Li 6.512 = 150,23–28 Joly-Byl), or hotter, e.g., Parm. (DK28) A52 (= Arist. *PA* 648a29–30) and *Mul.* I 1 (Li 8.12–14 = 90,5–10 Grensemann). A. Hanson 1992b.54–55 reconciles these views by arguing that the menstrual cycle was thought to determine whether females were hotter or colder.

[152] *Aer.* 19 (Li 2.72 = 234,11–14 Jouanna). Interestingly, the Scythians are not adversely affected by climate in Herodotus: see Jouanna 1999.225–31; Thomas 2000.54–74; Chiasson 2001.38–45, 56–69.

[153] *Aer.* 15 (Li 2.60–62 = 225,8–227,10 Jouanna); *Artic.* 52, *bis* (Li 4.232 = 193,10, 12 Kühlewein).

[154] *Epid.* VI 8.32 (Li 5.356 = 194,5–17 Manetti-Roselli). Sexual intercourse was seen as a way of keeping passages open and excess fluids moving in the female body (e.g., *Mul.* I 2, Li 8.14–16 = 90,30–92,2 Grensemann).

[155] See Dean-Jones 1994.136–47; H. King 1998.51–52, noting that (menstruating) women have an excess route to purge the *materia peccans*.

[156] See *Morb.* I 22 (Li 6.182–88 = 64,14–70,3 Wittern), where this principle is discussed in relation to the "diseased" bodies of old men.

[157] See also Pl. *R.* 3, 404a9-b2.

most threatening to both bare survival and living well. As A. E. Hanson has observed, the female's natural wetness is expressed in the male as pathological, corrosive fluxes, as we saw in the previous chapter.[158] The authors of *On the Sacred Disease* and *On Regimen* blame unstable perceptions and weakened intelligence, respectively, on excessive moisture. The watery nature of the *sōma* can also be seen as increasing its vulnerability to external stimuli: recall that, in *On Generation/ On the Nature of the Child*, the female body "senses" variations of temperature because it is moister than the male body, and this sensing agitates the blood.[159] In addition to wetness, the female body is defined by the womb, the archetypal cavity: unseen, receptive, nourishing.[160] The womb, moreover, is liable to wander if deprived of moisture, and its wanderings vividly enact the troubling automatism and the restlessness of the physical body and, in particular, sudden humoral fluxes.[161] Finally, the female body attracts heightened concern about cleanliness and damaging stuffs, requiring "more frequent and more radical cathartic interventions" than the male body.[162] In these various respects, female bodies model the problems that the physical body can create for men, problems that, at least for the medical writers, endanger both health and virtues such as intelligence, articulated form, and autarchy. Yet, whereas women are defined by these problems, men—or, rather, certain classes of men eligible for self-mastery—are capable of evading them, if they submit to the authority of medicine.

The divergence of female nature from an idealized norm places women in an ambiguous relationship to the dynamics of praise and blame, an ambiguity instructive for the larger ethical quandaries posed by the physical body. Insofar as women exhibit undesirable qualities, they would appear legitimate targets of disapproval. In Plato's *Timaeus*, for example, a man who has failed to conquer

---

[158] She observes that "writers in the Corpus feminized wetness and came to equate dominance by a bodily humor retained in excess with a feminine and sedentary lifestyle that resulted in fleshiness, weakness, fevers from accumulation, and general ill health" (1992b.51); see also Andò 2002.101. Paola Manuli takes menstruation as a pathological sign "che rappresenta il superamento di una *mesotes*, ed annuncia nello stesso tempo la crisi del male, il ristabilirsi di un nuovo e precario equilibrio" (1980.402); see also Dean-Jones 1994.43–45, 55–65, 124–25; Bodiou 2006.157–61; von Staden 2007a.48–49. Female embryos are likely to make their mothers sicker (*Steril.* 216 = Li 8.416), and most of the postpartum complications in the *Epidemics* follow the birth of a girl (A. Hanson 1992b.54).

[159] *Genit./Nat. Puer.* 15 (Li 7.494 = 57,18–24 Joly).

[160] See above, chapter 1, nn.115–16.

[161] On the wandering womb, especially in the classical medical texts, see Manuli 1980.398–99; Dean-Jones 1994.69–77, 135–36; Byl 2005. In the gynecological treatises, the womb's displacement is a mechanical response to its need for moisture. At Pl. *Ti.* 91b7–c7, however, it is a kind of animal. Hellenistic and imperial-age amulets designed to drive the womb back to its proper place attest the conceptualization of the womb as an indwelling demon in the first centuries CE: see Aubert 1989; A. Hanson 1995; Kotansky 1995.267; Faraone 2003; 2007. Lesley Dean-Jones argues that, because the Hippocratic physical theories did not require the mobile womb, belief in it "suggests that it fulfilled an important cultural role in characterizing the female sex" (1994.74).

[162] Von Staden 2007a.51. See also von Staden 1992a; 1992b. Carson 1990.158–60 considers the representation of women as polluting in nonmedical evidence.

the flood of sensations, pleasures, and desires that assail the body is fated to be reborn as a woman, an obvious fall down the chain of beings.[163] Yet, once he has been reborn, that failure is no longer evaluated in moral terms, because disordering motions naturally overpower women. As Aeschines says in the mid-fourth-century speech *Against Timarchus*, a man who blames a woman, "who errs by impulse of nature" (τῇ . . . κατὰ φύσιν ἁμαρτανούσῃ), lacks intelligence (1.185).[164] Plato arrives at a similar position later in the *Timaeus*, and extends it to anyone consigned by their body and their education to a life of disorder, declaring that incontinence cannot justly be reproached because it is due to some bad condition of the body (διὰ δὲ πονηρὰν ἕξιν τινὰ τοῦ σώματος) and poor upbringing.[165] To the extent that the condition of the body is fixed, it lies, like female nature, outside the scope of praise and blame.

Fixity in this last case, however, turns out to be more complex. On the one hand, Plato allows for the possibility that intemperance can be corrected in childhood (at least for some natures), a possibility that creates legitimate targets of blame: the parents who failed to take care. On the other hand, responsibility gravitates toward an ethical subject if it is within his power to change his disposition: "One must strive, however, as much as one can, through nourishment and study to flee badness and seize its contrary" (προθυμητέον μήν, ὅπῃ τις δύναται, καὶ διὰ τροφῆς καὶ δι᾽ ἐπιτηδευμάτων μαθημάτων τε φυγεῖν μὲν κακίαν, τοὐναντίον δὲ ἑλεῖν, Pl. *Ti.* 87b6–8). By deftly pairing a grammatical form that indicates necessity (the verbal adjective προθυμητέον, "one must strive") with the qualifying phrase "as much as one can" (ὅπῃ τις δύναται), Plato stakes out the crucial terrain between the realm of necessity and an ethics of care.

---

[163] Pl. *Ti.* 42b2–c1. See also *Leg.* 6, 780d9–781d1.

[164] The principle that one cannot blame people for things that happen through chance or nature is put forth as common knowledge by Protagoras in the eponymous dialogue (*Prt.* 323c8–d6). At the same time, being a slave to necessity can be reason for rebuke, as Just 1985 demonstrates.

[165] Pl. *Ti.* 86d5–e3: καὶ σχεδὸν δὴ πάντα ὁπόσα ἡδονῶν ἀκράτεια καὶ ὄνειδος ὡς ἑκόντων λέγεται τῶν κακῶν, οὐκ ὀρθῶς ὀνειδίζεται· κακὸς μὲν γὰρ ἑκὼν οὐδείς, διὰ δὲ πονηρὰν ἕξιν τινὰ τοῦ σώματος καὶ ἀπαίδευτον τροφὴν ὁ κακὸς γίγνεται κακός, παντὶ δὲ ταῦτα ἐχθρὰ καὶ ἄκοντι προσγίγνεται (We might almost say, indeed, of all that is called incontinence in pleasure, that it is not justly made a reproach, as if men were willingly bad. No one is willingly bad; the bad man becomes so because of some bad disposition of the body and poor upbringing, and these are hateful things that come against a man against his will). The *Timaeus* passage seems committed to the fact that the body can determine character: see C. Gill 2000; cf. Boys-Stones 2007.41–43, arguing that "it would not be right to say that the *natural* character of the irrational soul is determined by the body" (43, emphasis in original), because a bad bodily condition must combine with a lack of education to produce poor character. But, insofar as the irrational, that is, perverted soul has a natural character, this diseased state is caused by (διά) two psychosomatic factors that Plato weights equally, bad bodily constitution and lack of education; cf. *Phlb.* 45e5–7, where great pains and pleasures are due to the badness of both body and soul (ἔν τινι πονηρίᾳ ψυχῆς καὶ τοῦ σώματος). There is no hint in Plato's text of Boys-Stones's distinction between education's "natural" influence on the soul and the ("unnatural"?) influence of the body. Elsewhere, however, Plato does deny that the body can damage the soul (e.g., *R.* 10, 610a5–c1). See below, chapter 5, n.31. On the afterlife of the problems raised here in ancient philosophy, see Sorabji 2003.

I have suggested that the medical writers grant the person two basic positions vis-à-vis his body: he can either counter its natural volatility through vigilant mastery or suffer the vagaries of embodiment. Whether he is praised or blamed for the condition of his body seems to depend largely on his capacity for self-mastery. If the body itself, caught in the forces of necessity and nature, arrogates causal force, ethical judgments ebb away, and the self becomes just another symptom. Given that one must be naturally capable of controlling the physical body in order to take responsibility for it, the burden of taking care falls most heavily on those with the most to lose. Even a man born healthy and strong and raised well can be harmed by his regimen, cautions the author of *On Regimen*.[166] Xenophon tells us that Socrates never neglected the body and did not praise those who did.[167] We can imagine that it was because the physical body—volatile, unseen, and implicated in an automatized natural world—could seem so daemonic that entrusting life, both biological life and ethical life, to its dynamics could seem like ceding control of the human. The *tekhnē*, by restoring the conditions for agency, creates a domain where the care of one's own nature takes on ethical potential.

The rise of regimen, with its techniques for mastering "the diseased," however understood, latent within human nature, can be seen in part in terms of its larger cultural context: in this period—especially, but not only, at Athens—the idea of mastering the self was increasingly determining notions of freedom and the dynamics of praise and blame.[168] But we should be careful not to let the familiarity of this milieu, which has been the subject of much study in recent years, blind us to the historical and conceptual process through which human nature becomes an object of care. Part of this process, I have argued, involves the migration of responsibility to the physical body as a cause of suffering. This shift, rather than eliminating agents, divides causality between corporeal stuffs and forces and the person with the power to manage them. The result is a new kind of "ethical substance," a term that Foucault uses to talk about the part of the self that the subject targets reflexively through practices of care.[169]

It may be more accurate to speak of the emergence of ethical substance itself. Character and virtue, it is true, always require nurture in archaic ethics.[170] Yet these ethical goods are made newly malleable by physical models of the human.

---

[166] *Vict.* I 28 (Li 6.502 = 144,21–22 Joly-Byl).

[167] X. *Mem.* 1.2.4: ἀλλὰ μὴν καὶ τοῦ σώματος αὐτός τε οὐκ ἠμέλει τούς τ᾽ ἀμελοῦντας οὐκ ἐπῄνει; cf. 1.6.7, 2.7.7, and 3.12.8, where, because beauty and strength do not come automatically (αὐτόματα), not taking care, ἀμέλεια, is shameful. Care here primarily involves the restriction of pleasures: see further below, chapter 5.

[168] On self-mastery and freedom, see Foucault 1985.78–93; 1997.281–301. But see, too, Pericles' praise of *effortless* Athenian masculinity in the Funeral Oration, discussed at Wohl 2002.49–52.

[169] Foucault 1985.26–27. Foucault is working with a rather limited notion of ethical substance, namely *ta aphrodisia*, that is, things having to do with sexual pleasure, although he recognizes that food is often more important than sexual activity in the texts he examines (1985.110, 114).

[170] See esp. Pi. *N.* 8.40–42, with Halliwell 1990.32–33; Nussbaum 2001.1–3.

These models, at least in theory, put health and, to an extent, virtue, in reach of more people, while at the same time exaggerating the fragility of these goods by grounding them in the physical body. By recognizing the importance of the *sōma* to these changes, we can develop a more nuanced account of the ethical subject created out of techniques of care. Given how central this subject becomes in both philosophical ethics and popular morality, the consequences of widening our perspective are far reaching.

First, scholars have criticized Foucault's analysis of ancient Greek techniques of the care of the self, and particularly the "use of pleasures," for relying too heavily on norms and regulations and neglecting the messier dimensions of sexuality.[171] Foucault's critics identify a genuine lacuna in the second and third volumes of his *History of Sexuality*. But if we, in turn, rely on the psychoanalytic unconscious—or, now, the brain of cognitive science—to correct Foucault's error, we miss the opportunity to think about how techniques of care develop in classical Greece through the conceptualization of the physical body in terms of a daemonic space inside the self. Over the past two chapters, we have seen that, for the medical writers, the body is an ambiguous thing: not only an intelligible object of technical mastery but also a site of strange, unruly forces. The embodied subject, too, is caught in competing narratives of opposition and complicity, agency and suffering. In practice, most medical writers focus on how these narratives are realized at the level of natures and bodies. And, because they are under the care of physicians, most of the patients we encounter in the medical treatises are *not* subjects of self-knowledge and are thus outside the dynamics of praise and blame. Nevertheless, I have argued that medicine plays an important role in establishing the framework within which taking responsibility for the physical body becomes not just a necessity but an ethical obligation.

Second, scholars have tended to treat various techniques of caring for the self as different facets of a single cultural phenomenon. In truth, the nature of ethical substance is complicated by a growing rivalry between *sōma* and *psukhē*. The medical writers implicate character and ethical goods in both nature (*phusis*) and the body (*sōma*). The language of (human) nature emphasizes that the accounts they advance are inclusive, encompassing all aspects of a person. Nevertheless, *sōma*—the most common word in the Hippocratic Corpus, appearing more than fourteen hundred times—often functions as a metonym for human nature: what these texts show, then, is "that the body can be used to give an account of total experience."[172] By blurring the line between *phusis* and *sōma*,

---

[171] The criticism is often grounded in a psychoanalytic approach. See esp. Black 1998, for whom this unruliness can be seen as "all that is illusory, imaginary, and phantasmic about [sc. sexuality]" (59). Wohl 2002 aims to recover the erotic imaginary behind the (democratic) discourses of self-mastery in classical Athens: see esp. 12–20 for the critique of Foucauldian normativity. See also Goldhill 1995, who challenges Foucault's picture by looking to literary representations of sexuality. Cf. Nehamas 1998, who finds Foucault much richer than these critiques suggest.

[172] Singer 1992.142, reworking Simon's claim that, in these writers, "all diseases of the mind are diseases of the body" (1978.215). See also Beardslee 1918.35–36 (observing that *phusis* often simply

the medical writers confirm the significance of a body embedded in the dynamics of the physical world to their concepts of the human.

In other texts, however, we can see the role of the physical body in the production of selves coming under challenge. In *Republic* 3, as we have seen, Socrates complains that the excessive care of the *sōma* diverts attention from what really matters, namely learning and thinking—activities of the *psukhē*. If we look further, we see that he has even harsher words for regimen. He blames physicians for keeping patients alive without ensuring that they live well while, even worse, often enabling them to pursue lives of reckless pleasure (3, 405c8–d4). The problem of pleasure, it turns out, is not only, as Foucault assumes, a point of convergence for techniques of care. It is also a point where these techniques diverge to generate differing accounts of human nature and how best to protect it. In the late fifth century, we begin to find therapies of the *psukhē* advanced in self-conscious opposition to those advocated by physicians, yet indebted to medicine's conceptual-imaginative framework. Considering these therapies brings us to the gray zone where the physical body ends and the ethical subject begins.

---

means *sōma*); Gundert 2000.35. Even in *On Regimen*, the health of the *psukhē* is often dependent on the *sōma*, as at I 35 (Li 6.518 = 154,20–21 Joly-Byl): ἦν γὰρ ὑγιηρῶς ἔχῃ τὸ σῶμα καὶ μὴ ὑπ' ἄλλου τινὸς συνταράσσηται, τῆς ψυχῆς φρόνιμος [ἡ] σύγκρησις (for, if his body is in a healthy state and is not troubled from any source, the blend of his soul is intelligent). In the popular imagination, it became common to see physical explanations of cognitive disorders as dependent on *sōma* (e.g., Hdt. 3.33). By the early fourth century, "who doesn't know," asks Xenophon's Socrates, "that, in thinking, a grave many errors occur on account of the body not being healthy?" (*Mem.* 3.12.6).

CHAPTER FIVE

Beyond the *Sōma*: Therapies of the *Psukhē*

ut rediit, simulacra suae petit ille puellae
incumbensque toro dedit oscula; visa tepere est.
admovet os iterum, manibus quoque pectora temptat;
temptatum mollescit ebur positoque rigore
subsedit digitis ceditque, ut Hymettia sole
cera remollescit tractataque pollice multas
flectitur in facies ipsoque fit utilis usu.
dum stupet et dubie gaudet fallique veretur,
rursus amans rursusque manu sua vota retractat.
corpus erat; saliunt temptatae pollice venae.
tum vero Paphius plenissima concipit heros
verba quibus Veneri grates agit, oraque tandem
ore suo non falsa premit; dataque oscula virgo
sensit et erubuit, timidumque ad lumina lumen
attollens pariter cum caelo vidit amantem.
Ovid, *Metamorphoses* 10.280–94

And [Pygmalion] went home, seeking his reproduction of a girl;
sinking into bed he bestows kisses on her—she seems to kindle.
Once again he joins his mouth to hers, and with his hands tries her breast:
touched, the ivory grows supple and, its hardness laid aside,
gives itself over to his fingers—it yields, just as the wax of Hymettus
will soften in sun and, by the thumb worked, allows itself
bent to any shape, made useful by use itself.
Struck with wonder, cautiously joyous, and believing himself tricked,
again, with love, and yet again his hand queries his prayers—
she is body. Her pulse leaps to meet the thumb that takes it.
And then the Paphian hero tumbles word upon word
to render thanks to Venus, and, at last, lips not ersatz
he seizes with his own; and these kisses
the girl feels, and blushes. And raising her diffident gaze to his own,
she sees, in the same moment, the world and her lover.

IN THE *METAMORPHOSES*, Ovid traces over and again the disappearance of the human into another form. In the story of Galatea, however, he moves in the other direction, from a statue to a flesh-and-blood Roman woman. Pygmalion first perceives warmth where the statue was once cool; the ivory begins to yield, like wax, to the inquiring hand. The pulse that "leaps to meet the thumb that takes it" has become, in the time between classical Greek medical writing and Ovid, a sign of life central to medical diagnosis.[1] Yet the metamorphosis is realized only at the moment it is not the *corpus*, the "body," but the girl herself who senses and responds to Pygmalion's ardor with a blush. The blush takes the place of the mark that Pygmalion had earlier both hoped and feared he would make on the statue: the bruise.[2] But whereas the bruise would have simply registered the force of Pygmalion's desire—imposed, like a daemonic blow, from outside—the blush sweeps Galatea herself up in the dynamics of that desire. In the story immediately prior, Venus had punished the daughters of Propoetus for slandering her by condemning them to a life of prostitution. With their sense of shame they lose, too, the ability to blush, and their cheeks turn to stone (10.238–42). Galatea's blush signals the return of shame as a natural attribute of a woman (albeit one who is man-made).[3] At the same time, it raises the question of how ethically rich feelings, feelings that may constrain or encourage actions, are like or unlike a bruise or the pulse. The blush—provoked by an encounter between two people, subject to praise and blame, realized at the intersection of the voluntary and the involuntary—deftly captures the complexity of Galatea's change from object to subject.[4]

In this chapter, I take up the question of how the *sôma*—defined by innate heat, supple flesh, the pulse of life—differs from the person who experiences and responds to forces like desire and shame. We have seen the person represented both as a subject of medical knowledge, capable of taking care, and as a victim of events happening below his conscious control. But where do these two sides meet? The medical writers offer ambitious models of human nature, but if we look closely, we will see they have a hard time explaining why people act as they do. While they straightforwardly assume that someone with knowledge will turn it into efficacious action, they are more reticent about the beliefs and desires that motivate patients in ignorance or, indeed, sometimes in spite of knowledge. One possible motivation, pain, is the effect of a bodily state, rather than something that drives a person to act. And if speech matters to diagnosis, it matters only insofar as a patient is talking sense or nonsense.

---

[1] Kuriyama 1999.25–36.

[2] oscula dat reddique putat loquiturque tenetque / et credit tactis digitos insidere membris / et metuit pressos veniat ne livor in artus (Ov. *Met.* 10.256–58).

[3] That shame is acquired through culture is evidence used by the author of *On the Sacred Disease* to explain why children and adults react differently to the onset of an epileptic attack: children do not yet know how to be ashamed (*Morb. Sacr.* 12, Li 6.382–84 = 22,20–23,5 Jouanna). See also Democr. (DK68) B244.

[4] Insofar as "the blush could not be mastered" (C. Barton 1999.214), it was a valuable tool for diagnoses of character in the Roman period; on the relationship between bodily signs and truth in this period, see also Gleason 1999. Yet, as Barton goes on to show, the blush is more complicated. At *Am.* I 8.35–36, for example, Ovid has his alter ego Dipsas encourage her young charge to feign the blush.

I therefore move beyond the parameters of medical writing to consider how the emergence of the physical body might have influenced the ways in which people working in a broader cultural and intellectual milieu thought about human nature. I am interested in how that body, precisely because it is impersonal, works as a foil to the person. Yet I am also interested in the ways in which it becomes a resource for thinking about why people think, act, and suffer as they do, particularly in fifth- and fourth-century attempts to conceptualize diseases and therapies of the soul or the mind, attempts that explicitly draw on contemporary medicine.[5]

The idea that strong emotions like anger can be healed with words is as old as Greek poetry.[6] In the classical period, however, ideas about disease, health, and healing are acquiring new dimensions as physicians reorient their authority and expertise around the *sōma*. As a result, medicine comes to function as one of the most thorough applications of the inquiry into nature to human nature. To be sure, it is not the only area. Those who wrote on nature had things to say about humans that often overlap with extant medical writing; debates about *phusis* and *nomos* dwelt on social and political expressions of human nature.[7] Medicine is distinguished, however, by its desire to pursue a systematic inquiry into the workings of human nature in order to care for people, as well as by the priority it gives to the *sōma*, whose participation in the physical world, while by no means transparent, is more easily codified than that of the person. These characteristics give medicine a particular cultural authority.

Medical analogies acknowledge this authority. But they aim, too, to appropriate it. The medical analogy, after all, asserts difference and divergence. In many cases, it also openly declares the limits of medicine and, implicitly or explicitly, the body that figures so prominently in it. Those limits, we might imagine, were being felt more acutely as physicalized explanations of human nature grew more ambitious and robust, making the question of what these explanations leave out increasingly urgent. Socrates, legendary gadfly that he was, is often credited with raising this question.[8] In a famous passage, Plato has him recount becoming disillusioned with the inquiry into nature precisely because he believes that its causes—such as air and water, or sinews and bones—offer an impoverished account of why the world is as it is and people act as they do (*Phd.* 96a6–99d2). Behind the legend, however, lies a more complicated story. In the previous chapter, we began to detect fault lines between the person and his body in the course of considering how the former assumes responsibility for managing health. In this chapter, we can see these fault lines deepen as some thinkers explicitly lodge the responsibility for taking care in the *psukhē*,

[5] Medical analogies become increasingly sophisticated and complex in the Hellenistic and imperial periods: see Nussbaum 1994; Pigeaud 2006.

[6] For the idea that speech has both therapeutic and harmful properties, see *Il.* 9.507, 15.392–94, with Laín Entralgo 1970.1–31.

[7] See above, pp. 97–98.

[8] See Laks 2006.5–53.

imagined as the seat of reason, sensation-perception, emotion, desire, beliefs about and judgments of value, and intentional action—in short, the major components of ethical subjectivity.

The *psukhē* imagined in these terms attracts attention not only as the guardian of the *sōma* but as the seat of the rational and ethical subject. In such contexts, though the *sōma* remains a foil, it can also serve as a model for those wishing to probe more precisely how a "psychological" subject operates. As thinkers like Democritus and Plato begin to define the faculties that underwrite an ethics of praise and blame—a capacity to choose, to make rational judgments, to master desire—through the psychic conditions under which they are believed to flourish or fail, the specific vulnerability of the soul starts to come into focus. Each explains psychic malfunctioning in two basic ways: through a lack of knowledge; or through forces that, like those which cause bodily disease, have become uncoupled from daemonic agents—desires, emotions, and pleasures. These forces, even more than ignorance, threaten the *psukhē*'s identity as a rational agent capable of taking care of the self, creating a need for practices of care analogous to those applied to the *sōma*.

In light of the significance of this diagnostic and therapeutic context, I argue that the physical body functions not only as a foil but also as the dominant model for the *psukhē* as it emerges as the locus of the faculties that constitute ethical subjectivity.[9] I support, too, the related claim that what I have been calling the physical body crystallizes as a conceptual object in tandem with the emergence of this soul, which, at least for some thinkers, comes to mediate the body's relationship to the ethical subject.[10]

Ideas about the *sōma*, the *psukhē*, and human nature are messily proliferating in the late fifth and early fourth centuries BCE.[11] Too often, we try to resolve this messiness by reconstructing probable theories of mind, body, and soul.[12] Such approaches are undeniably useful, often clarifying the arguments that come to

---

[9] This is not to deny the importance of the eschatological context, which can justify the care of the *psukhē*, as at Pl. *Phd.* 82d1–7; see Bernabé 2007.34–36. See also *Chrm.* 156d4–157c6: the Thracian physicians taught by Zalmoxis both care for the *psukhē* and sometimes confer immortality. For Orphic-Pythagorean practices of care, see Foucault 2005.46–49. See also Kingsley 1995.283–86, on Pythagorean food taboos.

[10] The body is to some degree reintegrated with the ethical through the development of a more thorough teleology, such as that on display in Plato's account of the structure of the human body in the *Timaeus*. But even here, it is mind that organizes body: see Burgess 2000.

[11] On the particular messiness of body-soul dualism in general (in relation to other binaries), see the remarks of Lambek 1998.108–12. For the body-soul problematic in later Greco-Roman philosophical thought, see the recent essays in R. King 2006.

[12] There is the added problem that we sometimes mistake philosophical inquiry and debate for a widespread public conversation. See Winkler 1990b.17–20, who nevertheless goes too far, I think, in discrediting the influence of the new philosophical and physical inquiries on public debate. Allen 2006 demonstrates greater interaction between philosophy and oratory. See also Dover 1974.1–8, distinguishing between moral philosophy and popular morality (with useful observations on the nonsystematic nature of the latter); and 10–11 on popular attitudes toward philosophy.

shape the tradition of Greco-Roman philosophical ethics and the dualisms around which it forms. In this chapter, however, I approach *sōma* and *psukhē* as domains in the process of taking shape largely through the dynamics of analogy, with its mobile focus on both similarity and difference, concentrating on a handful of contexts where medicine's influence is explicit or likely.

I begin by defending the claim that the medical writers show little interest in motivations for action, focusing on their scant references to the workings of desire and pleasure. Their relative silence belies the easy association of the *sōma* with desire and pleasure in the late fifth and early fourth centuries, while also drawing attention to the difficulty of accounting for the desire-pleasure nexus solely in terms of the physical body. I then look at how making desire into a psychic problem helps to justify the care of the *psukhē*, sometimes over and above that of the *sōma*. Psychic care, I show, could also be independently defended on the grounds of its object's intrinsic worth, as in Plato's early dialogues. Nevertheless, in Plato's œuvre, speculation on why the *psukhē* errs ends up circling back to pleasures and pains and the powerful motivations to which they give rise. In the second half of the chapter, I look closely at Gorgias's *Helen* and Democritus's ethical fragments. Both authors give accounts of psychic disease that show affinities with contemporary medical explanations. These accounts allow us to see how the tension between a (nonhuman) object and a (human) subject finds its way into the *psukhē* at the very moment it is being defined against the *sōma*.

Bodily Needs

One of the problems with having a *sōma* is that it is strange and distant from the person: its inner life is mostly hidden from his senses; what he does sense does not readily disclose its causal mechanisms. Although we have approached this problem primarily in the context of symptoms, symptoms themselves can often be traced to an earlier stage in the person's estrangement from the *sōma*, namely to his difficulty in understanding and providing what it needs. If the person cannot implement his desires in the *sōma* directly but must rely on technical means—the manipulation of qualities, powers, or humors—we should not be surprised that what the *sōma* wants or needs does not typically surface in the person as desire. We can get a better sense of this situation by looking at a rare counterexample from *On Diseases* IV, where the needs of the *sōma* are seamlessly and uncannily transformed into the person's desires.

The author of this text assumes that the *sōma* is made up of four humors (or "juices"): bile, blood, phlegm, and water. Each humor is stored in a small *pēgē*, "reservoir," which, by storing and releasing the humor when necessary, regulates the ratio between the various humors.[13] If one of the reservoirs is exhausted,

---

[13] *Morb.* IV 39 (Li 7.556–60 = 92,12–94,9 Joly).

however, this autoregulation is extended to the person, who longs (ἱμείρεται ὁ ἄνθρωπος) to eat or drink whatever will restore the necessary resources, and he continues to desire this until balance is reestablished.[14] *Himeros,* "longing," then, is a mechanism that, at least in some cases, enables the person to operate as a perfect conduit between what the *sōma* needs and the fulfillment of those needs through voluntary action.[15]

But it is rare for the medical writers to represent the person as intuitively aware of bodily need. Such awareness is better seen as a haunting ideal that emerges in tandem with the physical body, akin to the preternatural awareness of a hero who understands exactly what the gods expect of him. It is true that hunger or thirst look like straightforward instances where the *sōma* communicates its needs.[16] But symbiosis between the *sōma* and the person can be achieved only if what the former needs appears to the latter as a specific object of desire. If the medical writers only rarely recognize this level of symbiosis, we should hardly be surprised. Effortless harmony between the person and his *sōma,* after all, erodes the authority of the physician, with his expert knowledge of *dunameis* and *phuseis.* At the same time, the very threat such harmony poses to medical authority only serves to emphasize the common ends of *phusis* and *tekhnē.* Although *On Diseases* IV seems unusual in representing the continuity between the *sōma* and the person as natural, its commitment to continuity is itself unremarkable. The basic assumption of naturalizing medicine, and especially regimen, is that technical knowledge enables people to give the physical body what it needs to thrive.

To thrive, the physician assumes, is what everyone naturally wants. That assumption, combined with the belief that health requires knowledge, leads to the idea that if people had knowledge, they would never fall ill in the first place.[17] On this principle, someone who intuitively knows what his body needs, as in *On Diseases* IV, should never fall ill, at least not from things under his

---

[14] *Morb.* IV 39 (Li 7.558–60 = 93,26–94,9 Joly).

[15] Cf. Emp. (DK31) A95 (= Aët. 5.28), where Empedocles is reported to have held that animals have appetites according to specific deficiencies. See also the puzzling passage at *Vict.* IV 93 (Li 6.660 = 228,26–27 Joly-Byl): dreaming of habitual food and drink signifies a lack of nourishment and a desire (?) of the soul (ἔνδειαν σημαίνει τροφῆς καὶ ψυχῆς ἐπιθυμίην [ἐπιθυμίην Littré Joly: ἀθυμίην θ M Jones]; cf. ψυχῆς ἐπιθυμίην, at 230,2 Joly-Byl). Yet dreaming of food also seems to indicate a surfeit, so that the proper response is to suppress food. In general, *On Regimen* IV holds that what the body needs can in some sense be communicated through dreams on the principle that, during sleep, the *psukhē* turns inward to "oversee its own household" (διοικεῖ τὸν ἑωυτῆς οἶκον, 86, Li 6.640 = 218,8 Joly-Byl). But dreams largely signal trouble that needs to be corrected: to know what to eat or do in the first place, one needs regimen. Moreover, when the *psukhē* looks inward, what it sees is a cosmological drama in which symbols take the place of symptoms. In other words, the body "speaks" in macrocosmic images. To understand these symbols, one needs a handbook like *On Regimen.* Thus, the information that filters from the *sōma* to the *psukhē* is not intuitively intelligible or automatically translated into desire but must be filtered through a medical framework of interpretation.

[16] See, e.g., Pl. *Phlb.* 31e6–32b4.

[17] *Art.* 11 (Li 6.20 = 238,1–2 Jouanna), cited above p. 177.

control, such as a humoral imbalance caused by food and drink. Indeed, when we look at the author's tripartite etiology of disease, we can see that the latter two classes of cause—environmental conditions and blunt trauma (e.g., a fall or a wound)—do fall outside the person's scope of action.[18] The first explanation, however, is more puzzling. If, when the *sōma* has a surfeit of food, the patient is not purged and continues to eat, disease develops.[19] How should we explain this situation? Is it that, in cases of surfeit, rather than depletion, the person loses touch with what the *sōma* needs to flourish?[20] Or does something drive him to eat *despite* a feeling that this is not what he, or, rather, his *sōma*, wants? The text offers little indication of which of these explanations is more likely to be true. On the principle that no one knowingly harms himself, we might conclude that the person simply does not know what he is doing. Even so, such a conclusion leaves us with the question of what motivates a person who neither senses his bodily needs nor has access to technical knowledge.

To consider these questions further, let us turn back to *On Ancient Medicine*, where pain plays a prominent role in acquainting people with their natures by leading them to reject foods that have caused harm in the past. The role of pain here suggests one way of thinking about motivation (i.e., as avoidance). Less obvious, but nonetheless present, is the factor of pleasure. On one occasion, the author considers cases where someone adopts a habit—say, eating one meal a day or two—that is not dictated by what his nature can tolerate (i.e., by pain). Habit here, he observes, is adopted either because of pleasure or for some other chance reason (δι' ἡδονὴν ἢ δι' ἄλλην τινὰ συγκυρίην, 10, Li 1.592 = 130,2 Jouanna). Can pleasure and chance also, perhaps, explain what the author calls *hamartēmata*, "errors," deviations in regimen that lead to disease?[21]

The factor of chance or accident in such deviations is left unexplored in the text. Pleasure, however, while not prominent, is subtly salient to the etiology of disease. In the *Kulturgeschichte*, the author observes:

> ἔτι γοῦν καὶ νῦν ὅσοι ἰητρικῇ μὴ χρέωνται, οἵ τε βάρβαροι καὶ τῶν Ἑλλήνων ἔνιοι, τὸν αὐτὸν τρόπον ὅνπερ οἱ ὑγιαίνοντες διαιτέονται πρὸς ἡδονὴν καὶ οὔτ' ἂν ἀπόσχοιντο οὐδενὸς ὧν ἐπιθυμέουσιν, οὐδ' ὑποστείλαιντο ἄν. (*VM* 5, Li 1.580 = 124,5–9 Jouanna)

---

[18] *Morb.* IV 50 (Li 7.582 = 106,16–23 Joly). See also Pl. *R.* 3, 405c8–d4, contrasting seasonal diseases and wounds with diseases of indulgence.

[19] *Morb.* IV 49 (Li 7.578–80 = 104,21–106,10 Joly).

[20] On the gap between what the person senses and what happens in the body in this treatise, see above, pp. 130–31.

[21] *Hamartēmata:VM* 12 (Li 1.596 = 132,11 Jouanna); see also *Prorrh.* II 3 (Li 9.10 = 224 Potter), of patients who depart from a prescribed regimen. Other errors in the treatise concern the physician, e.g., *VM* 9 (Li 1.588–90 = 127,15–129,13 Jouanna), where error does not imply culpability, because it arises from an unavoidable lack of knowledge: the author *praises* physicians who err only a little bit (ἐπαινέοιμι τὸν σμικρὰ ἁμαρτάνοντα), given the absence of precision in medical knowledge.

And what is certain is that even now all of those who do not use the medical *tekhnē*, barbarians and some of the Greeks, follow a regimen in the same way as the healthy do, for the sake of pleasure, and they could not hold themselves from anything they desire nor even reduce the amount.

As in the first passage, the author represents a diet unrestricted by the fear of pain as primarily motivated by pleasure.[22] We can detect, too, a new twist, insofar as he is also implicitly contrasting the indulgence of desire with the discipline imposed by medicine.[23] The contrast is echoed later in the treatise when the author notes that mild, well-blended foods are most beneficial to human nature, and then adds that these foods are also those most in use except for those seasoned and prepared "with a view to pleasure and satiety" (πρὸς ἡδονήν τε καὶ κόρον, 14, Li 1.604 = 137,5 Jouanna). What is most evident in this passage is the opposition between what is beneficial to human nature and what is merely pleasing. But, insofar as it is medicine that has discovered what is beneficial, we can discern, too, a latent tension between its guidelines and the pursuit of pleasure. Still, despite these glancing mentions of pleasure, the author stops short of implicating it in errors of regimen. He thus leaves the concept of blame untapped.

In one respect, by neglecting to fault pleasure for disease, the author of *On Ancient Medicine* departs from what was standard practice among his colleagues. Other writers regularly and with little fanfare trace disease to immoderate eating and drinking and sexual indulgence—the triad of what James Davidson has called the "consuming passions" of the classical Greek world.[24] In another respect, though, his approach to pleasure is typical. While *On Generation/On the Nature of the Child* shows it was possible to give a physiological account of pleasure, or at least sexual pleasure, the medical writers do not explain the *pursuit* of pleasure in terms of the physical body.[25] Their reticence in this respect can explain why, although they frequently treat the consuming passions as causal, they do not target them directly.[26] Thus, although the

---

[22] It is unclear whether these people do not suffer the consequences of pain, as earlier humans suffered less on account of their habituation to bestial foods (*VM* 3, Li 1.576 = 121,20–21,1 Jouanna), or whether pleasure overrides other considerations.

[23] On medical treatment that is painful but beneficial see, e.g., Pl. *Grg.* 478b7–c2.

[24] J. Davidson 1998.xvi, 139–82, with, e.g., Arist. *EN* 1118a29–32; Pl. *Leg.* 6, 782d10–783b1; *Phd.* 64d3–6; X. *Mem.* 2.1.1. On the indulgence of appetite as a cause of disease in medical etiology, see Foucault 1985.117–19, 125–39; Byl 2006.17–18.

[25] On the physiology of pleasure: *Genit./Nat. Puer.* 1 (Li 7.470 = 44,4–10 Joly), 4 (Li 7.474–76 = 46,21–47,19 Joly). But even this author declines to speak at length about erotic dreams (1, Li 7.472 = 45,8–10 Joly). See Dean-Jones 1992, arguing that the medical writers see sexual desire in men as stimulated by "something other than their bodies' requirements" and subject to their control (77). In contrast, female desire, as Dean-Jones persuasively argues, is represented as physiological and mechanical. See also Bodiou 2004.220–23.

[26] Emotions, however, have a more direct relationship to the humors. See *Morb. Sacr.* 10 (Li 6.380 = 20,1–5 Jouanna), where fear and weeping can induce an epileptic attack; cf. *Epid.* VI 5.5 (Li 5.316 = 108,5–110,2 Manetti-Roselli); *Hum.* 9 (Li 5.490 = 80 Jones). At *Epid.* II 4.4 (Li 5.126 = 72 Smith),

passions are recognized as damaging to health, they are largely neglected in medical writing.[27]

At the same time, by conceptualizing the physical body, physicians and medical writers are making a significant contribution to how desire—and especially the desire for pleasure—comes to be articulated as an ethical problem. Having a body, we have seen, does not entail knowing a body. Whereas a cow automatically eats whatever grasses supply needed nutrients, people must determine for themselves what to put into their bodies, with the result that there is room to make mistakes. Mistakes arise, in part, from ignorance. Yet ignorance is not the only problem produced by this arrangement. The fact that we are not compelled by our bodies' precise needs—understood as particular kinds of food and drink, rather than food and drink *tout court*—allows the formation of desires that have little or nothing to do with the needs on which bodily health depends.

The author of the treatise *On the Use of Liquids* makes just this assumption—namely, that because we are estranged from the cavity and its needs, other motivating forces, more intimately felt, surge up in the conscious field. The author has been observing that different parts of the *sōma* take pleasure in (ἥδομαι) or are vexed by (ἀγανακτέω, ἄχθομαι) heat and cold. He then turns to note that, although the cavity grows irritated when it is overpowered by cold, the person, being "very far from feeling it" (πλεῖστον ἀπέχει τοῦ παθεῖν), sometimes develops a desire for something cold. Given that this desire is most proximate, it is only to be expected that the person takes pleasure in his cold drink, oblivious, at least initially, to any distress caused to the cavity.[28] From one perspective, the (initially unfelt) conflict between the needs of the cavity and the needs of the person is just one possible example of conflict within the physical body's composite nature. At the same time, this conflict is singular, insofar as one "body part," that is, "the person," has the power to seek its pleasure at a significant cost to the pleasure of the other parts and, indeed, to the health of the whole. That conflict looms large in the contrast between mild, healthful diets and those prepared for the sake of pleasure in *On Ancient Medicine*, where pleasure is not correlated with any obvious need; it is assumed by etiologies that attribute disease to excessive eating or drinking.

The tension between (physical) need and desire comes to the foreground if we look outside medical writing. It is neatly laid out, for example, in Plato's *Gorgias*, when Socrates opposes the therapeutic arts of medicine and gymnastics to

---

inducing emotions can help balance the humors. Conversely, the regimens outlined in *Vict.* I 35 (Li 6.518 = 154,9–12 Joly-Byl) can stop people from weeping for no reason and fearing what is not fearful; see also *Virg.* 3 (Li 8.468–70 = 24,1–14 Lami), where sexual intercourse cures wild emotions.

[27] But cf. Pl. *Smp.* 186b8–d6, 187e1–6, where it is, indeed, the physician's job to produce desires in the *sōma* for the right kinds of things: Eryximachus, of course, is defending his authority in a discussion about *erōs*.

[28] *Liq.* 2 (Li 6.124 = 167,2–4 Joly).

fine cooking and cosmetics on the grounds that, whereas the former seek the good condition of the *sōma*, the latter peddle pleasures and deceptive beauty without giving any thought to what is properly beneficial (464b2–465c2).[29] Socrates' categorization assumes a principle that is fundamental to medicine, namely that bodies sometimes seem to be in a good condition even when they are not healthy; often only a physician or a trainer can perceive hidden trouble (464a2–b1). The concept of false seeming, grounded in the body's very nature, sheds some light on why people betray their health—presumably it is partly because the true condition of the body is so hard to perceive that "the beneficial" has such a weak motivational force. Its weakness leaves the door open to the deceptive promise of sensory pleasure. Indeed, Socrates observes that pleasure actively fosters misconceptions about which foods are beneficial for the *sōma* (464d2–e2).[30]

It would seem straightforward to assume that it is the person who both experiences these pleasures and forms beliefs about them. For, although the physical body has become a significant cause of human suffering by the end of the fifth century, its very nonhuman nature casts caregivers and embodied subjects—at least to the extent they can acquire knowledge and act—as its guardians, as we have seen. It comes as a surprise, then, that Socrates attributes misguided judgments about the pleasurable and the beneficial to the *sōma*. If the *sōma* were allowed to control itself, he says, it would choose on the basis of delight, mixing up the healthful, the medicinal, and the tasty in indiscriminate confusion (465c7–d6). Socrates seems to assume that the *sōma* is basically bipartite. It has an objective nature, of which medicine is the steward. It is also a subject of pleasure, who experiences, judges, and acts. We might question whether the claim that the *sōma* has such a subjective dimension is tenable, but Socrates is probably being playful here—elsewhere, those who choose on the basis of pleasure are children or men senseless as children (464d6–7). He is interested primarily in using the true and the false arts of the *sōma* to establish something about the *psukhē*—namely, that it, too, is endowed with a true nature, tended by the lawgiver and the judge, and a pleasure-seeking double, gratified by sophists. The analogy, then, ends up raising questions about the nature of the *psukhē*, rather than clarifying the relationship of the *sōma* to pleasure.

But the idea that pleasure is somatic is hardly unusual in this period. In Plato's *Phaedo*, the *sōma* is subjected to relentless censure for its love of pleasure, which blocks the proper pursuits of the *psukhē* and threatens to "nail" it to the

---

[29] Cf. *Grg.* 499d4–e1. On the contrast between what seems good and what is good in the later Greek ethical tradition, see Mitsis 1988.19–39.

[30] Cf. *Morb.* IV 39 (Li 7.558 = 93,23–25 Joly), where, in a context assuming harmony between the cavity and the person, feelings of pleasure confirm that something is beneficial: τούτων γὰρ ἡμῖν ὅ τι ἂν ἕκαστον πλεῖον τοῦ καιροῦ γίνηται καὶ ἐν τοῖσι ποτοῖσι καὶ ἐν τοῖσι βρωτοῖσι, κεῖνα οὐδὲ ἡδέα γίνεται· ἄσσα δὲ χατίζει μάλιστα κατὰ ταῦτα, κεῖνα ἡδέα ἐστίν (for if one of these [sc. humors-juices] is greater than it should be in our foods and our drinks, then these things are not pleasurable; but whatever is needed most in this regard, this is pleasurable).

morally degraded physical world.[31] In the *Memorabilia*, Xenophon casually
equates the gratification of desire with the gratification of the *sōma* (1.2.23).
And in Aeschines' *Against Timarchus*, a vicious attack on a political rival that
dates from the middle of the fourth century, the orator declares that the Furies
who drive humans to ruin on the tragic stage are nothing other than the rash
pleasures of the *sōma* (1.190–91).

   Yet the *sōma* of rash pleasures does not map precisely onto the *sōma* of the
medical writers. Nor does the daemonic force it arrogates from the Furies travel
the same channels as phlegm or bile. Indeed, if we attribute appetitive desire
and sensual pleasure to the *sōma*, it begins to look less like the *sōma* and more
like the person. In fact, when Socrates imagines the *sōma* choosing its own
pleasures, he treats the scenario as an unreal condition: "If the soul did not rule
over the body, but the body over itself . . . " (εἰ μὴ ἡ ψυχὴ τῷ σώματι ἐπεστάτει,
ἀλλ' αὐτὸ αὑτῷ, *Grg.* 465c7–d1).[32] Socrates implies that if the soul is in charge,
pleasures can be kept in check. But is it true that, if pleasures are not checked,
there is only the body to blame? What if we approach the problem of pleasure
in terms of not what the *sōma* wants but what the *psukhē* wants? What would
happen if we designate the *psukhē* not only as the locus of the responsibility to
take care of the *sōma* but also as the locus of desire?

PSYCHIC DESIRES

The *psukhē*'s culpability for what goes wrong in the *sōma* is vividly dramatized
in a scene that Plutarch tells us Democritus thought up:[33]

   εἰ τοῦ σώματος αὐτῇ δίκην λαχόντος, παρὰ πάντα τὸν βίον ὧν ὠδύνηται καὶ κακῶς
   πέπονθεν, αὐτὸς γένοιτο τοῦ ἐγκλήματος δικαστής, ἡδέως ἂν καταψηφίσασθαι
   τῆς ψυχῆς, ἐφ' οἷς τὰ μὲν ἀπώλεσε τοῦ σώματος ταῖς ἀμελείαις καὶ ἐξέλυσε ταῖς
   μέθαις, τὰ δὲ κατέφθειρε καὶ διέσπασε ταῖς φιληδονίαις, ὥσπερ ὀργάνου τινὸς ἢ
   σκεύους κακῶς ἔχοντος τὸν χρώμενον ἀφειδῶς αἰτιασάμενος. (DK68 B159)

---

[31] See *Phd.* 65a10, 66b7–67b2, 79c6–8, 80e2–81c6, 83d4–e2; see also, e.g., *R.* 10, 611b10–d6. Plato
repeatedly rethought the contours of the body and, more specifically, its role in pleasure and desire.
In the *Gorgias* and the *Phaedo*, where the tripartite soul is absent, the body tends to take the blame
for appetitive desires and pleasures. But with the introduction of the tripartite soul in the *Republic*,
desires are clearly located in the appetitive part of the soul without the body being absolved of responsibility (the *psukhē* appears to participate in disorderly motion *because* it is embedded in a
sōma at *Ti.* 42a3–4). The most complex psychosomatic explanation of sensory pleasures is found in
the *Philebus*. For further discussion, see Holmes, forthcoming (b). On dualism and the tripartite
soul, see T. Robinson 2000.42–47.

[32] Socrates goes on to locate all desires in the soul: see *Grg.* 493a3–5. The context is Orphic-
Pythagorean, but he does not indicate that he disagrees with the view presented.

[33] Plut. *Lib.* 2; see also Plut. *Mor.* 135E. (In both places, Theophrastus, responding to Democritus, is
credited with the opposing view—namely, that the soul is blamed unfairly for the evils of the body:
see frr. 440A, 440B FHSG.)

If the body were to bring suit against [sc. the soul] on account of all the sufferings and pains that it had undergone its whole life, and one was the judge of the charge, one would happily find the soul guilty of having destroyed aspects of the body through lack of care and dissipated it through drink and corrupted it and broken it down through love of pleasures, just as if a tool or a utensil were in a bad state one would blame the person who used it recklessly.

It is clear from this passage that Democritus accepts that a person, and more specifically, here, the soul, exercises power over the body.[34] Indeed, in another fragment, he offers a variation on the call to "help oneself" familiar from *On Regimen*: "People request health from the gods through prayer, not knowing that they hold the *dunamis* to achieve this in themselves [ἐν ἑαυτοῖς]" (DK68 B234). At the same time, in acknowledging the power of the soul, Democritus eliminates the responsibility of the body for its suffering. The body becomes the docile instrument of a psychic agent capable of both care and abuse.

By granting the soul so much power over health, Democritus is, in one sense, taking the physicians very seriously. They tend, after all, to invest significant causal weight in the things they and their patients can control, like diet and physical training; from Democritus's perspective, the soul is simply the locus of this control. At the same time, Democritus's diagnosis of suffering leads him to see control rather differently. Whereas the author of *On Regimen* fears people will fail to take care because they lack knowledge or sufficient time, in the courtroom fragment, Democritus attributes *ameleia*, "lack of care," to the love of pleasure. This stance is consistent with the second half of B234, where he correlates our capacity to achieve health with our capacity for self-mastery, understood as mastery over our appetitive desires.[35] Democritus thus makes health dependent on whether we can manage our desires, rather than on medical expertise or a complex regimen. In another fragment, he declares that it is easy to satisfy the body's needs once the misguided desires produced by faulty judgment are eliminated.[36] If the physicians encourage the patient

---

[34] In addition to contrasting *sōma* and *psukhē*, Democritus also opposes *sōma* to *nous* (B105). The relationship of *psukhē* to *nous* has long been an object of debate on the basis of Aristotle's comments at *De an.* 404a27–31, 405a9 that Democritus does not distinguish *nous* from *psukhē* (because, says Aristotle, he held that appearance is truth, a criticism related to his critique of the physicalism of Democritus's psychology: see further above, chapter 2, n.133). For modern versions of this position, see Kahn 1985.10; C. Taylor 2007.77–78. In the fragments, Democritus seems to make *psukhē* responsible for thought, perception-sensation, desire, and voluntary motion; *nous* is probably restricted to rational judgment and perhaps several other faculties.

[35] DK68 B234: ἀκρασίῃ δὲ τἀναντία πρήσσοντες αὐτοὶ προδόται τῆς ὑγιείης τῇσιν ἐπιθυμίῃσιν γίνονται (but by doing the opposite things through lack of self-control, [people] betray their health to their desires).

[36] DK68 B223: ὧν τὸ σκῆνος χρῄζει, πᾶσι πάρεστιν εὐμαρέως ἄτερ μόχθου καὶ ταλαιπωρίης· ὁκόσα δὲ μόχθου καὶ ταλαιπωρίης χρῄζει καὶ βίον ἀλγύνει, τούτων οὐκ ἱμείρεται τὸ σκῆνος, ἀλλ' ἡ τῆς γνώμης κακοθιγίη [κακοθιγίη Diels-Kranz: κακοθηγίη καθοδιγίη MSS: κακοηθίη Wilamowitz Taylor] (What the body requires can easily be acquired by everybody without effort and misery; the things that require effort and misery and make one's life painful are desired not by the body but by

to adopt an "objective" position on the body akin to their own, a position isolated from the turmoil of physicality, Democritus cordons off a place for intelligent agency *inside the person*. At the same time, he introduces the problem of desire into the very place from which that agency arises. By contaminating this agency with the potential for turmoil, he creates a model of psychic disease.

Despite curtailing the body's role in disease in order to shift responsibility to the soul, Democritus does not seem to have rejected the legitimacy or the value of contemporary medicine. Indeed, he is credited with quite a few biological, physiological, and medical titles, including works on dietetics and prognosis.[37] He was interested, rather, in imposing limits on medicine's expertise: "Medicine heals the sickness of the body," reads one programmatic fragment, "while wisdom rids the soul of its suffering" (ἰατρικὴ μὲν γὰρ σώματος νόσους ἀκέεται, σοφίη δὲ ψυχὴν παθῶν ἀφαιρεῖται, B31).[38] Others, too, in the fifth and fourth centuries were fashioning therapies analogous to those in medicine but directed at the mind or the emotions or the soul.[39] As I suggested at the beginning of this chapter, although the language of healing had long been used of emotional or mental distress, we should approach a project like Democritus's from within its historical context, in which medicine and related techniques of caring for the body had achieved newfound cultural authority. That authority looks like the

---

aimless judgment). Note that what I translate as "body" here is the word σκῆνος, "tent." See also B37; B187 (cited below); B288. On the use of this term, see Peixoto 2001.192–96, who argues that it refers to "le corps en tant qu'enveloppe corporelle, c'est-à-dire en tant qu'enveloppe du complexe psychosomatique" (195).

[37] See DK68 B26b–d and the overviews in Guthrie 1962–69, 2:465–71 and Leszl 2007.40. At *Ep.* 17 (Li 9.352 = 74,22–27 Smith), one of the apocryphal Hippocratic letters from the Hellenistic period, the great physician finds Democritus surrounded by the bodies of half-dissected animals.

[38] The use of πάθος to mean "affection" here seemed suspiciously Stoic to Diels; see also Kahn 1985.24 n.50. But the gist of the fragment, at least, is central to Democritus. See also B281; B288: νόσος οἴκου καὶ βίου γίνεται ὅκωσπερ καὶ σκήνεος (there is disease of the household and of life in the same way as of the body). J. Warren 2002.46, referring specifically to B191, speculates that Democritus offers the earliest philosophical example of therapeutic argument. The healer-philosopher figure, however, is also important to Pythagoreanism (with which Democritus is sometimes associated): see Kingsley 1995.327–28, 335–47; for Pythagoreanism and medicine more generally, see Burkert 1972.262–64, 292–95. Empedocles, too, presents himself as a healer: see DK31 B111.1–2; B112, with Burkert 1972.153–54; Kingsley 1995.217–27, 247–48; Vegetti 1998; Hoessly 2001.188–97.

[39] See, e.g., Isoc. 8 (*On the Peace*) 39–40. See also Antiphon Soph. T6a–d (Pendrick) for reports from later antiquity that Antiphon created a *tekhnē* for removing sorrow just like the therapy set up by physicians for the sick, except reliant on words. Pendrick 2002.240–42 is probably rightly skeptical about the reliability of these reports (see also 1–2 nn.4–5 on the unreliability of [Plut.] *Vitae X or.* 833C–D, one of the main sources for the anecdote), though they may have originated in late fifth-century comedy on the basis of Antiphon's practices. On "mental" disease, see also Emp. (DK31) A98 (= Cael. Aur. *Chron.* 1.5.145). Music could also form the basis of a therapy of the soul: see, e.g., Pl. *Prt.* 326a4–b6; *R.* 3, 400a5–b4, with Woerther 2008. On the training of the soul as analogous to the training of the body: X. *Mem.* 1.2.19, 2.1.19–20.

target of a fragment in which Democritus tries to establish the *psukhē*'s priority vis-à-vis the *sōma*:[40]

ἀνθρώποις ἁρμόδιον ψυχῆς μᾶλλον ἢ σώματος λόγον ποιεῖσθαι· ψυχῆς μὲν γὰρ τελεότης σκήνεος μοχθηρίην ὀρθοῖ, σκήνεος δὲ ἰσχὺς ἄνευ λογισμοῦ ψυχὴν οὐδέν τι ἀμείνω τίθησιν. (DK68 B187)

It is appropriate for people to take the soul rather than the body into account. For the perfection of the soul puts right the corruption of the "tent," while the strength of the "tent" without reasoning does not make the soul the least bit better.

Much as some physicians were trying to free themselves from a more global inquiry into nature, then, others in the fifth century were working to delineate a target of care not only beyond the reach of humoral medicine but also more worthy of attention than its target, the physical body.

Democritus's attempt to establish the priority of the *psukhē* and its care recalls Plato's critique of regimen and the excessive care of the *sōma* in *Republic* 3. In fact, Plato's arguments, though harsher, dovetail quite neatly with those found in the Democritean fragments. Like Democritus, Plato accepts that the capacity to be well lies in us.[41] He, too, argues that a healthy body, by means of its own virtue (τῇ αὑτοῦ ἀρετῇ), cannot improve a soul—thereby tacitly denying or at least minimizing the body's role in the full spectrum of human faculties— although, the opposite is true, that is, a good soul can make the body as good as possible.[42] On these grounds, he has Socrates advocate caring for our *dianoia*, "capacity for thought," and entrusting it with the supervision of the body (3, 403d1–e2).[43] It might be that this supervision, if it requires specialized knowledge, is taken up in cooperation with a physician—Socrates does not say. What he does make clear is that the physician-patient partnership in its current form is a failure: physicians are simply treating the symptoms of diseases that can be traced to a breakdown in a population's mastery of its desires.[44] The *sōma*

[40] See also DK68 B57.

[41] See Pl. *R.* 2, 379c2–7: the gods do not, as the masses believe, cause bad things. The gods do cause good things, but this never obviates the need for a complex set of human institutions and practices designed to guide the soul to its true nature.

[42] See also Pl. *R.* 3, 408e2–5: οὐ γάρ, οἶμαι, σώματι σῶμα θεραπεύουσιν . . . ἀλλὰ ψυχῇ σῶμα (For I do not think that [sc. physicians] treat a body with a body. . . . But it is with a soul that a body is treated). In the *Philebus*, both the body and the soul require measure for health, but only the soul can impose it. For the soul entrusted with bodily care, see also X. *Mem.* 1.4.13: the gods give humans a soul in part so they can protect themselves against the elements, relieve sickness, and foster health.

[43] Much as Democritus declares that it is easy to supply the body's needs, Socrates assumes there is no need to go on at length (μὴ μακρολογῶμεν, 3, 403e1) about what the body needs—an implicit rebuke, presumably, to regimen's detailed prescriptions.

[44] For the representation of new diseases of affluence: Pl. *R.* 3, 405c7–d5; cf. 404b11–404e6, with J. Davidson 1998.33. Cf. Pl. *La.* 195c9–11: physicians do not know whether health or illness is the more terrible thing for a man. Elsewhere, physicians know bodies without knowing themselves (*Alc.* I 131a5–7; *Chrm.* 164a9–c2).

is a casualty of this crisis. The real problem, as in Democritus, lies with a soul that indulges its desires.

Even Aeschines, who equates the tragic Furies with the "rash pleasures of the *sōma*," turns out to see the body more as a victim than an aggressor. In his attack on Timarchus, a field day of moral censure, he gives the idea of erring against the body a different cast than it had in *On Ancient Medicine*.[45] The most important of these errors are sexual—prostitution, passive homosexuality, voracious appetite—but they include, too, gluttony and extravagance at the table (1.42). These lawless desires are, in Aeschines' mind, properly feminine. But whereas, as we have seen, women have no way of mastering these desires and, hence, cannot be blamed for them, Timarchus, as a man, could have acted otherwise once he was old enough to know the laws, making him a legitimate target of blame.[46] The (visible) body is introduced as supporting evidence for these accusations. Aeschines recalls a time when Timarchus, speaking before the assembly, threw off his cloak, revealing a physique wasted by depravity. The surface of the body serves not so much as a place where symptoms erupt, as in medicine, but as a tableau on which years of failing to take care have hardened into an indictment of Timarchus's *bios*, his way of life (1.26–27).

Aeschines no doubt hopes that this vicarious glance at Timarchus's body will lead his audience to fault Timarchus as readily as Democritus blames the soul for the body's suffering in B159. Yet it is worth observing a difference in their respective allegations. While Democritus simply charges the soul for damage to the body, Aeschines is accusing Timarchus of something else, namely his corruption *qua* elite citizen qualified to advise the *polis* and, more broadly, *qua* free man.[47] On closer inspection, however, Democritus, too, understands the consequences of indulgence to be far greater than bodily harm, as we will see later, as does Plato. Indeed, Plato makes the intrinsic worth of the *psukhē* the primary justification for its care in his early "Socratic" dialogues, perhaps adopting this position from the historical Socrates.[48] In the *Apology*, Plato's own account of Socrates' trial, the defendant declares:

οὐδὲν γὰρ ἄλλο πράττων ἐγὼ περιέρχομαι ἢ πείθων ὑμῶν καὶ νεωτέρους καὶ πρεσβυτέρους μήτε σωμάτων ἐπιμελεῖσθαι μήτε χρημάτων πρότερον μηδὲ οὕτω σφόδρα ὡς τῆς ψυχῆς ὅπως ὡς ἀρίστη ἔσται. (Pl. *Ap.* 30a7–b2)

---

[45] See Aeschines 1.39, 185.

[46] Aeschines 1.39. On the culpability of ethical ignorance, see Arist. *EN* 1110b31–1111a1. See also X. *Mem.* 1.1.16: Socrates thought the ignorant should be called slavish.

[47] See Winkler 1990b.54–64 on the "testing of speakers," of which *Against Timarchus* is our surviving example.

[48] For my purposes, it is not necessary that the dialogues usually referred to as "Socratic" (*Apology, Charmides, Crito, Euthydemus, Euthyphro, Hippias Minor, Ion, Laches, Menexenus, Protagoras, Republic* I; also often included are *Alcibiades* I and *The Lovers*: see below, n.50) reflect the views of the historical Socrates. Burnet 1916 makes the care of the soul a Socratic "invention." See also Havelock 1972; Claus 1981.157–59.

For I go around doing nothing but trying to persuade you, young and old, to care neither for your bodies nor for your possessions before [your soul], nor even so much as you care for your soul, that it is as good as possible.

On what grounds, though, should the welfare of the soul be elevated over bodies and possessions?

Throughout the *Apology*, Socrates speaks of the soul in relation to *phronēsis*, "thought." At the same time, as Eric Havelock points out, he uses the expression "to care for the soul" interchangeably with the expression "to care for oneself," suggesting that he sees the soul as equivalent to, if not synonymous with, the reflexive pronoun.[49] His language implicitly justifies the soul's priority through its importance to the defining activity of the person, namely thought.

That justification becomes more explicit in *Alcibiades* I, perhaps one of the earliest of Plato's dialogues, where Socrates undertakes a more systematic equation of the soul with the self.[50] Socrates is here shown in action, exhorting the dialogue's namesake to care for himself. What this care entails, however, is not clear to Alcibiades. So Socrates explains what he means by running through a range of candidates whose care is potentially equivalent to self-care, systematically eliminating them until he arrives at the soul. He begins with objects within the orbit of the self but far from its center (shoes, rings), each of which is abandoned on the grounds that it merely belongs to a part of the body (127e–128d). But, although in this first phase the body and its parts stand in contrast to instruments, caring for the body does not qualify as an art of caring for oneself. In the next phase of the argument, we learn why. By introducing a second opposition between user and used—recall that Democritus, too, has exploited these terms—Socrates succeeds in moving body parts (hands, eyes) into the same class as inanimate objects (tools, harps). The last of these objects to be *heteron*, "other," than the person is the body (129e7).[51] Transformed into an instrument, the body serves as a foil against which the person can be defined as a user and, hence, on the undefended premise that the user of the body just *is* the soul, as the soul. Socrates then takes the argument one step further. The soul not only uses the body but also rules over it, because, as Socrates asserts and Alcibiades concedes, the body cannot rule itself.[52] Given the soul's role as user and master of the body, its neglect incurs shame in a community that prizes the

---

[49] Havelock 1972.6–9. See also Foucault 2005.52–54.

[50] The dialogue's authenticity has been questioned, in part because the soul is seen as the ruler of the body, but see Annas 1985.111–15, defending it as genuine. The idea of the soul ruling the body is presented as Socratic at X. *Mem.* 1.4.8–9, 4.3.14; cf. 1.4.17 (ὁ σὸς νοῦς ἐνὼν τὸ σὸν σῶμα ὅπως βούλεται μεταχειρίζεται). See also the discussion of *Alcibiades* I in Foucault 1997.228–31.

[51] Cf. *Alc.* I 131a2–3: ὅστις ἄρα τῶν τοῦ σώματός τι γιγνώσκει, τὰ αὑτοῦ ἀλλ᾽ οὐχ αὑτὸν ἔγνωκεν (anyone who gets to know something of the body knows the things that are his, but not himself).

[52] Claus 1981.169–70 thinks that there may be an implicit contrast with medical definitions of the soul here. I agree that physiological definitions of a human being are a plausible subtext for Socrates' arguments here, though it would seem, *pace* Claus, that these definitions have more to do with *phusis* than with the *psukhē qua* life-force.

capacity to act and to rule: "I fear," says a chastened Alcibiades, "that I have escaped my own notice for a long time now, *most shamefully*" (κινδυνεύω δὲ καὶ πάλαι λεληθέναι ἐμαυτὸν αἴσχιστα ἔχων, 127d7–8).[53]

More than once in the early dialogues we find Plato defining the worth of the soul *qua* ethical self against the body. Far from marginalizing the arts of the body, however, Plato often uses them as models for a *tekhnē* of soul care. In the opening scenes of the *Protagoras*, we find Socrates again with a young man, aptly named Hippocrates, who is eager to become a student of Protagoras. Socrates cautions that before seeking the great sophist's teachings, he should consider the risk he is taking with his soul, "through which we conduct our own affairs well or poorly" (ἐν ᾧ πάντ᾽ ἐστὶν τὰ σὰ ἢ εὖ ἢ κακῶς πράττειν, *Prt.* 313a7–8; cf. 313e2–314a1). For the sophist, like a merchant of foodstuffs who does not know what the effects of his wares will be on the body, cannot say "whether his teachings will be beneficial or harmful for the soul" (ὅτι χρηστὸν ἢ πονηρὸν πρὸς τὴν ψυχήν, 313d8–e1; cf. 334a3–5), with the result that his client is risking his soul in unknown territory. The young Hippocrates would not take such odds with his body, Socrates argues; he would most probably consult a physician before swallowing foods whose effects he cannot predict.[54] How, then, can he gamble with the soul, which is far more valuable?[55] Should he not seek expert knowledge here, too? Plato makes the case for the worth of "whatever there is in us which justice and injustice concern" (ὅτι ποτ᾽ ἐστὶ τῶν ἡμετέρων, περὶ ὃ ἥ τε ἀδικία καὶ ἡ δικαιοσύνη ἐστίν)—the soul is not named—even more forcefully in the *Crito*, again using as his model the body whose nature is known only to experts. The athlete, he points out, must listen to his trainer and his physician and ignore the advice of the crowds if he wants to avoid destroying his body. So, too, then, must we shut out the opinions of the many if we do not want to ruin that part of us that is most valuable and makes life most worth living (*Cri.* 47d6–48a4).[56]

Even this cursory glance at some of the earlier Platonic dialogues suggests two basic uses for the *sōma*. It serves, on the one hand, as a foil to that part of us that thinks, acts, and exercises mastery; determines whether we conduct our affairs well or poorly; and is concerned with what is just and unjust. Plato consistently calls this part of us *psukhē*. On the other hand, the *sōma* is not simply the object that defines a psychological subject. In medical contexts, Plato also casts it as a physical object embedded in a web of unseen forces that can be channeled toward benefit or harm by those with expert knowledge. Seen in these terms, the *sōma* becomes a model for the *psukhē*, through which it

---

[53] See also *Grg.* 477b8–e6, 479b4–c4: the value of the soul means that psychic disease is most shameful.

[54] On the expertise of the physician about the beneficial, see also *Cri.* 47b1–3; *Grg.* 490b1–7, 517d6–518a1. For the analogy between nourishment and teachings, see *Phdr.* 270b4–9; *R.* 9, 585a8–586b4; *Ti.* 44b8–c2. For medicine as a model *tekhnē*, see Reeve 2000; M. Gill 2003.

[55] *Prt.* 313a6–7; cf. 313e5–314a1.

[56] On the medical analogy, see also *Grg.* 505a2–b6, 512a2–b2; *Hp. Mi.* 372e6–373a2.

acquires its own principle of flourishing, nourished by teachings and suscepti-ble to benefit and damage.[57] It is possible that physiological ideas about life and health played a significant role in how Plato (or Socrates before him) conceptu-alized what we might call a principle of ethical life, realized through actions that constitute "doing well" or "living well" and based in the soul. Such a princi-ple seems to be present later in the *Protagoras*, where Socrates makes it a tenet of human nature that we desire and pursue those things which we believe to be good.[58] The similarities between these two principles, biological and ethical, can explain the affinities of Socrates' position—we fail to flourish because we lack knowledge about the good—with the idea that health depends on acquir-ing expert knowledge about what helps and harms the *sōma*.

In valorizing knowledge, moreover, the Socrates of Plato's early dialogues develops a silence not unlike that observed earlier in the Hippocratic writers. Recall that, although those writers not infrequently trace disease to desires for food and sex, they are rather reticent about what motivates a patient who nei-ther forms desires on the basis of bodily needs nor acquires knowledge about how to achieve health from his physician. Plato's Socrates, too, is rather vague about why we act as we do in our ignorance. Or, rather, while he is clear that we act on the basis of false beliefs about the good, he does not elaborate how these beliefs form.[59] In the so-called middle dialogues, such as the *Gorgias*, the *Phaedo*, and the *Republic*, however, Plato begins to explore in greater detail why our natural tendency to seek the good goes astray.[60] In so doing, he ex-pands the analogy between health and virtue from the early dialogues in order to develop a notion of psychic disease in which appetitive desires and pleasures become analogous to the things inside the body that hurt it.[61] These psychic

[57] On the soul's flourishing, see also discussions in Havelock 1972.5–7; Nussbaum 2001.97–98; Rus-sell 2005.28–43. On the analogy, see also Claus 1981.109–10, 182–83.

[58] See *Prt.* 358c7–d2: οὐδ᾽ ἔστι τοῦτο, ὡς ἔοικεν, ἐν ἀνθρώπου φύσει, ἐπὶ ἃ οἴεται κακὰ εἶναι ἐθέλειν ἰέναι ἀντὶ τῶν ἀγαθῶν (To want to go toward those things that one considers bad instead of [things considered] good is not, it seems, in human nature); cf. *Grg.* 468b1–4. According to psychological eudaemonism, our only motivation for our actions is a belief about the good: see Irwin 1995.52–53. Yet this state of motivation can be classified as unnatural or, rather, "diseased" if our beliefs are mis-aligned with the truth. That is, only when we know the good do we desire naturally. The topic de-serves more attention than I can give it here.

[59] The closest he comes to explaining the origins of false belief is *Prt.* 356c8–e2, although interpreta-tions of this passage range widely: see Holmes, forthcoming (b), with further bibliography. The conventional story, which has Socrates eliminate the role of nonrational or "good-indifferent" de-sires in human action, has recently come under challenge. Bobonich and Destrée 2007.xviii–xxiii give a brief overview of these developments.

[60] For the *Gorgias* as a transitional dialogue, see Claus 1981.175–80 (though he sees in it a transition to a less psychosomatic, more "abstract" inquiry into the soul); Woolf 2000.

[61] On the "medical" or "scientific" treatment of pleasures and desires in the *Philebus*, in particular, see D. Frede 1992.435, 450, 456; Peponi 2002. On the virtue-health/vice-disease analogy, see Jaeger 1944.21–26; Tracy 1969.90–96, 120–36; Lidz 1995; Gocer 1999.24–33; T. Robinson 2000.39–41; G. Lloyd 2003.142–52. Cf. concerns about the application of a medical model to virtue and vice in MacKenzie 1981, esp. 158–78; Stalley 1981; 1996; Ruttenberg 1986.

"things" can answer the question of what motivates us in the absence of clear information from the cavity about what it needs for health. But even more important, they can be faulted for turning us from the true nature of the soul. For our true nature, unlike the nature of the body, *can* form a continuum with our motivations if we acquire the appropriate knowledge and manage our appetites. In other words, if we have knowledge, we can desire just what the soul needs.[62]

Plato's growing interest in the nature of desire makes his exploration of psychic disease increasingly complex, too complex to tackle further here. It is worth keeping in mind, however, that although this exploration unfolds in Plato's œuvre as a development in his own thinking, the problem of pleasure, and specifically the mastery of pleasures, was already widely recognized in the late fifth and early fourth centuries. Indeed, Socrates admits he is swimming against the tide of popular opinion when, in the *Protagoras*, he categorically denies that someone can "be bested by pleasures" (ὑπὸ τῶν ἡδονῶν ἡττᾶσθαι, 352e6–353a1) in order to argue that people act in ignorance of what is beneficial.[63] Most people, he says, think that knowledge is "nothing strong, no ruling or hegemonic part" (οὐκ ἰσχυρὸν οὐδ᾽ ἡγεμονικὸν οὐδ᾽ ἀρχικόν):

> οὐδὲ ὡς περὶ τοιούτου αὐτοῦ ὄντος διανοοῦνται, ἀλλ᾽ ἐνούσης πολλάκις ἀνθρώπῳ ἐπιστήμης οὐ τὴν ἐπιστήμην αὐτοῦ ἄρχειν ἀλλ᾽ ἄλλο τι, τοτὲ μὲν θυμόν, τοτὲ δὲ ἡδονήν, τοτὲ δὲ λύπην, ἐνίοτε δὲ ἔρωτα, πολλάκις δὲ φόβον, ἀτεχνῶς διανοούμενοι περὶ τῆς ἐπιστήμης ὥσπερ περὶ ἀνδραπόδου, περιελκομένης ὑπὸ τῶν ἄλλων ἁπάντων. (*Prt.* 352b5–c2)

> They don't see it as something like that, but they think that, although a person often has knowledge within him, knowledge does not rule him, but something else—now anger, now pleasure, now pain, sometimes sexual desire, and frequently fear. They just think of knowledge as a slave, pushed around by all the other things.

It is hard to know when the language of mastery, sometimes expressed quantitatively as being "greater" or "lesser" than pleasures or emotions, became widespread. Its popularity, however, can explain why, in cases where the *psukhē* is seen as the seat of knowing, believing, judging, perceiving, and voluntary action, the threat to these faculties—over and above any threat to physical

---

[62] See Segvic 2000, esp. 9, who, defending a similar claim, calls this "Socratic wanting."

[63] See also *Grg.* 491d10–e1: when pressed as to what he means by governing oneself, Socrates replies he is speaking of the popular notion of being temperate and mastering one's own pleasures and appetites (σώφρονα ὄντα καὶ ἐγκρατῆ αὐτὸν ἑαυτοῦ, τῶν ἡδονῶν καὶ ἐπιθυμιῶν ἄρχοντα τῶν ἐν ἑαυτῷ). On being "less than" pleasure or Aphrodite, see Ar. *Nu.* 1081; Democr. (DK68) B214; E. *Andr.* 629–31; *Hipp.* 475, 727; frr. 187.6K (= *Antiope* fr. 11 J.-V.L.), 282.5K (= *Autolycus* fr. 1 J.-V.L.). See also Antiphon Soph. fr. 58 (Pendrick), on conquering oneself by resisting pleasures. While the idea of mastering or being "stronger than" pleasures is central to Xenophon's portrait of Socrates (e.g., *Mem.* 1.1.20, 1.2.14), Plato was far more wary of the idea, as Dorion 2007 demonstrates. On the mastery of pleasure, see also Foucault 1985.63–77; Winkler 1990b.49–50.

health—often takes the shape of desires and pleasures. One way of articulating this threat, as Plato's dialogues indicate, is to appropriate figures of disease from contemporary medicine, turning medicine into a significant conceptual and imaginative resource for the theorization of pleasures, desires, and false beliefs as the Furies that drive humans to ruin.

Yet, if the soul is vulnerable to forces that behave like those in the body, its defining power, intelligent agency, is compromised, as we saw above. It is true that that agency is already under threat during disease in the medical writers. Nevertheless, despite the emphasis in some texts on regimen and compliance, in medicine there is a sense that intelligence and agency, while neither omnipotent nor infallible, are safely vested with a physician. When these faculties are located in a soul responsible for self-reflexive care, however, they become more vulnerable, not only to somatic forces but also to psychic ones. Psychic disease, that is, with its warping of motivation and belief, complicates the possibility of adopting the position of the physician vis-à-vis oneself. If the internal threats to psychic order (desires, beliefs, thoughts) work analogously to forces inside the body, how can a space of intelligent agency be maintained?

We possess a late fifth-century text that deftly exploits just this difficulty. In his *Encomium to Helen*, Gorgias gives an account of psychic compulsion that turns on a provocative translation of daemonic agency into the dynamics of physicality—*logos*, for example, "accomplishes the most godlike things by means of a very small and invisible body" (σμικροτάτῳ σώματι καὶ ἀφανεστάτῳ θειότατα ἔργα ἀποτελεῖ, 8). Let us inquire more closely, then, into how contemporary models of bodily disease inform Gorgias's speech and the consequences of these models for his representation of the soul. Having examined Gorgias's challenge to the legitimacy of praise and blame, I will return to Democritus's fragments on psychic disease in order to see how, in adapting the idea of technical agency to the care of the soul, he recuperates a place for praise and blame and, hence, for ethical subjectivity.

GORGIAS'S *ENCOMIUM TO HELEN* AND HUMAN DISEASES

The *Encomium to Helen* is, as its title suggests and as Gorgias declares outright in the final lines of the speech, an exercise in denying blame. What makes it particularly fascinating for our purposes is that Gorgias is interested in defending Helen's innocence not simply on conventional grounds but also in terms of impersonal forces that operate through nature, necessity, and chance. In fact, the common axiom of the four causal scenarios he outlines, while valid for each of them, rings of the inquiry into nature:

πέφυκε γὰρ οὐ τὸ κρεῖσσον ὑπὸ τοῦ ἥσσονος κωλύεσθαι, ἀλλὰ τὸ ἥσσον ὑπὸ τοῦ κρείσσονος ἄρχεσθαι καὶ ἄγεσθαι, καὶ τὸ μὲν κρεῖσσον ἡγεῖσθαι, τὸ δὲ ἥσσον ἕπεσθαι. (Gorg. *Hel.* 6)

For it is the nature of things, not for the strong to be hindered by the weak, but for the weaker to be ruled and drawn by the stronger, and for the stronger to lead and the weaker to follow.

Gorgias begins exonerating Helen by invoking, then quickly setting aside, the first possible cause: the familiar triad of the gods' plans, Chance, and Necessity (the last two *qua* quasi-daemonic forces whose workings are not open to examination).[64] *Bia*, "brute force," also requires little explanation. The last two cases, however, *logos* and *erōs*, demand further discussion. If *logos* is a *dunastēs megas*, a "great ruler" (8), for example, we need to know *how* it exercises its power. In fact, Gorgias spends the rest of the speech responding to just this question, namely, how are people forced to act by the words and images that strike their souls?

When Gorgias says that *logos* accomplishes great things "with a very small invisible body" (8), he is not imagining a homunculus.[65] Having a body, rather, means having the power to act: the word can (δύναται) stop fear, take away grief, and create joy, precisely because, like other physical stuffs, it has a *dunamis*.[66] To explain this power, Gorgias will eventually invoke a medical model, arguing that the power of speech over the ordering of the soul, *psukhē*, has "the same logic" (τὸν αὐτὸν δὲ λόγον) as the power of drugs over the nature of bodies: "For just like some kinds of drugs take some humors [χυμούς] from the body, and some stop illness, others life, in this way do some words harm those listening, and others delight them" (14).[67] The analogy is anticipated earlier in the speech when Gorgias describes persuasion by marrying the traditional language of enchantment to that of physical change (ἔθελξε, μετέστησεν, 10). And while the *dunamis* of *erōs*, sparked by *opsis*, "vision," works in a slightly different way, Gorgias represents its effects, too, as a "human disease" (ἀνθρώπινον νόσημα) and psychic ignorance (19).[68] Gorgias thus seems to adopt the physical body to help represent a transition from power understood anthropomorphically to power envisioned in terms of impersonal stuffs.

---

[64] Ford 2002.175 n.57 sees the near conflation of this triad as indicative of an enlightened view of the "divine." See also de Romilly 1976.319; Spatharas 2002.169–70.

[65] Guthrie 1962–69, 2:111 n.2, assuming that *logos* is personified here, excludes *Hel.* 8 from his list of fifth-century examples of inanimate *sōma*.

[66] See *Hel.* 10: ἡ δύναμις τῆς ἐπῳδῆς; 14: ἥ τε τοῦ λόγου δύναμις.

[67] On Gorgias's medical analogy, see Segal 1962.104–6, 133; Ford 2002.162, 184. The analogy does not imply that the soul or speech is not physical, although commentators tend to insert qualifiers (e.g., "quasi-physical," Segal 1962.106; "near-physical," Worman 1997.173; cf. Ford 2002.177 n.61; Horky 2006). Nevertheless, as Porter 1993.287–88 observes, "Gorgias simply fails to spell out the physiology by and through which language is presumed to operate psychologically." Vision, though, receives more attention.

[68] In elucidating the power of *erōs*, which works through the image, most commentators have looked at the effluence theory of perception ascribed to both Empedocles and Gorgias at Pl. *Men.* 76c7–e3: see Segal 1962.99–102; Kerferd 1985; Ford 2002.179–82. Ford also points to the depiction of air as a μέγιστος δυνάστης at *Flat.* 3 (Li 6.94 = 106,2–3 Jouanna); see also Buchheim 1989.164; Jouanna 1999.82–83, and above, p. 135.

Yet how should we understand the word "like" on which Gorgias's comparison between the body and the soul rests? How is the soul that receives words and images like the body manipulated by the physician? How are they different? One point of similarity is that Gorgias sees force building up through a causal chain in the soul much as it does in the body. In some cases, he treats *opsis* or *logos* as the simple mechanism through which the soul is affected by outside forces: shivering, tearful pity, and love of mourning arise through words (διὰ τῶν λόγων, 9); pleasure and pain are produced because of words (διὰ λόγων, 10); the soul is imprinted by the image on account of vision (διὰ τῆς ὄψεως, 15).[69] In this last example, however, Gorgias goes on to provide a more detailed account of what can happen in the soul between the impact of the image and its perceptible effects. His account, responding to the implicit how question that arises when daemonic agents are eliminated, has affinities with contemporary explanations of how disease arises in a body through an increasingly dangerous series of actions and reactions.

Gorgias begins by stating that if the vision—notice the substitution of the faculty for the person[70]—sees bodies arrayed for battle, it is thrown into disorder: the verb for disordering, *tarassō*, is standard for humoral disturbance. Indeed, much as bile and phlegm, once disturbed, disturb the rest of the body, the disturbed vision disturbs the *psukhē*, with the result that those struck (ἐκπλαγέντες) by fearful images often flee (16).[71] Seeing fearful things, moreover, can turn people away from their present purpose (τοῦ παρόντος ἐν τῷ παρόντι χρόνῳ φρονήματος ἐξέστησαν): "Fear," Gorgias says bluntly, "thus extinguishes and drives out thinking" (οὕτως ἀπέσβεσε καὶ ἐξήλασεν ὁ φόβος τὸ νόημα, 17). The impact of the image does not necessarily end even here. Seeing fearful things, many people, Gorgias goes on, have fallen into fruitless troubles and terrible diseases and incurable madness, because "vision engraves in thought [ἡ ὄψις ἐνέγραψεν ἐν τῷ φρονήματι] images of the things seen" (17).

---

[69] Persuasion, too, "stamps" the soul (τὴν ψυχὴν ἐτυπώσατο, 13). For the idea of mental imprinting, see A. *Pr.* 788–89 and esp. Pl. *Tht.* 193b9–d2, with Horky 2006.

[70] See also *Hel.* 13 (τοῖς τῆς δόξης ὄμμασιν); 15 (διὰ τῆς ὄψεως); 16 (εἰ θεάσεται ἡ ὄψις; ἀπὸ τῆς ὄψεως); 17 (ἡ ὄψις ἐνέγραψεν); 18 (τέρπουσι τὴν ὄψιν; τοῖς ὄμμασιν; τὴν ὄψιν); 19 (τὸ τῆς Ἑλένης ὄμμα).

[71] The sentence in the latter half of chapter 16 may be corrupt. It is difficult, in any event, to reconcile the transmitted text with its context. DK82 B11 reads: ἰσχυρὰ γὰρ ἡ συνήθεια [MSS. ἀλήθεια] τοῦ νόμου διὰ τὸν φόβον ἐξῳκίσθη [MSS. εἰσῳκίσθη] τὸν ἀπὸ τῆς ὄψεως, ἥτις ἐλθοῦσα ἐποίησεν ἀμελῆσαι [MSS. ἀσμενίσαι] καὶ τοῦ καλοῦ τοῦ διὰ τὸν νόμον κρινομένου καὶ τοῦ ἀγαθοῦ τοῦ διὰ τὴν νίκην [MSS. δίκην] γινομένου. On this reading, fear drives out respect for law and makes the person neglect what is good and beautiful by custom and law. The sense goes nicely with the context; see also X. *Mem.* 1.2.22, where appetitive desire precludes caring, ἐπιμελεῖσθαι, about what is right. Cf. Donadi 1978.53–55, concluding that both εἰσῳκίσθη and ἀσμενίσαι must be retained (see also Donadi 1982). Nevertheless, Donadi's own interpretation of the passage is strained. Buchheim prints εἰσῳκίσθη and ἀσμενίσαι but concedes that the sentence is hard to fit into the context (1989.172). See also the emendations of MacDowell 1961.121 (retained at MacDowell 1982.24–26). The translation at Kennedy 1991.287 neglects a crucial γάρ.

By treating images as seeds capable of generating increasingly serious conditions, Gorgias strengthens the ties between his account of psychic affections and contemporary nosologies, where trouble often gathers bit by bit. Like the medical writers, he distributes the daemonic power symbolized by the hand across a spatiotemporal process, leading us through an internalized series of cascading effects triggered, here, by a single image.

These effects unfold in the realm of physical realities, unaffected by our wishes. First, "what we see does not have the nature we want it to have but what each happens to have" (ἃ γὰρ ὁρῶμεν, ἔχει φύσιν οὐχ ἣν ἡμεῖς θέλομεν, ἀλλ᾽ ἣν ἕκαστον ἔτυχε, 15).[72] Moreover, once things have been set in motion, there seems to be no stopping them. Yet we might recognize the very appearance of necessity here as a rhetorical strategy. We have seen that the medical writers understand disease as a process realized in and through an individual *sōma*, which is interposed between an external catalyst and a (visible) outcome. The "intervallic" status of the *sōma* opens up the possibility of different outcomes: the force rushing in might be conquered if the body's *dunamis* is strong; the person, sensing the beginning of trouble, might take measures to correct the problem before it gets out of hand; an ill-chosen meal the day before might turn that force into a full-fledged disease. In fact, the soul, too, may be a kind of interval, Gorgias implies.[73] Though he takes for granted that under certain circumstances the vision and the soul will always be disturbed, once we reach the result clause, where those struck by fearful images flee, he introduces the adverb *pollakis*, "often." Moreover, it is only *some* people who, seeing fearful things, go out of their minds. Many (but not all) fall into disease and madness. But what, we might ask, determines who flees and who goes mad? Is there a way to avoid these outcomes?

In asking these questions, we are led to reflect on what an individual soul, either as the locus of a certain kind of character or as a possible agent of intervention in the process, contributes to the outcome of its initial disturbance. And this is precisely why Gorgias, committed to defending Helen's innocence, would prefer that we not ask them. While he does allow that different people will be affected differently by terrifying images, he remains focused on impersonal causes loosely clustered around the triad of nature, necessity, and chance and operating independently of the person. Desire and fear, for example, are natural phenomena: "It is natural [πέφυκε] for the vision to be pained at some things and long for others"; indeed, many things produce in us a longing and desire for things and bodies (18). Moreover, *erōs* is *not* an error, *hamartēma*, but an *atukhēma*, a "misfortune" (19): if Helen was persuaded, "she did no wrong, but was simply unfortunate" (οὐκ ἠδίκησεν ἀλλ᾽ ἠτύχησεν, 15). Finally, by stressing physical reactions to speech like shuddering and crying, Gorgias infects

---

[72] Persuasion, however, imprints "whatever *it* wants" (ὅπως ἐβούλετο, 13).

[73] See Horky 2006.377, reading ἴδιόν τι πάθημα at *Hel.* 9 in this way ("souls become individuated according to the particular reception of the general *logos*").

emotions and actions with the automatism of the *sōma*.[74] Seen in this context, his use of the humoral body as an analogue to the soul looks like another tactic to cast psychic disease as a process beyond the scope of ethical subjects.

Nevertheless, the soul is not the same as the body—more is at stake in fear or desire. When a medical model, under which the body betrays its own health in response to a powerful catalyst, is adapted to the psychic domain, it becomes scandalous. If a chance encounter with beauty can so easily annul the jurisdiction of *nomos*, the ethics of praise and blame are so contingent as to be worthless, secured neither by reason nor by the gods. It is a very bleak scenario, made bleaker by the fact that Gorgias withholds any hope of resistance.

But it is not simply the troubling consequences of psychic disease that set it apart. The mechanisms themselves are ambiguous: speech is only *like* a drug; the persuader is only *like* one acting with force (ὡς ἀναγκάσας), while the persuaded is *like* one forced (ὡς ἀναγκασθεῖσα, 12).[75] The "like" of the *Helen* can be read against a passage from the *Philebus*, where Plato says that Gorgias distinguished between violence and persuasion by arguing that persuasion "makes all things its slaves not through force, but because they are willing [δι' ἑκόντων ἀλλ' οὐ διὰ βίας, 58b1]." In *Helen*, Gorgias may, indeed, be implying that, in the interval between word (or image) and action, lies a moment of acquiescence. That is to say, his breezy confidence in conflating the mechanics of the physical body with what happens in the soul may very well be a challenge to the alibis created out of the new physics, a wink at an audience too easily transfixed by its desires and its fears. Helen, of course, incarnates the problem of desire, both through her power to attract other bodies (4) and in her own attraction to the body of Paris.[76] She would thus seem to raise difficult questions about objects that, by promising pleasures and pains, co-opt our very capacity to choose what is good, leading us toward ruin. These difficult questions, however, are deftly sidestepped by Gorgias in his denial that psychic disease can be evaluated within a rubric of praise and blame.[77]

Given this refusal of blame, it is not surprising that Gorgias does not think hard, at least in this speech, about the possibility that different souls respond to stimuli differently. He does not ask what kind of soul it would take to stand firm

---

[74] See Segal 1962.107.

[75] Porter 1993.288 reads in that "like" a "metaphor of materialism": "The mechanisms by which *logos* is translated into its effects are anything but self-evident, and they seem to advertise their fictional or metaphorical status. Their crossing-over into other domains is literally a category mistake. Is Gorgias's materialism a metaphor? If not, then his account has too many shortcomings to name. If it is, then this makes Gorgias's own account a metaphor—but of what?"

[76] Porter 1993.282–83, 294; Worman 1997.171; 2002.156–59.

[77] See also Kallet 1999 on Thucydides' use of contemporary ideas about disease to complicate ideas of moral responsibility. Compare, too, Socrates' explanation of why people err in regard to pleasure at Pl. *Prt.* 356c8–e2, also focused on the deceiving power of the image. In the *Protagoras*, however, people can acquire, through *tekhnē*, the capacity to choose rightly (although Plato accepts elsewhere that some natures cannot be cured of psychic disease: see Scott 1999; C. Gill 2000; Brickhouse and Smith 2002). On Gorgias and Socrates, see Calogero 1957.

in battle or resist Paris but keeps his focus on the power of images and words to act on a soul. At the other extreme, in *Against Timarchus*, Aeschines, despite equating the tragic Furies with the rash pleasures of the body, sees in his opponent's actions only individual depravity, nothing of its catalysts or mechanisms. I would like to turn now to a position between these two poles of ethical judgment. Democritus, as we have seen, attributes suffering to the soul's capitulation to pleasure. But because he also accepts that people hold the *dunamis* of wellness in themselves, he does not deny the possibility of blame. We saw in chapter 4 that the potential subject of medical knowledge is delicately poised between being the initiating cause of action or being merely a symptom. Democritus expresses that delicate balance in a new idiom. Despite the limits of the evidence, we can glimpse in his fragments a sketch of psychic disease, as well as strategies for protecting not simply bare life but also the eudaemonic life, the life of the soul.[78]

PSYCHIC DISORDER IN DEMOCRITUS

In the *Helen*, Gorgias is vague about the physical status of words and images: what matters is that they do things in the soul. Democritus, however, is credited with developing atomism, one of the most influential physical theories from antiquity. We may expect, then, that if Democritus wanted to explain why and how humans go astray in a world where gods do not cause bad things, he might look to the atomic underpinnings of their actions.

In fact, although scholars largely concur that Democritus viewed the soul (*psukhē*) and the mind (*noos*) in physical terms, they have not always accepted that his ethics is informed by his physics.[79] Some of this skepticism can be attributed to contemporary concerns about reducing psychological states to physical ones.[80] Scholars have been wary, too, of an apparent contradiction between a physical theory that has been interpreted since antiquity as rigidly determinist and an ethics premised on praise and blame and, hence, implicitly,

---

[78] On *eudaimoniē*, see DK68 B170: εὐδαιμονίη ψυχῆς καὶ κακοδαιμονίη; see also B171. The sources for Democritus's ethical views pose some problems. Fragments B35–115, from the "Democrates" collection, are usually seen as the most unreliable, while those from Stobaeus (B169–297), and particularly the longer fragments from this collection, tend to be preferred: see Procopé 1989.307–8; 1990.22–23; C. Taylor 1999a.222–27; J. Warren 2002.30–32. Leszl 2007.65–69 challenges the skepticism about the shorter sentences, pointing out that we do not know if Democritus compiled maxims rather than writing continuous works on ethics. On the ethical writings ascribed to Democritus, see Leszl 2007.28–29, 52–56, and esp. 64–76.

[79] For thought as physical alteration, see Thphr. *De sens.* 58 (DK68 A135), with J. Warren 2002.64–71. See also B158 and Arist. *De an.* 404a27–31 (A101) and above, chapter 2, nn.131,133,137.

[80] See esp. C. Taylor 1967 and 1999a.232–34, responding to Vlastos 1945 and 1946, and J. Warren 2002.59–60 n.91; 2007a.87–90 on the debate.

voluntary action.[81] Finally, because we have only fragments, many of which are aphoristic and reminiscent of traditional gnomic wisdom, it has been easy to deny that Democritus had an overarching ethical system or, at the very least, an innovative one.[82]

Let us begin with the last objection. There is an undeniable overlap between popular morality and the fragments. When Democritus writes that "such things as are bad and harmful and useless, neither in the past nor now do the gods bestow such things on people, but people run into them themselves through blindness of mind and lack of judgment [διὰ νοῦ τυφλότητα καὶ ἀγνωμοσύνην]" (B175), he would seem to be revisiting Zeus's remarks at the start of the *Odyssey*: while people blame the gods for their troubles, the truth is that they incur pains beyond what is fated "through their own folly" (σφῆσιν ἀτασθαλίῃσιν, 1.32–34).[83] Upon inspection, however, the fragments suggest that Democritus was trying to conceptualize mental blindness as an objective state of human nature, with specific causes and outcomes, and thus as a legitimate target of inquiry. It is presumably because he believed such a state could be described in causal terms that he held out the possibility of remedying it, thereby both preserving and justifying the conditions of praise and blame that Zeus simply assumes.

But how can we modulate our desires if they belong to a class of physical causes that unfold a chain of necessary outcomes? The question of how we intercede in such a chain does seem to become a concern in later (Epicurean) atomism, with its notorious concept of the swerve. But on the basis of the fragments we have from Democritus, the challenge of ethical agency appears to be formulated rather differently. The relevant model, I suggest, is the one we saw in the previous chapter of a subject who can be categorized *either* as someone who takes care of himself *or* as a kind of complex symptom produced by forces within the cavity. Like a physician vis-à-vis the body, Democritus sees the soul as a physical entity whose flourishing is imperiled by disordering tendencies within it. Yet there are practices within the scope of our power that can keep these tendencies in check. Such practices are, thus, indispensable to living well.

Despite the relevance of a medical model of care, however, Democritus seems to recognize a categorical difference between flesh and humors and, say, desires

---

[81] See, e.g., Kahn 1985.10–11. For Aristotle's concerns about Democritus's account of how the soul initiates motion, see *De an.* 406b15–22 (DK68 A104), 409a31–b4 (A104a). Cf. the account of Democritus's relationship to determinism in Farrar 1988.215–41, with which I am in broad sympathy.

[82] See Annas 2002, esp. 170–71. Cf. J. Warren 2007a.87 n.1, defending the view that the eudaemonist reading is anachronistic. Regardless of this debate, in recent decades, Democritus's ethics have received more attention: see, in addition to the pioneering Vlastos 1945 and 1946, C. Taylor 1967; Tortora 1983; 1984; Kahn 1985; Farrar 1988.192–264; Procopé 1989; Peixoto 2001; Annas 2002; J. Warren 2002; and the essays in Brancacci and Morel 2007.

[83] Note that, at the beginning of the fragment, Democritus says that the gods do give all *good* things to men (though, as for Plato, this does not eliminate the need for our agency). See also DK68 B217. On Democritus's theology, see C. Taylor 1999a.211–16.

and emotions. This difference does not, strictly speaking, have to do with atoms, for all these things are atomic. Rather, the difference between humors and desires appears to depend on a categorical difference between bodies and souls that, while traceable to atomic difference, cannot be adequately understood in atomic terms.[84] That may not seem like it helps much. It may be more useful to explore in greater detail how thoughts and desires and emotions work differently from humors or other such stuffs. Let us begin with the longest extant ethical fragment as an entry point to the question of how Democritus represents the causal factors of psychic wellness and disease, keeping in mind the concerns that have been raised about the consistency of Democritus's explanation of error.

B191 is a particularly valuable fragment, drawing together themes that pepper the shorter fragments into a single, sustained account that is worth quoting at length.

ἀνθρώποισι γὰρ εὐθυμίη γίνεται μετριότητι τέρψιος καὶ βίου συμμετρίη· τὰ δ᾽ ἐλλείποντα καὶ ὑπερβάλλοντα μεταπίπτειν τε φιλεῖ καὶ μεγάλας κινήσιας ἐμποιεῖν τῇ ψυχῇ. αἱ δ᾽ ἐκ μεγάλων διαστημάτων κινούμεναι τῶν ψυχέων οὔτε εὐσταθέες εἰσιν οὔτε εὔθυμοι. ἐπὶ τοῖς δυνατοῖς οὖν δεῖ ἔχειν τὴν γνώμην καὶ τοῖς παρεοῦσιν ἀρκέεσθαι τῶν μὲν ζηλουμένων καὶ θαυμαζομένων ὀλίγην μνήμην ἔχοντα καὶ τῇ διανοίᾳ μὴ προσεδρεύοντα, τῶν δὲ ταλαιπωρεόντων τοὺς βίους θεωρέειν, ἐννοούμενον ἃ πάσχουσι κάρτα, ὅκως ἂν τὰ παρεόντα σοι καὶ ὑπάρχοντα μεγάλα καὶ ζηλωτὰ φαίνηται, καὶ μηκέτι πλειόνων ἐπιθυμέοντι συμβαίνῃ κακοπαθεῖν τῇ ψυχῇ. ὁ γὰρ θαυμάζων τοὺς ἔχοντας καὶ μακαριζομένους ὑπὸ τῶν ἄλλων ἀνθρώπων καὶ τῇ μνήμῃ πᾶσαν ὥραν προσεδρεύων ἀεὶ ἐπικαινουργεῖν ἀναγκάζεται καὶ ἐπιβάλλεσθαι δι᾽ ἐπιθυμίην τοῦ τι πρήσσειν ἀνήκεστον ὧν νόμοι κωλύουσιν. διόπερ τὰ μὲν μὴ δίζεσθαι χρεών, ἐπὶ δὲ τοῖς εὐθυμέεσθαι χρεών, παραβάλλοντα τὸν ἑαυτοῦ βίον πρὸς τὸν τῶν φαυλότερον πρησσόντων καὶ μακαρίζειν ἑωυτὸν ἐνθυμεύμενον ἃ πάσχουσιν, ὁκόσῳ αὐτέων βέλτιον πρήσσει τε καὶ διάγει. ταύτης γὰρ ἐχόμενος τῆς γνώμης εὐθυμότερόν τε διάξεις καὶ οὐκ ὀλίγας κῆρας ἐν τῷ βίῳ διώσεαι, φθόνον καὶ ζῆλον καὶ δυσμενίην. (DK68 191)

Happiness belongs to men through the moderation of joy and balance in life. Deficiencies and excesses tend to change into one another and create great motions in the soul. Those souls that are moved out of large intervals are neither well settled nor *euthumoi*. You must, then, set your mind on what is possible and be content with what is present, paying little heed to and not dwelling on those who are envied or marveled at. But you should consider the lives of people in trouble, thinking about what they are suffering so that what you have at present seems great and enviable, and it no longer happens that you are in a bad state in the soul through desire for more. For whoever wonders at the wealthy and those thought blessed by other men and constantly dwells on it in his memory finds it necessary to keep

---

[84] Soul atoms, importantly, are reportedly fine and spherical, which makes them capable of causing motion (Arist. *De an.* 405a8–13 [DK 68 A101]). Psychic disease, in a sense, elaborates what can go wrong with atoms that cause humans to move.

discovering new schemes and, on account of the desire to do something, to attempt a desperate deed which the laws forbid. Therefore, you should not seek some things, but be happy with others, comparing your life with the lives of those who are doing worse, and, thinking about what they are suffering and how much better your life is proceeding than theirs, you should consider yourself blessed. Holding to this thought you will live your life more happily and you will drive back not a few troubles from it, namely envy, jealousy, and ill-will.

Democritus's stated subject is *euthumiē*, psychic wellness.[85] In the course of learning what this is and how to achieve it, we also find out a good deal about the things that imperil it. Democritus explains psychic suffering first in terms of what look like physical events that arise when measure is not observed and the balance inside the soul is lost: a seesawing between excesses and deficiencies that provokes "great motions."[86] Two adjectives are then denied to souls that are "moved out of large intervals": *eustathees*, "well settled," and *euthumoi*, "content," perhaps denoting an objective perspective and a subjective one, respectively.[87] But the primary cause of psychic suffering is not a movement but a mental action, that is, desiring more, here expressed as dwelling on what others have. The outcome of such desire, moreover, is expressed not in physical terms but in terms of psychic states (envy, ill will) and actions (seeking new things, transgressing the laws). Democritus thus appears to recognize two different levels of description in the soul, although he leaves their relationship vague.[88] Each level offers resources for locating suffering in a causal chain that unfolds inside the soul over time. The person not only *can* intervene in this chain by thinking about the right kinds of things, like other people's pain or what is possible: he ought (δεῖ, χρεών) to do so.

It is possible here, as it was in Gorgias, to see affinities with medical accounts of disease. Although those features that look medical may have developed independently, Democritus's own reference to a medical analogy, together with his work in medicine, makes it not unlikely that he was drawing in part on contemporary accounts of bodily diseases when he developed his views on psychic disease. For just as the physicians are developing the idea that things inside the body hurt it, Democritus is elaborating a model that refers psychic trouble to things inside the soul. A passage from Plutarch suggests that Democritus described the soul as "a storehouse and treasury of ills, subject to all kinds of affections" (ποικίλον τι καὶ πολυπαθὲς κακῶν ταμιεῖον ... καὶ

---

[85] On the concept of *euthumiē* in Democritus, see J. Warren 2002.32–72.

[86] For balance (συμμετρίη) as a harmonious bodily state, see, e.g., *Vict.* I 32 (Li 6.510 = 148,29–31 Joly-Byl). On the mechanics of soul movements—best understood in physical terms, given not only the dynamics on which atomism depends but also the significant role of flux in humoral disorder— see Vlastos 1945.583–85. Cf. C. Taylor 1967.13, 26–27; 1999a.232–33, arguing that these motions are simply metaphorical.

[87] See J. Warren 2002.60–71 on the expression "moved out of large intervals." The adjective εὐσταθής, "settled, stable," means "well built" in Homer (e.g., *Il.* 18.374; *Od.* 20.258).

[88] See Farrar 1988.199–204.

θησαύρισμα, B149).[89] Foremost among these ills, it is easy to imagine, are the desires in B191 that, by outstripping what is possible, drive a person to harm himself and others.

One of the reasons Democritus may be so interested in desire is because it seems to mark for him our distance from knowing what our nature needs. One fragment runs, "the thing that is in need knows how much it needs, but the person who is in need does not know" (τὸ χρῆζον οἶδεν, ὁκόσον χρήζει, ὁ δὲ χρῆζων οὐ γινώσκει, B198).[90] It is because we lack this knowledge and, with it, any clear sense of measure that desire spirals out of control. In this respect, desire is much like a humor, or like those fluxes inside the body that, as we saw at the end of chapter 3, are so difficult to harness. At the same time, insofar as the soul is responsible for both health and psychic wellness, we might see desires not simply as analogues of humors but as more serious threats. The problem of desire restages the problems posed by the humors in the domain of the soul, perverting not just our health but also our drive to live well.[91]

The fragments suggest at least two ways of conceptualizing how desires get out of control. On the one hand, Democritus discusses how the indulgence of desire creates ever more violent appetites.[92]

ὅσοι ἀπὸ γαστρὸς τὰς ἡδονὰς ποιέονται ὑπερβεβληκότες τὸν καιρὸν ἐπὶ βρώσεσιν ἢ πόσεσιν ἢ ἀφροδισίοισιν, τοῖσι πᾶσιν αἱ μὲν ἡδοναὶ βραχεῖαί τε καὶ δι᾽ ὀλίγου γίνονται, ὁκόσον ἂν χρόνον ἐσθίωσιν ἢ πίνωσιν, αἱ δὲ λῦπαι πολλαί. τοῦτο μὲν γὰρ τὸ ἐπιθυμεῖν ἀεὶ τῶν αὐτῶν πάρεστι καὶ ὁκόταν γένηται ὁκοίων ἐπιθυμέουσι, διὰ ταχέος τε ἡ ἡδονὴ παροίχεται, καὶ οὐδὲν ἐν αὐτοῖσι χρηστόν ἐστιν ἀλλ᾽ ἢ τέρψις βραχεῖα, καὶ αὖθις τῶν αὐτῶν δεῖ. (DK68 B235)

Those who take their pleasures from the belly, going beyond what is appropriate in their food and drink and sexual indulgences, for all of these people the pleasures are small and last a short time, for however long they are eating and drinking, but the pains are many. For the desire for the same things is always present, even when they get what they desire, and the pleasure shortly passes, and there is nothing useful left to them save this fleeting joy, and then there is need of the same things all over again.

The paradox of pleasures of the belly is that, by coming and going quickly (διὰ ταχέος, δι᾽ ὀλίγου) without delivering satisfaction, they increase desire, rather than sating it. What is more, they leave pains in their wake. Reading these pains in light of the body's suit against the soul at B159, we can see them as arising

---

[89] The passage continues: ". . . [ills] which do not flow in from outside, but have, as it were, native and autochthonous springs, which badness, widely diffused and abundantly supplied with affections, sends forth." These lines are probably not a direct quotation from Democritus, but they shed light on the original context of the fragment.

[90] Compare DK68 B223; see also Motte 1984 and Foucault 1985.49–50 on the "hyperbolic" potential of the sexual drive in Greek ethics.

[91] Democritus specifically distinguishes between living and living well: see, e.g., DK68 B200; B201.

[92] Violent appetites: see DK68 B72 (from "Democrates").

from the conflict, which we saw above, between the person's pleasures and what is beneficial to the body. These pains, however terrible, cannot deter future indulgence, presumably because of desire's powerful impetus.

But indulgence incurs a greater cost than bodily damage. The serial satisfaction of desires, after all, seems like a good candidate for causing the excesses and deficiencies responsible for psychic instability in B191.[93] In other fragments, Democritus is clear about the costs of indulging appetitive desires at the level of emotions, character, and behavior: immoderation is the worst teacher of the young, for example, because it "gives birth to those pleasures from which badness arises" (τίκτει τὰς ἡδονὰς ταύτας, ἐξ ὧν ἡ κακότης γίνεται, B178); taking pleasures in "mortal things" is a recipe for distress (B189). Desire, by giving rise to pleasures that generate more desires, would thus seem to create a downward spiral in which one bad thing adds to another "automatically," as it were, until not just the body but the soul is thoroughly ruined.[94]

But people drive this process not simply by indulging their desires but also by the mental activity of desiring. As we saw in B191, dwelling on the honor of others causes psychic distress by stirring up envy and enmity.[95] These emotional states, in turn, lead to further trouble. Envy, for example, gives rise to strife (B245), in part, as Plutarch reports, by being transmitted through vision—which is triggered, in atomism, by tiny *eidōla*, "films"—from the envious person to the souls of others.[96] And if we always think about those who are more fortunate we will be compelled to go looking for new things and to attempt crimes. These transgressions, in turn, provoke even greater psychic distress, as the wrongdoer is plagued by fear of punishment and shame.[97] Emotions, thoughts, and memories, by feeding desire and by their own power to upset the soul, are thus all active causes of both psychic and somatic distress.

It is possible to avoid such cycles only if one achieves "self-sufficiency."[98] But how can the tendency of the soul toward disorder be countered? Democritus

---

[93] See DK68 B219, where greater appetites, being insatiable, create greater lacks (μέζονες γὰρ ὀρέξεις μέζονας ἐνδείας ποιεῦσιν); B224. On the effect of bodily troubles on the soul, see also Thphr. *De sens.* 58 (DK68 A135). At X. *Mem.* 1.3.5, 1.5.3–5, 3.14.7, Socrates is alert to the psychophysical consequences of indulgence.

[94] See DK68 B182: τὰ δ' αἰσχρὰ ἄνευ πόνων αὐτόματα καρποῦται (shameful things bear fruit automatically without any labors).

[95] In fact, the transition in B191 between the description of unstable souls and Democritus's advice is marked by οὖν (therefore), indicating that one should not, for example, think about what others have precisely *because* it produces great movements. On the power of thoughts, see also DK68 B62; B68; B89 (all from "Democrates").

[96] See Plut. *Mor.* 682F–683A; cf. 734F–735C (DK68 A77), with J. Warren 2007a.

[97] DK68 B174: ὃς δ' ἂν καὶ δίκης ἀλογῇ καὶ τὰ χρὴ ἐόντα μὴ ἔρδῃ, τούτῳ πάντα τὰ τοιαῦτα ἀτερπείη, ὅταν τευ ἀναμνησθῇ, καὶ δέδοικε καὶ ἑωυτὸν κακίζει (Whoever disregards justice and does not do what should be done—for this man, all such things are a cause of unpleasure, whenever he thinks back to any of them, and he is afraid and reproaches himself). On fear, see also DK68 B199; B205–6; B215; B297, with Procopé 1989; 1990. See also B45 (from "Democrates"), where the wrongdoer's unhappiness is probably due to fear of retribution.

[98] See DK68 B209 (αὐταρκείη τροφῆς). See also B210; B246. Cf. X. *Mem.* 1.3.5.

makes a repeated call in the fragments for simple moderation.[99] Yet is this all there is to it? One problem we have seen is that no one intuitively knows what he needs or what is beneficial to him. Another is the power of desires to stir up escalating cycles of psychic distress that would seem to preclude the kinds of thinking crucial to reestablishing order. Democritus seems to have strategies to counteract both of these problems.

One of the difficulties presented by sensory pleasure is that it is not consistently or even regularly aligned with what is beneficial. Democritus is well aware of this problem. But he also recognizes another kind of pleasure, one that does correspond to what is beneficial for both the soul and the body. He frequently refers to this beneficial pleasure as *terpsis,* while reserving *hēdonē* for sensory pleasure.[100] In a famous fragment, *terpsis* allows us to recognize the beneficial: "The measure of what is suitable and what is not suitable is pleasure and unpleasure" (ὅρος συμφόρων καὶ ἀσυμφόρων τέρψις καὶ ἀτερπίη, B188; cf. B4). In claiming that measure can (retroactively) be discerned through a particular kind of pleasure and pain, Democritus, as Vlastos observed, adopts a position similar to that of the author of *On Ancient Medicine*, who emphasizes the *aisthēsis* of the body as the most important criterion in medicine.[101] Moreover, Democritus recognizes, again like the Hippocratic author, that natures both differ from one another and show variation under different circumstances (e.g., sickness and health). Thus, if someone wants to discover the *kairos,* the "right time and measure," for his needs and desires, he must be well acquainted with what is beneficial.[102] Part of the challenge of harmonizing one's own nature with the world is that, as in medicine, the very things that harm can also help. "Evils for people," for example, "grow out of good things, when someone does not know how to guide and keep them resourcefully" (ἀνθρώποισι κακὰ ἐξ ἀγαθῶν φύεται, ἐπὴν τις τἀγαθὰ μὴ 'πιστῆται ποδηγετεῖν μηδὲ ὀχεῖν εὐπόρως, B173). Or, as Democritus puts it in another fragment, though deep water may have benefits, one can also drown—hence, the invention of a "strategy," teaching people to swim (B172). The image of a boundary marker emphasizes the need to impose measure on the soul. The reference to teaching people to swim underscores the fact that people must impose measure on themselves, especially by becoming sensitive to the pleasure produced by what is beneficial. It is

---

[99] E.g., DK68 B3; B210; B219; B233.

[100] E.g., at DK68 B74, what is pleasant should also be beneficial. See J. Warren 2002.48–58, esp. 50. See also Farrar 1988.219–21; Annas 2002.176. Cf. C. Taylor 1967.17, contrasting *terpsis* as an ongoing state to *hēdonai* as ephemeral pleasures. B194 and B232, however, imply episodic *terpsis*. Nevertheless, the "objective good" interpretation of *terpsis* also has its difficulties: if *terpsis* is objectively good, it makes little sense to moderate it, as B191 advises (see J. Warren 2002.51); see also B223. Conversely, at B207, a *hēdonē* in what is fine is choiceworthy. J. Warren 2002.52 concludes that the vocabulary is not rigid enough to encompass all the evidence. But then Taylor's distinction may still be relevant.

[101] Vlastos 1945.586–87.

[102] On *kairos,* see DK68 B229, with Tortora 1983; J. Warren 2002.52–54. See also, more generally, Foucault 1985.57–59.

thus because human beings can "listen" to feedback from the soul that they have the potential to bridge the schism between what they need to flourish and what they desire.

Yet, if people could achieve psychic health simply by registering what feels good, it would be hard to know why they err. To understand this erring, we need to remember that there are two kinds of pleasure: competing with our feelings of the beneficial is the pleasure that we feel when we satisfy our appetites. Moderation itself can quiet this interference, because the less we indulge, the smaller our desires and our sensory pleasures become. But to break the cycle of indulgence, we also need to know how to think about our needs. Thoughts interact dynamically with the physical state of the soul, not only feeding desires but also keeping order. As we saw in B191, one ought to concentrate on what is possible and think about those with less. By thinking rightly, we can refrain from transgressing the limits of our natures, as well as the limits of society as a whole: as one fragment reads, one must "set up this law in the soul [τοῦτον νόμον τῇ ψυχῇ καθεστάναι], to do nothing unfitting" (B264).[103] In this context, what is unfitting appears less like something we discover through experience and more like something we avoid through knowledge and right thinking.

If thoughts can act, as it were, as drugs against potentially damaging desires in the soul, how should we imagine their force? Does right thinking or knowledge always trump desire? Or should we envision a struggle along the lines of those we see in the body, where the outcome is determined by what has more power at any given moment, or what prevails in a certain type of body? Democritus does use the language of being "stronger than pleasures" (ὁ τῶν ἡδονῶν κρείσσων, B214). But it is hazardous to hang too much weight on a phrase that, while plausibly informed by contemporary debates about the "law of the stronger," is too common to clarify how Democritus imagined the agonistic world of the soul, and our evidence is simply too sparse to know how—or even whether—Democritus developed a model of psychic struggle.[104] Nevertheless, these questions touch on an important problem: if wisdom or right thinking secures protection against desire, what secures wisdom? The fragments suggest two possible answers, each showing affinities with contemporary technical strategies of caring for the body.

First, Democritus occasionally uses the language of prophylaxis that is common in *On Regimen*. One must, for example, *ekhein phulakēn*, "be on guard," lest a stroke of good fortune impel one to start thinking *es to pleon*, "to the more," and attempt the impossible (B3). Until now, we have focused on the place

---

[103] Farrar 1988.241–42 sees Democritus as reconciling the *phusis-nomos* opposition here.

[104] Even in Plato, for whom we have far more evidence, the logistics of psychic struggle are ambiguous. Two basic problems recur. First, are desires beliefs or nonrational forces (and, the corollary, are they subject to persuasion or force)? Second, is reason strengthened by the acquisition of knowledge alone or must desires be tamed—either by some kind of bodily therapy or through therapy directed at the appetitive part of the soul—for reason to flourish? For some recent work on these problems, see Bobonich 1994; 2007; and the essays in Bobonich and Destrée 2007.

of things inside the person in Democritus's descriptions of psychic distress. Here, however, we can see that, much as in diseases of the body, these things can be stirred up by external factors, like unexpected success. One of the reasons that even good fortune can have a negative effect, it would seem, is that, by disrupting the soul's sense of the proper limits of pleasure, it causes desires and hopes to expand beyond what kind of future satisfaction one can reasonably expect. *Tukhē* may be a giver of great gifts, but it is unreliable; "nature, on the other hand, is autarchic" (φύσις δὲ αὐτάρκης, B176).[105] Yet, precisely because it is in the soul's nature to err in the absence of limits, self-sufficiency must be actively upheld, much as it is in dietetics. That is, if souls are to stay strong in the face of the impinging world and their own tendencies toward disorder, we must actively care for them by thinking rightly, for example, and acting with moderation.[106] Indeed, "more people become good from practice [ἐξ ἀσκήσιος]," Democritus claims, "than from nature [ἢ ἀπὸ φύσιος]" (B242).[107]

Given that our responses to *tukhē* are not simply natural but "up to us"—to borrow a phrase that becomes standard in Aristotle and the later philosophical tradition—they are open to ethical meaning. Whereas Gorgias uses chance to deny responsibility, Democritus sees it as mostly a mirage that disappears in the face of clear-sighted prudence, much as it does for the medical writers in the face of *tekhnē*.

> ἄνθρωποι τύχης εἴδωλον ἐπλάσαντο πρόφασιν ἰδίης ἀβουλίης. βαιὰ γὰρ φρονήσει
> τύχη μάχεται, τὰ δὲ πλεῖστα ἐν βίῳ εὐξύνετος ὀξυδερκείη κατιθύνει. (DK68 B119)
>
> People fashioned an image of fortune as an excuse for their own folly. For, in a few cases, fortune battles with prudence, but with most things in life intelligent clear-sightedness steers rightly.

Thus, even if thoughtlessness is initiated by the vagaries of fortune, the fact that we can resist the drive to desire "to the more" makes thoughtlessness something that must be owned. Whereas "the unwise are shaped by the gifts of fortune" (ἀνοήμονες ῥυσμοῦνται τοῖς τῆς τύχης κέρδεσιν), those who know are shaped by wisdom (B197).

The idea of being molded by knowledge, which has attracted considerable scholarly attention, occurs elsewhere in Democritus. In one of the most famous fragments, he declares: "Nature and teaching are similar; teaching reshapes a man, and in reshaping fashions his nature" (ἡ φύσις καὶ ἡ διδαχὴ παραπλήσιόν ἐστι. καὶ γὰρ ἡ διδαχὴ μεταρυσμοῖ τὸν ἄνθρωπον, μεταρυσμοῦσα δὲ φυσιοποιεῖ,

---

[105] See also DK68 B146: the sage is "accustomed to derive his joys from himself" (ἐξ ἑαυτοῦ), with Farrar 1988.230–35; J. Warren 2002.55–57. Recall the contrast in *On Places in a Human Being* between *tukhē*, which is self-ruled, and knowledge.

[106] See esp. Vlastos 1945.585; 1946.59–60.

[107] Conversely, "continuous association with the wicked increases a bad character" (φαύλων ὁμιλίη συνεχὴς ἕξιν κακίης συναύξει, DK68 B184). On *ponos* and *askēsis*, see also B157; B179; B182; B241–43.

B33). Vlastos is almost certainly right that the verbs *rhusmoō* and *metarhusmoō*, "to fashion," in B33 and B197 refer to the arrangement of the atoms in the soul.[108] These two fragments, then, bolster the idea that both mental acts and external influences dynamically interact with the soul *qua* physical thing. The nature-molding influence of teaching, however, is particularly interesting insofar as it resembles the practices of self-fashioning that we have seen: "learning accomplishes fine things through labors" (τὰ μὲν καλὰ χρήματα τοῖς πόνοις ἡ μάθησις ἐξεργάζεται), while bad things proliferate of their own accord (B182).[109] Whether we choose to pursue such learning seems to be up to us. Nevertheless, by stressing the role of teaching, Democritus reminds us that it can be difficult to develop an intuitive grasp of our nature, whether of the soul or the body, and the knowledge of how to care for it without being educated. Education may play a role analogous to right thinking, instilling the proper conditions for moderation before damaging cycles of desiring become entrenched—recall that immoderation is a bad teacher for the young because it breeds the pleasures that give rise to badness (B178).

Despite the state of the evidence, then, it is possible to discern in Democritus's fragments an understanding of psychic distress and wellness that recurs in various forms in later centuries. If we are to help ourselves through thought and action, he argues, we need to acquire and, indeed, to be physically transformed by knowledge of our nature, or at least practices that support that nature, rather than appealing to gods or trying to constrain daemonic agents. By failing to take care, we allow the stuffs and powers within us to be increasingly diverted toward suffering and self-destruction until we are conquered by vice. It is easy to lose sight of the basic assumptions of Democritus's account, given the lively debates that characterize the tradition of philosophical ethics in Greco-Roman antiquity. But if we do so, we fail to notice that this tradition develops out of a far-reaching reconceptualization of the ethical subject in the classical period, a reconceptualization that, I have argued, develops both in response to and in tandem with the emergence of the physical body. Let us briefly review the basic aspects of their relationship.

First, the physical body acts as a foil against which the person, understood as a social and ethical agent endowed with intentions, desires, emotions, and thoughts, comes into focus. It is true that as early as Theognis, *sōma* and *noos* can designate separate aspects of a person (frr. 649–50 W²). Nevertheless, as the body emerges as an object affected by both physical forces and technical manipulation, what is simply difference in Theognis becomes, in some late fifth-century thinkers, an electrified field within which *sōma* and *psukhē* are being reciprocally defined and opposed. One common strategy is to represent the

---

[108] Vlastos 1946.57 n.14. C.C.W. Taylor, initially skeptical, accepts this interpretation at 1999a.233.
[109] See also DK68 B180. For Vlastos, the power of the soul "to move itself in the 'subtler' inquiry of reason" (1946.57), which we might correlate with the emphasis on learning (*mathēsis, paideia*) in the fragments, distinguishes autarchic *phusis* from the self formed by chance; see also Tortora 1984.

sōma as the mere instrument of a soul or an ensouled subject who assumes responsibility for its use, as in Democritus B159 or Plato's *Alcibiades* I. Plato offers a striking portrayal of the *sōma* in just these terms in *Republic* 5, where Socrates mocks the warrior who would abuse the *sōma* of an enemy who has fluttered away, "leaving behind that with which he fought [ᾧ ἐπολέμει]." "Do you think," Socrates asks, "that people who do this are any different from dogs who get angry with the stones that strike them but leave the person throwing them alone?" (5, 469d7–e2). The warrior who violates the corpse in this instance is bestialized not because he denies the corpse burial and reduces it to "mute earth," like Achilles with Hector's body in the *Iliad*. Rather, he is dog-like because he makes a category mistake, confusing the thing, the body, with the agent.

Those writers who foreground the instrumentality of the physical body tend to act as though it is inert without the guiding soul. That body, however, can also be represented as an object on the basis of its participation in a world governed by nature and necessity, a world where actions and reactions are both predictable (and, hence, manageable) and uncannily alien to the emotions, desires, beliefs, and thoughts characteristic of ethical subjects. From this latter angle, the body is no longer simply a foil to the soul, its passivity clarifying psychic agency. Rather, insofar as it is understood as a physical object that can be known and manipulated, it provides a model for the thinkers interested in pinning down the soul as an object of knowledge and care. As these thinkers develop explanations of psychic health and suffering that do not rely on the gods as causal factors, the conceptual resources developed in contemporary medicine to explain health and disease become increasingly important. Foremost among these resources is the idea that the physical body harbors both vital tendencies and tendencies toward perversion and death, an idea that allows the disruptive, daemonic force of symptoms to be explained through stuffs and powers inside the body that we do not always understand and that often operate below the threshold of consciousness and thought. Transposed to the soul, such a model of disease comes to encompass our very faculties of sensation, perception, agency, cognition, and judgment.

By extending medicine's model of disease to the seat of ethical subjectivity, where goods like virtue and health are secured by intelligent agency, thinkers like Gorgias, Democritus, and Plato would appear to be undermining the very definition of the soul as an ethical agent by exposing it to forces that, like those in the body, are subject to chance and natural necessity.[110] In response to this threat, we can see practices of psychic care developing, practices that recognize the soul's very capacity for self-mastery as contingent on conditions that must be managed if they are to remain conducive to the flourishing of ethical agency.

Care of the soul, of course, does not cancel out the need for care of the body.[111] The two are often intertwined, whether a writer sees the soul as

---

[110] For concerns about vulnerability to chance within Greek ethics, see Nussbaum 2001.

[111] The intimacy of psychology and physiology, loosely structured along an analogy, explains why medicine never fully relinquishes therapeutic power over the ethical substance in classical antiquity

dependent on the condition of the body; whether he takes the care of the body to be one benefit of a healthy soul; or whether he sees the care of the body and the care of the soul as complementary.[112] In recent years, scholars have been exploring the close relationship between body and soul that we find even in a textbook dualist like Plato. In rediscovering their surprising intimacy, we may wonder whether dualist language is misleading. It is worth remembering, however, that the very idea of two entities to be related, body and soul, of which one is somehow *not quite you*, reflects changes to how a human being—and, more specifically, an ethical subject—is being conceptualized in the fifth and fourth centuries. These changes can be understood only if we stop treating "the" body as a timeless physical object that is simply "other" than the person and recognize that the emergence of the physical body changes how otherness, once equated with gods and *daimones*, is understood. Moreover, though most closely associated with the body, this otherness is also infecting the terrain of the person or the soul, *even as the person-soul continues to be defined against the body*.

Explanations of human nature and human suffering organized around the physical body thus enter the cultural imagination not only in their specific details—bile and phlegm, for example, or the importance of diet—but also as a bundle of conceptual and imaginative resources that must be understood more broadly. In this broader sense, the physical body becomes relevant to representations of disease in tragedy, and particularly in Euripides. Euripides, of course, does not forgo daemonic agency. Rather, symptoms, because they point to hidden worlds without revealing them, allow him to explore the implications of both traditional and novel ways of explaining suffering. In tragedy, we discover the most searching interrogations of what it *means* to interpret symptoms in terms of a daemonic space inside the self.

---

and why those who do advocate therapies of the soul continue to draw on medicine: Galen, for example, wrote treatises like "The Soul's Dependence on the Body" (Kühn 4.767–822) and "The Affections and Errors of the Soul" (Kühn 5.1–103).

[112] On the complementary care of body and soul, see, e.g., Antisth. fr. 163 (Giannantoni); X. *Mem.* 1.3.5.

CHAPTER SIX

Forces of Nature, Acts of Gods: Euripides' Symptoms

THE STORY OF GALATEA in Ovid's *Metamorphoses* moves from cold ivory to a sentient, acculturated Roman woman. Helen's story in Gorgias's *Encomium* travels in the opposite direction: she sees Paris, and all her plans—indeed, her very capacity to think—are driven from her soul; she becomes putty in his hands. In view of the fact that the chain reaction triggered in Helen by the sight of Paris and his persuasive words is governed by necessity and the law of the stronger, Gorgias argues, she is entirely passive and, hence, cannot be blamed.

In Euripides' *Troades*, we again encounter the question of Helen's guilt. This time, however, we are dealing not with a *paignion*, "game," as Gorgias describes his speech, but with an *agōn*, a "contest," to determine whether she will live or die.[1] The *agōn*, in which characters engage in a debate thick with the language and the tactics of the lawcourt and other arenas of public argument, is a distinctive feature of tragedy. In the *Troades*, it allows Euripides to take two scenarios that Gorgias conflates in his speech—one where the gods are responsible, another where beauty and seductive speech are blamed—and pit them against one another. Helen, speaking in her own defense, focuses on the role of the gods in her fate, beginning with Aphrodite's decision to pledge her as the prize in the Judgment of Paris and ending with Paris's arrival at Sparta "with no small goddess at his side" (*Tro.* 940–41).[2] Hecuba, her opponent, has no patience for such explanations. She discredits Helen's alleged motivation for the Judgment of Paris (971–81) before arguing that the gods do not dirty their hands with the stupidity of mortals (981–82).[3] After contesting Helen's claim to be a victim of Zeus's plans and mocking the idea that gods whisk mortals away in clouds, she plays these two models of daemonic agency against one another: "Could [Aphrodite] not have stayed quietly in heaven and led you and all of Amyclae to Ilium?" (985–86).

In her own account of Helen's crime, Hecuba foregrounds the power of vision. The moment you saw Paris, she tells her daughter-in-law, "your mind was

---

[1] Gorgias's *Helen* probably dates to the last quarter of the fifth century: see Basta Donzelli 1985.402–4; Orsini 1956; Donadi 1978.76 (positing a very late [405 BCE] date). Because we cannot date the speech precisely, it is impossible to determine if Gorgias influenced Euripides or vice versa. Helen's guilt, in any event, seems to have been a popular topic of debate. See Adkins 1960.124–27; Croally 1994.155–56; Worman 2002.123–35, all reading *Troades* against the backdrop of Gorgias's *Encomium*.

[2] On Helen's line of argument, see de Romilly 1976.318–19; Croally 1994.138–45. Pasiphae offers a similar "sophistic" defense at E. fr. 472eK (= *Cretans* fr. 5 J.-V.L.): see Rivier 1958; Reckford 1974.319–22.

[3] See also E. frr. 254K (= *Archelaus* fr. 23 J.-V.L.), 1078K.

made Kupris" (ὁ σὸς δ᾽ ἰδών νιν νοῦς ἐποιήθη Κύπρις, 988); seeing the brilliance of his beautiful clothing, "you went mad" (ἐξεμαργώθης φρένας, 992). Hecuba's focus on seeing reflects the close association between *erōs* and the eyes already evident in archaic poetry.[4] By presenting seeing in terms of its consequences for the mind, she may also be cuing contemporary speculation about the mechanics of desire as a kind of "human disease," to adopt Gorgias's phrasing. Indeed, she dismisses Aphrodite as a name that mortals wrongly give to their own *aphrosunē*, "folly" (989–90). Because that folly belongs to them, she holds, much as Democritus does, they ought to be held responsible for it. In this case, that means that Helen should be put to death as the cause of the Trojan War.

The exchange between Helen and Hecuba offers a fascinating perspective on the question raised in the previous chapter: why do we err? Before the tragedy's spectators stand indisputable facts: Paris came to Sparta; Helen fled to Troy; catastrophe followed. These facts give rise to two competing stories: one in which a god is held responsible, releasing the victim from blame; another in which the goddess Aphrodite is replaced by folly. It is true that the latter story still represents Helen as passive: your mind, Hecuba says to her, *was made* (ἐποιήθη) Kupris.[5] But, although Hecuba seems confident that her account secures Helen's responsibility, she does not spell out the grounds for blame. Blame may come to rest on Helen simply because the gods are absent as masterminds. Or it may be that Helen is to blame for being overpowered not by outside forces but by her own desires. In any event, the contest neatly severs "double determination" into competing accounts of culpability.[6]

In this chapter, I argue that tragic symptoms, a category comprising both phenomena *and* acts blamed on daemonic forces, behave very much like Helen's crime in the *Troades*.[7] First, like that crime, they attract different types of explanations that, implicitly or explicitly, compete against each other. It is because symptoms support such different explanations that they so effectively straddle medical and magico-religious paradigms in tragedy. Of all the genres we have explored, tragedy most thoroughly realizes the potential of the symptom to generate meaning, rather than simply revealing "facts." Erupting on the tragic

[4] Spatharas 2002 uses this association to exclude claims that Euripides is influenced by contemporary theories of vision: on *erōs* and vision in early poetry, see Pearson 1909; Calame 1999.20–21. On the importance of vision and desire more generally in the *agōn*, see Worman 2002.125–35.

[5] Once Helen is in Troy, however, Hecuba seems confident about introducing her as the subject of wanting and following fortune (1008–9, 1021). On this aspect of Helen's hedonism, see Croally 1994.150–52.

[6] On the *agōn*, see Croally 1994.134–62; Worman 1997.180–97. The *agōn* by its nature is suited to producing clear-cut positions on cause and blame: see, e.g., S. *El.* 566–76. But Euripides seems to exploit it as a way of polarizing questions of mortal and immortal responsibility (M. Lloyd 1992.15–18). On double determination, see above, chapter 1, n.119.

[7] There are, of course, important differences between phenomena like rolling eyes or foam at the mouth and acts. Yet they also exist on a continuum of effects provoked by the encounter between the person and daemonic force. See below, n.54, on active and passive diseases.

stage, symptoms allow the implications of different worldviews to be probed and the limits to different explanations of suffering exposed. I close this study by looking at tragedy because, unlike a magico-religious explanation or a medical treatise or an ethical text, tragedy is capable of engaging not only the conceptual but also the moral complexity of what it means to be a subject of the symptom in the late fifth century.

Second, the contest between Helen and Hecuba reminds us that tragedy as a genre was committed to the problem of responsibility in a world uncertain about ethical agency. In the formulation of Vernant:

> For there to be tragic action it is necessary that a concept of human nature with its own characteristics should have already emerged and that the human and divine spheres should have become sufficiently distinct from each other for them to stand in opposition; yet at the same time they must continue to appear as inseparable. The tragic sense of responsibility makes its appearance at the point when, in human action, a place is given to internal debate on the part of the subject, to intention and pre-meditation, but when this human action has still not acquired enough consistency and autonomy to be entirely self-sufficient.[8]

These concerns about autonomy, however, are articulated not only vis-à-vis an externalized divine but also vis-à-vis forces within the tragic subject. One way a tragedian could represent the hero's ambiguous relationship to the divine-daemonic plane was to explore varying interpretations of the symptom. These interpretations often differ with respect to the weight they assign to internal and external factors, with a greater focus on internal factors tending to correspond to the fading of the gods as agents, if not their elimination altogether, as in the *Troades*. In making this observation, I am not denying that from Homer to Euripides and beyond, the gods work through the innermost part of the person. Nor am I claiming that when tragedy does focus on internal factors, these factors are necessarily "medical" or physical. I am suggesting, rather, that medicine was particularly relevant to tragedy because it was developing conceptual and imaginative resources to describe struggles for power in the inner recesses of a human being. "Tragedy," writes Williams, "is formed round ideas it does not expound, and to understand its history is in some part to understand those ideas and their place in the society that produced it."[9] The function of those ideas, Vernant observes, "once they are taken out of their technical context . . . to some extent changes."[10] Having vested daemonic power in the physical body, medicine does not determine tragedy's representation of disease, but, rather,

---

[8] Vernant 1988a.46–47.

[9] Williams 1993.15.

[10] Vernant 1988a.32, speaking about the influence of contemporary legal theory and practice on tragedy. He goes on: "In the hands of the tragic writers, intermingled with and opposed to other terms, [sc. these ideas] become elements in a general clash of values and in a reappraisal of all norms that are part of an inquiry that is no longer concerned with the law but is focused upon man himself."

enriches its resources for representing the conundrum of responsibility while also complicating that conundrum.

In exploring the influence of medicine, and more specifically the physical body, on tragedy, I have chosen to focus on several works by Euripides. Of the three tragedians, Euripides is widely recognized to have been most engaged with contemporary intellectual developments.[11] He is also arguably the tragedian most intrigued by the shadowy regions of the daemonic.[12] On both these issues, however, scholars have been historically polarized, casting Euripides as both an iconoclast deeply sympathetic to the sophists and a staunch traditionalist.[13] Nowhere has this polarization been more pronounced than in discussions of how he represents the gods.[14] Many scholars have speculated that the playwright himself adhered to the heterodox ideas about the gods sometimes advanced by his characters, pointing to how he appears in the comedies of his contemporary Aristophanes.[15] Others have vigorously contested Euripides' alleged atheism.[16] It is true that in recent years many critics have tried to develop a more nuanced approach to Euripides' gods by distinguishing between authorial belief, thematic motifs across a literary œuvre, and the views of individual characters.[17] Prevailing trends in literary criticism have also made scholars more tolerant of ambiguity and open-endedness.[18] Nevertheless, it is still often assumed that the plays ultimately endorse a theological vision that can be attributed to the playwright, an assumption particularly prevalent in work on medical influence. While usually accepting Euripides' interest in contemporary medicine, scholars remain wary of making claims about causality that would marginalize the gods' power in his plays.[19]

---

[11] On Euripides and the sophists, see Reinhardt 1957; Winnington-Ingram 1969; Kerferd 1981. 169–72; Diggle 1999; Allan 1999–2000; 2005a; Assaël 2001.

[12] See [Long.] De subl. 15.3 (Euripides is particularly interested in love and madness) and Rivier 1960.

[13] See esp. Michelini 1987.3–51 on polarization in Euripidean scholarship.

[14] See Schlesier 1983 and 1985 on modern debates about Euripides' gods.

[15] See Ar. Th. 14–15 (Euripides spins cosmogonies around Ether), 450–51 (a wreathseller laments that Euripides has persuaded men that the gods do not exist); Ra. 888–93 (the playwright is shown praying to gods like the "pivot of the tongue" or sunesis, "comprehension").

[16] E.g., Lloyd-Jones 1983.151–55; Burnett 1985; Lefkowitz 1987; 1989; Yunis 1988; Mikalson 1991, esp. 225–36; Sourvinou-Inwood 2003.291–300.

[17] Wildberg 1999–2000.238, for example, asks, "What do the tragedies tell us about religious concepts and preconceptions which the authorial character seems to employ in his dramatic plot?"

[18] E.g., Easterling 1993, arguing that the gods foster multiple perspectives; Dunn 1996.

[19] See, e.g., Papadopoulou 2005.59: "As a general rule, medical works substituted natural causes for divine causation in any type of bodily or mental disorder. Greek tragedy, on the contrary, is a literary genre that dramatizes myths; it may indeed be enriched by the vocabulary of ancient medicine, it may even at times seem, especially in the case of Euripides, to present its audience with almost clinical cases of madness, yet it retains the notion of divine causation of madness as established in literary tradition from Homer onwards." See also the classification of medical influence outlined at Jouanna 1987.120 (terminology, representation or description of pathological cases, allusions to

Strong presuppositions about Euripides' theology have, unsurprisingly, influenced how his tragedies are read. Scholars trying to demonstrate Euripides' piety often bracket large swathes of his plays as extradramatic or irrelevant to the theological vision of the work.[20] The idea of such a vision is predicated on the belief that the plays offer a final word on cause and culpability, often in the form of a *deus ex machina*.[21] But, in many cases, no such final word can be assumed. A tragedy like the *Orestes* seems to mock the very convention of the *deus ex machina* capable of restoring order and meaning. In the *Heracles*, epiphany is "used up" prematurely without clarifying matters for either the internal audience or, arguably, the external one. At the same time, the opposite approach, which treats Euripides' gods as flagrant fictions in the service of an enlightened theology, is no more satisfactory.[22] Euripides, as his most perceptive critics have observed, is not a philosopher. If, however, "philosophy and science can only begin when a set of questions is substituted for a set of vaguely assumed certainties,"[23] he is one of our most valuable witnesses to the ways in which the emergence of the physical body could transform conventional narratives about suffering. In that capacity, he shows us the ethical crisis that is created when disease is decoupled from daemonic agents. By using the symptom as a magnet for different worldviews, a node where narratives of disease clash and cross-pollinate, Euripides makes it a privileged tool in his dramatization of questions about otherness, the self, and the meaning of suffering.[24]

In this chapter, I defend my approach against other ways of interpreting tragic symptoms vis-à-vis contemporary medicine and then illustrate this approach in short readings of three plays where the problem of disease figures prominently: *Hippolytus*, *Heracles*, and *Orestes*. In developing these readings, I have been aware of the challenges inherent in trying both to prove the influence of medicine and to gauge its importance. Scholars of Greek tragedy sometimes seem to

---

medical theories), adopted by Guardasole 2000. But cf. W. Smith 1967, on the *Orestes*: "Medical concepts are useful vehicles for [Euripides'] thought and expression not only because they offer a controlled description of the mechanism of mental aberration, but also because they deal in complex processes of reaction and compensation which cause both health and disease" (306).

[20] Choral laments are sometimes dismissed on the grounds that they do not drive the action of the play (e.g., Wildberg 1999–2000.241). Fragments are also often viewed as inadmissible evidence for understanding Euripides' approach to the gods because they appear out of context: see, e.g., Yunis 1988.94; Mikalson 1991.5–8. These strategies of interpretation assume that skepticism about the gods is introduced only to be superseded, ignored, or dismissed (e.g., "any character in Euripides who expresses 'philosophical' notions about the gods does so out of desperation," Lefkowitz 1989.72). Yet trust in myths can be seen as just as much of an emotional response or character-revealing trait as skepticism. What matters are the kinds of questions that Euripides introduces.

[21] "Ultimately, the gods in that play will prove—not always to the characters' satisfaction—that the gods still retain their traditional powers" (Lefkowitz 1989.72).

[22] See, e.g., Verrall 1905; Greenwood 1953; Conacher 1967.

[23] G. Lloyd 1979.266. On Euripides' capacity to raise questions about cause and suffering, see also Ciani 1974.92; Ferrini 1978.60; Schlesier 1985.14–16, 34; Kosak 2004.

[24] Classic midcentury readings of this friction are Reinhardt 1957; Arrowsmith 1963. See, more recently, Pucci 2005.

view claims of medical influence as threatening the sanctity of religion or adulterating the spirit of tragedy. That fear may be assuaged by Gillian Beer's incisive reflections on the imaginative repercussions of evolutionary narrative in the nineteenth century:

> The acquired cultural language of science, like that of neo-classical allusion, offers a controlled range of imaginative consequences shared by writer and first readers. It offers an imaginative shift in the valency of words, new spaces for experience to occupy in language, confirmation of some kinds of vocabulary, increased prowess of punning, in which diverse senses are held in equipoise within the surveillance of consciousness. These effects register a moment when a particular discourse has reached its fullest range. It can then suggest new bearings for experiences which had earlier seemed quite separate from each other. At such moments of transposition emotion can find its full extent in language.[25]

It is always a challenge for a reading, which is inherently impoverished with regard to its parent text, to capture the full range of a particular discourse. This is even truer when we are dealing with a culture about which we still know far too little and a genre that was meant to be performed. Nevertheless, in the end what matters is whether a reading remains faithful to the text's complexity without resorting to empty appeals to indeterminacy. If, then, the symptom invites and sustains different interpretive frameworks, we need to try to understand how these differences make dramatic sense. Although I do not have the space to develop extensive readings, I hope to make a case that both our appreciation of Euripidean tragedy and our understanding of the physical body's emergence can be deepened by reading them in light of each other.

THE POLYSEMY OF THE SYMPTOM

Scholars have long been trying to map the contact between tragedy and contemporary medical explanations of disease.[26] In considering this contact in Aeschylus, who worked in the early and middle decades of the fifth century, we must contend with the problem that we lack secure evidence of medical writing before about 440 or 430 BCE, though the inquiry into nature and the biological inquiries associated with it date from the sixth century.[27] While concerns about dating the rise of naturalizing medicine become less pressing when we look at the later plays of Sophocles, Sophocles' relationship to the new medicine remains

---

[25] Beer 2000.140–41. Contrast Willink 1986.xxvi, arguing that sophistic and medical language and ideas in the *Orestes* constitute merely an "aesthetic" addition to "essentially mythical dramas."

[26] Medical influence on comedy has also been explored (H. Miller 1945; Byl 1990), although, given the relative absence of theological difficulties, the stakes are not as high.

[27] On Aeschylus, see Jouanna 1987.123–24; Guardasole 2000.40–58, 160–76 (Guardasole's work supersedes the problematic Dumortier 1935); Craik 2001a.82.

controversial.[28] When we come to Euripides, however, we are on more stable ground. His interest in contemporary medicine was already recognized in antiquity and remains generally accepted today.[29] Technical terms frequently appear in his plays,[30] for example, and his characters regularly voice opinions about health and healing in the idiom of physicians and trainers.[31]

Inquiries into the relationship between tragedy and medicine, and particularly between Euripides and medicine, have often converged on the symptom.[32] Heracles' symptoms in Euripides' eponymous play, for example, have been read in light of contemporary medical descriptions of disease, particularly the portrait of the epileptic in *On the Sacred Disease*: both texts refer to rolling eyes, foam at the mouth, and irregular breathing.[33] Yet the practice of using symptoms to prove the influence of contemporary medicine on the *Heracles* or on any other tragedy has not gone unchallenged, and there are, indeed, difficulties involved in this approach.

[28] According to the *Vita*, Sophocles was a priest of Asclepius, and a paean to the healing god is credited to him (S. fr. 737 *PMG*); see Guardasole 2000.58–62. On his familiarity with Hippocratic writing, opinions range: see Psichari 1908.98–99, 108–13; Nestle 1938.23–24; Collinge 1962; Curiazi 1997–2000; Guardasole 2000.58–76, 107–15, 176–92; Ceschi 2003; Craik 2003.

[29] See esp. E. frr. 282K (= *Autolycus* fr. 1 J.-V.L.), 286bK (= *Bellerophon* fr. 9 J.-V.L.), 682K (= *Scyrians* fr. 2 J.-V.L.), 981K, 1072K, 1086K. On the basis of fr. 917K, which Clement of Alexandria pairs with *Aph.* I.2 (Li 4.458 = 98 Jones), Nestle asserts that Euripides had read *Airs, Waters, Places* (1938.24–27). Few scholars have been so bold, but they have repeatedly noted affinities between Euripides and the medical writers. See Musitelli 1968; Mattes 1970.8, 76; Pigeaud 1976; 2006.376–439; Ferrini 1978; Jouanna 1987.124–26; Garzya 1992.511–12; Guardasole 2000.76–86, 192–230; Craik 2001a; Kosak 2004. Cf. Collinge 1962.45, 49: Euripides is an "outsider" who does not seem "instinctively medical" (although Collinge recognizes his familiarity with medical culture).

[30] Craik 2001a.92–94. Words are usually called medical if they appear in the corpus. Yet vocabulary shared by medicine and tragedy may be drawn from a common Ionic stock (Jouanna and Demont 1981; Jouanna 1987.124), and it can be difficult to determine how technical a word would have seemed to a fifth-century audience. See the methodological remarks at Collinge 1962; Guardasole 2000.29–30; Craik 2001a.83–86, 89–90. See also Langslow 1999 on medical language in Latin poetry.

[31] See citations in n.29.

[32] Harries 1891; Psichari 1908, esp. 120–28 on *Philoctetes*; Baumann-Oosterbeek 1932.309–10 on *Prometheus Bound*; Dumortier 1935.69–83 on Aeschylus; Nestle 1938.27; Musitelli 1968 on the *Bacchae* (esp. 97–99, 113); Ferrini 1978; Garzya 1992 on the *Orestes*; Barra 1993 on the *Agamemnon*; Guardasole 2000.159–251; Ceschi 2003 on the *Trachiniae*. See also Vasquez 1972.433–46, exploring how pathological conditions that are described in medical texts influence the portrayal of tragic symptoms. Other scholars have used tragic symptoms to generate diagnoses in modern clinical terms, e.g., Baumann-Oosterbeek 1932.310–12; Collinge 1962.48–52; Gourevitch and Gourevitch 1979. For arguments against retrospective diagnosis: Starobinski 1974.16–18; Padel 1981.117–18; 1995.229–32.

[33] See Harries 1891.19; O'Brien-Moore 1924.126–29; Ferrini 1978.51–52; Guardasole 2000.198–201. Cf. the cautionary remarks in Jouanna 1987.121–23; von Staden 1992d.138–40. Pigeaud 1987.38 notes the parallels between Heracles' symptoms and those in *Int.* 48 (Li 7.284–88 = 230–36 Potter). Some authors have argued that medical symptoms are influenced by literature: Lanata 1968; Mauri 1990.51–53. For the impact of tragedy on later literary and nonliterary representations of madness, see Klibansky, Panofsky, and Saxl 1964.15–16; Padel 1981.115.

One problem is that Heracles' symptoms, for example, are much like those of other tragic characters under duress.[34] Clytemnestra speaks of Cassandra foaming with rage and confusion like a wild animal (A. *Ag.* 1064–67); Io is driven offstage by a sudden attack of madness, her eyes twisting in their sockets (A. *Pr.* 877–86). Rolling eyes appear as early as the *Iliad*, when Apollo strikes a blow to Patroclus (16.792), suggesting a long literary tradition of signs of daemonic attack. In tragedy, however, these symptoms take on particular importance. Tragic plots often turn on manifestations of unseen, divine power, which is spectacularly realized by symptoms in dramatic space. Moreover, because the audience of a tragedy lacks an omniscient narrator (with the exception of the *deus ex machina*), the genre necessarily develops resources to communicate characters' inner struggles onstage.[35] The "new music" that becomes popular toward the end of the century, in part through Euripidean drama, appears to have been particularly well suited to expressing pathos.[36] Meter could mark off scenes of suffering, which often exhibited a lyric core surrounded by "framing scenes."[37] We know little about tragic gestures, but they undoubtedly helped to communicate pain and distress, as did masks.[38] Symptoms belong among these resources. Though characters may describe symptoms that erupt offstage—in the *Heracles*, Lussa enumerates the effects of her madness as she provokes them— more often tragedians use symptoms in combination with other dramatic conventions to help the audience understand what it is "witnessing" onstage. Just as tragedy recognizes "a topography of the body . . . structured around the places of death,"[39] it recognizes a topography of the body structured around the sites that manifest daemonic attack. Given both the symptom's organic relationship to what tragedy aims to express and the venerable tradition of poetic symptoms, it seems too simple to refer tragic symptoms to medical texts.

Against claims of medical influence at the level of symptoms, one might argue further that, unlike theories about cause, symptoms are there for anyone

---

[34] On the literary tradition behind tragic symptoms, which comes to include tragedy's own conventions, see Mattes 1970.74–92; Vasquez 1972.411–15; Ciani 1974.79, 107; Jouanna 1987.121; von Staden 1992d.139–40.

[35] See esp. the comprehensive study of Vasquez 1972 on the tragic conventions of suffering. Ciani 1974, on madness, is more restricted.

[36] On Euripides' prominent role in the New Music, see Csapo 1999–2000, esp. 414, 424–26 on its expression of emotional crisis.

[37] Vasquez 1972.68–103 on the scene structure; on meter, see 105–11, 476–88. See also Moreau 1989.106–7; Padel 1995.139–40.

[38] On gesture, see Pickard-Cambridge 1968.171–76. Padel draws a comparison with Noh drama (1981.107; 1995.140). On dance in tragedy: Kitto 1955; Vasquez 1972.191–96; J. F. Davidson 1986; Golder 1996; Henrichs 1996. Masks, at least in the Hellenistic period, could communicate illness, such as by depicting a sallow skin color (Pollux 4.135, 137). Pickard-Cambridge speculates that Orestes may have worn the mask identified as *pinaros* in Pollux (1968.192; see, too, Donadi 1974.113–14). McDermott 2000.248–49, following a suggestion from Marilyn Skinner, indicates that the reference to the cloud on Phaedra's brow at *Hipp.* 172 may refer to her mask.

[39] Loraux 1987.49.

to see and to describe.[40] Euripides, on this view, was an unusually gifted observer of pathological conditions. It is possible to counter that what gets noticed is what one is looking for: medicine may have codified a way of looking at the body that is then used to present tragic disease. But because tragedians tend to focus on the most spectacular symptoms, rather than on, say, symptoms that signal a crisis in the *Epidemics*, this argument can be taken only so far. Moreover, if we can identify habits of seeing, such as heightened attention to the eyes as sites of meaning, these habits are likely due to the cultural context shared by the poet and the medical writers.

In fact, this shared context poses the most powerful challenge to narrow characterizations of Euripides as an adept of contemporary medicine or a strict realist or a traditional poet. Critics who look to the treatise *On the Sacred Disease* as a model for tragic symptoms often fail to note that the very symptoms identified as Hippocratic are targeted by competing explanations in that text. We can recall that when symptoms like bellowing or frothing at the mouth are first introduced, the author correlates them with what his *opponents*, that is, the magico-religious healers who place blame on "the divine and the daemonic," say about them: if a patient leaps up out of bed, Hecate or the heroes are attacking; if he foams at the mouth and kicks, Ares is to blame, and so on.[41] The diverse symptoms, which are taken for granted as part of a common vocabulary, are easily accommodated to a polytheistic etiology. The Hippocratic author later systematically repeats these symptoms in order to supply his own phlegm-based explanation to each of them.[42] That repetition suggests he is not innovating in his identification of symptoms but appropriating a shared set of signs for his own explanatory system.

What the evidence from *On the Sacred Disease* indicates is that symptoms, particularly theatrical ones, have become *contested sites of interpretation* in the latter part of the fifth century. In the historians, too, we witness proliferating explanations for the symptom. Herodotus, for example, attributes Cambyses' madness *either* to his treatment of Apis *or* to any of the evils that overtake humans (εἴτε δὴ διὰ τὸν Ἄπιν εἴτε καὶ ἄλλως, οἷα πολλὰ ἔωθε ἀνθρώπους κακὰ καταλαμβάνειν, 3.33).[43] According to some people, Cambyses had suffered from birth a serious disease "which some people call sacred" (τὴν ἱρὴν ὀνομάζουσί τινες), an explanation Herodotus finds plausible: "And there is nothing strange in the fact that, his body suffering a serious disease, his *phrenes* should not be healthy" (οὐ νύν τοι ἀεικὲς οὐδὲν ἦν τοῦ σώματος νοῦσον μεγάλην νοσέοντος

---

[40] Blaiklock 1952.125–26; Mattes 1970.60–61, 83–84. Attention to the body in tragedy is regularly deemed "realist": see, e.g., de Romilly 1958.19; Musitelli 1968.93; Mattes 1970.91; Ferrini 1978.53; Jouanna 1987.121; Guardasole 2000.31, 162, 175–76, 193.

[41] See above, p. 55.

[42] *Morb. Sacr.* 7 (Li 6.372–74 = 14,21–16,23 Jouanna).

[43] See, too, Hdt. 6.84 on the madness of Cleomenes, who is either punished for sacrilege or suffers the effects of drinking too much unmixed wine. For Herodotus's interaction with fifth-century medical culture, see Lateiner 1986; Thomas 2000, esp. 28–74, 34–35 on Cambyses.

μηδὲ τὰς φρένας ὑγιαίνειν). The *sōma* acts here as a counterweight to divine vengeance (though Herodotus still uses the idea of godsent retribution when it suits him).[44] Over the course of the fifth century, then, tragedy's use of symptoms to stage encounters between gods and humans increasingly dovetails with a lively public debate about how symptoms should be interpreted and the nature of the world that produces them.[45] When the same symptoms participate in competing stories, it is likely that one story can be screened behind or challenge another.

Looking to symptoms in tragedy, we can see that they regularly occasion questions without confirming answers.[46] The Chorus of Sophocles' *Ajax*, for example, responds to the news of his mad rampage by asking which of the gods is responsible: "Can it have been wild, bull-consorting Artemis . . . that stirred you . . . to move against the flocks? . . . Or was it Enualios, the bronze-cased Lord of War?" (172–81). In the *Medea*, Glauke's nurse first responds to the sight of her mistress going pale and collapsing into a chair by raising a ritual cry. The messenger infers that she believes that the sudden attack was caused by a frenzy sent by Pan.[47] Yet, as soon as the nurse sees the rolling eyes and the foaming mouth—prime tragic symptoms of disaster—she realizes that matters are serious and gives up the ritual cry for a shout of terror (1171–77). In the *Hippolytus*, the Chorus, speculating on Phaedra's symptoms, entertains not only different gods as causes but also jealousy, sorrow, and pregnancy, the last-named cause expressive of the female body's "unstable" or "ill-fitted" mixture (141–69; cf. 237–38). In the *Orestes*, the title character gives a series of answers to Menelaus's question, "What sickness assails you?": *sunesis*, which means something like "conscience"; *lupē*, "grief" or "sorrow"; and the Furies of his mother's blood (396–400). Note that in these last two tragedies, the gods are joined as causes by emotions, knowledge, and the nature of the (female) body.

Euripides deliberately and regularly exaggerates uncertainty about which story to attach to symptoms. He blurs the boundaries around conventional disease scenes, which, in isolating the attack of disease, usually associate it with the

---

[44] Magic is also coming to occupy a crucial place in the public sphere in this period, as Graf 1997 argues. In the *Hippolytus* and the *Trachiniae*, the logic of the magical *pharmakon* figures prominently in the circulation of harm (Faraone 1994; Fountoulakis 1999).

[45] We can also assume that in this period some medical explanations are becoming accepted in day-to-day life: see, e.g., E. fr. 682K (*Scyrians* fr. 2 J.-V.L.), dating from a play probably performed between 445 and 435 BCE: an attendant tells the king that his daughter is sick and dying, to which the king replies, "What's the matter? . . . Is a chill of bile affecting her lungs?" On the relationship between bile and pleurisy in the medical writers, see Guardasole 2000.231–32. S. fr. 507R speaks of a quotidian fever, as well as a tertian fever, which brings a chill to the jaws. On these fevers in the medical writers, see Guardasole 2000.232–34.

[46] See Mikalson 1991.17–29; Mastronarde 2002.34–42, on the difficulties of inferring divine presence in tragedy. On the range of causes in tragedy, see Kosak 2004.1–2, 93–99.

[47] On Pan, see above, chapter 1, n.45. Borgeaud 1988.107 believes that Pan's agency could probably have been identified through "visible signs and unambiguous symptoms," but this passage and that from the *Hippolytus* suggest more potential for ambiguity.

gods. Characters often voice competing explanations of events, which are then undercut by other sources of meaning. If people know stories about the gods, they anxiously wonder whether they are true.[48] Of course, the purposes and the actions of the gods are always opaque in tragedy. The plays of Aeschylus and Sophocles, however, seem based on the assumption that screened behind suffering there is some divine truth, some deep reserve of meaning. For example, Aeschylus's characters, as Jacqueline de Romilly and others have observed, often describe, with startling concreteness, vague feelings of fear and foreboding that travel like fluxes in the cavity, lacerating and attacking the innards.[49] Even if these fears are imprecise, they appear to be stirred by the gods. Or consider that, at the end of the *Trachiniae*, Heracles' suffering turns out to have been foretold by oracles sent by his father Zeus (1159–71), while *Oedipus Rex* closes with the promise that Oedipus is destined for great things (1455–57), a promise fulfilled decades later in the *Oedipus at Colonus*.[50] But, in Euripides' plays, the symptom is unmoored from the gods. That is not to say these plays eliminate the gods, but, rather, that they cultivate uncertainty about divine agency, thereby opening up space to explore other possibilities, as in Phaedra's Great Speech about the pursuit of the good in the *Hippolytus* or in the last scene of the *Heracles*.[51]

Even in cases where *we* know very well which of the gods has acted, Euripides' multiple explanations make us aware of the risk of insufficiency within the common conceptualization of tragic irony, that is, the idea that the audience knows what the characters do not. It may turn out that one answer *is not enough.* The "right" answer may be recoded by one of the "wrong" ones. The version of the female body advanced by the Chorus in the *Hippolytus* parodos, for example, troubles the thematization of *erōs* as godsent and extrinsic.[52] In the *Orestes*, each of Orestes' self-diagnoses remains viable for the length of the play, despite appearing to reference different interpretive frameworks. Characters take on necessity not only in the form of a god's will or daemonic wrath but *qua phusis*.[53] In Euripides, then, symptoms are not citations of specific Hippocratic texts

---

[48] E. *El.* 737–45, cited above in chapter 2. On myths as the writings and songs of the ancients, see *Hipp.* 451–52; see also the remarks about "metamythology" at M. Wright 2006.37–39.

[49] De Romilly 1958. See also Webster 1957.152–53; Maloney 1983.74–75. Flux: A. *Ch.* 183–84; *Eu.* 832. Laceration: *Ag.* 791; *Pers.* 115–16. See also *Ag.* 1121–23, with Guardasole 2000.118–30. On the relationship of innards to prophecy, see Padel 1992.12–18, 68–75; on their relationship to the divine, 114–37.

[50] The involvement of the gods in Sophocles does not imply that the hero himself is not implicated in his disease. See Biggs 1966 on disease and character in the *Trachiniae*, *Ajax*, and *Philoctetes*; on *Ajax*, Starobinski 1974. Cf. Padel 1995.242–44.

[51] Contrast Lloyd-Jones 1983.146 ("the inscrutability of the divine purpose is an ancient commonplace of Greek religion, whose content is not altered by describing it in modern terms").

[52] See Zeitlin 1996.237. See also Reckford 1974.322–23 n.22, observing that other guesses, for example, about Theseus's sexual infidelities and Phaedra's Cretan past, open other possible story lines that may still haunt the drama; the former, for example, is developed by Seneca and Racine. Jouanna sees a stronger break between religious and medical explanation here (1987.114–17).

[53] See E. frr. 840K (*Chrysippus* fr. 3 J.-V.L.), 904K.

but loci where questions of tragic responsibility converge and become dramatically productive. The symptom, in other words, is a tragic convention that Euripides exploits with uncommon skill to engage not only a poetic-tragic tradition of representing suffering but also medical and ethical ideas about pain, distress, and antinomian desires and acts.

But, in what form do these ideas enter the tragic imagination? Disease in tragedy is always corporeal, insofar as cases sometimes fastidiously classified by modern critics as physical suffering, madness, or mental anguish share a pattern of symptoms realized through the body and the voice.[54] Yet, if we speak of the body here, it cannot be simply equated with the physical body of the medical writers. Nor am I arguing that tragedy adopts medicine's diseases (e.g., pleurisy, suppuration) to the letter, any more than Gorgias and Democritus do. How, then, can we understand the impact of the physical body on tragedy?

One strategy would be to see the influence of the body as entailing the internalization of cause, a process that has often been identified in the name of Euripidean "psychology" (usually without clarification of what it means for Euripides to have a *logos* of the *psukhē*). It is because medicine has conventionally been associated with a shift toward internal causes that some critics have sought to limit or deny its impact on tragedy. Yet we cannot too quickly assume the amalgamation of "medical" and "internal." For the tragedians themselves were deeply interested in "internal" as well as "external" causes, an interest often seen in terms of double determination. Moreover, the medical writers, as we saw in chapter 3, do not limit their explanations to things inside the cavity but explore, too, the various forces that have an impact on the *sōma* from outside. They thus formulate their own kind of double determination by explaining symptoms in terms of both an exciting cause and the constituent stuffs of the physical body, a model that, as we have seen, is taken up by therapies of the soul. Let us look more closely, then, at how the physical body and its diseases might have been fruitful for tragic ideas about interiority.

Tragedy and the Interval

For all its carnage, tragedy, unlike epic, is drawn to violence that happens out of sight. It is a genre that seeks to track the *coming to light* of damage done behind closed doors or under the voluminous folds of the tragic costume. Often the revelation of damage takes the form of a corpse. But whereas the corpse appears after the fact, symptoms index the unseen attack as it unfolds: spasms and

---

[54] Vasquez 1972.19–28. The salient difference is whether the sufferer is passive or aggressive. The active diseases usually result in harm to others and are accompanied by a lack of understanding, as well as joy and pride (E. *Ba.* 1168–1258; *HF* 935–63; S. *Aj.* 271–76). "Passive" diseases often allow the victim some awareness of what is happening to him and may involve a struggle. On the importance of recognizing a "sliding scale" of madness, see C. Gill 1996b.60–61.

inarticulate speech spectacularly reveal the hero's loss of control; apostrophe or cries announce unseen blows as they strike.[55] The embodied hero becomes a site where concealed forces—understood as instruments of a god's anger or a coiled family curse or impersonal powers like desire, necessity, or nature—first materialize onstage. Tragic performances of sickness express that force more powerfully than perhaps any other damage witnessed onstage, turning the hero into a live conduit of daemonic power.[56]

By representing daemonic attack as a blow to the innards manifested through symptoms, the tragedians are working with an inherited model that, while poetic, no doubt had deep roots in archaic culture, as we saw in chapter 1.[57] But because tragedy is a genre oriented around spectacle and thus attuned not only to what can be seen but also to what lies beyond the seen, tragic performance draws attention to the fact that the hero's encounter with the daemonic is something that the perceiver is not shown and *cannot ever be shown*. The interest in seen and unseen distinguishes the tragedian from the magico-religious healers in *On the Sacred Disease*, who simply correlate symptoms with the god who is *aitios*, or the epic poet, who pays equal attention to the gods and their victim, using the dactylic hexameter to stitch together the mortal and immortal worlds. In tragedy, then, symptoms mark the threshold of a daemonism that is powerfully present while remaining beyond the spectators' field of vision.[58]

Tragic symptoms, in short, are surrounded by a nimbus of uncertainty. What is uncertain may be the god who is *aitios*, as we have seen. Equally uncertain, however, is how much weight we should assign external forces. For, by serving as the hidden passage between causes (e.g., Aphrodite's power and intentions) and effects (e.g., Phaedra's symptoms or Helen's flight to Troy), the embodied actor also offers a specifically tragic model of what I have been calling the interval, that is, the space between catalyst and symptom. We might even say that one of the distinguishing features of tragedy, whose heroes are so entangled in their errors and their sufferings, is its interest in the interval. It is true that the archaic poets already have a flexible notion of the person as a conduit for divine

---

[55] Vasquez 1972.104–53, 186–239.

[56] Power exhausts its capacity to harm in the dead body: as Aeschylus's Philoctetes says, "pain in no way touches a corpse" (fr. 255R; see also E. *Hipp.* 1373; S. *Ph.* 797–98).

[57] For continuities and changes between the tragic language of innards and earlier poetry, see Webster 1957; Solmsen 1984; Capone Ciollaro 1987. See also, more generally, Padel 1992.18–48. Aeschylus's vivid descriptions of fear (above, n.49), which have been seen as presenting "una immagine priva di delimitazione assoluta fra il terrore e la malattia" (Guardasole 2000.119; see also de Romilly 1958.78–79), develop the inner body as dramatic space, perhaps under the influence of contemporary medicine. Nevertheless, the innards continue to respond primarily to the domain of the gods in Aeschylus.

[58] On the inside-outside dichotomy in tragedy, see Loraux 1987.21–24; Padel 1990; 1992.47–48; Zeitlin 1996.353–56; Wohl 1998.43–46. Cf. Rehm 2002.21–22, 54–57, contesting its importance. On the use of the *ekkuklēma* to represent a hidden interior, see Dale 1956; Gould 1978.49–50. House and body may stand in for each other: for example, Lussa's raging in the breast of Heracles becomes the collapse of the house witnessed by the Chorus; see also Wohlberg 1968.

power, as we have seen. They can emphasize either the god as the source of power and knowledge or the person through whom these things are made manifest. In his famous Apology (*Il.* 19.86–138), for example, Agamemnon blames Zeus for *atē* while still accepting responsibility for the damage done through his blindness; fear, on the other hand, is a daemonic and external force that nevertheless can reveal something about a warrior's *aretē*.[59] In tragedy, however, the friction in these mortal-immortal relationships comes to the fore. The tragedians are fascinated by cases where daemonic pressure appears to compel action. The *Seven Against Thebes* is animated by the mad decision of Oedipus's sons to embrace the Labdacid curse; Agamemnon in Aeschylus is said by the Chorus to take on the yoke of necessity (*Ag.* 218) when he enters the state of frenzy that allows him to commit infanticide. Cooperation between mortal and immortal, emphasized in Alcinous's description of Demodocus's poetic inspiration (*Od.* 8.44–45), can turn combative: the *theophorētos*, "god-driven" (A. *Ag.* 1140; cf. 1150), Cassandra in Aeschylus's *Agamemnon* describes her revelation of truth as a *deinos ponos*, "terrible labor" (1215), that pits her against Apollo.[60] In the *Troades*, Hecuba turns Helen's lack of resistance, not to a god but to the beautiful image, into an occasion for blame; while, in the *Hippolytus*, Euripides questions whether one can, in fact, resist daemonic force by portraying Phaedra as a woman struggling to overcome *erōs* through self-starvation. Whereas the polysemy of the symptom describes the possibility of multiple explanations for a rupture in the fabric of the subject, the unseen interval between catalyst and symptom draws attention to the incalculable role of the subject in his or her own undoing.

Yet, if double determination is part of tragedy's patrimony, it is also the case that tragic approaches to the place of the subject in disease and its aftermath are dynamic over the course of the fifth century. In Euripides, in particular, we can see the concept of double determination fracturing under a number of pressures: medical and sophistic explanations of human behavior in terms of impersonal, internal forces; the rise of the courts together with a rhetoric of responsibility in Athens; and the staging and restaging of tragedy itself. In the *Troades*, Hecuba's clever substitution of *aphrosunē* for Aphrodite suggests that Euripides is responding to contemporary speculation about the conditions internal to human nature that lead it astray. In a tantalizing fragment from his *Bellerophon*, diseases are divided into those that are *authairetoi*, "self-incurred," and those that are godsent (fr. 286bK = *Bellerophon* fr. 9 J.-V.L.).[61]

---

[59] The classic discussion is Dodds 1951.1–27. Williams 1993.50–55 contrasts *Od.* 22.154–56 to Agamemnon's Apology: Telemachus, while admitting a mistake, claims that he is *aitios* as a way of accepting blame. On fear, see above, pp. 69–72.

[60] On Cassandra, see above, chapter 1, n.116. On the idea of being *theomachos*, see Kamerbeek 1948.

[61] See also E. fr. 339K (= *Dictys* fr. 7 J.-V.L.): καὶ γὰρ οὐκ αὐθαίρετοι / βροτοῖς ἔρωτες οὐδ᾽ ἑκουσία νόσος. It is possible in fr. 286bK that the category "godsent" is qualified by the statement "if the gods do something shameful, they are not gods." A number of scholars have argued there are several lines missing before the phrase "if the gods do . . .": Müller 1993 hypothesizes that the lost lines

It may be precisely because Euripides is so interested in the tragic subject as an interval between catalyst and damage that interpretations of the symptom in his plays are open to medicine, with its interest in the daemonic space inside the person.

Symptoms thus offer an entry point into tragic stories of suffering that do not simply bring together mortal and immortal but invoke different ways of understanding humans and the inhuman, and particularly the space of the inhuman within the human. I turn now to the tragedies themselves. First, to demonstrate the polysemy of the symptom, I consider how symptoms interact with different interpretive frameworks in two tragedies traditionally located at opposite poles of the godsent to "self-caused" continuum: the *Heracles* and the *Orestes*.[62] Then, moving from the *Orestes* to the *Hippolytus*, I reflect on how Euripides represents disease as something realized within and through the tragic subject in dramatic time, considering, too, how he explores the possibility that disease can be resisted. I close by returning to the *Heracles* in order to reflect on what the presence of different models of suffering can contribute to a tragedy's dramatic force, as well as what tragedy suggests of the imaginative impact of the physical body on late fifth-century ideas about the ethical subject.

EURIPIDES' CAUSES: THE MADNESS OF HERACLES

Euripides is particularly fond of the *deus ex machina*, making its significance in his plays difficult to explain away.[63] Attempts to do so, such as A. W. Verrall's argument that the Chorus of the *Heracles* hallucinates Iris and Lussa and then promptly suffers amnesia, have few adherents today.[64] Even without dismissing the *deus ex machina*, though, we can recognize that Verrall's reading holds a kernel of insight about the epiphany of Lussa and Iris in the *Heracles*. For after the two goddesses appear to the Chorus, midway through the tragedy, they are essentially forgotten. The main characters are never informed of their appearance, and the Chorus never mentions them again. The epiphany's limited impact presents us with something of a quandary. On the one hand, Euripides stages Heracles' madness as unambiguously godsent. On the other hand, with the gods nowhere to be seen in the last half of the play, the characters are left to speculate

---

dealt with gods helping the pious, meaning the failure to help would be the "shameful thing." But we cannot rule out that the shameful thing may simply be sending diseases: see *Morb. Sacr.* 1 (Li 6.362 = 9,8–10 Jouanna), where gods are too pure to defile the body. Harries 1891.15–16 relates the Hippocratic texts to both the *Heracles* (discussed below) and fr. 286bK; see also Nestle 1938.27–28; Mesturini 1981.

[62] I have offered a more detailed reading of the *Heracles* in Holmes 2008.

[63] On epiphanies in Euripides: Michelini 1987.102–11; Wildberg 1999–2000.245–56.

[64] Verrall 1905.168–74. It is true that Lussa appears to strike a kind of madness in the Chorus (ἆρ' ἐς τὸν αὐτὸν πίτυλον ἥκομεν φόβου, / γέροντες, οἷον φάσμ' ὑπὲρ δόμων ὁρῶ, 816–17). On πίτυλος, cf. E. *Alc.* 798; *HF* 1187; *IT* 307.

about what has been done to Heracles and what he, in turn, has done. The Lussa scene, then, is a good starting point for thinking about how the dramatic presence of the gods can coexist with the polysemy of the tragic symptom.

Although in many respects conventional, Lussa's appearance displays some curious features.[65] Euripides' gods usually appear in prologues, where they provide background information, or at the end of his plays, where they extend the repercussions of the tragic event into the future. The goddesses' arrival is, then, rather like the symptom itself: sudden, shocking, disruptive.[66] Even stranger is the nature of these divinities. Lussa, by trying to reason with the gods who have sent her—"I advise both you and Hera now to hear me out," she warns, trying to spare Heracles, "lest I see you err" (847–48)—undermines her own identity as the personification of madness. By introducing this paradoxical Lussa, Euripides creates a palpable discontinuity between the two levels of madness: the level of personified gods and the level of its outbreak.

As soon as she accepts her task, however, Lussa's identity narrows back to the familiar. She commands Iris to retire to Olympus and declares that she herself "will sink unseen into the house of Heracles" (ἐς δόμους δ᾽ ἡμεῖς ἄφαντοι δυσόμεσθ᾽ Ἡρακλέους, 874).[67] The verb *duō* may simply mean "to go" or "to sink into." Homer uses it with weapons (*Il.* 16.340), as well as with powerful forces that enter a person, such as *odunai* (*Il.* 11.272), *kholos* (*Il.* 19.16), and *lussa* (*Il.* 9.239). Sinking into the house coincides with Lussa's entry into Heracles himself—"such races I will run into the breast of Heracles" (οἵ᾽ ἐγὼ στάδια δραμοῦμαι στέρνον εἰς Ἡρακλέους, 863)—just as the destruction of the house later mirrors the collapse of Heracles' *demas*.[68]

We should hesitate, though, before imagining that Lussa enters Heracles *qua* indwelling demon,[69] for the descent into the house muddies Lussa's status as an embodied actor: "I will break through the roof and I will fall upon the house, having first killed the children" (καὶ καταρρήξω μέλαθρα καὶ δόμους ἐπεμβαλῶ, / τέκν᾽ ἀποκτείνασα πρῶτον, 864–65) turns into "but he killing will not know that he is slaughtering the children whom he begat, before he lets go of my madness" (ὁ δὲ κανὼν οὐκ εἴσεται / παῖδας οὓς ἔτικτεν ἐναρῶν, πρὶν ἂν ἐμὰς λύσσας ἀφῇ, 865–66). Having descended into the house, Lussa belongs to Heracles as much as he belongs to her, and madness takes on a uniquely Heracleian

[65] See also A. fr. 169R, from the *Xantriae*, where Lussa has a speaking part. On Lussa in tragedy and vase painting, see Duchemin 1967; Jouan 1970.317–19; Sutton 1975; Shapiro 1993.168–70; Padel 1995.17–20, 141–43.

[66] Kroeker 1938.59; Bond 1981.279–80; Lee 1982.44.

[67] The most plausible staging would have Iris exit via the *mēchanē* and Lussa step down either behind the *skēnē* or through a trapdoor in the roof, as Mastronarde 1990.268–69 argues; see also Lee 1982.45.

[68] Ἡράκλειον δέμας: *HF* 1036–37. While similar periphrases with δέμας are found elsewhere in tragedy (e.g., S. *Ant.* 944–45), this "is more than a mere periphrasis for Heracles . . . the emphasis on Heracles' body is obvious" (Bond 1981.331).

[69] Franzino 1995.62–63 emphasizes the dual aspect of personification and abstraction.

expression.[70] Those activities which define Heracles elsewhere in myth and poetry as violent and voracious figure prominently in the messenger speech: city-
sacking (943–46, 998–1000), eating (955–57), wrestling (959–62), and clubbing
heads (990–94). Collectively, they give the impression of deranged labor, thereby
perverting the image of the hero developed in the play's first half, where Heracles' labors are repeatedly, excessively lauded by the Chorus and his family.[71] The
series culminates, after Athena's intervention, with Heracles' binding, a potent
image of enslavement that conditions the audience's introduction to the "new"
Heracles. Thus, while it is true that tragic gods conventionally stand apart from
the point of their impact, Lussa's isolation on the *theologeion* need not be mere
tragic convention. Euripides, rather, seems to exploit this convention to emphasize that, however extrinsic the goad to madness, it is realized onstage only once
it has entered Heracles and erupted through symptoms of his mythic passions.

Because madness enters the tragic action through Heracles' symptoms, it
gives rise to multiple interpretations, rather than straightforwardly pointing to
Hera. The polysemy of the symptom is fostered by the displacement of the daemonic, poeticized filter from the experience of those who witness Heracles'
rampage. Conversely, those with access to the divine plane do not see madness
realized except through Lussa's performative speech:

> ἦν ἰδού· καὶ δὴ τινάσσει κρᾶτα βαλβίδων ἄπο
> καὶ διαστρόφους ἑλίσσει σῖγα γοργωποὺς κόρας,
> ἀμπνοὰς δ' οὐ σωφρονίζει, ταῦρος ὣς ἐς ἐμβολήν,
> δεινὰ μυκᾶται δέ Κῆρας ἀνακαλῶν τὰς Ταρτάρου.
> τάχα σ' ἐγὼ μᾶλλον χορεύσω καὶ καταυλήσω φόβῳ.

(867–71)

See! He shakes his head at the race's start; he silently rolls his Gorgon eyes from side
to side, and he breathes uncontrollably; like a bull ready to charge he lets forth an
awful bellow, calling up the Furies of Tartarus. Soon I will cause you to dance more
still; I will charm you with a dreadful flute.

Instead of the mad Heracles, we are given choral song that is rich in the conventional imagery of madness, such as the goad and Bacchic perversions (889–
90, 896–97; cf. 1119), and punctuated by the cries of Amphitryon from the
house.[72] While the details of what happens inside are restored to us by the messenger speech—a paragon of Euripidean "realism" focused on the seen, rather
than the unseen, aspects of Heracles' madness—the Chorus never speaks of
Lussa again.[73] When Hera's name recurs, it is under a cloud of confusion.

---

[70] On the madness as a perversion of Heracles' mythic identity: Barlow 1982.121–23; Burnett 1985.
170–71; Hartigan 1987.128; Fitzgerald 1991.91–93; Worman 1999.100–101; Papadopoulou 2004.
[71] Deranged labor: 943–46, 978, 992, 999.
[72] Cf. A. *Eu.* 307–96, where the song of the Furies is part of the main action.
[73] See esp. Barlow 1982.120–22 on the romantic mode of the first stasimon (and the Chorus's reaction to Lussa) and the "realist" tone of the messenger speech. See also Harries 1891.5–7; de Romilly
1961.20–21; Ciani 1974.88–89. On different registers of tragic disease, see Vasquez 1972.82–91.

For those inside the house see Heracles but not Lussa. As a result, when symptoms erupt inside the house, they give rise to uncertainty and speculation. The first confused reaction is that of the servants, who do not know whether they should feel fear or amusement (διπλοῦς δ᾽ ὀπαδοῖς ἦν γέλως φόβος θ᾽ ὁμοῦ, 950), or whether their master is playing or mad (παίζει πρὸς ἡμᾶς δεσπότης ἢ μαίνεται; 952).[74] The second response is Amphitryon's. Once it is clear that his son's transformation is no game, he lays blame on the bloodshed from the recent murders on Heracles' hands (966–67).[75] The specter of Athena that hurls a rock at Heracles as he is about to commit patricide offers another explanation. Someone, Amphitryon or possibly Heracles,[76] blames *her* for sending a *taragma tartareion*, "hellish whirlwind," against the house (906–9).[77] Hera's mandate is thus contaminated with the uncertainty that first appeared in the prologue, where Amphitryon blames the labors on *either* Hera *or* necessity (20–21).

The different perspectives on the madness and its cause converge on the symptom. In Lussa's speech, the head shakes, the eyes roll, the voice disappears and is reborn as a bellow, and Heracles' breathing becomes uneven (867–71). The rolling eyes and the sudden silence reappear in the messenger speech, which adds foaming at the mouth, blood-gorged veins in the eyes, mad laughter, and visual hallucinations. But perhaps most important, symptoms form a bridge between the attack and a third framework of interpretation that begins to unfold at the moment Heracles is wheeled out from the palace asleep, covered in blood, and tied to a broken column.

Heracles' reappearance marks a turning point in the tragedy. The appearance of Lussa and Hera begins to fade, and the tragedy comes to fix on Heracles' massive body. Over the course of a slow and halting awakening, Heracles confronts this strange thing through the subsiding *taragma*, "upheaval," in his *phrenes* and his hot, unsteady breath.[78] Nothing is familiar (1108). Whereas, in the *Bacchae*, Agave has a dim awareness of her crimes, Heracles' knowledge of what he has done can arrive only from his father: his self-alienation is total.[79] Nevertheless,

[74] The servants' response has a metatheatrical element, as Heracles' symptoms are those of tragic madness. On the homologous relationship between madness and theatrical performance, see Bassi 1998.12–31, 192–244; Kraus 1998.151–56 on the *Heracles*.

[75] On the relationship between fresh bloodshed and madness, see R. Parker 1983.128–30; Padel 1992.172–75. On *miasma*, see further below, pp. 271–73.

[76] Lines 1002–3 suggest that Athena appears to Heracles. Nevertheless, it is possible that Amphitryon speaks at 906–9: see Bond 1981.304–5.

[77] Kosak 2004.159–62 follows the word ταραγμός, which the medical writers use to describe internal imbalance, from the *polis* (e.g., 533) to Heracles' *phrenes* over the course of the play. See also Padel 1995.131–32.

[78] Kovacs 1996.142–43 argues that πέπτωκα and πνέω cannot refer to Heracles' present experience, because, when Heracles awakes, the madness is over: thus Heracles cannot say, "I have fallen into a dreadful wave of mental confusion" while reasoning calmly about his present state. This complaint, however, disregards tragic convention. Characters are often capable of reporting on their experience in the midst of their illness or, here, during the aftershock of madness.

[79] On Agave, see Devereux 1970.42.

this body belongs to Heracles, for once madness is realized, it is no longer autonomous or external. If the *tukhē* of Hera strikes a single blow (1393),[80] that blow reveals a body vulnerable to daemonic forces that erupt from within. In tears, Heracles gauges his distance from his former self: "Never have I shed water from my eyes, nor did I ever even consider that it would come to this, tears fallen from my eyes" (οὔτ᾽ ἀπ᾽ ὀμμάτων / ἔσταξα πηγάς, οὐδ᾽ ἂν ᾠόμην ποτὲ / ἐς τοῦθ᾽ ἱκέσθαι, δάκρυ᾽ ἀπ᾽ ὀμμάτων βαλεῖν, 1354–56). Tears demonstrate that *tukhē* is not under the control of the autarchic archer, but is internal to his identity: "I see, then, that we are necessarily enslaved to *tukhē*" (νῦν δ᾽, ὡς ἔοικε, τῇ τύχῃ δουλευτέον, 1357).[81]

Despite Lussa's dramatic appearance, our attention shifts to the eruption of the symptom. The gods do not disappear from the explanations offered by the characters who confront Heracles' madness. Yet in the final scene, the debate about the role of Hera and the nature of the gods develops against the backdrop of Heracles' newfound vulnerability in a world where the expectation of epiphanies has passed. I return to the final scene at the end of the chapter in order to explore in more detail the multiple meanings of madness developed there. First, however, having sketched a case for the polysemy of the symptom in a tragedy where disease is often seen by critics as unambiguously godsent, I would like to look at a play whose relationship to the new medicine and contemporary intellectual culture is relatively uncontroversial: *Orestes*.[82]

EURIPIDES' CAUSES: THE MADNESS OF ORESTES

Euripides' *Orestes* opens on the title character asleep in his sickbed. Ravaged by disease, he has been confined here, we soon learn, since killing his mother six days earlier. The opening visual tableau cues where Euripides' telling of the myth is headed. Half a century earlier, in his *Eumenides*, Aeschylus had introduced the Furies onstage as the personified agents of Orestes' madness.[83] Euripides, however, restricts our access to the Furies, showing them only as they are refracted through Orestes' symptoms and thus inviting the audience to wonder whether they are invisibly present or simply the product of Orestes' visual hallucinations. Over the course of the play, this causal uncertainty spreads to the matricide itself. While Apollo is said to have commanded the murder, his

---

[80] On this "single blow," see Schlesier 1985.35, with n.97.

[81] On being enslaved to fate or the gods, see also E. *Ba.* 366; *HF* 1396; *Or.* 418.

[82] For the contrast between the *Heracles* and the *Orestes*, see Hartigan 1987; Theodorou 1993. On contemporary medical motifs in the *Orestes*: W. Smith 1967; Parry 1969; Willink 1986; Hoessly 2001.132–43; Kosak 2004.131–50. On the play's relationship to a broader intellectual culture, see also Greenberg 1962; M. Wright 2006.

[83] See Theodorou 1993.39–41 for a detailed comparison of the two tragedies; see also Burnett 1985.205–22.

increasingly conspicuous absence leaves Orestes' motives for killing open to speculation. Orestes' very willingness to trust ostensibly divine orders ("we are enslaved to the gods, whatever the gods are," *Or.* 418) comes to appear suspect as he tries to repeat the matricide by murdering Helen—not simply the cause of the Trojan War but a double of her sister Clytemnestra—in an even more perverse defense of patriarchy. Our sense that what drives Orestes may not be a god is strengthened when Apollo is finally forced to step in and avert Helen's death. For, while Apollo uses the opportunity to assure the audience that he did sanction the original murder, the very occasion of his epiphany—Orestes' attempt at a second—undercuts our sense that Orestes was ever fulfilling a divine plan. In any event, if Lussa and Iris appear too soon in the *Heracles*, leaving the characters to interpret madness in their own terms, Apollo arrives too late. The god's belatedness allows Orestes' disease to become increasingly complex, fostering multiple explanations of what is driving its expression.

From the beginning of the play, cause is presented from multiple angles.[84] Electra starts the prologue with a gnomic statement: "There is no word so terrible to utter, no *pathos*, no godsent misfortune [ξυμφορὰ θεήλατος], whose burden human nature could not bear" (1–3). Holding two of these perspectives, *pathos* and godsent misfortune, in perfect equipoise across a single line, Electra's maxim sets up the classic tragic complication of her ancestors' troubles that immediately follows—Tantalus, for example, suffered a terrible fate at the hands of the gods, but he was driven to it by his unbridled tongue, "a most shameful *nosos*" (10)—while anticipating a family curse in the terms of contemporary anthropological inquiry.[85] Euripides thus establishes the tragedy at the outset as both a new take on the last generation of the House of Atreus and a study of human nature under duress.[86]

When Electra turns to her brother's trouble, however, she shifts fully into the language of disease (νόσος, 43), cataloging in detail his multifarious symptoms (not eating, not bathing, leaping from bed, hiding beneath the covers) and his swings between delirium and grief. While she unambiguously traces all their sufferings back to Apollo and blames the Furies of her mother's blood for Orestes' madness, in flagging the symptom as the threshold of what the audience and the characters can see, she primes us for the dramatic presentation of

[84] Greenberg 1962, esp. 166–67; W. Smith 1967.306 ("Euripides' clinical approach is less interested in passing obvious judgments than in exploring causes"); Theodorou 1993.41. Zeitlin speaks of the play as a "palimpsestic text" (1980.54). See also M. Wright 2006.46: *Orestes* problematizes what we can know, making moral judgments unstable.

[85] See also Electra's apostrophe to *phusis* following Helen's departure: ὦ φύσις, ἐν ἀνθρώποισιν ὡς μέγ' εἶ κακόν, / σωτήριον δὲ τοῖς καλῶς κεκτημένοις (126–27). Most editors (including Kovacs) bracket 127. On ἀνθρώπου φύσις, Willink 1986.79 cites natural philosophy, as well as other Euripidean passages (*Hec.* 296; *Ion* 1004; frr. 170K [= *Antigone* fr. 18 J.-V.L.], 834K [= *Phrixus* fr. 18 J.-V.L.]). The figure of Tantalus was perhaps linked to contemporary physicists (Willink 1983), especially Anaxagoras (Scodel 1984).

[86] On the mythic innovations, see esp. Zeitlin 1980. See also Euben 1986.237–51 on the play's distance from its mythic models and earlier tragedy.

Orestes as the conduit for daemonic power onstage. That preparation is unusually extensive here: whereas Euripides often sets the prologue apart from the main action, here he extends the framework that it establishes into the play's first exchanges.[87] These exchanges, in turn, elaborate the idea of disease at the expense of the gods ambiguously lying behind it.

The first stage entrance gives us a brief glimpse of Helen who, seeing the sorry lot of her sister's children, attributes fault for the matricide to Apollo (76). Yet her displacement of culpability onto the gods is immediately made problematic by her blithe dismissal of her own crime as godsent madness (θεομανεῖ πότμῳ, 79): thinking back to Gorgias's *Encomium* and Euripides' own *Troades*, we may expect that Helen was hardly the best mouthpiece for claims of divine compulsion.[88] Her deft evasion of blame puts Electra's naming of Apollo *qua* cause in a more troubling light and looks forward to Orestes' own, more conflicted attempts to exonerate himself by shifting responsibility to the god (285–87; cf. 579–80, 591–99).

If Helen poisons the attribution of cause to the gods, Orestes' madness is staged in such a way as to strengthen the representation of his disease as a developing affliction that feeds on things inside him. The scene is dominated, as soon as the patient awakes, by an acute attack of delirium. Yet the disease is not contained by the fits of mania but presses on Orestes even when he is ostensibly *emphrōn*, "in his right mind."[89] Limp and *anarthros*, "weak" or "disarticulated" (228), Orestes requires his sister to prop him up, turn him around, and help him to walk (218–19, 231–34). Other symptoms, too, testify to the degree to which Orestes has diverged from a normal state: his sense of disorientation (215–16), the crust of foam around his eyes and mouth (219–20)—perhaps represented through a "squalid" mask—the matted, unwashed hair (223–26). When Menelaus first encounters Orestes, he notes his fearsome stare, his parched eyes (389), and his collapse into *amorphia*, "formlessness" (391).

By emphasizing the deepening entrenchment of disease, Euripides blurs the boundaries between Orestes and what is assailing him, allowing us to imagine causes that, as the play develops, move beyond the Furies and Apollo *qua* instigator of the crime. Orestes himself responds to Menelaus's request for a diagnosis ("what are you suffering, what disease destroys you?") by proposing a series of causes. He begins his tripartite etiology with *sunesis*, which he glosses with the phrase "I know [σύνοιδα] that I have done terrible things" (396), a gloss that cues his explanation as self-consciously sophisticated. The word itself has a modern ring: Aristophanes mocks *sunesis* as one of Euripides' new gods (*Ra.* 892–93),

---

[87] Burnett 1985.195–96 discusses the unusually long opening sequence.

[88] She goes so far as to ask Clytemnestra to be gracious to her murderers, the children "whom the god destroyed" (οὓς ἀπώλεσεν θεός, 121). R. Parker 1983.311 sees the denial of blame as an expression of "her glib moral laxity."

[89] See Theodorou 1993.36–38. Cf. Kovacs 2002, arguing that it is only during Orestes' fit that he is sane, because only then does he accept the reality of the Furies.

while the author of *On the Sacred Disease* uses the word to describe our alert awareness of the world.[90] Later, Orestes uses it again, with maximum irony, to describe the Phrygian slave's canny avoidance of death (σῴζει σε σύνεσις, 1524).[91] In the exchange with Menelaus, it presumably means something like "conscience" or "remorse."[92] To this explanation, Orestes adds two more: *lupē* and madness or, more specifically, "the avengers of my mother's blood" (398–400).[93]

While Orestes' etiology can be seen as a series of parallel explanations, it also draws a conflicted portrait of his disease and suggests that his mad fits may be the eruption of a bitter struggle between different forces within him—guilt and sorrow, but also hatred and a thirst for vengeance.[94] Consider the opening scene, with its focus on the sleeping Orestes. Whereas, in Aeschylus's *Eumenides*, whose first scene shows the sleeping Furies, Orestes' respite depends on his assailants' momentary oblivion, in Euripides' play the enchantment of sleep is the "savior of the sick" (ἐπίκουρον νόσου, 211) only if *Orestes himself* is allowed to forget his troubles.[95] And, when Euripides stages the madness scene, he uses Orestes' *own* memory to catalyze the attack, rather than the memory of the Furies.[96] Whereas Aeschylus had used the ghost of Clytemnestra to stir the Furies to action, in the *Orestes*, another "ghostly" Clytemnestra, this time the mother that Orestes remembers, sets off the madness in a rather different way. Electra has reported Helen's return to Argos to her brother; she then denounces both her aunt and her mother. In response, Orestes urges his sister not to imitate her female relatives. As he does so, his eyes grow agitated (ὄμμα σὸν ταράσσεται, 253), he believes he sees the Furies approaching, and he leaps from the bed. By making Electra's words trigger Orestes' attack, Euripides aligns the unexpected violence of the symptom with Orestes' fraught relationship to Clytemnestra and Helen, rather than with the Furies. The scene gives us a glimpse of the fear and loathing that Orestes feels toward these women—the countercurrent to the horrified shame he

---

[90] See *Morb. Sacr.* 16 (Li 6.390 = 29,11–12 Jouanna), 17 (Li 6.392 = 30,4 Jouanna), with Garzya 1992; Guardasole 2000.211–19.

[91] On the slave as a mirror to Orestes, see Euben 1986.231–32.

[92] See W. Smith 1967.297; Rodgers 1969; Assaël 1996; Pigeaud 2006.418–19. Cf. Democr. (DK68) B181.

[93] On *lupē* as a disease, see below, n.157.

[94] We see this conflict staged immediately after his delirium recedes, when he confesses to Electra that he no longer believes that Agamemnon would have sanctioned the murder, although the reasons for his disapproval—Clytemnestra's death could never bring Agamemnon back to life; the suffering it caused Orestes outweighs any profit (288–93)—do not include a sense of the act as lawless.

[95] On this point, see Zeitlin 1980.55. Sleep, of course, is a conventional element in scenes of suffering, appearing, for example, in the *Heracles* and Sophocles' *Philoctetes*: see Jouanna 1983b. Yet the shift from sleeping Furies to the sleeping Orestes, with the implication that the forces in need of quieting lie within the patient, finds confirmation in the act's final lines, spoken by Electra: "Even if you are not ill, but you are imagining you are ill, it is a dead-end toil for mortals" (314–15), which we can read as something like "for when people *think* they are ill, even when they are not, they really become ill" (Willink 1986.136; emphasis in original).

[96] For the Erinyes as keepers of memory: Padel 1992.168–85.

also exhibits.[97] The hatred that implicates Orestes in his mother's murder will erupt again, unmotivated by a god's voice, to aim for the murder of Helen.[98] The onset of his madness thus looks forward as much as it looks backward to the matricide.

By placing dramatic weight on the potency of Orestes' emotions, Euripides conditions how we view not only his disease but also his deeds: the matricide and the attempt on Helen's life. In so doing, he raises questions about the nature of Apollo himself and his shocking orders. Menelaus, for example, deems Apollo's command "completely ignorant of the good and the just" (417),[99] implying that the very illegitimacy of the command attributed to Apollo weakens the likelihood of its divine provenance. His skepticism surfaces immediately afterward in his questions about Apollo's failure to rescue Orestes from the consequences of his action (423). Tyndareus is more direct. His blistering speech shifts the ignorance of right and wrong onto Orestes, who is both the most *unaware* of men (τίς ἀνδρῶν ... ἀσυνετώτερος; 493) and a "sick-eyed" snake (δράκων / στίλβει νοσώδεις ἀστραπάς, 479–80).[100] Orestes, he alleges, has failed to seize "what is wise" and betrayed the common law of the Greeks by forgoing a legal solution to his father's murder (502–4). With such a charge, Euripides exploits fully the anachronistic transposition of the *Oresteia* myth into a "historical" Argos. Because the matricide now postdates the establishment of a legal solution to vendetta killing—the triumph, we might say, of *nomos* over *phusis*—it is Orestes, in the eyes of Tyndareus, who is regressively aligned with a law of blood. Indeed, his grandfather denounces him as *to thēriōdes*, "something bestial," using a word common in contemporary intellectual circles to describe the subhuman state before the establishment of law and society.[101] Tyndareus thus

---

[97] Rodgers 1969.250–52 argues for Orestes' general "horror of the deed," rather than any moral guilt. But Euripides is vague on whether this horror is motivated by shame, a sense of justice, or, perhaps, the realization that matricide has made him into his mother's son.

[98] E.g., 572: μισῶν δὲ μητέρ' ἐνδίκως ἀπώλεσα (hating my mother, I killed her justly).

[99] Euripides' characters are often anxious about the perceived lawlessness of the gods. Ion, for example, is indignant that Apollo would abuse his power to rape virgins, so that "you who write the laws for mortals incur yourselves a charge of lawlessness" (*Ion* 440–41). In the *Heracles*, Amphitryon, enraged at Zeus's inaction, concludes, "either you are an ignorant god or you are not, by nature, just" (ἀμαθής τις εἶ θεὸς ἢ δίκαιος οὐκ ἔφυς, 347). See also frr. 645K (= *Polyidus* fr. 10 J.-V.L.), 832K (= *Phrixus* fr. 16 J.-V.L.). Despair about the lack of cosmic justice may cause doubt as to whether there are gods at all. See, e.g., *El.* 583–84; further evidence at Riedweg 1990.40–42. Moreover, the gods' desires are often represented by Euripides as too petty or unseemly to explain anything satisfactorily: see *Ba.* 1346–48; *HF* 1307–8; *Hipp.* 120; *IT* 380; *Tro.* 67–68; fr. 210K [= *Antiope* fr. 34 J.-V.L.].

[100] Tyndareus's interlacing of magico-religious and medical language is perfectly expressed in the conjunction δράκων... νοσώδεις ἀστραπάς, which combines the serpent-figure of the Aeschylean Clytemnestra's godsent nightmare with an adjective modeled on technical medical terms. Euripides is fond of –ώδης compounds, for example, λυσσώδης (*Ba.* 981), ἀφρώδης (*Or.* 220), ἑλκώδης (*Hipp.* 1359)—all in "medical" contexts. Orestes calls the Furies δρακοντώδεις at 256.

[101] See Democr. (DK68) B5 (D.S. 1.8.1); Critias (DK88) B25.2. See also Boulter 1962 and, more generally, Jouanna 1988a; 1990a.

firmly distances Orestes' act from the Olympian order, condemning him to the "same *daimōn*" as his mother and attributing his madness to the retributive power of just gods (531–33).

Apollo will appear *ex machina* over a thousand lines later to confirm Orestes' defense that he was divinely compelled to kill his mother (1665).[102] The belated arrival of that authoritative narrative, as we have seen, allows a range of perspectives on culpability to be introduced and the audience to form its own ideas about blame. These ideas are influenced not only by the remarks of individual characters but also by the development of Orestes' disease in dramatic time. In staging disease as a complex event, Euripides may be drawing on contemporary medical ideas about inner space, impersonal forces, and the complicity of human nature with disease. Euripides, in other words, can be seen as working out his own kind of medical analogy.

One concept that may be salient to this analogy is the fracturing of the human into seen and unseen space in medical writing, through which the archaic boundary between radically other daemonic space and the terrain of the self is internalized. From this perspective, we might refer Orestes' sudden attack of madness to emotions that erupt from a hidden space inside him. At the same time, his disease is not contained by such attacks: his eyes flash dragon-like even when he is lucid. These two facets of the disease complicate the medical analogy. In staging delirious fits, uncontrolled movement, and other nearly automatic behaviors, Euripides may be cuing the daemonic physical body of contemporary medicine, suggesting that submerged below the threshold of conscious control are not only impersonal stuffs like bile and phlegm but also emotions like hatred or desire. When Orestes is "in his right mind," however, these emotions, like desires and emotions in thinkers like Democritus and Plato, inhabit the more intimate space of deliberation, reflection, and agency that, against the foil of the *sōma*, was taking shape as the *psukhē* in the late fifth century. By allowing the dynamics of disease to infiltrate Orestes' "right thinking," Euripides makes us increasingly wonder just how foreign the forces assailing him are.

The more the forces behind disease move into the domain of the person, the more the idea of theomachy seems strained, even as the figure of disease keeps the notion of compulsion in play. No one in tragedy fights a god and wins—that is why blaming the gods is a certain route to innocence. But, when the tragic subject appears to be struggling to master things inside him (e.g., love, hate, sorrow, guilt) whose force is triggered by nondivine or impersonal catalysts (e.g., beautiful bodies, the threat of death), theomachy merges with the contemporary idioms of autarchy and being "stronger than" pleasure or fear. What are the implications of this shift for the idea of struggle? Is capitulation still inevitable and, if so, at what point? How might expanding the importance of an interval

---

[102] At which point, Orestes *himself* admits that he feared he had heard the voice of some *alastōr* speaking at Delphi, rather than Apollo himself (1668–69). Most critics read Apollo's reassurances as hollow, but see Kovacs 2002; Lefkowitz 2002.

between catalyst and act or symptom influence the role of character or nature in the staging of outcomes?

In the *Orestes*, Euripides turns Orestes' acquiescence to Apollo's command into a problem. The play can be seen as returning to a classic moment from Aeschylus's *Agamemnon*—the moment when Orestes' father assumed the force of Necessity as his *own* furious desire to kill his daughter—in order to elaborate, through the figure of disease, Agamemnon's assumption of necessity (where necessity encompasses both a long family curse and the anger of the gods). In the *Orestes*, murderous desires continue to animate Orestes even after Necessity and the gods' intentions have fallen away, rendering the figure of "double determination" irrelevant. At the same time, he begins to suffer from surges of sorrow and guilt that work from within, rather than arriving from an externalized daemonic space, like the Furies or Clytemnestra *qua* avenger of Agamemnon's wrong. In acquiescing to Apollo's command, then, Orestes seems to internalize the strife that has defined his genealogical line, a back-and-forth of violence and vengeance further complicated by his own raw desire for self-preservation.[103] In becoming the god's slave, he is also, in a sense, giving in to the restless agonism of human nature itself, played out through the volatile desires, emotions, intentions, and beliefs of his disease. We find a quite different depiction of divine compulsion in the *Hippolytus*, a play that engages the question of whether anyone can resist realizing a god's plan by interrogating contemporary strategies of self-mastery.

Realizing Disease in the *Hippolytus*

In the *Hippolytus*, we are introduced first to the god's plan, then to the disease it triggers.[104] In the prologue, Aphrodite explains her intention to "trip up" the young Hippolytus, who has neglected to pay her honor, through a triangulated scheme that turns her victim into the object of another's love.[105] The lover is Phaedra, Hippolytus's otherwise innocent stepmother, who is entangled in Aphrodite's revenge plot through an act of vision: seeing Hippolytus, Phaedra is seized in her heart *with* a terrible desire (ἔρωτι δεινῷ) *through* the plotting of Aphrodite (τοῖς ἐμοῖς βουλεύμασιν, *Hipp.* 24–28). The two datives, which

---

[103] For the theme of exchange, see 842–43: σφάγιον ἔθετο / ματέρα, πατρῴων παθέων ἀμοιβάν (he slaughtered his mother / a trade for paternal sufferings). Moreover, the tragedy abounds in *polyptota*: deaths are traded for deaths (θανάτους θανάτων, 1007), murders for murders (φόνῳ φόνος, 510, 816 [Kovacs reads πόνῳ πόνος here, following Willink]). On the family curse, see, e.g., 996–97.

[104] The words νοσέω (186, 279, 293, 463, 477), νοσερός (131, 179), and νόσος (40, 176, 205, 269, 283, 294, 394, 405, 477, 479, 512, 597, 698, 730, 766) occur twenty-two times before Phaedra's death is announced, halfway through the tragedy. By contrast, there are only two examples in the latter half of the tragedy: νοσοῦμεν at 933 (the single reference to Hippolytus) and νόσον at 1306 (Phaedra's *erōs*).

[105] See Zeitlin 1996.278–84, with bibliography on Aphrodite's wrath at 278 n.107. See also Calame 1999.24–25.

together fill the line, correspond to two modalities of action in the tragedy. At one level, we find the angry goddess, whose plans bear an ambiguous relationship to the tragic action; at another, we find "something more than a god" (τι μεῖζον ἄλλο ... θεοῦ, 360) that works through Phaedra.[106] But, while the tragic narrative is launched from Phaedra's body—her clouded brow (172), pallid skin (175), and weak and wasted form (274)—the symptoms of *erōs* erupt from a space uncharted by the medical writers.

We might dismiss the use of Phaedra to reveal what is unseen, that is, the power of Aphrodite, as a dramatic necessity. Yet, much as Euripides plays with the personified *deus ex machina* in the *Heracles*, he complicates Phaedra's role as a conduit by having her resist the revelation of *erōs*. She not only conceals the cause of her suffering but tries, too, to keep from betraying her secret by starving herself to death. Her attempts to conquer Aphrodite present an inscrutable tableau to those around her: "We *see* the wretched sufferings of Phaedra," says the Chorus, "but whatever disease this is, that is unclear to us" (ἄσημα δ᾽ ἡμῖν ἥτις ἐστὶν ἡ νόσος, 268–69; cf. 173–75, 236, 346). This defiant Phaedra is a departure from other Euripidean heroines conquered by *erōs*, such as Pasiphae and the headstrong Phaedra of the tragedian's other (lost) *Hippolytus* play, who bears similarities to the title character of Sophocles' *Phaedra*.[107] Whereas Euripides' earlier Phaedra seems to have readily capitulated to *erōs*,[108] this Phaedra tries to (re)write the story of her suffering as one of heroic self-mastery. In our

---

[106] See esp. Rivier 1960; Winnington-Ingram 1960; cf. Sourvinou-Inwood 2003.330–32. For *erōs* as madness, see frr. 161K (= *Antigone* fr. 10 J.-V.L.), 331K (= *Dictys* fr. 5 J.-V.L.). See also Pi. *N.* 11.48; Prodicus (DK84) B7. *Erōs* is a particularly volatile force in Euripides: see *HF* 66; *IA* 808; *Med.* 529–30, 714; *Pho.* 622; *Supp.* 178; frr. 138K (= *Andromeda* fr. 32 J.-V.L.), 322K (= *Danae* fr. 17 J.-V.L.), 358K (= *Erectheus* fr. 17 J.-V.L.), 430K (= *Hipp. Kal.* fr. 4 J.-V.L.), 663K (= *Stheneboa* fr. 3 J.-V.L.), 816K (= *Phoenix* fr. 14 J.-V.L.), 895K, 897K, 898K, 1076K. See Borthwick 1997 for the marked increase in the use of *erōs* in Euripides—eighty-seven instances versus sixteen in Aeschylus and eighteen in Sophocles—as well as related terms like "Kupris" and "Aphrodite."

[107] On Pasiphae, see Rivier 1958. On Sophocles' Phaedra, see esp. frr. 679–80R. Scholars have long seen the extant *Hippolytus* play as the second of two, performed in 428, on the basis of the Aristophanic hypothesis: see W. Barrett 1964.11–45; Snell 1964.23–69; Reckford 1974.309–19; Dunn 1996.98–100; Mills 1997.195–207; and McDermott 2000, offering a clever reading of our play as a rewriting of the lost first version. Gibert 1997 raises important objections to the standard view without making a compelling case for the alternative. The publication of new papyri evidence, however, has suggested that the lost version may be more different from our play than was previously believed, thereby inviting further speculation about the order of the plays. Hutchinson 2004, discussing the papyri evidence, builds on the uncertainty the new evidence creates to argue on metrical grounds that our *Hippolytus* is earlier than 428 (and, hence, the earlier version); cf. the objections in Cropp and Fick 2005. See also Luppe 2005, who argues (on the basis of textual corruption in the Aristophanes' hypothesis) that both plays are earlier and concludes that the traditional order (our *Hippolytus* as second) is most probable.

[108] See esp. fr. 444K (= *Hipp. Kal.* fr. 17 J.-V.L.): ὦ δαῖμον, ὡς οὐκ ἔστ᾽ ἀποστροφὴ βροτοῖς / τῶν ἐμφύτων τε καὶ θεηλάτων κακῶν (O daemon, there is no recourse for mortals against inborn and godsent evils). It is generally agreed that the Phaedra of the other *Hippolytus* tried to seduce her stepson directly (see esp. fr. 430K = *Hipp. Kal.* fr. 4 J.-V.L.). References to Phaedra in Aristophanes (*Ra.* 1043–52; *Th.* 497–98, 547; fr. 469 PCG) presumably target this Phaedra.

Hippolytus, *erōs* does not set off the chain of dominoes that Gorgias describes in his *Helen*. Rather, Aphrodite's blow opens up a space of deliberation: "When *erōs* wounded me," Phaedra says, "I *pondered* how best to bear it" (392–93). Thus, caught between concealment and revelation, between Aphrodite's power and Phaedra's, the symptom becomes the crux of the tragedy's first half.[109]

In archaic poetry, *erōs* lodges in the *phrenes* or curls up under the *kradiē*.[110] In Euripides' play, the idea that *erōs* develops in hidden inner space is elaborated through the staging of its intermittent eruption. Phaedra's first entrance is itself a spectacular act of revelation—the Chorus tells us in the parodos that the queen has been keeping her *demas* inside the palace, wasting away in a "sick lying" and "covering her golden head in fine-spun robes" (131–34).[111] In her first moments onstage, the process of unveiling initiated by her entrance continues: "My headdress weighs on my head—take it off!" she commands her attendants; "Let my hair fall over my shoulders" (201–2). Revelation culminates in language, as Phaedra declares her desire to go to the mountains, to hunt stags, and to race horses on the beach—in short, to engage in the very Artemisian pursuits that occupy Hippolytus.[112] Coming to her senses, she is shamed by her outburst and desperately tries to cover herself back up. Those around her recognize that something daemonic has broken the surface without understanding what it means: the Nurse thinks much divination is needed to know "which of the gods is drawing you off course and striking your *phrenes* askance" (ὅστις σε θεῶν ἀνασειράζει / καὶ παρακόπτει φρένας, 237–38). The audience, on the other hand, recognizes the first flash of *erōs* escaping from Phaedra into the dramatic space of the mortal world.

If, however, Phaedra's body and her words serve as parallel sites for the revelation of disease, they also reveal different kinds of forces. It is *erōs* that surfaces in her words. But the question posed by the Chorus as to why the queen's complexion is marred (δεδήληται, 174) has as its most obvious answer not *erōs* but Phaedra's refusal to eat. Her refusal becomes the most immediate cause of the symptoms—loosened limbs, pallor, wasting, and irritability—that might otherwise be mistaken for *erōs*.[113] By actively using starvation to reproduce the suf-

---

[109] On concealment and revelation in the tragedy, see Segal 1988; Goff 1990.12–20; Zeitlin 1996.243–57, 264–78. Note the violent enjambment of the key adverb "in silence" (ἡ τάλαιν' ἀπόλλυται / σιγῇ, 39–40) in Aphrodite's description of Phaedra's suffering; this may cue the key change of a second version (W. Barrett 1964.163; McDermott 2000.246).

[110] One Euripidean character lodges *erōs* "in the worst part of the *phrenes*" (fr. 1054K).

[111] The extravagant quality of her entrance is strongly marked by the anomalous choral commentary on it. Other Euripidean uses of anapestic commentary on otherwise conventional entrances mark the arrival of chariots and corpses, as McDermott 2000.248 observes.

[112] On desire in language in the play, see Goff 1990.7, 27–54; Zeitlin 1996.244–45.

[113] "How could she not" be wasted, asks the Nurse, "when she has not eaten for three days?" (πῶς δ' οὔ, τριταίαν γ' οὖσ' ἄσιτος ἡμέραν; 275). A lack of appetite could be a symptom of *erōs* in the classical period (e.g., Pl. *Smp.* 191b1–2), but it does not help the Chorus or the Nurse make a diagnosis. The wasted lover becomes a trope in Hellenistic poetry (e.g., Theoc. *Id.* 11.69), then Roman love elegy. The refusal to eat might also express anxiety, grief, or madness, e.g., *Il.* 19.205–10; E. *Med.* 24;

fering body traditionally created by desire, Phaedra overdetermines the figure of *nosos*. Her success in redrawing the symptoms' referential field turns the central question taxing everyone onstage into a question of her own agency: is she driven by *atē* or is she trying to die (276)?[114] Phaedra's attempt to "keep her body in purity from the grain of Demeter" (138)[115] thus crystallizes the central problem of the *Hippolytus*, a problem that seems to have fascinated Euripides more generally: is resistance to Aphrodite possible?

Phaedra believes that it is. Once she has betrayed the fatal name "Hippolytus" to the Nurse, after a long series of delays and false starts, she gives a detailed exposition of her dilemma. We learn that her decision to die is the last in a series of attempts to master *erōs*. Yet, if Phaedra wants to die, why does she drag things out? The simple answer is that if Phaedra were prematurely beached on death's shore, *erōs* would never reach Hippolytus. A more satisfying one might recognize the symbiosis of *erōs* and *sophrosunē*, "modesty," Aphrodite's power and Phaedra's.[116] For, while the disease is shameful, Phaedra's resistance to it, which her chosen form of suicide allows her to perform in dramatic time, should bring her *timē* (329). At the same time, if Phaedra's wish is "would that I not escape notice when acting well, nor find many witnesses when acting shamefully" (403–4), she faces a problem. Showing, she shows too much; concealing, no one can know that she is "contriving honorable things from shameful ones" (ἐκ τῶν γὰρ αἰσχρῶν ἐσθλὰ μηχανώμεθα, 331). As long as *erōs* remains a secret, no one can understand the context of her destructive self-mastery through starvation.[117] Symptoms, as we have seen, require stories.

The long speech that Phaedra offers to the women onstage is one version of the story she wants to tell, an account of "the pathway of [her] deliberation" (τῆς ἐμῆς γνώμης ὁδόν, 391; cf. 290) embedded in a series of generalizing reflections on pleasure, shame, and the good. Phaedra accepts that she has been struck by *erōs*, an event that, until this point, both she (315, 319) and the Nurse (358–60) have described in terms of overwhelming force. Here, she changes tack to map out what she sees as the scope of ethical action in the face of disease. She says that she first resolved to hide her disease through silence. When

---

S. *Aj.* 324; see also Martinez 1995.343–44. In the medical writers, being ἄσιτος is simply another symptom of a mechanical cause, e.g., *Aff.* 15 (Li 6.222 = 26 Potter); *Mul.* I 9 (Li 8.38 = 106,20–21 Grensemann).

[114] In the parodos, the opposition collapses into the syntax of double determination: "because of a hidden grief, wishing to ground her ship at death's unhappy terminus" (κρυπτῷ πένθει θανάτου θέλουσ-/αν κέλσαι ποτὶ τέρμα δύστανον, 139–40; cf. 322).

[115] The idea of purity is closely associated with Hippolytus (102, 1003): see Segal 1970.278–83; 1978.135.

[116] The final explanation that Artemis gives of events makes clear the entanglement of shame and honor: speaking to Theseus, she wishes to make clear "the maddened passion of your wife or, in a way, her nobility" (σῆς γυναικὸς οἶστρον ἢ τρόπον τινὰ / γενναιότητα, 1300–1301). Cf. 1429–30, where it is simply Phaedra's *erōs* that lives on in ritual, with Loraux 1979.53–54; Dunn 1996.95–96.

[117] Winnington-Ingram 1960.179–80; Loraux 1979.52; Rabinowitz 1986.131; Goff 1990.15; Cairns 1993.331.

that failed, she tried to bear her madness "by conquering through being
sophrōn" (τῷ σωφρονεῖν νικῶσα, 399). But this, too, failed to overpower Kupris, leaving suicide as her remaining option, the best, "most powerful" of plans
(κράτιστον ... βουλευμάτων, 402).

In describing her struggle with *erōs*, Phaedra offers a series of gnomic remarks couched as the fruit of long reflection on the question of how people
ruin their lives. It is here that she first translates the language of daemonic compulsion into what looks like contemporary ethical debate.[118]

> καί μοι δοκοῦσιν οὐ κατὰ γνώμης φύσιν
> πράσσειν κάκιον· ἔστι γὰρ τό γ᾽ εὖ φρονεῖν
> πολλοῖσιν· ἀλλὰ τῇδ᾽ ἀθρητέον τόδε·
> ἃ χρήστ᾽ ἐπιστάμεσθα καὶ γιγνώσκομεν
> οὐκ ἐκπονοῦμεν, οἱ μὲν ἀργίας ὕπο,
> οἱ δ᾽ ἡδονὴν προθέντες ἀντὶ τοῦ καλοῦ
> ἄλλην τιν᾽.

(E. *Hipp.* 377–83)

And in my opinion it is not because of the nature of their judgment that people end
up worse off; for thinking well is possible for many of them. But we should look at
it this way instead: what we know and understand to be noble, we fail to carry out,
some because of laziness, others by giving preference, in place of the good, to some
other pleasure.

While Phaedra's reflections relate to her own situation on a number of levels, it
is difficult to know the precise nature of these relationships. Does Euripides intend us to place Phaedra among those who choose some other pleasure in place
of the good?[119] Phaedra, in any case, seems to use these opening lines as a way
of framing her *own* attempt to resist *erōs* as the pursuit of *to kalon*, "the good."
Most important, her syntax recovers a place for the ethical subject who chooses
(προθέντες) some pleasure over the good. That phrasing emphasizes that Phaedra places neither god nor nature in the way of the good, but qualities and actions, which, like Democritus, she finds worthy of moral censure. She takes a
remarkable stand, then, against all the Helens and the Stheneboas and the Pa-
siphaes who use compulsion to deny culpability. It is left to the Nurse, in her response to Phaedra's speech (433–81), to lay out the standard exculpatory arguments about omnipotent gods and the futility of resistance.

The belief that one can overpower Aphrodite is as old as Homer, who shows
it to be illusory (*Il.* 3.399–420). Indeed, the Nurse sees Phaedra's desire to be

---

[118] On the intellectual-ethical language of the speech, see Moline 1975.54; Craik 1993.49–52, 55–59
on its relationship to fifth-century debates on pleasure. Cf. Willink 1968.11–26.

[119] Commentators have been quick to see *aidōs* as implicated in a downfall *of which Phaedra herself
is not aware*. Her strange list of pleasures (long talks, leisure, and the infamous two kinds of *aidōs*)
has been seen as indicating her own susceptibility to *erōs*: see Winnington-Ingram 1960.176–77;
W. Barrett 1964.229–30; Willink 1968.14–17; Moline 1975.58–62; cf. Solmsen 1973.420–22.

stronger than the *daimones* as reckless hubris (οὐ γὰρ ἄλλο πλὴν ὕβρις / τάδ᾽ ἐστί, κρείσσω δαιμόνων εἶναι θέλειν, 474–75). The impossibility of fighting gods explains why rhetorical challenges to the "god" defense often secularize force: by casting the defendant as stronger or weaker than external pressures and internal passions, the accuser introduces the possibility of blame. Phaedra, surprisingly, seems to agree with a stance that locates the problem with the nature of the person, at least insofar as she energetically denounces those women who shame the beds of their husbands.[120] By appropriating the language of power and honor for herself, on the other hand, she inhabits the heroic, *masculine* position on pleasure so central to contemporary ethical debates.[121]

Nevertheless, in the end, Phaedra's long speech becomes a testament to the impossibility of striking at *erōs* through either silence or *sophrosunē*. Her opening lines make clear that even her current plan, starvation, cannot contain *erōs*.[122] The reason, we might say, is that her refusal to eat misses the mark, insofar as the unspeakable ills that she suffers do not belong to the body (which is why speaking about them to physicians, as the Nurse proposes early in the tragedy—"but, if your problem may be brought forth to men, speak, so that this matter might be revealed to doctors" [εἰ δ᾽ ἔκφορός σοι συμφορὰ πρὸς ἄρσενας, / λέγ᾽, ὡς ἰατροῖς πρᾶγμα μηνυθῇ τόδε, 295–96]—will do no good). They are unspeakable precisely because they exist within the realm of speech, even as they challenge the moral codes it helps uphold. Desire travels via language and images, making it a disease of the *phrēn*, the *kardia*, and the *psukhē*. The mouth that Phaedra needs to close, then, leads to a different kind of inner space, one that she has failed to master by willing herself into *sophrosunē* or by refusing food,[123] a space captured by a line already notorious in antiquity: "My hands are

---

[120] See also *Ba.* 314–18, where Tiresias refutes the claim that Dionysus makes women lascivious by arguing that a woman's chastity has nothing to do with the god: whether she transgresses in a Bacchic ritual depends, rather, on her *phusis*. The text is problematic, but the sense is clear. Kovacs prints: οὐχ ὁ Διόνυσος † σωφρονεῖν † ἀναγκάσει / γυναῖκας ἐς τὴν Κύπριν, ἀλλ᾽ ἐν τῇ φύσει / [τὸ σωφρονεῖν ἔνεστιν ἐς τὰ πάντ᾽ ἀεί] / τοῦτο· σκοπεῖν χρή· καὶ γὰρ ἐν βακχεύμασιν / οὖσ᾽ ἥ γε σώφρων οὐ διαφθαρήσεται. After Pentheus's assertion that the Bacchants are interested only in sex (221–25), we would expect Tiresias to say that Dionysus does *not* make women misbehave. In Stobaeus, a μή is inserted before σωφρονεῖν, and this may be the correct reading: see Kovacs 2003.122; cf. Dodds 1960.111–12.

[121] See Loraux 1979.

[122] The refusal to eat may have weight as a symbolic gesture related to ritual chastity (W. Barrett 1964.187; see also Kingsley 1995.350–52; Martinez 1995.342–43), as well as a medical resonance. The medical writers thought the female body had two mouths, the second being the *stoma* of the womb, which opened at puberty and was thought to close only in cases of pregnancy and ill health (Dean-Jones 1994.62, with n.70); the idea probably had its origins in folk belief (Armstrong and Hanson 1986). Phaedra's closing of one mouth may be, then, a symbolic reenactment of the sealing of the lower mouth.

[123] For the use of *stoma* with respect to dangerous speech or the secret, see 100, 498, 660, 882, 1060, 1167, 1412. On silence and starvation, see Rabinowitz 1986.130; Goff 1990.5; Sissa 1990a.60–62. For the dynamic between speech and silence in the play, see Knox 1952; Goff 1990; Montiglio 2000.233–38.

pure, but my *phrēn* holds some miasma" (χεῖρες μὲν ἁγναί, φρὴν δ' ἔχει μίασμά τι, 317; cf. *Or.* 1604).

But, although the *phrēn* does not coincide with the inside of the physical body, Euripides, in locating it beyond the reach of Phaedra's best intentions, casts it as a space analogous to the cavity, part of Phaedra and yet outside her control. Moreover, the disease that Phaedra harbors, *erōs*, bears similarities to the diseases that develop in the medical writers' cavity. Like peccant humors, for example, immoderate affections and attachments become dangerously entrenched in the soul. The Nurse, though she speaks in ignorance of Phaedra's true disease, remarks:

> χρῆν γὰρ μετρίας εἰς ἀλλήλους
> φιλίας θνητοὺς ἀνακίρνασθαι
> καὶ μὴ πρὸς ἄκρον μυελὸν ψυχῆς,
> εὔλυτα δ᾽ εἶναι στέργηθρα φρενῶν
> ἀπό τ᾽ ὤσασθαι καὶ ξυντεῖναι·

(E. *Hipp.* 253–57)

Mortals ought to mix a cup of affection toward one another in moderation and not reach the deepest marrow of the soul; but the loves of the *phrenes* should be easy to loosen, easy to push away and to bind together.

Of particular interest in the Nurse's remark is the expression "the marrow of the soul." In epic and early fifth-century tragedy, the word I translated "marrow," *muelos*, exhibits both "seen" (the marrow of the bones, *Il.* 20.482) and "felt" (vital force, A. *Ag.* 76) aspects. The medical writers, unsurprisingly, give the word a physical sense (bone nutrient, spinal fluid).[124] The single time Sophocles uses it, in the *Trachiniae*, it has a similarly "seen" meaning, describing Lichas's spattered brain (781). It may be because the word takes on such a physical connotation that Euripides can use it with a recognizably metaphorical sense in the *Hippolytus*, transferring it from the interior of the bones to the interior of the soul, which presumably has no *muelos*. Whereas emotion moves in an indifferently corporeal space in Homer and Aeschylus, here it lodges in a space only *like* the chambered, hidden world of *On the Tekhnē* that we saw at the beginning of chapter 3.

The innermost space of the soul is distinguished from the territory of the humors and their *pharmaka* because it is vulnerable to words and images, just as we saw in the texts in the previous chapter. It is when Phaedra is "touched" by the name of Hippolytus that she betrays her secret (310); the Nurse, in turn, is "struck" by her words (342). The pathway to Hippolytus's "virgin soul" is through the ear, which he longs to purge after the Nurse's revelation of Phaedra's desire (653–54). The figure of *erōs* as a force fed by words, thoughts, and

---

[124] *Carn.* 4 (Li 8.588 = 191,1–7 Joly); *Morb.* II 5 (Li 7.14 = 137,2–4 Jouanna). See also Guardasole 2000.91–97. On the affections that "bind hearts," see Burgess 2000.47, who reads the *phrenes* here in terms of contemporary physiological ideas about sinews and *harmonia*.

memories emerges most powerfully in the exchange that follows the two long speeches by Phaedra and the Nurse, an exchange in which the crisp positions on ethical agency and daemonic compulsion delineated in those speeches begin to blur together. The Phaedra who so boldly declares that no *pharmakon* can make her change her mind about the good turns out to be deathly afraid of the Nurse's "too beautiful words" (οἱ καλοὶ λίαν λόγοι, 487). Whereas, in her speech, she had claimed that one *chooses* pleasure over the good, she now fears that the Nurse's promise of pleasure will sway her in her already weakened state: because she has already been "plowed up" in her soul by *erōs* (ὑπείργασμαι μὲν εὖ / ψυχὴν ἔρωτι, 504–5), the wrong word might push her toward disease. As she tells the Nurse, "If you keep speaking beautifully about what is shameful, I will be fully spent on what I now flee" (τἀσχρὰ δ᾿ ἢν λέγῃς καλῶς, / ἐς τοῦθ᾿ ὃ φεύγω νῦν ἀναλωθήσομαι, 505–6). With the unusual verb *analiskomai*, "to be spent, to be consumed," Phaedra replaces the logic of ethical choice with an economy of force, leaving us to wonder whether the power she has invested in mastering desire will be diverted toward its satisfaction: having proved weaker than *erōs*, she would become complicit with it.

Phaedra's seduction by the Nurse, more than any Euripidean character's rhetorical defense of daemonic compulsion, brilliantly casts doubt on the viability of an ethics of desire predicated on simple self-mastery or knowledge of the good.[125] At the same time, the scene upholds the idea of the *psukhē* (or, here, also *phrēn*) as an intervallic space, that is, a space where outcomes are not necessary but sited at the convergence of multiple forces: entrenched *erōs*, Phaedra's attempts at resistance, the Nurse's seductive speech, and the very nature of a woman who comes from a long line of women cursed in love.[126] As in the *Orestes*, in the *Hippolytus* Euripides focuses not on the moment of daemonic attack but on the unfolding of the causal chain through Phaedra, dramatizing actions and reactions that confuse the relationship between compulsion, culpable error, and deliberate attempts at self-mastery. That uncertainty is the climate of Phaedra's fatal decision to allow the Nurse to seek a "*pharmakon*" for her disease, which turns out to be Hippolytus himself. For the scene is staged in such a way as to suggest that Phaedra both knows and does not know what the Nurse will do (518, 520) when she cloudily assents to her plea that she give up her self-destructive commitment to virtue (507–8). At the end of the play, Artemis, appearing *ex machina*, will declare that Phaedra "was destroyed by the stratagems of her nurse *unwillingly*" (τροφοῦ διώλετ᾿ οὐχ ἑκοῦσα μηχαναῖς, 1305).

[125] Phaedra's position in her *rhēsis* has been seen as Euripidean polemic against the Socratic Paradox: Dodds 1929.103; 1951.186–87; Snell 1964.59–69; Irwin 1983; Cairns 1993.322–23 n.214; Craik 1993.49. I find this thesis compelling, though ultimately unprovable. Cf. W. Barrett 1964.227–28; Claus 1972; Moline 1975. Pigeaud 1976 and C. Gill 1990a speak more generally of the relationship between self-knowledge in the *Hippolytus* and Plato's work; see also Wildberg 2006 on the evidence for, and implications of, interaction between Euripides and Socrates.
[126] On Phaedra's Cretan past, see Winnington-Ingram 1960.175–76; Reckford 1974; Goff 1990.37; Mills 1997.199–200.

The very simplicity of such an explanation, like the stark words of Apollo at the end of the *Orestes*, leaves those who have witnessed Phaedra's capitulation to keep reflecting on its complications.

DAEMONIC *PHUSIS*

The prologue of the *Hippolytus* rules out in advance the possibility of Phaedra conquering *erōs*. Yet the little bit of work that remains to Aphrodite (οὐ πόνου πολλοῦ με δεῖ, 23) becomes the tragic window of time in which we watch Phaedra struggle to carry out (ἐκπονοῦμεν, 381) the good in the face of *erōs*. We have seen that in her speech she adopts the (masculine) language of self-mastery to describe her battle with Aphrodite. Yet what gives the speech its power is its speaker's bitter recognition that the battle is already lost. Phaedra's hidden *erōs* makes her hatred of women who are chaste in words but audacious behind closed doors a form of self-hatred that has found its final expression in her attempt to induce an *apostasis* of her very life (ἀσιτεῖ δ' εἰς ἀπόστασιν βίου, 277). The medical writers, we can recall, use the term *apostasis* to describe the isolation and expulsion of corrupted humors. Deftly adopted by Euripides, it describes a life that can no longer be separated from the disease—it is only after Phaedra's suicide that she can be said to have "removed painful *erōs* from her *phrenes*" (ἀπαλλάσ- / σουσά τ' ἀλγεινὸν φρενῶν ἔρωτα, 774–75).[127] The deep entrenchment of disease in Phaedra yokes the timing of the play's first half to a process of revelation, which unveils (ἐξέφην', 428) not simply *erōs* but Phaedra herself as one of the "worst of mortals." Phaedra signals this process by invoking the figure of a young girl, a *parthenos*, before whom time sets up the mirror (428–30).[128] For what time eventually reveals to the *parthenos* is that she is, in fact, a woman, and a woman, as Phaedra declares, is a *misēma*, an "object of hatred," to all (407).

Women attract hatred, Phaedra indicates, precisely because they are enslaved to sexual pleasure. She appropriates the traditionally misogynist language of blame to excoriate women as traitors within the house, an invective that will be picked up by her stepson and hurled back at her. For, the moment Hippolytus learns of Phaedra's love, he launches into a long diatribe, cursing women as a great evil (627) in whom intelligence can be nothing more than a handmaiden

---

[127] See Kosak 2004.57, also observing the medical connection. The verbs ἀπαλλάσσω and especially ἀπαλλάσσομαι (with the genitive) are often used by the Hippocratics to describe either simply recovery or more specifically a patient "freeing" himself or his body from disease or symptoms, e.g., *Art.* 3 (Li 6.4 = 226,13–14 Jouanna); *Morb.* II 40 (Li 7.56 = 171,16 Jouanna); *Mul.* II 116 (Li 8.252); *Prorrh.* II 11 (Li 9.32 = 246 Potter).

[128] See esp. Zeitlin 1996.269–78, on the mirror's ability to grant the woman access to the image by which she is judged in the public domain. From this point, Zeitlin argues, Phaedra becomes the mirror image accessible to Hippolytus through which he learns the lesson of the divided self. For other readings of the mirror, see Pigeaud 1976; Luschnig 1988; Goff 1990.23–24, 72.

to sexual intemperance (643–44), a race whose wickedness is eternal (664–66). Elsewhere in the *Hippolytus*, women are given a nature that forecloses the mastery of desire. In the parodos, the Chorus laments the *dustropos harmonia*, the "ill-fitted composition," that makes women naturally (φιλεῖ) prone to helplessness and folly, *aphrosunē* (161–64)—a pun on Aphrodite that anticipates Hecuba's biting wordplay in the *Troades*.[129] Theseus later observes that licentiousness is innate (ἐμπέφυκεν) in women, presumably because Kupris "disturbs" (ταράξῃ) their *phrēn* as easily as she stirs that of a young man (966–70), a characterization that recalls the medical writers' depiction of female bodies as wetter and thus more "sensitive" to outside forces.[130] "If women are not *by nature* just," observes one Euripidean character, "why bother continuing to try to hold them in check? The whole thing is bound to fail" (fr. 1061K).

Negative views of women appear in our earliest Greek texts.[131] In recent years, moreover, the representation of women as prone to suffering and passion has been shown to play an important role in tragedy's interrogation of Athenian ideals of the male citizen self. As Froma Zeitlin and Nicole Loraux have argued, tragedy is fundamentally a genre that stages men's confrontation with the feminine, frequently in terms of suffering and bodily vulnerability.[132] Women are associated with bodily processes and the natural world in a number of cultures and historical periods.[133] Yet concepts like nature or "the body" are never given or stable, particularly, as we have seen, in late fifth-century Athens. I have argued that the emergence of the physical body, while not crowding out existing ideas about women's relationship to suffering, transforms the representational potential of the (mature) female body. In discussions of what women are "by nature," necessity is shifted from the gods to the fixity of nature. In chapter 4, I suggested that female bodies exaggerate the most troubling aspects of the physical body: its hidden inner space, its volatility and propensity toward disorder, its daemonic automatism, its openness to external influences, its need for

---

[129] The expression δύστροπος ἁρμονία works on multiple levels. The word ἁρμονία, "joint," in Homer (*Od.* 5.248), comes to play an important role in Presocratics like Heraclitus and Philolaus as "a principle that explains the connection between things that differ or are unlike" (Huffman 1993.139). Empedocles uses it to describe the principle that binds the elements in a composite body, e.g., DK31 B96.3–4; see further Ierodiakonou 2005.6–8. See also *Vict.* I 8 (Li 6.482 = 132,6 Joly-Byl, 132,8 Joly-Byl) and 9 (Li 6.482 = 132,13 Joly-Byl), where the word is used in the context of embryological development. The word δύστροπος is rare. It seems to mean something like "troublesome," as at Democr. (DK68) B100.

[130] See above, pp. 185–187. Carson 1990.138–43 discusses the relationship between wantonness and wetness; see also Just 1989.157–63 on women and sexual incontinence. For female folly (τὸ μῶρον) in tragedy, see also E. *Andr.* 674; *El.* 1035; *Hipp.* 644; *Tro.* 1059; fr. 331K (= *Dictys* fr. 5 J.-V.L.).

[131] See, e.g., Padel 1983; Carson 1990.

[132] Bodiliness defines woman, as Zeitlin argues, "in the cultural system that associates her with physical processes of birth and death and emphasizes the material dimensions of her existence" (1996.351). On the importance of the female body to the *Hippolytus*, see 237–57. Loraux 1995.37–43 stresses the importance of childbirth as a paradigm of tragic suffering; see also Holmes 2007.71–80.

[133] See Ortner 1974.

constant cleansing. They thus illustrate the threat posed by male bodies in the absence of technical mastery, not only to health but also to broader ideals of ethical subjectivity, particularly in classical Athens, a culture committed to the mastery of the self as the precondition of empire and the right to speak in the public sphere. The *Hippolytus*, too, seems to approach female nature as a model for the daemonism that is buried in human nature. The base helplessness lamented by the women of the Chorus as the lot of their sex (161–64) thus returns with a vengeance as the fate of Phaedra, most unfortunate of women, who, in the end, lacks a *tekhnē* to free herself from *erōs* (670–71).

When Phaedra appropriates the language of blame to attack *other* women as traitors within the home, she is trying to distance herself from them, to keep herself from becoming what her culture, her genealogy, and the tragic tradition demand that she be. Yet, in the end, she fails both to conquer her desire and to keep it secret—far from going unnoticed, her passion is memorialized in ritual. Should we read this failure as confirming the Nurse's speech on daemonic compulsion? Or is Aphrodite's power a means of channeling the weight of poetic tradition to eventually bring Phaedra in line with Euripides' other wanton women, a means, that is, of compelling her fidelity to the myth? Is Phaedra's capitulation an indictment of what looks like a contemporary ethical belief, perhaps associated with Socrates, that one can choose the good over the pleasurable? Or is Euripides being absurd in putting the discourse of self-mastery in the mouth of a woman, the paragon of intemperance?

The *Hippolytus* is far too rich a play to constrain us to a single line of interpretation. It is the nature of the symptom, after all, to foster the convergence of multiple interpretative frameworks—magico-religious, medical, ethical. Before leaving the *Hippolytus*, I would like to consider one more angle on daemonic *phusis*, one that encompasses not only Phaedra but Hippolytus as well. If Phaedra swears that Hippolytus "will learn *sophrosunē* by sharing in my disease" (τῆς νόσου δὲ τῆσδέ μοι / κοινῇ μετασχὼν σωφρονεῖν μαθήσεται, 730–31), what lesson does her experience model?[134]

One way of answering this question is to inquire into an intriguing detail in Phaedra's first entrance that is echoed at the end of the tragedy. When Phaedra first appears onstage, she commands her attendants to raise her up, "for," as she says, "I have been loosened in the binding together of my dear limbs" (λέλυμαι μελέων σύνδεσμα φίλων, 199). The word that I translated with both "my" and "dear," *philos*, is often used by Homer with parts of the self, not only the limbs but also *ētor* and *thumos*.[135] So common are such collocations that some mod-

---

[134] Phaedra's "lesson" is too complex to analyze in full here. See esp. Zeitlin 1996.219–84: the lesson of Aphrodite is an initiation into divided selfhood. Cf. Kurke 1999, critiquing Zeitlin for adopting a Snellian model of tragic subjectivity and, hence, failing to recognize "the Greek tragic self not as our origin and kin, but as alienated and different, intimately related to the materiality of practices" (336, with n.12). I am arguing that the concept of inner conflict in the *Hippolytus* is, indeed, shaped by practices—the practices of caring for the *sōma* and the *psukhē* in this period.

[135] E.g., *Il.* 5.155, 11.342, 20.412; *Od.* 14.405, 16.428. See also Hes. *Op.* 608.

ern commentators have posited a secondary, "possessive" meaning for the word in epic poetry. In recent years, however, others have challenged this meaning on both etymological and conceptual grounds. David Robinson has argued, for example, that parts of the self are naturally dear to their owner, particularly when they are threatened or suffering, as is the case in the majority of Homeric examples.[136] Phaedra's use of *philos* at the moment her limbs are in distress leads Robinson to classify this as a Homerism.[137]

Interestingly, the *Hippolytus* offers a second example of this "Homeric" use of *philos*, this time with respect to Hippolytus. With Hippolytus's death, *erōs*, which has long simmered beneath the surface of the tragedy, explodes into violence. Exiled and cursed by his father, Hippolytus is driving his mares along the beach when the monstrous bull of Poseidon charges out of the sea.[138] Just as the sight of Hippolytus is too powerful for Phaedra to resist, the bull is "stronger than any looks" (κρεῖσσον ... δεργμάτων, 1217), and a terrible, awesome fear falls on the horses. Once nourished at Hippolytus's hand, they suddenly threaten to destroy their master. He, in turn, straps his body into the leather thongs and pulls back against them, but he cannot check their frenzy of fear and also, perhaps, of desire.[139] The mares are driven this way and that until they capsize the chariot against a rock, at which point the distinction between master and mastered grows confused:

> αὐτὸς δ᾽ ὁ τλήμων ἡνίαισιν ἐμπλακεὶς
> δεσμὸν δυσεξέλικτον ἕλκεται δεθείς,
> σποδούμενος μὲν πρὸς πέτραις φίλον κάρα
> θραύων τε σάρκας, δεινὰ δ᾽ ἐξαυδῶν κλυεῖν.
>
> (E. *Hipp.* 1236–39)

And the wretched man himself, entangled in reins, bound in a hard-to-unravel bind, was dragged, smashing his dear head against the rocks and breaking his flesh, crying out things terrible to hear.

Hippolytus cries out to his mares not to destroy him. Yet nearly every participle in the messenger's report is in the active or the middle voice, with Hippolytus as its subject. To judge from the grammar, then, Hippolytus is destroying Hippolytus. Entangled in the reins he once used to control his horses, he ends up smashing himself against the rocks.[140]

---

[136] D. Robinson 1990. See also Hooker 1987.

[137] D. Robinson 1990.108.

[138] Segal 1978.138 reads the bull as a sign of paternal, phallic authority and repressed sexuality. See also Goff 1990.74–75.

[139] Mares often appear in erotic contexts, e.g., Anacr. fr. 346 (*PMG*); Sappho fr. 2 (L-P); Thgn. frr. 1249–52 (W²): see Zeitlin 1996.279–80.

[140] W. Barrett 1964.389 reads σποδούμενος in the middle voice, pointing to the parallel active participles. He supports his reading further by pointing to φίλος, which he takes in the "possessive" sense. D. Robinson 1990.108 sees φίλος at 1238 as a possible "Homeric" construction.

It is obvious that Hippolytus's head is in danger at the moment that it is called *philos*. The adjective may, then, capture the dearness of a part of the self as it comes under threat, as Robinson's analysis of the Homeric examples would suggest. Euripides' use of the word, however, may be more complex. He emphasizes the dearness of these parts at a moment when the danger posed to them comes from the subject himself as he loses control over himself. The adjective *philos*, which in Homer appears related to an external threat, may participate in the tragedy's general thematization of the threat posed by what is most intimate, a threat first signaled by the collapse of Phaedra's limbs ("the point," observes W. S. Barrett, "is that the familiar obedience of her own body has deserted her").[141] On the verge of revealing her secret, Phaedra tells the Nurse, "a *philos* is unwillingly destroying me, unwilling" (φίλος μ᾽ ἀπόλλυσ᾽ οὐχ ἑκοῦσαν οὐχ ἑκών, 319). While Hippolytus is the most obvious aggressor here, this intrafamilial violence also exists inside the self on account of the powerful, competing forces with which one dwells.[142] The uses of *philos* that bookend the *Hippolytus* thus trouble the difference between inside and outside, victim and aggressor, friendly and unfriendly, intimacy and alienation. The wrecked body dragged onstage at the end of the tragedy becomes a mirror that reveals the inner conflict hidden by Phaedra's apparently inviolate corpse, just as her disease had prefigured the struggle that time brings to light in Hippolytus's "virgin soul."[143]

What is particularly striking is that the most decisive acts of aggression against the self in the play do not arise from the erotic energies represented by Phaedra's delirious speech or Hippolytus's mares. Aggression erupts, rather, out of the tragic subject's efforts to control these energies. Phaedra's limbs collapse because she seeks to starve her disease of its power. Failing to quell it, she resorts to suicide, an act through which she forces body and voice to submit, once and for all, to the story that she wishes to tell of her *sophrosunē*. And while Hippolytus is dragged to the rocks by his frenzied mares, he is broken because, entrapped in his reins, he seems to turn on himself. The forces that wreck these characters not only express dangerous, subhuman energies that must be checked by reason or moderation, but encompass, too, the drive to mastery inherent in reason and moderation (a drive that looks forward to Pentheus in the *Bacchae*). The tragedy thus seems to cast the desire to resist Aphrodite as a force no less powerful and destructive than Aphrodite herself.

---

[141] W. Barrett 1964.200.

[142] Hippolytus "dwells with [ξυνοικῶν] horses' ways" (1219–20), much as resourcelessness is wont to dwell with (συνοικεῖν) the *discordia concors* of women (161–63).

[143] Euripides represents Hippolytus's suffering in terms that recall Phaedra's disease and female bodies more generally. The pains that "dart" or "shoot" (ᾄσσουσ᾽, 1351) through his head echo the breath that darts (ᾖξεν, 165) through the belly in pregnancy: see Loraux 1979; 1995.38–39; Zeitlin 1996.247–48, 351. Conversely, Phaedra tries to reclaim the bodily integrity of the *parthenos* in death—hanging was associated with virgins: see Loraux 1995.109–15; Zeitlin 1996.238–43; H. King 1998.80–84.

The Semantics of Suffering

The concept of disease in the *Hippolytus* is, as we have seen, highly overdetermined. While the body is not the primary locus of attention, Euripides, in scripting *erōs* as a disease, seems to be drawing on the conceptual resources being developed in contemporary medicine to describe the body: the triggering of disease by an external physical stimulus; the body's strange complicity in its destruction; the cavity as the origin of the symptom; and the entrenchment of the disease over time. Much like early proponents of a medical analogy, Euripides does not adopt these resources wholesale, but uses them to explore the daemonic recesses of the ethical subject. Unlike them, he seems skeptical about whether these recesses can be mastered and alert to the strange power of the desire for mastery itself. Nevertheless, he is not deaf to the ethical complexities created by the idea that we are implicated in the necessities of nature through our own natures. I close by examining how Euripides takes up the question of autarchy at the crossroads of different worldviews in the final scene of the *Heracles*.

Like Hippolytus, Euripides' Heracles finds his control over himself destroyed by the eruption of powerful daemonic forces after having been cast as a model of corporeal integrity. His autarchic identity is captured well by Amphitryon's description of his son as the consummate archer:

ἀνὴρ ὁπλίτης δοῦλός ἐστι τῶν ὅπλων	190
θραύσας τε λόγχην οὐκ ἔχει τῷ σώματι	193
θάνατον ἀμῦναι, μίαν ἔχων ἀλκὴν μόνον·	194
καὶ τοῖσι συνταχθεῖσιν οὖσι μὴ ἀγαθοῖς	191
αὐτὸς τέθνηκε δειλίᾳ τῇ τῶν πέλας.[144]	192
ὅσοι δὲ τόξοις χεῖρ' ἔχουσιν εὔστοχον,	195
ἐν μὲν τὸ λῷστον, μυρίους οἰστοὺς ἀφεὶς	
ἄλλοις τὸ σῶμα ῥύεται μὴ κατθανεῖν,	
ἑκὰς δ' ἀφεστὼς πολεμίους ἀμύνεται	
τυφλοῖς ὁρῶντας οὐτάσας τοξεύμασιν	
τὸ σῶμά τ' οὐ δίδωσι τοῖς ἐναντίοις,	
ἐν εὐφυλάκτῳ δ' ἐστί. τοῦτο δ' ἐν μάχῃ	
σοφὸν μάλιστα, δρῶντα πολεμίους κακῶς	
σῴζειν τὸ σῶμα, μὴ 'κ τύχης ὡρμισμένον.	

(E. *HF* 190–203)

The spearman is the slave of his weapons, since, breaking his spear, he is not able from his body to ward off death, having only a single defense; and on account of his fellow soldiers, if they are not brave, he dies himself, because of the cowardice of his neighbors. But the man whose hand can aim the bow well holds the one best

---

[144] 191–92 post 194 trai. Wilamowitz. The transposition has been accepted by recent editors (Diggle, Kovacs), but see Renehan 1985.151–52 and Kovacs 2003.169–71 for the difficulties with the passage.

thing: having shot a thousand arrows, by others still he protects his body from death; positioned at a distance, he guards himself against enemies who, though they are looking, are wounded by unseen arrows, and he does not betray his body to his opponents, but keeps it well protected. This, in battle, is the wisest plan: while harming your enemies, to safeguard your body, unmoored to *tukhē*.

The bow allows Heracles to wound without being wounded, to attack the many without needing the many for protection.[145] Amphitryon's description of the archer who controls the fates of others, not through force but through an epistemic advantage, recalls the discussion of archers in chapter 1, where we saw that the asymmetrical relationship of the archer to his victim mimics the asymmetry between mortals and immortals that is part of what enables the gods to inflict pain.[146] To the extent that the wound caused by the unseen arrow arises from a place unobserved and unassailable, it is like the damage caused by gods, that is, the symptom. But, on Amphitryon's view, the archer himself, equated with a *sōma* outside the martial law of reciprocity and beyond the reach of *tukhē*, does not suffer symptoms. He is fully autarchic.[147]

Euripides' Heracles is a strikingly unfamiliar take on a familiar myth. In the mythic and poetic tradition, Heracles is virtually synonymous with what is eventually seen as his body—its strength, but also its appetites, labors, suffering, and passions.[148] It is not surprising, then, that the only two tragedies known to have featured Heracles as a protagonist, Sophocles' *Trachiniae* and Euripides' *Heracles*, construct his tragic identity through the figure of disease, thereby placing his body, with its enormous capacity to inflict and suffer pain, center stage. Yet the two tragedians represent Heracles and his disease in markedly different ways. Sophocles' Heracles is preceded onstage by legends of boundless

---

[145] For Heracles as an archer, see also 179, 366–67, 392, 422–24, 472–73, 571. Some attribute the prominence of archery to recent military events, but Foley 1985.169 n.43 rightly insists on the importance of literary *topoi* of the archer (for Heracles as an archer in myth: *Il.* 5.392–404; *Od.* 8.225, 11.601–26). For discussion of these *topoi* in the *Heracles*, see Foley 1985.169–75; Hamilton 1985; Michelini 1987.242–46; Padilla 1992; George 1994; Cerri 1997.241–44; Dunn 1997.96–98; Papadopoulou 2005.137–51. At the same time, we can assume that the idea of an archer Heracles underwent changes over time: Cohen 1994, for example, argues that representations of Heracles as an archer were largely suppressed after the Persian Wars in favor of representations of him with a club.

[146] See above, pp. 49–51. Euripides regularly associates the τοξ- stem with the gods (Padilla 1992.3). On the godlike status of Heracles *qua* archer, see Padilla 1992; George 1994.

[147] Cf. Th. 2.41–42, for whom it is the citizen-hoplite who is autarchic (αὐτάρκης) insofar as he freely consigns his *sōma* to *tukhē* on the battlefield. See also 1.70. On Heracles' autarchy, see Wilamowitz 1909.127–28; Rohdich 1968.80–81; Desch 1986.13–14; Cerri 1997.237–41; Griffiths 2002. Papadopoulou 1999.303 sees the first part of the play as setting up "the idea of the sovereignty of the subject."

[148] Heracles was always defined by his physical strength: in epic he is referred to as βίη Ἡρακληείη (e.g., *Il.* 2.658; Hes. *Th.* 289), and he could later represent the law of might makes right (Pl. *Grg.* 484b1–c3). On the various diseases associated with Heracles, see von Staden 1992d; see also Filhol 1989. His diseases may explain why he was a popular cult healer: see above, chapter 1, n.169. On his appetites and his belly, see Loraux 1995.124, 297 n.42.

passions and enslavement: Omphale, the queen whom Heracles was compelled to serve, is mentioned early on (*Tr.* 69–70, 252–57), as is the murder of Iphitas (38), thus preparing the way for a hero vanquished by his diseased love for Iole (488–89) and the murder of Lichas (777–82).[149] His labors are couched as service to another man.[150] His strength comes from the stalwart hands, back, chest, and arms that he apostrophizes as the erstwhile conquerors of monsters when they are finally devoured by *atē* (1089–1100; cf. 1046–47).[151] Conversely, the Heracles who dominates the first half of Euripides' tragedy is a civilizer and a savior. In the prologue, Amphitryon says his labors were motivated by filial piety (17–18); these "noble" labors (γενναίων . . . πόνων, 357) are said to tame and purify the earth (20, 225–26, 698–700, 851–52), bringing freedom and calm in their wake (221, 400–402). Euripides' Heracles is thus closer to sophistic reassessments of the hero, which emphasized the labors as freely chosen and civilizing, than to the archaic warrior.[152] Moreover, although Heracles' threatened revenge against Lycus gives us a glimpse of his antinomian tendencies, his passions are initially withheld from view. His relationship to Megara exudes domesticity, rather than *erōs*, and when his wife does mention the sack of Oechalia (473), she is silent about Iole. Finally, whereas, in the *Trachiniae*, Heracles fights with bare hands, in the *Heracles* he relies on a hand with good aim (χεῖρ' . . . εὔστοχον, 195), a sign of efficacious agency. Indeed, the villain Lycus charges that Heracles used nets, rather than his own arms, to catch the hydra and the Nemean lion (151–54)—*tekhnē*, that is, in place of raw strength.[153] The Euripidean hero's intelligent mastery of bestial threats to calm and civilization thus implies self-mastery. The Heracles of the play's first half recalls the hero of the Prodikean Choice, who rejects his trademark pleasures to pursue a life of virtue, submitting his *sōma* to *gnōmē* and a rigorous regimen.[154] He who brings freedom to the peoples of the world is the slave of no one and nothing.

---

[149] On *erōs* and *nosos* in the play, see Vasquez 1972.349–50; Holt 1981; Ryzman 1993; Schlesier 1993.106; Wohl 1998.6–11. On disease in the play more generally, see Biggs 1966; Ceschi 2003.

[150] The verb is λατρεύω (34–35; cf. 70, 357, 830): see Jourdain-Annequin 1985.497–522; Loraux 1995.120–21.

[151] On devouring pain, see also *Tr.* 769–71, 778, 805, 831–40, 987, 999, 1010, 1053–57, 1083–84, 1253–54. On devouring diseases in tragedy, see Jouanna 1988a; 1990a; Guardasole 2000.240–49. On the brute strength of Heracles' hands in the play, see also 488, 517, 1047, 1089, 1102, 1133.

[152] On the trend toward moralizing and humanizing Heracles in the latter part of the fifth century, see Woodford 1966; Kuntz 1994 (on Prodicus). Amphitryon does speak of Heracles as being mastered by Hera or necessity in undertaking the labors (20–21); see also 387–88, 580 (references to serving Eurystheus). Yet characters do not speak of Heracles as enslaved, nor is Omphale mentioned. The opposition freedom-slavery is played out, rather, between Lycus and the Thebans (e.g., 251, 270), which strengthens the portrait of Heracles as a liberator of the city.

[153] For similar rationalizations of mythic heroism, see Papadopoulou 2005.135–37.

[154] On Heracles' Choice, see X. *Mem.* 2.1.21–34, esp. 28: εἰ δὲ καὶ τῷ σώματι βούλει δυνατὸς εἶναι, τῇ γνώμῃ ὑπηρετεῖν ἐθιστέον τὸ σῶμα καὶ γυμναστέον σὺν πόνοις καὶ ἱδρῶτι (if you wish to be powerful in body, then you must submit the body to the mind and train with labor and sweat). Although Xenophon's telling of the story owes much to the thematic concerns of the *Memorabilia*, it

Euripides' brilliant plotting in the *Heracles*, however, creates a loophole in his hero's civilizing career. By having Heracles stable the monstrous guardian of the underworld, Cerberus, at Hermione in order to return to Thebes, he leaves just enough space to introduce Hera's series-canceling "last labor" (1279). Euripides seems to correlate Heracles' success until this point with the protection of his *sōma*, a word that appears four times in quick succession in Amphitryon's paean to the archer. Indeed, Heracles realizes that the boundaries of his *sōma* have been breached when, awaking from his madness, he sees his scattered arrows, which before stood by his arms and preserved his flanks (ἃ πρὶν παρασπίζοντ᾽ ἐμοῖς βραχίοσιν / ἔσῳζε πλευρὰς, 1099–1100). Protected by his arrows, Heracles' body had been invulnerable. He wakes up in a world transformed by its violation.

With the arrival of Lussa, the Heracles of myth—the hero who suffers, the hero open to daemonic arrows, the hero enslaved—is introduced in a single stroke. Having entered the house confident in his powers, Heracles returns as a figure crumpled in sleep, his hands bound to a column fragment. As it was for Hippolytus, tragedy is a lesson in suffering. Yet, in the closing scene of the play, this lesson is open to multiple interpretations, interpretations that are not easily classified by the adjectives "religious" and "secular." As Heracles begins to try to make sense of the "new thing" (τι καινόν, 1118) inscribed into his life, his guest-friend Theseus arrives and, hearing of Heracles' plight, invites him to settle in Athens. The scene has long been celebrated for its valorization of friendship between men, its image of a benevolent and enlightened Athens, and its bitter-sweet humanism.[155] Heracles can be recuperated as an Athenian hero only if he trades his dead sons for civic sons and disavows his "feminine" suffering—in short, if he forgets his encounter with the daemonic.[156] Through his mourning and his fixation on *miasma*, however, Heracles makes visible his resistance to Theseus's solution. In the struggle for closure, the last scene of the *Heracles* dramatizes how the meaning of tragic suffering can gain in complexity and richness through the crossing of interpretive paradigms.

Heracles' madness arrives and departs suddenly. Yet its eruption transforms the life to be lived henceforth. The final scene exhibits a cyclical structure— Heracles laments, recovers, and laments again, before departing—that seems to restage disease as a struggle with *lupē*.[157] This struggle, though visible in his

---

seems clear that the Prodikean Choice placed Heracles' infamous body in the service of ethical, mind-based *aretē* and assimilated the labors to the practice of such virtue.

[155] For readings that view Heracles' incorporation into the *polis* in a quasi-Hegelian light, see Foley 1985.165–67, 174–75, 192–200 (though see 199–200 on "remaining contradictions"); Mills 1997.129–59, esp. 145–46; Worman 1999.102–3; Assaël 2001.184–86. See also the optimistic reading at Griffiths 2002.655–56 and the bibliography at Schlesier 1985.32 n.87. Cf. Pucci 1980.182–87; Dunn 1997. For what I mean by humanism, see Holmes 2008.232 n.3.

[156] This is a particularly fascinating situation if we remember that Heracles played this role for Admetus in Euripides' *Alcestis* more than twenty years earlier, counseling him to lay aside his excessive grief (794) and accept the gift of a *xenos*: see esp. *Alc.* 1077–87. On the two Heracles, see Fitzgerald 1991.

[157] For *lupē* and *nosos*, see E. fr. 1071K: λῦπαι γὰρ ἀνθρώποισι τίκτουσιν νόσους (for sorrows breed sufferings diseases for humans); see also frr. 1070K, 1079K. Elsewhere in Euripides, *lupē* corrodes

initial exchanges with Theseus, surfaces at the moment Heracles returns to the point in his labors where he had left off before the start of the tragic action. Having left Hades' hound Cerberus at Hermione, Heracles had been free to summon Lussa's dogs (860) for his mad "trip" to Mycenae. At the end of the play, he must undertake that trip again in order to complete his labors, this time in reality. Yet his sense of distance from the former Heracles is palpable. He is anxious about going to Mycenae alone, "lest, bereft of my sons, I suffer something on account of my sorrow" (λύπῃ τι παίδων μὴ πάθω μονούμενος, 1388). Is Heracles worried that *lupē* will overtake him as madness once did, exposing him to Cerberus's power? Is he fearful at the possibility that he is no longer able to tame the forces of Hades, whose Bacchant he has now been?[158] Sorrow threatens to bind him to suffering, to keep him open to forces he cannot control.

These forces appear, in fact, to be resurging right before our eyes. Having expressed his fear of *lupē*, Heracles suddenly turns away from Theseus and exhorts the city to grieve with him (κείρασθε, συμπενθήσατ᾽, 1390). By using a *sun-* compound with the Thebans instead of reciprocating the inclusive civic language used earlier by Theseus (1202), Heracles establishes an alliance proper to women—for there are no women left to mourn. His lament is cut short by Theseus, who demands that he get up and put an end to his tears (1394, 1398). Theseus's demand is spoken in the name of *philia*, "friendship," which is presented in the final scene as the panacea for Heracles' ills, offering an alternative to actual death, that is, Heracles' threatened suicide, as well as to the symbolic death of heroic identity. By promising to restore Heracles' *timē* and, together with it, the old culture hero, Theseus answers Heracles' argument that his misfortunes will isolate him from the civilized and even the natural worlds (1281–1302). At the same time, Theseus recognizes that *philia* must strategically counter the threat posed by *lupē* to heroic autarchy. Faced with the resurgence of Heracles' grief, Theseus tries to steer his friend in the direction of Athens.

Yet *philia* does not resolve the tragedy's problems so easily. Even after Heracles has accepted Theseus's offer of support, named him as a surrogate son, and begun to move again in the direction of Athens, his movement forward stalls. Amphitryon, saying goodbye, praises Athens as a land *euteknos*, "lucky in sons," as Thebes manifestly is not; Heracles, like Orestes hearing of his mother and his aunt, is struck by his father's words and, stopping in his tracks, he demands to see the corpses of his own sons again.[159] Looking upon the dead is literally a

---

the *phrenes* (*Hel.* 1192); the *kardia* is bitten by it (*Alc.* 1100); it may induce a chill (*Hipp.* 803). It is among the self-diagnoses Orestes offers (*Or.* 398). In Sophocles' *Ajax*, *lupē* extends the hero's madness: both are described with *nosos*-language (59, 66, 271, 274, 452, 625, 635; see also 581). On the *Ajax* in relation to the *Heracles*, see Barlow 1981. For *lupē* in the medical writers, see, e.g., *Acut. Sp.* 40 (Li 2.476, ch. 16 = 87,11–12 Joly); *Hum.* 9 (Li 5.488 = 80 Jones).

[158] On the pervasiveness of Hades and the forces of Night in the tragedy, see Assaël 1994.

[159] On Thebes as an "anti-Athens," see Zeitlin 1990, though she does not include Heracles in her analysis on the grounds that he is a Panhellenic hero and, hence, insufficiently Theban (144 n.16).

turning back (πάλιν με στρέψον, 1406), which can explain why Theseus balks at Heracles' request, asking, "Why? Will this charm [φίλτρον] make you feel better?"[160] Heracles' response, "I long to," confirms the magnetism of *lupē* and the threat that it poses to tragic closure. His desire to embrace his father again recalls Amphitryon's earlier, lyric supplication of Heracles (1203–13), which had been superseded by Theseus's measured argumentation against suicide, threatening to undo the "yoke of friendship" (ζεῦγός γε φίλιον, 1403) that Theseus had forged with Heracles *qua* hero.

Heracles' desire to see his sons and embrace his father attests the tenacity of his refusal to forget his misfortune. Faced with this resistance, Theseus tries to force his friend to remember differently: "Have you no longer any memory of your labors?" (οὕτω πόνων σῶν οὐκέτι μνήμην ἔχεις; 1410).[161] Yet Heracles answers Theseus's demand by defiantly investing the word *ponos* with the weight of his suffering (1411; cf. 1279–80), leading the Athenian king to charge him with "being womanly" (θῆλυν ὄντ', 1412)—an accusation for which evidence has been building from the moment the Heracleian body first erupted into visibility, through Heracles' Bacchic frenzy, his subjection to a goddess, his covering of his head, and his tears and lamentation.[162] The conflation of blame, suffering, and female nature turns the ideal of the earlier Heracles, the autarchic civilizer, on its head. What is surprising is *this* Heracles' resistance to Theseus's logic: "Does my life seem lowly to you? Yet it did not seem so before" (ζῶ σοι ταπεινός; ἀλλὰ πρόσθεν οὐ δοκῶ, 1413). When Theseus responds, "The famous Heracles did not suffer [νοσῶν],"[163] Heracles invites his friend to remem-

---

Cf. Bernardini 1997, arguing against a clear Thebes-Athens opposition in the play (though he is focused on the *polis* itself); Cerri 1997.

[160] A φίλτρον is a "love charm" (e.g., E. *Andr.* 207; *Hipp.* 509; *IT* 1182), something that incites love and affection. Children provoke such attachments, which may be fierce (e.g., E. fr. 103K = *Alcmene* fr. 17 J.-V.L.): the corpse of the fallen son is an ἄγαλμα for the mother (*Supp.* 370–71; cf. 69–70, 941–46). For Theseus as *iatros*, see Kosak 2004.172–73, who notes that "to feel better" (ῥάων εἶναι) in the medical writers concerns treatment that may ease pain but does not cure the disease.

[161] Bond 1981.417–18 argues that 1410–17 should fit between 1253 and 1254, noting the jarring tone they create at the end; cf. Michelini 1987.260–62. Bond's means of explaining them at the end is to emphasize Heracles' delay tactic and to assume excessive lamentation between father and son, but he is uncomfortable with this reading—hence, the suggested transposition. Yet both aspects of this explanation, the delaying and the lamentation, are central to the final scene. The prolonged farewell participates in Heracles' overall feminization: see E. fr. 362K (= *Erechtheus* fr. 19.32–34 J.-V.L.).

[162] The feminization of the Sophoclean Heracles has received far more attention: Faraone 1994; Pozzi 1994; Loraux 1995.39–42, 53–58; Zeitlin 1996.350; Wohl 1998.6–11. See Loraux 1995.116–39 on the feminized Heracles more generally. See also Sourvinou-Inwood 2003.367–68 on the *Heracles*. On Bacchic frenzy and women, see Schlesier 1993. As is well known, Plato makes the indulgence of grief and excessive lamentation feminine types of behavior, which should not be imitated by men on the tragic stage (*R.* 3, 395d5–e2; see also Archil. frr. 11, 13 W²). On the political marginalization of mourning women, see Foley 1993 (in tragedy); Loraux 1998 (more generally).

[163] ὁ κλεινὸς Ἡρακλῆς οὐκ εἶ νοσῶν [οὐκ εἶ νοσῶν Wilamowitz: ποῦ κεῖνος ὤν L].

ber the misfórtune he himself suffered in Hades ("What were you like when you were in trouble underground?" σὺ ποῖος ἦσθα νέρθεν ἐν κακοῖσιν ὤν; 1415). Theseus is forced to confess his own lapsed masculinity (ἥσσων ἀνήρ, 1416), leading Heracles to a final question—"How, then, can you say that I am reduced by my ills?" (πῶς οὖν †ἔτ᾽ εἴπῃς† ὅτι συνέσταλμαι κακοῖς; 1417)—that Theseus is unable to answer. He responds only with a command: "Move onward!" (πρόβαινε).

Heracles' refusal to disavow his sufferings not only challenges Theseus's civic model of ethical subjectivity. It unsettles, too, how Theseus understands the place of the gods in Heracles' misfortune. Earlier, struggling against his friend's attempt to shift culpability to Hera, Heracles declares: "God, if he is truly god, needs nothing" (δεῖται γὰρ ὁ θεός, εἴπερ ἔστ᾽ ὀρθῶς θεός, / οὐδενός, 1345–46),[164] a sentiment that evokes ideas about the gods found in the fragments of Xenophanes and contemporary thinkers.[165] Although he questions the gods' desire as a cause and refuses to see himself as a legitimate target of divine anger (1310), Heracles cannot be said to be advocating a secular explanation of his suffering, if by this we mean an account consistent with contemporary medical and ethical concepts of diseased bodies and souls. One point of difference worth noting is Heracles' commitment to the idea of *miasma*.[166]

Let us begin by considering Theseus's stance on *miasma*. For, quite surprisingly, he denies it any power, mocking the hooded Heracles' attempts to protect him from pollution—at one point, he even invites him to smear blood on his cloak (ἔκμασσε, φείδου μηδέν, 1400). But what is it exactly that Theseus is denying? In response to Heracles' initial resistance to making potentially polluting

---

[164] These lines have been very troublesome, particularly for critics committed to defending the divine nature of Heracles' madness. Some have credited them to the playwright speaking *in propria persona*. See Greenwood 1953.64–91; A. Brown 1978; cf. Halleran 1986.173; Michelini 1987.275–76; Lawrence 1998.132–33. Others have dismissed the lines as the ad hoc arguments of a desperate man. Bond, for example, is adamant that they not be logically connected to anything else in the play, namely, Heracles' birth or Hera's anger (1981.399). See also Gregory 1977.273–74; Burnett 1985.174–77. Cf. Halleran 1986.177–80; Lawrence 1998.130–31. Still others have seen Heracles' words as expressing mere disapproval, rather than outright rejection, e.g., Stinton 1976.82–84; Foley 1985.163–65. Yunis 1988.157–66, for example, argues that, while the existence of a being Hera is not in doubt, Heracles refuses to acknowledge her as a god; see also Desch 1986; Papadopoulou 2005.114–16; cf. Lawrence 1998.136–37. For a more detailed discussion of these various interpretations, see Lawrence 1998. On my reading, the force of these lines cannot be neutralized. My sympathies are thus with the readings offered by Kroeker 1938.100–102, 122–24; Arrowsmith 1956; Lawrence 1998.138–46.

[165] See Xenoph. (DK21) B11; A32 (= [Plut.] *Strom.* 4), cited at Bond 1981.400, with further references. At X. *Mem.* 1.4.10–11, the idea that the gods need nothing from us is part of the standard position for a critic of traditional religion.

[166] Although Theseus does say he will purify Heracles of *miasma* at Athens (1324), he mentions this almost as a technicality: it is his disregard for pollution that is dramatically effective. In rites of purification, the washing off of the blood would be followed by appeasement: see R. Parker 1983.107–8. On Hippocratic notions of *miasma*, see above, chapter 3, n.45.

contact with his guest-friend, he says, "There is no *alastōr* for *philoi* from *philoi*" (οὐδεὶς ἀλάστωρ τοῖς φίλοις ἐκ τῶν φίλων, 1234). The *alastōr* in archaic and classical Greek culture is the one who refuses to forget, nonoblivion, the figure of perpetual mourning and perpetual anger, victim and avenger.[167] Clytemnestra, emerging from the palace with Agamemnon's blood on her hands, sees herself as the *alastōr* of the house of Atreus (A. *Ag.* 1501); Oedipus announces in the *Oedipus as Colonus*, a tragedy that looks forward to the decimation of the last generation of Labdacids, that he will forever reign as an *alastōr* in Thebes (S. *OC* 788). Each is an *alastōr* for *philoi* from *philoi*. But among *philoi* in the *polis*, Theseus insists, there is no *alastōr*. He thus ejects those forces that compel a return to tragic trauma both from the city and from *philia* among men.

Theseus's "enlightened" approach to *miasma* would appear to contradict his belief in vengeful gods. The apparent incoherence of his position, however, makes it clear that tragedy never adopts one worldview (divine-mythic or "secular") over another but, rather, plays them off of one another to explore their implications. Theseus's strategy turns out to make perfect sense. He is interested, after all, in extricating Heracles from what he has done, thereby recovering the identity of the civilizing hero as it stood before being resignified by his perverted labor.[168] Theseus isolates the disease from the divine in such a way that the cause falls to the gods—the war is Hera's (1189)—but the effects cannot touch them: "You, being mortal, cannot stain divine things" (οὐ μιαίνεις θνητὸς ὢν τὰ τῶν θεῶν, 1232).[169] The crime is thus liberated from the body that commits it. Theseus works to externalize *tukhai* in order that they might be exchanged like honors within the mutual support system of *philia* without interfering in the construction of the public self. In such a world, there is no *alastōr*, because the divine cannot be stained and, hence, forced to remember.

Heracles' position shows the same surface incoherence as Theseus's. By insisting that "god, if he is truly god, needs nothing," he challenges the logic of divine anger and retribution. But were we to attribute a doctrine of "enlightened" theology to Heracles, it would appear incompatible with his belief in *miasma*. Here again, however, Euripides creates a perspective on symptoms that cuts across our analytical categories. Heracles, like Phaedra, refuses to blame the gods for his misfortune. Yet, like her, he also refuses to give up blame altogether, as Gorgias seems to suggest might be possible in a mechanistic world where souls chance upon the wrong words and images. In its disregard for intentionality, the "regressive" notion of *miasma* manages to bridge two worlds by ac-

---

[167] Loraux 1998.99–102. On the active and passive dimensions of *alastōr*, see R. Parker 1983.108–9; Jouanna 2003.63–64.

[168] Theseus continues to recognize the gods, on the one hand, in order to demonstrate the impossibility of resisting *tukhē*, an argument familiar from the Nurse's attempts to keep Phaedra alive in the *Hippolytus* (433–81). On the other hand, he uses them to eliminate human responsibility altogether, a position familiar from the *Troades* and other Euripidean plays.

[169] See also S. *Ant.* 1041–44; cf. *OT* 1424–28. See Bond 1981.376, who sees in Theseus's answer a "new rationalistic spirit"; R. Parker 1983.145–46.

commodating the helplessness of a body caught in a causal chain alongside the need to make someone pay for the damage.[170] *Miasma*, in other words, may be working here as physical stuff that remembers human crimes and suffering. To give it up would be to concede that the daemonic has no bearing on the human, the impersonal on the personal—that the deaths of Heracles' wife and sons are without meaning.[171] By memorializing these deaths, *miasma* inscribes them into a physical economy where humans have value over and above the sum of their elements. Clinging to the hands, *miasma* insists on human responsibility despite the instrumentalization of those hands by inhuman force.

It is a delicate task to assign responsibility to an event occurring at the intersection of the human and the inhuman. Yet the pressure to do so is overwhelming when someone gets hurt.[172] On the face of things, there is no difference between calling the inhuman Aphrodite or *erōs*, Apollo or bile, Zeus or "the hot." Nevertheless, I have sought to show how the friction between self and other grows stronger and more problematic as contemporary concepts of cause, disease, and embodiment enter the tragic vocabulary. By staging tragedies like *Heracles*, *Hippolytus*, *Orestes*, and *Troades*, Euripides asks what it means for us to be intimately implicated in an order that is indifferent to the distinctions between what is good and what is shameful. The unhinging of this order from a logic of cosmic justice sensitive to human wrongdoing and goodness leaves uncertain what might be learned from suffering.

What is perhaps most powerful in so many of these tragedies is their eventual uncoupling of responsibility and blame. In the *Heracles*, remembering the rift created by the symptom, together with the trauma it leaves behind, undermines the heroic subject of the play's first half. Nevertheless, in the final scene of the tragedy, Heracles resists the urge to recover a sense of autarchic integrity through calculated amnesia or the displacement of blame. He rejects, that is, both the forgetfulness of becoming that Socrates believes can make one godlike in the *Philebus* and the feminization of vulnerability that comes to structure the ethical tradition—the subject *qua* master and the subject *qua* symptom. He challenges the physicians, too, and their beliefs in the power of the *tekhnē* to manage *tukhē*. This is not to say that Heracles repudiates technical agency. At the end of the tragedy, he picks up the arrows that he once believed could ward off death. In doing so, however, he recognizes the arrows' indifference to ends. He recognizes, too, the limits to his field of vision, outside which lie not only the Lussas and the Heras of myth, but also the ceaseless exchanges and negotiations of a world as indifferent to human greatness as to the death of a child. In such a world, reclaiming responsibility can be understood as simply the pursuit of

---

[170] On the absence of intention in *miasma*, see Adkins 1960.86–115; R. Parker 1983.111; Williams 1993.59–60.

[171] Compare S. *El*. 245–50: if the dead are no more than "earth and nothingness" (γᾱ τε καὶ οὐδὲν), then the reverence and piety (αἰδὼς . . . τ᾽ εὐσέβεια) of mortals is lost.

[172] Williams 1993.70.

meaning adequate to the complexity of suffering. What must be recognized, however, is that this challenge to create meaning takes shape in different ways in response to contemporary perceptions of the causes of suffering. Euripidean tragedy powerfully attests how generative the physical body had become for questions of suffering and ethical subjectivity in the late fifth century.

Near the beginning of Plato's *Timaeus*, the dialogue's eponymous narrator sets out to describe how the world was created. After going on about the creation of the world *sōma*, he realizes that he is mixed up. Naturally, he says, the divine demiurge did not make the *sōma* before the *psukhē*, the younger before the older, the ruled before the ruler. Timaeus blames his confusion on the fact that we are subject to chance, inhabiting bodies whose participation in a haphazard world casts our words adrift, skewing the stories we tell (34b10–35a1).

Over the course of this book, I have defended the possibility that in "erring" Timaeus may be closer to a likely story than he believes. Whereas most accounts of the development of dualism in fifth-century Greece have focused attention on the soul, I have argued that the emergence of the physical body as a conceptual object plays a significant role in shaping the notions of soul and ethical subjectivity that become central to dualism in the West. The crux of my argument has been that the physical body is not an ahistorical thing that the Greeks eventually learn to think past. Rather, as the *sōma* comes to be "seen" as a physical thing and, more specifically, as the impersonal and largely unfelt substratum of the human being, the question of where it meets the person (or the soul or the mind) is invested with increasing significance and urgency.

In emphasizing the importance of mental seeing, I am not saying that the physical body is a historical or cultural construction. Indeed, some experience of dualism, or at least our sense of ourselves as physical objects distinct from the awareness of a conscious field, is probably part of being human. My claim, rather, has been that the idea of human nature begins to encompass an unseen previously allied with the divine and the daemonic under particular conceptual and historical conditions. Having incorporated much of this unseen world, the physical body becomes a site of inhuman otherness within the self. At the same time, it begins to shape the understanding of the self in its full spectrum of traits and faculties. "Seen" as such, it acquires significant conceptual, imaginative, and cultural power.

In telling this story, I have paid particular attention to naturalizing medicine in the classical period. My interest is due in part to the fact that the medical writers give us access to the kinds of ideas and claims that were being vigorously debated about human nature, the body, and disease in the late fifth and early fourth centuries, thereby allowing us to see how the causes of suffering were being realized through impersonal stuffs and forces. It is difficult to know, of course, how deeply these ideas and claims had penetrated the Greek-speaking world in this period, and even more difficult to gauge the impact they had on how people experienced their bodies. It is hard not to suspect, with Plato, that a carpenter would have had no time for the recommendations of *On Regimen*. But regardless of the social impact of naturalizing medicine in the ancient Mediterranean world, its conceptual impact was shaped by its aspirations not only to *think* about the physical body but also to *act* on it and to cultivate authority for those actions. The body that appears in medicine's field of vision is understood not only as an object of knowledge but also an object of control, both in disease and, increasingly in the fifth century, in health. The idea of control emphasizes that the body is an economy of forces governed by laws and, hence, subject to technical agency. It also points to the need to manage this potentially dangerous part of us. Taken together, these two aspects lay the groundwork for new forms of ethical subjectivity and, more specifically, an ethics of care. The possibility of taking responsibility for the body reconfigures the social and ethical meanings of disease. At the same time, because it is so difficult to know where the physical body turns into the person, disease destabilizes the very ideas of praise and blame.

These complications unfold from a physiological-medical approach to human nature. Yet they are not elaborated by the medical writers—at least from what we can see. They arise, rather, as thinkers outside medicine develop the concept of the mind or the soul within the context of a medical analogy that assumes there are diseases specific to the soul, often understood in terms of false belief and desire. By displacing the possibility of daemonic disorder to the soul itself, thinkers like Plato and Democritus make the need for practices of care all the more urgent. But despite the shift to the soul, the physical body remains present as both a model object of care—by turns daemonic and docile—and, at least at times in Plato, the origin of psychic disorder.

We can get a sense of the influential and complex role of the physical body in the developing ethics of care by looking at two medical analogies from a famous discussion in Aristotle's *Nicomachean Ethics*:

ἔτι δ' ἄλογον τὸν ἀδικοῦντα μὴ βούλεσθαι ἄδικον εἶναι ἢ τὸν ἀκολασταίνοντα ἀκόλαστον. εἰ δὲ μὴ ἀγνοῶν τις πράττει ἐξ ὧν ἔσται ἄδικος, ἑκὼν ἄδικος ἂν εἴη, οὐ μὴν ἐάν γε βούληται, ἄδικος ὢν παύσεται καὶ ἔσται δίκαιος. οὐδὲ γὰρ ὁ νοσῶν ὑγιής. καὶ εἰ οὕτως ἔτυχεν, ἑκὼν νοσεῖ, ἀκρατῶς βιοτεύων καὶ ἀπειθῶν τοῖς ἰατροῖς. τότε μὲν οὖν ἐξῆν αὐτῷ μὴ νοσεῖν, προεμένῳ δ' οὐκέτι, ὥσπερ οὐδ' ἀφέντι λίθον ἔτ' αὐτὸν δυνατὸν ἀναλαβεῖν· ἀλλ' ὅμως ἐπ' αὐτῷ τὸ βαλεῖν [καὶ ῥῖψαι]· ἡ γὰρ ἀρχὴ ἐν αὐτῷ. οὕτω δὲ καὶ τῷ ἀδίκῳ καὶ τῷ ἀκολάστῳ ἐξ ἀρχῆς μὲν ἐξῆν τοιούτοις μὴ γενέσθαι, διὸ ἑκόντες εἰσίν· γενομένοις δ' οὐκέτι ἔστι μὴ εἶναι. (Arist. *EN* 1114a11–21)

Again, it is unreasonable to suppose that a man who acts unjustly or licentiously does not wish to be unjust or licentious; and if anyone, without being in ignorance, acts, he will be voluntarily unjust; but it does not follow that he can stop being unjust and be just if he wants to—no more than a sick man can become healthy, even though (it may be) his sickness is voluntary, being the result of incontinent living and disobeying his doctors. There was a time when it was open to him not to be ill; but when he had once thrown away his chance, it was gone; just as when one has once let go of a stone, it is too late to get it back—but the agent was responsible for throwing it, because the origin of the action was in himself. So too it was at first open to the unjust and licentious persons not to become such, and therefore they are voluntarily what they are; but now that they have become what they are, it is no longer open to them not to be such. (trans. Thomson)

Aristotle is speaking about the voluntary and the involuntary under conditions that would appear to negate the possibility of praise and blame, specifically cases where, through negligence, a person commits a blameworthy act. He introduces the medical patient as part of his attempt to recuperate, in the context of such errors, the concept of the voluntary.[1] Aristotle declares that the patient once had the chance to take care by exercising mastery over himself and complying with his physicians.[2] As soon as he throws that chance away, however, he becomes a mere symptom of his disease: his health is like a stone that cannot be recovered.[3] Character formation, Aristotle argues, works the same way. If vice can eventually destroy the conditions of ethical agency, this does not nullify praise and blame, for it was once in the corrupt person's power to take care.[4]

Aristotle's choice of a medical analogy to illustrate this point appears calculated. Within the analogy, we can identify points of contact beyond a straightforward parallel between vice and bodily disease, suggesting more complex roles for both the body and the soul. On the one hand, if a person lives *akratōs*, "without mastery," the problem would seem to be at the level of the soul, although the repercussions are felt in the body. On the other hand, the body helps Aristotle model the forces of necessity at work within us: once disease has taken hold, he says, no amount of wishing can make us healthy.

The relationship between wishing and health, in truth, is always complex, insofar as health is realized inside a space that we cannot engage directly. For the

[1] On the medical analogy in Aristotle, see Nussbaum 1994.53–101, esp. 58–76: Nussbaum is more focused on the therapeutic aspects of the analogy. See also Jaeger 1957; Tracy 1969.157–333.

[2] Aristotle also admits the possibility of people who become sick or disabled through no fault of their own (1114a25–27). In these cases, praise and blame are illegitimate, as at Pl. *Ti.* 86d5–e3.

[3] The irreversibility of disease is closely related to the purpose of the analogy. While, strictly speaking, in bodily disease there might be a possibility of recovering, provided one complies with the physician's recommendations, in vice, it would seem, the disease is beyond remedy once it is entrenched.

[4] Aristotle uses the language of care at 1113b33–1114a3: people are ignorant because of lack of care (δι᾽ ἀμέλειαν), though it is in their power to take care (τοῦ γὰρ ἐπιμεληθῆναι κύριοι). Note that there are significant differences between Democritus's apparent views on the scope of care and Aristotle's more pessimistic views. As the above passage suggests, both Plato and Aristotle lean toward limiting the time in which a soul can be molded to a window in youth. They also limit the kinds of natures subject to molding. See esp. *EN* 1179b4–18, refuting the idea that *anyone* can be "remolded"—Aristotle uses the verb μεταρρυθμίζω, suggesting a direct engagement with Democritus—by argument.

medical writers, it is in the interval between intentions, on the one hand, and symptoms, on the other, that disease develops "bit by bit" before suddenly overtaking the person, at which point it may be too late. Aristotle adopts a similar model—with specific reference to the body—later in 3.5 to clarify the difference between actions and dispositions, whose individual stages of development, just as in diseases, are unnoticeable. Like a disease, vice grows through repeated acts of injustice below the threshold of our awareness, accumulating force until it destroys the possibility of improvement.[5] Vice, here, is not a disease of the physical body. Yet even when that body does not threaten the voluntary directly, it is appropriated to describe the kernel of nontransparency and automatism—perhaps something like what Aristotle elsewhere calls "daemonic nature" (δαιμονία φύσις)—within the ethical subject.[6]

Aristotle thus uses the physical body to develop the idea of the involuntary, while using the possibility of care to establish the parameters of the voluntary. The work performed by the body in this context suggests that it may have played a role in shaping not only the soul but also new concepts of the voluntary or, more problematically, the "will."[7] That is not to say that, in the archaic period, people were puppets. Rather, I mean to say that, against the foil of physical causes, which threaten to erupt from within if left on their own, the idea of agency begins to looks like something that has to be secured and upheld. What I have sought to recover are the conditions under which the physical body, together with the embodied subject to which it gives rise, fosters a different kind of otherness capable of undermining the integrity of the human, turning human nature into a target of concern.

Both Platonic and Cartesian dualism are today seen largely as discarded notions. But the physical body continues to function in ways that have become familiar over the course of this book, identified more than ever as an object of biomedical mastery while largely excluded from much twentieth-century critical theory as a figure of absolute otherness—pure daemonism, outside language

---

[5] οὐχ ὁμοίως δὲ αἱ πράξεις ἑκούσιοί εἰσι καὶ αἱ ἕξεις· τῶν μὲν γὰρ πράξεων ἀπ᾽ ἀρχῆς μέχρι τοῦ τέλους κύριοί ἐσμεν, εἰδότες τὰ καθ᾽ ἕκαστα, τῶν ἕξεων δὲ τῆς ἀρχῆς, καθ᾽ ἕκαστα δὲ ἡ πρόσθεσις οὐ γνώριμος, ὥσπερ ἐπὶ τῶν ἀρρωστιῶν· ἀλλ᾽ ὅτι ἐφ᾽ ἡμῖν ἦν οὕτως ἢ μὴ οὕτω χρήσασθαι, διὰ τοῦτο ἑκούσιοι (But our dispositions are not voluntary in the same sense that our actions are. Our actions are under our control from beginning to end, because we are aware of the individual stages, but we only control the beginning of our dispositions; the individual stages of their development, as in the case of illness, are unnoticeable. They are, however, voluntary in the sense that it was originally in our power to exercise them one way or the other; trans. Thomson, *EN* 1114b30–1115a3).

[6] See Arist. *Div. somn.* 463b14, with van der Eijk 2005b.246–47 and n.30. As for Plato, the body is not simply a model for the soul for Aristotle but also sometimes seems to be a cause of its disorder: see van der Eijk 2005b.139–275, esp. 206–37.

[7] On differences between ancient and modern notions of the will, see Vernant 1988b, esp. 57–60. For Vernant, the will is "not a datum of human nature," but, rather, "a complex construction whose history appears to be as difficult, multiple, and incomplete as that of the self, of which it is to a great extent an integral part."

and culture. These tendencies over the past decades have converged on the notion of the physical body as real, the natural counterpart to cultural constructions. By tracking the symptomatic emergence of a body defined by its *phusis*, we may gain insight into a problem no less urgent today, namely how we negotiate our own understanding of—and implication in—physicality.

BIBLIOGRAPHY

Primary Texts

Oxford Classical Texts are used when they are available. In other cases, I use the standard edition cited in the *Oxford Classical Dictionary*, rev. 3rd ed., ed. S. Hornblower and A. Spawforth (Oxford, 2003). For the Presocratics, I have used H. Diels, ed., *Die Fragmente der Vorsokratiker*, 6th ed., revised by W. Kranz (Berlin, 1951–52). While in many cases Diels-Kranz has been superseded by modern editions of fragments, I have continued to use it for simplicity of reference, noting modern editions, which appear in the bibliography, where they have particular relevance to my argument. For all "A" testimonia, I have indicated the source. Note, however, that there is not always an exact correspondence between the source citation and the "A" entry in DK. Note, too, that for Gorgias and Antiphon the Sophist, I have used T. Buchheim, ed. and trans., *Gorgias von Leontini. Reden, Fragmente und Testimonien* (Hamburg, 1989); and G. J. Pendrick, ed. and trans., *Antiphon the Sophist: The Fragments* (Cambridge, 2002). For the medical writers, see the list of abbreviations at the beginning of the book. For Euripides, unless otherwise noted, I have used D. Kovacs, ed. and trans., *Euripides*, 6 vols. (Cambridge, Mass., 1994–2002), with the occasional minor modification.

Secondary Sources

Adkins, A.W.H. 1960. *Merit and Responsibility: A Study in Greek Values*. Oxford.

Agamben, G. 2004. *The Open: Man and Animal*. Trans. K. Attell. Stanford. [*L'aperto: l'uomo e l'animale*. Turin, 2002.]

Alessi, R. 2008. "Bodily Features in the Corpus Hippocraticum: Remarks about the Method of Classification of Individuals into Groups." Presented at the XIIIth Colloquium Hippocraticum, Austin, Texas, August 11–13.

Alexanderson, B., ed. 1963. *Die hippokratische Schrift "Prognostikon."* Göteborg.

Algra, K. 1999. "The Beginnings of Cosmology." In Long 1999a, 45–65.

Allan, W. 1999–2000. "Euripides and the Sophists: Society and the Theatre of War." In Cropp, Lee, and Sansone 1999–2000, 145–56.

———. 2005a. "Tragedy and the Early Greek Philosophical Tradition." In *A Companion to Greek Tragedy*, ed. J. Gregory, 71–82. Malden, Mass.

———. 2005b. "Arms and the Man: Euphorbus, Hector, and the Death of Patroclus." *CQ* 55:1–16.

Allen, D. 2000. "Envisaging the Body of the Condemned: The Power of Platonic Symbols." *CP* 95:133–50.

———. 2006. "Talking about Revolution: On Political Change in Fourth-Century Athens and Historiographic Method." In Goldhill and Osborne 2006, 183–217.

Amundsen, D. W., and G. B. Ferngren. 1977. "The Physician as an Expert Witness in Athenian Law." *BHM* 51:202–13.

Andò, V. 1999. "Alla ricerca della physis: uomo e natura nella Grecia antica." In *Natura e . . . esplorazione polifonica di un'idea*, ed. L. Mortari, 183–211. Milan.

———. 2002. "La φύσις tra normale e patologico." In Thivel and Zucker 2002, 97–122.

Andriopoulos, D. Z. 1972. "Empedocles' Theory of Perception." *Platon* 24:290–98.

Annas, J. 1985. "Self-Knowledge in Early Plato." In *Platonic Investigations*, ed. D. J. O'Meara, 111–38. Washington, D.C.

———. 2002. "Democritus and Eudaimonism." In Caston and Graham 2002, 169–81.

Annoni, J. M., and V. Barras. 1993. "La découpe du corps humain et ses justifications dans l'Antiquité." *Canadian Bulletin for Medical History* 10:185–227.

Armstrong, D., and A. E. Hanson. 1986. "Two Notes on Greek Tragedy." *BICS* 33:97–102.

Arnott, R. 1996. "Healing and Medicine in the Aegean Bronze Age." *Journal of the Royal Society of Medicine* 89:265–70.

———. 2004. "Minoan and Mycenaean Medicine and Its Near Eastern Contacts." In Horstmanshoff and Stol 2004, 153–73.

Arrowsmith, W. 1956. Introduction to the translation of *Heracles*. In *The Complete Greek Tragedies*, vol. 2, ed. D. Grene and R. Lattimore. Chicago.

———. 1963. "A Greek Theater of Ideas." *Arion* 2:32–56.

Assaël, J. 1994. "*L'Héraclès* d'Euripide et les ténèbres infernales." *Les études classiques* 62:313–26.

———. 1996. "*Synesis* dans *Oreste* d'Euripide." *L'Antiquité classique* 65:53–69.

———. 2001. *Euripide, philosophe et poète tragique*. Brussels.

Aubert, J. J. 1989. "Threatened Wombs: Aspects of Ancient Uterine Magic." *GRBS* 30:421–49.

Austin, N. 1999. "Anger and Disease in Homer's *Iliad*." In *Euphrosyne: Studies in Ancient Epic and Its Legacy in Honor of Dimitris N. Maronitis*, ed. J. N. Kazazis and A. Rengakos, 11–49. Stuttgart.

Ayache, L. 1992. "Hippocrate laissait-t-il la nature agir?" In López Férez 1992, 19–35.

———. 1997. "L'animal, les hommes et l'ancienne médecine." In *L'animal dans l'Antiquité*, ed. B. Cassin and J. L. Labarrière, 55–74. Paris.

Aydede, M. 2005. "Introduction: A Critical and Quasi-Historical Essay on Theories of Pain." In *Pain: New Essays on Its Nature and the Methodology of Its Study*, ed. M. Aydede, 1–58. Cambridge, Mass.

Baader, G., and R. Winau, eds. 1989. *Die hippokratischen Epidemien: Theorie-Praxis-Tradition; Verhandlungen des Ve Colloque international hippocratique*. Stuttgart.

Bailey, C. 1928. *The Greek Atomists and Epicurus: A Study*. Oxford.

Bakhtin, M. M. 1986. "The Problem of Speech Genres." In *Speech Genres and Other Late Essays*, trans. V. McGee, ed. C. Emerson and M. Holquist, 60–102. Austin. [*Éstetika slovesnogo tvorchestva*. Moscow, 1979.]

Baltussen, H. 2000. *Theophrastus against the Presocratics and Plato: Peripatetic Dialectic in the "De sensibus."* Leiden.

Barlow, S. A. 1981. "Sophocles' *Ajax* and Euripides' *Heracles*." *Ramus* 10:112–28.

———. 1982. "Structure and Dramatic Realism in Euripides' *Heracles*." *G & R* 29:115–25.

Barra, E. 1993. "'Un dio ti fa cantare' (*Ag.* 1175/76): la Cassandra di Eschilo fra Ippocrate e la Pizia." *Mythos* 5:5–43.

Barrett, J. L. 2007. "Cognitive Science of Religion: What Is It and Why Is It?" *Religion Compass* 1:768–86.

Barrett, W. S., ed. 1964. *Euripides, Hippolytos*. Oxford.

Barthes, R. 1972. "Sémiologie et médecine." In *Les sciences de la folie*, ed. R. Bastide, 37–46. Paris.

Barton, C. 1999. "The Roman Blush: The Delicate Matter of Self-Control." In Porter 1999a, 212–34.

Barton, T. S. 1994. *Power and Knowledge: Astrology, Physiognomics, and Medicine under the Roman Empire*. Ann Arbor.

Bassi, K. 1998. *Acting like Men: Gender, Drama, and Nostalgia in Ancient Greece*. Ann Arbor.

———. 2003. "The Semantics of Manliness in Ancient Greece." In Rosen and Sluiter 2003, 25–58.

Basta Donzelli, G. 1985. "La colpa di Elena: Gorgia ed Euripide a confronto." In Montoneri and Romano 1985, 389–409.

Bates, D., ed. 1995. *Knowledge and the Scholarly Medical Traditions*. Cambridge.

Baumann-Oosterbeek, E. D. 1932. "Der Wahnsinn der Io." *Archiv für Geschichte der Medizin* 25:307–14.

Beardslee, J. W. 1918. *The Use of ΦΥΣΙΣ in Fifth-Century Greek Literature*. Chicago.

Beer, G. 2000. *Darwin's Plots: Evolutionary Narrative in Darwin, George Eliot and Nineteenth-Century Fiction*. 2nd ed. Cambridge.

Benakēs, L. G., ed. 1984. *Proceedings of the First International Congress on Democritus, Xanthi 6–9 October 1983*, 2 vols. Xanthi.

Benveniste, E. 1945. "La doctrine médicale des Indo-Européens." *Revue de l'histoire des religions* 130:5–12.

Bernabé, A. 2007. "L'âme après la mort: modèles orphiques et transposition platonicienne." *Études platoniciennes* 4:25–44.

Bernardini, P. A. 1997a. "La città di Tebe nell'*Eracle* di Euripide." In Bernardini 1997b, 219–32.

———, ed. 1997b. *Presenza e funzione della città di Tebe nella cultura Greca: atti del Convegno Internazionale (Urbino 7–9 luglio 1997)*. Pisa.

Bernheim, F., and A. A. Zener. 1978. "The Sminthian Apollo and the Epidemic among the Achaeans at Troy." *TAPA* 108:11–14.

Bernheimer, C., ed. 1995. *Comparative Literature in the Age of Multiculturalism*. Baltimore.

Bett, R. 2002. "Is There a Sophistic Ethics?" *AncPhil* 22:235–62.

Biggs, P. 1966. "The Disease Theme in Sophocles' *Ajax, Philoctetes* and *Trachiniae*." *CP* 61:223–35.

Bird-David, N. 1999. "'Animism' Revisited: Personhood, Environment, and Relational Epistemology." *Current Anthropology*, suppl., 40:67–91.

Black, J. 1998. "Taking the Sex Out of Sexuality: Foucault's Failed History." In Larmour, Miller, and Platter 1998, 42–60.

Blaiklock, E. M. 1952. *The Male Characters of Euripides: A Study in Realism*. Wellington.

Blickman, D. R. 1987. "The Role of the Plague in the *Iliad*." *ClAnt* 6:1–10.

Bobonich, C. 1994. "*Akrasia* and Agency in Plato's *Laws* and *Republic*." *Archiv für Geschichte der Philosophie* 76:3–36. Reprinted in *Essays on Plato's Psychology*, ed. E. Wagner, 203–37. Lanham, Md., 2001.

———. 2007. "Plato on *Akrasia* and Knowing Your Own Mind." In Bobonich and Destrée 2007, 41–60.

Bobonich, C., and P. Destrée, eds. 2007. *Akrasia in Greek Philosophy: From Socrates to Plotinus*. Leiden.

Bodiou, L. 2004. "Désordres et malheurs du corps féminin en Grèce classique d'après les écrits médicaux et biologiques." In *Au jardin des Hespérides: histoire, société et épigraphie des mondes anciens; mélanges offerts à Alain Tranoy*, ed. C. Auliard and L. Bodiou, 217–32. Rennes.

Bodiou, L. 2006. "De l'utilité du ventre des femmes: lectures médicales du corps féminin." In Prost and Wilgaux 2006, 153–66.

Boehm, I. 2002. "Inconscience et insensibilité dans la *Collection hippocratique*." In Thivel and Zucker 2002, 257–69.

———. 2003. "Toucher du doigt: le vocabulaire du toucher dans les textes médicaux grecs et latins." In *Manus medica: actions et gestes de l'officiant dans les textes médicaux latins; questions de thérapeutique et de lexique; actes du colloque tenu à l'Université Lumière-Lyon II, les 18 et 19 septembre 2001*, ed. F. Gaide and F. Biville, 229–40. Aix-en-Provence.

Böhme, J. 1929. *Die Seele und das Ich im homerischen Epos*. Leipzig.

Bolelli, T. 1948. "Il valore semasiologico delle voci ἦτορ, κῆρ e κραδίη nell'epos omerico." *Annali della Scuola Normale Superiore di Pisa: Lettere, storia e filosofia* 17:66–75.

Bolens, G. 1999. "Homeric Joints and the Marrow in Plato's *Timaeus*: Two Logics of the Body." *Multilingua* 18:149–57.

———. 2000. *La logique du corps articulaire: les articulations du corps humain dans la littérature occidentale*. Rennes.

Boncompagni, R. 1972. "Concezione della malattia e senso dell'individualità nei testi cnidi del *Corpus Hippocraticum*." *La parola del passato* 27:209–38.

Bond, G. W. 1981. *Euripides, Heracles*. Oxford.

Bonnard, J. B. 2007. "La construction des genres dans la Collection hippocratique." In *Problèmes du genre en Grèce ancienne*, ed. V. Sebillotte Cuchet and N. Ernoult, 159–70. Paris.

Borgeaud, P. 1988. *The Cult of Pan in Ancient Greece*, trans. K. Atlass and J. Redfield. Chicago. [*Recherches sur le dieu Pan*. Geneva, 1979.]

Borthwick, E. K. 1997. "Euripides Erotodidaskalos?: A Note on Aristophanes *Frogs* 957." *CP* 92:363–67.

Boudon, V. 1994. "Le rôle de l'eau dans les prescriptions médicales d'Asclépios chez Galien et Aelius Aristide." In Ginouvès et al. 1994, 157–68.

Boulter, P. N. 1962. "The Theme of ἄγρια in Euripides' *Orestes*." *Phoenix* 16:102–6.

Bourbon, F., ed. and trans. 2008. *Hippocrate, Nature de la femme*. CUF t. 12.1. Paris.

Bourdieu, P. 1977. *Outline of a Theory of Practice*, trans. R. Nice. Cambridge. [*Esquisse d'une théorie de la pratique: précédé de trois études d'ethnologie kabyle*. Paris, 1972.]

———. 1990. *The Logic of Practice*, trans. R. Nice. Stanford. [*Le sens pratique*. Paris, 1980.]

Bourgey, L. 1953. *Observation et expérience chez les médecins de la Collection hippocratique*. Paris.

———. 1975. "La relation du médecin au malade dans les écrits de l'école de Cos." In Bourgey and Jouanna 1975, 209–27.

Bourgey, L., and J. Jouanna, eds. 1975. *La Collection hippocratique et son rôle dans l'histoire de la médecine: Colloque de Strasbourg, 23–27 octobre 1972*. Leiden.

Bouvier, D. 2005. "La fascination du cadavre dans la poésie homérique." In *Antigone et le devoir de sépulture: actes du colloque international de l'Université de Lausanne (mai 2005)*, ed. F. Ansermet and M. Gilbert, 70–84. Geneva.

Boyer, P. 1996. "What Makes Anthropomorphism Natural: Intuitive Ontology and Cultural Representations." *Journal of the Royal Anthropological Institute* 2:83–97.

———. 2001. *Religion Explained: The Evolutionary Origins of Religious Thought*. New York.

Boys-Stones, G. 2007. "Physiognomy and Ancient Psychological Theory." In *Seeing the Face, Seeing the Soul: Polemon's Physiognomy from Classical Antiquity to Medieval Islam*, ed. S. Swain, 19–124. Oxford.

Brancacci, A., and P.-M. Morel, eds. 2007. *Democritus: Science, the Arts, and the Care of the Soul; Proceedings of the International Colloquium on Democritus (Paris, 18–20 September 2003)*. Leiden.

Bratescu, G. 1975. "Éléments archaïques dans la médecine hippocratique." In Bourgey and Jouanna 1975, 41–49.

———. 1983. "Le problème de la mesure dans la *Collection hippocratique*." In Lasserre and Mudry 1983, 137–44.

———. 1990. "Les facteurs endogènes et exogènes dans l'étio-pathogénie hippocratique." In Potter, Maloney, and Desautels 1990, 267–78.

———. 2002. "Rapports entre le naturel, le normal et le divin hippocratiques." In Thivel and Zucker 2002, 13–22.

Brelich, A. 1958. *Gli eroi greci: un problema storico-religioso*. Rome.

Bremmer, J. N. 1983. *The Early Greek Concept of the Soul*. Princeton.

Brenk, F. 1986. "In the Light of the Moon: Demonology in the Early Imperial Period." *Aufstieg und Niedergang der römischen Welt* 2.16.3:2068–2145. Berlin.

Brickhouse, T. C., and N. D. Smith. 2002. "Incurable Souls in Socratic Psychology." *Anc-Phil* 22:21–36.

Broadie, S. 1999. "Rational Theology." In Long 1999a, 205–24.

Brown, A. L. 1978. "Wretched Tales of Poets: Euripides, *Heracles* 1340–6." *PCPS* 24:22–30.

Brown, P. 1988. *The Body and Society: Men, Women, and Sexual Renunciation in Early Christianity*. New York.

Buchheim, T. 1989. *Gorgias von Leontini. Reden, Fragmente und Testimonien*. Hamburg.

Burgess, S. 2000. "How to Build a Human Body: An Idealist's Guide." In M. R. Wright 2000, 43–58.

Burkert, W. 1972. *Lore and Science in Ancient Pythagoreanism*. Trans. E. L. Minar Jr. Cambridge, Mass. [*Weisheit und Wissenschaft. Studien zu Pythagoras, Philolaos und Plato*. Nürnberg, 1962.]

———. 1983. "Itinerant Diviners and Magicians: A Neglected Element in Cultural Contacts." In *The Greek Renaissance of the Eighth Century B.C.: Tradition and Innovation; Proceedings of the Second International Symposium at the Swedish Institute in Athens, 1–5 June 1981*, ed. R. Hägg, 115–19. Stockholm.

———. 1992. *The Orientalizing Revolution: Near Eastern Influence on Greek Culture in the Early Archaic Age*. Trans. W. Burkert and M. E. Pinder. Cambridge, Mass. [*Die orientalisierende Epoche in griechischen Religion und Literatur*. Heidelberg, 1984.]

Burnet, J. 1916. "The Socratic Doctrine of the Soul." *Proceedings of the British Academy*, 235–59.

Burnett, A. P. 1985. *Catastrophe Survived: Euripides' Plays of Mixed Reversal*. 2nd ed. Oxford.

Burnyeat, M. F. 1982. "The Origins of Non-Deductive Inference." In *Science and Speculation: Studies in Hellenistic Theory and Practice*, ed. J. Barnes et al., 193–238. Cambridge.

Butler, J. 1993. *Bodies That Matter: On the Discursive Limits of "Sex."* New York.

———. 2005. *Giving an Account of Oneself*. New York.

Byl, S. 1990. "Le vocabulaire hippocratique dans les comédies d'Aristophane et particulièrement dans les deux dernières." *Revue de philologie* 64:151–62.

———. 1992. "Le traitement de la douleur dans le *Corpus* hippocratique." In López Férez 1992, 203–13.

———. 1998. "Sommeil et insomnie dans le *Corpus Hippocraticum.*" *RBPh* 76:31–36.

———. 2002. "Liste de fréquence de φύσις et classement des œuvres hippocratiques." In Thivel and Zucker 2002, 45–54.

———. 2005. "L'anthropomorphisme de la matrice dans la médecine de la Grèce ancienne." In *Histoire de la médecine: leçons méthodologiques*, ed. D. Gourevitch, 115–29. Paris.

———. 2006. "Le délire hippocratique dans son contexte." *RBPh* 84:5–24.

Bynum, C. W. 1991. *Fragmentation and Redemption: Essays on Gender and the Human Body in Medieval Religion.* New York.

———. 1995. "Why All the Fuss about the Body?: A Medievalist's Perspective." *Critical Inquiry* 22:1–33.

Caciola, N. 2000. "Mystics, Demoniacs, and the Physiology of Spirit Possession in Medieval Europe." *Comparative Studies in Society and History* 42:268–306.

Cairns, D. L. 1993. *Aidōs: The Psychology and Ethics of Honour and Shame in Ancient Greek Literature.* Oxford.

Calame, C. 1999. *The Poetics of Eros in Ancient Greece.* Trans. J. Lloyd. Princeton. [*L'éros dans la Grèce antique.* Paris, 1996.]

———. 2005. "Uttering Human Nature by Constructing the Inhabited World: The Well-Tempered Racism of Hippocrates." In *Masks of Authority: Fiction and Pragmatics in Ancient Greek Poetics*, trans. P. M. Burk, 135–56. Ithaca. [*Masques d'autorité: fiction et pragmatique dans la poétique grecque antique.* Paris, 2005.]

Calasso, R. 2001. *Literature and the Gods.* Trans. T. Parks. New York. [*La letteratura e gli dèi.* Milan, 2001.]

Calogero, G. 1957. "Gorgias and the Socratic Principle *nemo sua sponte peccat.*" *JHS* 77:12–17.

Cambiano, G. 1980. "Une interprétation 'matérialiste' des rêves: du *Régime IV.*" In Grmek 1980, 87–96.

———. 1983. "Pathologie et analogie politique." In Lasserre and Mudry 1983, 441–58.

Canguilhem, G. 1963. "The Role of Analogies and Models in Biological Discovery." In Crombie 1963, 507–20.

Čapek, M. 1992. "Microphysical Indeterminacy and Freedom: Bergson and Peirce." In *The Crisis in Modernism: Bergson and the Vitalist Controversy*, ed. F. Burwick and P. Douglass, 171–89. Cambridge.

Capone Ciollaro, M. 1987. "Relazioni psicofisiche nella tragedia greca: la semantica di ἧπαρ, σπλάγχνον, στέρνον, πλεύμων." In Ταλαρίσκος: *studia graeca Antonio Garzya sexagenario a discipulis oblata*, ed. U. Criscuolo, 7–24. Naples.

Carone, G. R. 2005a. "Mind and Body in Late Plato." *Archiv für Geschichte der Philosophie* 87:227–69.

———. 2005b. *Plato's Cosmology and Its Ethical Dimensions.* New York.

Carson, A. 1990. "Putting Her in Her Place: Woman, Dirt, and Desire." In Halperin, Winkler, and Zeitlin 1990, 135–69. Revised version reprinted as "Dirt and Desire: The Phenomenology of Female Pollution in Antiquity." In Porter 1999a, 77–100.

Caston, V., and D. W. Graham, eds. 2002. *Presocratic Philosophy: Essays in Honour of Alexander Mourelatos.* Aldershot.

Caswell, C. P. 1990. *A Study of THUMOS in Early Greek Epic.* Leiden.

Cerri, G. 1997. "L'etica di Simonide nell'*Eracle* di Euripide: l'opposizione mitica Atene-Tebe." In Bernardini 1997b, 233–63.

Ceschi, G. 2003. "Il caso clinico di Eracle nelle *Trachinie* di Sofocle." *Atti dell'Istituto Veneto di Scienze, Lettere ed Arti: Classe di scienze morali, lettere ed arti* 161:65–93.

Chaniotis, A. 1995. "Illness and Cures in the Greek Propitiatory Inscriptions and Dedications of Lydia and Phrygia." In van der Eijk, Horstmanshoff, and Schrijvers 1995, 323–44.

Cheah, P. 1996. "Mattering." *Diacritics* 26:108–39.

Cherniss, H. 1935. *Aristotle's Criticism of Presocratic Philosophy.* Baltimore.

Cheyns, A. 1980. "La notion de φρένες dans l'*Iliade* et l'*Odyssée* I." *Cahiers de l'Institut de linguistique* 6:121–202.

———. 1985. "Recherche sur l'emploi des synonymes ἦτορ, κῆρ et κραδίη dans l'*Iliade* et l'*Odyssée.*" *RBPh* 63:15–73.

Chiasson, C. 2001. "Scythian Androgyny and Environmental Determinism in Herodotus and the Hippocratic περὶ ἀέρων ὑδάτων τόπων." *Syllecta classica* 12:33–73.

Ciani, M. G. 1974. "Lessico e funzione della follia nella tragedia greca." *Bollettino dell'Istituto di filologia greca* 1:70–110.

———. 1987. "The Silences of the Body: Defect and Absence of Voice in Hippocrates." In *The Regions of Silence: Studies on the Difficulty of Communicating,* ed. M. G. Ciani, 145–60. Amsterdam.

Clarke, M. 1995. "The Wisdom of Thales and the Problem of the Word ΙΕΡΟΣ." *CQ* 45:296–317.

———. 1999. *Flesh and Spirit in the Songs of Homer: A Study of Words and Myths.* Oxford.

Claus, D. B. 1972. "Phaedra and the Socratic Paradox." *YCS* 22:223–38.

———. 1981. *Toward the Soul: An Inquiry into the Meaning of ψυχή before Plato.* New Haven.

Clay, J. 1974. "*Demas* and *Aude*: The Nature of Divine Transformation in Homer." *Hermes* 102:129–36.

Cohen, B. 1994. "From Bowman to Clubman: Herakles and Olympia." *Art Bulletin* 76:695–715.

Cole, T. 1990. *Democritus and the Sources of Greek Anthropology.* 2nd ed. Atlanta.

Collinge, N. E. 1962. "Medical Terms and Clinical Attitudes in the Tragedians." *BICS* 9:43–55.

Collins, D. 1998. *Immortal Armor: The Concept of Alkē in Archaic Greek Poetry.* Lanham, Md.

———. 2003. "Nature, Cause, and Agency in Greek Magic." *TAPA* 133:17–49.

Collobert, C. 2002. "Aristotle's Review of the Presocratics: Is Aristotle Finally a Historian of Philosophy?" *Journal of the History of Philosophy* 40:281–95.

Conacher, D. J. 1967. *Euripidean Drama: Myth, Theme and Structure.* Toronto.

Cooper, J. M. 2004. "Method and Science in *On Ancient Medicine.*" In *Knowledge, Nature, and the Good: Essays on Ancient Philosophy,* 3–42. Princeton. Revised and expanded version of an article first published in *Interpretation und Argument,* ed. H. Linneweber-Lammerskitten and G. Mohr, 25–57. Würzburg, 2002.

Cordes, P. 1991. "Innere Medizin bei Homer?" *Rheinisches Museum* 134:113–20.

Covotti, A. 1898. "Melissi Samii reliquiae." *Studi italiani di filologia classica* 6:213–27.

Craik, E. M. 1993. "ΑΙΔΩΣ in Euripides' *Hippolytus* 373–430: Review and Reinterpretation." *JHS* 113:45–59.

———, ed. and trans. 1998. *Hippocrates, Places in Man*. Oxford.

———. 2001a. "Medical Reference in Euripides." *BICS* 45:81–95.

———. 2001b. "Thucydides on the Plague: Physiology of Flux and Fixation." *CQ* 51:102–8.

———. 2001c. "Plato and Medical Texts: *Symposium* 185c–193d." *CQ* 51:109–14.

———. 2003. "Medical Language in the Sophoklean Fragments." In *Shards from Kolonos: Studies in Sophoclean Fragments*, ed. A. H. Sommerstein, 45–56. Bari.

Crippa, S. 2006. "La voce quale luogo di sperimentazione del corpo nella tragedia greca." In *Il corpo teatrale fra testi e messinscena*, ed. A. M. Andrisano, 87–98. Rome.

Croally, N. T. 1994. *Euripidean Polemic: The "Trojan Women" and the Function of Tragedy*. Cambridge.

Crombie, A. C., ed. 1963. *Scientific Change: Historical Studies in the Intellectual, Social, and Technical Conditions for Scientific Discovery and Technical Invention, from Antiquity to the Present*. New York.

Cropp, M., and G. Fick. 2005. "On the Date of the Extant *Hippolytus*." *ZPE* 154:43–45.

Cropp M., K. Lee, and D. Sansone, eds. 1999–2000. "Euripides and Tragic Theatre in the Late Fifth Century." Special issue: *ICS* 24–25.

Csapo, E. 1999–2000. "Later Euripidean Music." In Cropp, Lee, and Sansone 1999–2000, 399–426.

Csordas, T. 1990. "Embodiment as a Paradigm for Anthropology." *Ethos* 18:5–47.

———. 1993. "Somatic Modes of Attention." *Cultural Anthropology* 8:135–56.

Cuny, D. 2002. "Le corps souffrant chez Sophocle: *Les Trachiniennes* et *Philoctète*." *Kentron* 18:69–78.

Curd, P. 1993. "Eleatic Monism in Zeno and Melissus." *AncPhil* 13:1–22.

———. 1998. *The Legacy of Parmenides: Eleatic Monism and Later Presocratic Thought*. Princeton.

———. 2001. "Why Democritus Was Not a Skeptic." In *Essays in Greek Philosophy VI: Before Plato*, ed. A. Preus, 149–69. Albany.

———. 2002. "The Metaphysics of Physics: Mixture and Separation in Empedocles and Anaxagoras." In Caston and Graham 2002, 139–58.

———, ed. and trans. 2007. *Anaxagoras of Clazomenae: Fragments and Testimonia*. Toronto.

Curiazi, D. 1997–2000. "Presenze ippocratiche nell'*Edipo re* di Sofocle." *Museum Criticum* 32–35:51–60.

Cyrino, M. S. 1995. *In Pandora's Jar: Lovesickness in Early Greek Poetry*. Lanham, Md.

Dale, A. M. 1956. "Seen and Unseen on the Greek Stage." *Wiener Studien* 69:96–106. Reprinted in *Collected Papers*, 119–29. Cambridge, 1969.

Darcus, S. M. 1979a. "A Person's Relation to ψυχή in Homer, Hesiod, and the Greek Lyric Poets." *Glotta* 57:30–39.

———. 1979b. "A Person's Relation to φρήν in Homer, Hesiod, and the Greek Lyric Poets." *Glotta* 57:159–73.

———. 1980. "How a Person Relates to θυμός in Homer." *Indogermanische Forschung* 85:138–50.

———. 1981. "The Function of θυμός in Hesiod and the Greek Lyric Poets." *Glotta* 59:147–55.

Daremberg, C. 1865. *La médecine dans Homère*. Paris.

Daston, L. 2000. "The Coming into Being of Scientific Objects." In *Biographies of Scientific Objects*, ed. L. Daston, 1–14. Chicago.

Daudet, A. 2002. *In the Land of Pain*. Ed. and trans. Julian Barnes. London. [*La doulou*. Paris, 1930.]

Davidson, J. 1998. *Courtesans and Fishcakes: The Consuming Passions of Classical Athens*. New York.

———. 2001. "Dover, Foucault and Greek Homosexuality: Penetration and the Truth of Sex." *Past and Present* 170:3–51.

Davidson, J. F. 1986. "The Circle and the Tragic Chorus." *G & R* 33:38–46.

Davies, M. 1989. *The Epic Cycle*. Bristol.

Dean-Jones, L. 1991. "The Cultural Construct of the Female Body in Classical Greek Science." In Pomeroy 1991, 111–37.

———. 1992. "The Politics of Pleasure: Female Sexual Appetite in the Hippocratic Corpus." *Helios* 19:72–91.

———. 1994. *Women's Bodies in Classical Greek Science*. Oxford.

———. 1995. "*Autopsia, Historia* and What Women Know: The Authority of Women in Hippocratic Gynaecology." In Bates 1995, 41–59.

———. 2003. "Literacy and the Charlatan in Ancient Greek Medicine." In *Written Texts and the Rise of Literate Culture in Ancient Greece*, ed. H. Yunis, 97–121. Cambridge.

De Hart, S. M. 1999. "Hippocratic Medicine and the Greek Body Image." *Perspectives on Science* 7:349–82.

Deichgräber, K. 1933. "Zu Hippokrates' ΠΕΡΙ ΑΡΧΑΙΗΣ ΙΗΤΡΙΚΗΣ 9." *Hermes* 68:356–58.

———, ed. 1935. *Hippokrates über Entstehung und Aufbau des menschlichen Körpers*: ΠΕΡΙ ΣΑΡΚΩΝ. Leipzig.

Delcourt, M. 1938. *Stérilités mystérieuses et naissances maléfiques dans l'Antiquité classique*. Liège.

Deleuze, G. 1988. *Foucault*. Trans. S. Hand. Minneapolis. [*Foucault*. Paris, 1986.]

———. 2000. *Proust and Signs: The Complete Text*. Trans. R. Howard. Minneapolis. [*Proust et les signes*. Paris, 1964.]

Demont, P. 2002. "Équilibre et déséquilibre des 'penchants' et 'tendances' dans la médecine hippocratique." In Thivel and Zucker 2002, 245–56.

———. 2005. "About Philosophy and Humoural Medicine." In van der Eijk 2005a, 271–86.

Deonna, W. 1939. "Le genou, siège de force et de vie et sa protection magique." *Revue archéologique* 13:224–35.

de Romilly, J. 1958. *La crainte et l'angoisse dans le théâtre d'Eschyle*. Paris.

———. 1961. *L'évolution du pathétique d'Eschyle à Euripide*. Paris.

———. 1976. "L'excuse de l'invincible amour dans la tragédie grecque." In *Miscellanea tragica in honorem J.C. Kamerbeek*, ed. J. M. Bremer, S. L. Radt, and C. J. Ruijgh, 309–21. Amsterdam.

Desch, W. 1986. "Der 'Herakles' des Euripides und die Götter." *Philologus* 130:8–23.

Desclos, M.-L. 2007. "Le vocabulaire de l'analyse psychologique chez les sophistes." *Études platoniciennes* 4:13–23.

Detienne, M. 1973. "Ébauche de la personne dans la Grèce archaïque." In *Problèmes de la personne*, ed. I. Meyerson, 46–54. Paris.

———. 1996. *The Masters of Truth in Archaic Greece*. Trans. J. Lloyd. New York. [*Les maîtres de vérité dans la Grèce archaïque*. Paris, 1967.]

Dettori, E. 1990–93. "Alcmae. fr. 1 D.-K." *Museum Criticum* 25–28:45–57.

Devereux, G. 1970. "The Psychotherapy Scene in Euripides' *Bacchae*." *JHS* 90:35–48.

di Benedetto. 1966. "Tendenza e probabilità nell'antica medicina greca." *Critica storia* 3:315–68.

———. 1986. *Il medico e la malattia: la scienza di Ippocrate.* Turin.

Dickie, M. W. 1999. "Bonds and Headless Demons in Greco-Roman Magic." *GRBS* 40:99–104.

Diggle, J. 1999. "Euripides the Psychologist." In Patsalidis and Sakellaridou 1999, 287–96.

Dilcher, R. 2006. "Parmenides on the Place of Mind." In R. King 2006, 31–48.

Diller, H. 1932. "ΟΨΙΣ ΑΔΗΛΩΝ ΤΑ ΦΑΙΝΟΜΕΝΑ." *Hermes* 67:14–42. Reprinted in *Kleine Schriften zur antiken Literatur*, 119–43. Munich, 1971.

———. 1964. "Ausdrucksformen des methodischen Bewusstseins in den hippokratischen *Epidemien*." *Archiv für Begriffsgeschichte* 9:133–50. Reprinted in *Kleine Schriften zur antiken Medizin*, 106–28. Berlin, 1973.

———, ed. and trans. 1970. *Hippokrates. Über die Umwelt. (De aere aquis locis). CMG* I.1.2. Berlin.

Dillon, J. 1995. "Rejecting the Body, Refining the Body: Some Remarks on the Development of Platonist Asceticism." In *Asceticism*, ed. V. L. Wimbush and R. Valantasis, 80–87. Oxford.

Dodds, E. R. 1929. "Euripides the Irrationalist." *Classical Review* 43:97–104. Reprinted in *The Ancient Concept of Progress and Other Essays on Greek Literature and Belief*, 1–25. Oxford, 1973.

———. 1951. *The Greeks and the Irrational.* Berkeley.

———, ed. 1960. *Euripides, Bacchae.* 2nd ed. Oxford.

Donadi, F. 1974. "In margine alla follia di Oreste." *Bollettino dell'Istituto di filologia greca* 1:111–27.

———. 1978. "Gorgia, Elena 16 (Quel quattrocentocinque)." *Bollettino dell'Istituto di filologia greca* 4:48–77.

———, ed. 1982. *Gorgia, Encomio di Elena.* Rome.

Dorion, L. A. 2007. "Plato and *Enkrateia*." In Bobonich and Destrée 2007, 119–38.

Dover, K. J. 1974. *Greek Popular Morality in the Time of Plato and Aristotle.* Oxford.

———. 1976. "The Freedom of the Intellectual in Greek Society." *Talanta* 7:24–54. Reprinted in *Greek and the Greeks: Collected Papers*, 2 vols., 2:135–58. Oxford, 1987–88.

Doyle, R. E. 1984. *ΑΤΗ: Its Use and Meaning; A Study in the Greek Poetic Tradition from Homer to Euripides.* New York.

Drossaart Lulofs, H. J., and E.L.J. Poortman, eds. and trans. 1989. *Nicolaus Damascenus, De plantis: Five Translations.* Amsterdam.

duBois, P. 1988. *Sowing the Body: Psychoanalysis and Ancient Representations of Women.* Chicago.

———. 1991. *Torture and Truth.* New York.

Ducatillon, J. 1969. "Collection hippocratique, *Du régime*, Livre III: les deux publics." *REG* 82:33–42.

———. 1977. *Polémiques dans la Collection hippocratique.* Paris.

———. 1990. "Le facteur divin dans les maladies d'après le *Pronostic*." In Potter, Maloney, and Desautels 1990, 61–73.

Duchemin, J. 1967. "Le personnage de Lyssa dans l'*Héraclès furieux* d'Euripide." *REG* 80:130–39.

Duden, B. 1991. *The Woman beneath the Skin: A Doctor's Patients in Eighteenth-Century Germany.* Trans. T. Dunlap. Cambridge, Mass. [*Geschichte unter der Haut. Ein Eisenacher Arzt und seine Patientinnen um 1730.* Stuttgart, 1987.]

Dumézil, G. 1983. "'Fouge' et 'rage' dans l'*Iliade*." In *La courtisane et les seigneurs colorés et autres essais,* 181–91. Paris.

Duminil, M. P. 1992. "Les malades 'frappés.'" In López Férez 1992, 215–24.

———, ed. and trans. 1998. *Hippocrate, Plaies; Nature des os; Cœur; Anatomie.* CUF t. 8. Paris.

Dumortier, J. 1935. *Le vocabulaire médical d'Eschyle et les écrits hippocratiques.* Paris.

Dunbar, N., ed. 1995. *Aristophanes, Birds.* Oxford.

Dunn, F. M. 1996. *Tragedy's End: Closure and Innovation in Euripidean Drama.* New York.

———. 1997. "Ends and Means in Euripides' *Heracles*." In *Classical Closure: Reading the End in Greek and Latin Literature,* ed. D. H. Roberts, F. M. Dunn, and D. Fowler, 83–111. Princeton.

———. 2005. "*On Ancient Medicine* and Its Intellectual Context." In van der Eijk 2005a, 49–67.

Dupréel, E. 1933. *La cause et l'intervalle; ou, ordre et probabilité.* Brussels.

Easterling, P. E. 1993. "Gods on Stage in Greek Tragedy." In *Religio Graeco-Romana. Festschrift für Walter Pötscher,* ed. J. Dalfen, G. Petersmann, and F. F. Schwartz, 77–86. Horn.

Edelstein, L. 1967a. *Ancient Medicine: Selected Papers of Ludwig Edelstein.* Trans. C. L. Temkin. Ed. O. Temkin and C. L. Temkin. Baltimore.

———. 1967b. "Hippocratic Prognosis." In Edelstein 1967a, 65–85. [*ΠΕΡΙ ΑΕΡΩΝ und die Sammlung der hippokratischen Schriften,* 60–88. Berlin, 1931.]

———. 1967c. "The Genuine Works of Hippocrates." In Edelstein 1967a, 133–44. [Orig. pub. in *BHM* 7 (1939): 236–48.]

———. 1967d. "Greek Medicine in Its Relation to Religion and Magic." In Edelstein 1967a, 205–46. [Orig. pub. in *BHM* 5 (1937): 201–46.]

———. 1967e. "The History of Anatomy in Antiquity." In Edelstein 1967a, 247–301. ["Die Geschichte der Sektion in der Antike." In *Quellen und Studien zur Geschichte der Naturwissenschaften und der Medizin,* 3.2, 50–106. Berlin, 1932.]

———. 1967f. "The Dietetics of Antiquity." In Edelstein 1967a, 303–16. ["Antike Diätetik." *Die Antike* 7 (1931): 255–70.]

Edelstein L., and E. J. Edelstein. 1998. *Asclepius: Collection and Interpretation of the Testimonies.* 2 vols. Baltimore. [Orig. pub. 1945.]

Eliade, M. 1968. "Notes on the Symbolism of the Arrow." In *Religions in Antiquity: Essays in Memory of Erwin Ramsdell Goodenough,* ed. J. Neusner, 463–75. Leiden.

Elsner, J. 2006. "Reflections on the 'Greek Revolution' in Art: From Changes in Viewing to the Transformation of Subjectivity." In Goldhill and Osborne 2006, 68–95.

Engmann, J. 1991. "Cosmic Justice in Anaximander." *Phronesis* 36:1–25.

Euben, J. P. 1986. "Political Corruption in Euripides' *Orestes*." In *Greek Tragedy and Political Theory,* ed. J. P. Euben, 222–51. Berkeley.

Evans, E. C. 1969. *Physiognomics in the Ancient World.* Philadelphia.

Evans, M. 2007. "Plato and the Meaning of Pain." *Apeiron* 40:71–93.

Everson, S., ed. 1991. *Psychology.* Cambridge.

Fadiman, A. 1997. *The Spirit Catches You and You Fall Down: A Hmong Child, Her American Doctors, and the Collision of Two Cultures.* New York.

Falcon, A. 2005. *Aristotle and the Science of Nature: Unity without Uniformity.* Cambridge.

Faranda, L. 1993. "De-scrivere la sofferenza, patire la scrittura: metafore del corpo dell'universo femminile greco." In *"Il mio nome è sofferenza": le forme e la rappresentazione del dolore,* ed. F. Rosa, 59–78. Trento.

Faraone, C. A. 1992. *Talismans and Trojan Horses: Guardian Statues in Ancient Greek Myth and Ritual.* New York.

———. 1994. "Deianira's Mistake and the Demise of Heracles: Erotic Magic in Sophocles' *Trachiniae*." *Helios* 21:115–35.

———. 1999. *Ancient Greek Love Magic.* Cambridge, Mass.

———. 2001. "The Undercutter, the Woodcutter, and Greek Demon Names Ending in -*tomos* (Hom. *Hymn to Dem* 228–29)." *AJP* 122:1–10.

———. 2003. "New Light on Ancient Greek Exorcisms of the Wandering Womb." *ZPE* 144:189–97.

———. 2007. "The Rise of the Demon Womb in Greco-Roman Antiquity." In *Finding Persephone: Women's Rituals in the Ancient Mediterranean,* ed. M. Parca and A. Tzanetou, 154–64. Bloomington, Ind.

Farnell, L. R. 1896–1909. *The Cults of the Greek States.* 5 vols. Oxford.

Farrar, C. 1988. *The Origins of Democratic Thinking: The Invention of Politics in Classical Athens.* Cambridge.

Fausti, D. 2002. "Malattia e normalità: il medico ippocratico e l'inferenza dei segni non verbali." In Thivel and Zucker 2002, 229–44.

Ferrari, F. 2005. "Melisso et la scuola eleatica." In *Da Elea a Samo: filosofi e politici di fronte all'impero ateniese; atti del convegno di studi, Santa Maria Capua Vetere, 4–5 giugno 2003,* ed. L. Breglia and M. Lupi, 85–94. Naples.

Ferrini, F. 1978. "Tragedia e patologia: lessico ippocratico in Euripide." *QUCC* 29:49–62.

Ferwerda, R. 1986. "The Meaning of the Word σῶμα (Body) in the Axial Age: An Interpretation of Plato's *Cratylus* 400C." In *The Origins and Diversity of Axial Age Civilizations,* ed. S. N. Eisenstadt, 111–24. Albany.

Festugière, A. J., ed. and trans. 1948. *Hippocrate, L'ancienne médecine.* Paris.

Filhol, E. 1989. "Hérakleiè nosos: l'épilepsie d'Héraclès." *Revue de l'histoire des religions* 206:3–20.

Fine, G., ed. 2000. *Plato.* Oxford.

Finkelberg, A. 1998. "On the History of the Greek ΚΟΣΜΟΣ." *HSCP* 98:103–36.

Fitzgerald, G. J. 1991. "The Euripidean Heracles: An Intellectual and a Coward?" *Mnemosyne* 44:85–95.

Flemming, R. 2000. *Medicine and the Making of Roman Women.* Oxford.

Flemming, R., and A. E. Hanson, ed. and trans. 1998. "Hippocrates' *Peri Parthenión* ('Diseases of Young Girls'): Text and Translation." *Early Science and Medicine* 3:241–52.

Fletcher, J. 1999. "Sacrificial Bodies and the Body of the Text in Aristophanes' *Lysistrata*." *Ramus* 28:108–25.

Foley, H. 1985. *Ritual Irony: Poetry and Sacrifice in Euripides.* Ithaca.

———. 1993. "The Politics of Tragic Lamentation." In *Tragedy, Comedy, and the Polis: Papers from the Greek Drama Conference, Nottingham, 18–20 July 1990,* ed. A. Sommerstein et al., 101–45. Bari.

———. 2000. "The Comic Body in Greek Art and Drama." In *Not the Classical Ideal: Athens and the Construction of the Other in Greek Art,* ed. B. Cohen, 275–311. Leiden.

Ford, A. 2002. *The Origins of Criticism: Literary Culture and Poetic Theory in Classical Greece*. Princeton.

Foucault, M. 1973. *The Birth of the Clinic: An Archaeology of Medical Perception*. Trans. A. M. Sheridan Smith. New York. [*Naissance de la clinique: une archéologie du regard médical*. Paris, 1963.]

———. 1977a. *Discipline and Punish: The Birth of the Prison*. Trans. A. Sheridan. New York. [*Surveiller et punir: naissance de la prison*. Paris, 1975.]

———. 1977b. "Nietzsche, Genealogy, History." In *Language, Counter-Memory, Practice: Selected Essays and Interviews*, trans. D. F. Bouchard and S. Simon, 139–64. Ithaca. ["Nietzsche, l'histoire, la généalogie." In *Hommage à Jean Hyppolite*, 145–72. Paris, 1971.]

———. 1985. *The History of Sexuality*. Vol. 2: *The Use of Pleasure*. Trans. R. Hurley. New York. [*Histoire de la sexualité, 2: L'usage des plaisirs*. Paris, 1984.]

———. 1986. *The History of Sexuality*. Vol. 3: *The Care of the Self*. Trans. R. Hurley. New York. [*Histoire de la sexualité, 3: Le souci de soi*. Paris, 1984.]

———. 1997. *Ethics: Subjectivity and Truth*. Ed. P. Rabinow. New York. [Selections from *Dits et écrits: 1954–1988*. 2 vols. Paris, 1994.]

———. 2005. *The Hermeneutics of the Subject: Lectures at the Collège de France, 1981–82*. Trans. G. Burchell. Ed. F. Gros. New York. [*L'herméneutique du sujet: cours au Collège de France, 1981–1982*. Paris, 2001.]

Fountoulakis, A. 1999. "Οὐσία in Euripides, *Hippolytus* 514 and the Greek Magical Papyri." *Maia* 51:193–204.

Foxhall, L. 1998. "Pandora Unbound: A Feminist Critique of Foucault's *History of Sexuality*." In Larmour, Miller, and Platter 1998, 122–37.

Foxhall, L., and J. Salmon, eds. 1998a. *Thinking Men: Masculinity and Its Self-Representation in the Classical Tradition*. London.

———, eds. 1998b. *When Men Were Men: Masculinity, Power and Identity in Classical Antiquity*. London.

Fränkel, H. 1975. *Early Greek Poetry and Philosophy*. Trans. M. Hadas and J. Willis. New York. [*Dichtung und Philosophie des frühen Griechentums. Eine Geschichte der griechischen Epik, Lyrik und Prosa bis zur Mitte des fünften Jahrhunderts*. 2nd ed. Munich, 1962.]

Franzino, E. 1995. "Euripides' *Heracles* 858–73." *ICS* 20:57–63.

Frede, D. 1992. "Disintegration and Restoration: Pleasure and Pain in Plato's *Philebus*." In *The Cambridge Companion to Plato*, ed. R. Kraut, 425–63. Cambridge.

Frede, M. 1987. "The Original Notion of Cause." In *Essays in Ancient Philosophy*, 125–50. Minneapolis.

———. 1988. "The Empiricist Attitude towards Reason and Theory." In "Method, Medicine and Metaphysics: Studies in the Philosophy of Ancient Science," ed. R. J. Hankinson, 70–97. Special issue: *Apeiron* 21.

———. 2004. "Aristotle's Account of the Origins of Philosophy." *Rhizai: A Journal for Ancient Philosophy and Science* 1:9–44.

Freud, S. 1919. "The 'Uncanny.' " In *The Standard Edition of the Complete Psychological Works of Sigmund Freud*, ed. J. Strachey, 17:217–56. London, 1953–74.

———. 1923. "The Ego and the Id." In *The Standard Edition of the Complete Psychological Works of Sigmund Freud*, ed. J. Strachey, 19:1–66. London, 1953–74.

Friedrich, W. H. 2003. *Wounding and Death in the "Iliad": Homeric Techniques of Description*. Trans. P. Jones and G. Wright. London. [*Verwundung und Tod in der Ilias. Homerische Darstellungsweisen*. Göttingen, 1956.]

Furley, D. J. 1956. "The Early History of the Concept of Soul." *BICS* 3:1–18.

———. 1967. *Two Studies in the Greek Atomists*. Princeton.

———. 1989. "Melissus of Samos." In *Ionian Philosophy*, ed. K. J. Boudouris, 114–22. Athens.

Gagarin, M. 2002. "Greek Law and the Presocratics." In Caston and Graham 2002, 19–24.

Gallego Pérez, M. T. 1996. "*Physis* dans la Collection hippocratique." In *Hippokratische Medizin und antike Philosophie: Verhandlungen des VIII. Internationalen Hippokrates-Kolloquiums in Kloster Banz/Staffelstein vom 23.–28. Sept. 1993*, ed. R. Wittern and P. Pellegrin, 419–36. Hildesheim.

Garofalo, I., et al., eds. 1999. *Aspetti della terapia nel "Corpus Hippocraticum": atti del IXᵉ Colloque international hippocratique, Pisa, 25–29 settembre 1996*. Florence.

Garzya, A. 1992. "Σύνεσις come malattia: Euripide e Ippocrate." In López Férez 1992, 505–12.

Gaskin, R. 1990. "Do Homeric Heroes Make Real Decisions?" *CQ* 40:1–15.

Gell, A. 1998. *Art and Agency: An Anthropological Theory*. Oxford.

Geller, M. J. 2004. "West Meets East: Early Greek and Babylonian Diagnosis." In Horstmanshoff and Stol 2004, 11–61.

George, D. B. 1994. "Euripides' *Heracles* 140–235: Staging and the Stage Iconography of Heracles' Bow." *GRBS* 35:145–57.

Giacomelli, A. 1980. "Aphrodite and After." *Phoenix* 34:1–19.

Giambalvo, M. 2002. "Normale versus Anormale?: lo statuto del patologico nella *Collezione Ippocratica*." In Thivel and Zucker 2002, 55–96.

Gibert, J. C. 1997. "Euripides' Hippolytus Plays: Which Came First?" *CQ* 47:85–97.

Gill, C. 1990a. "The Articulation of the Self in Euripides' *Hippolytus*." In *Euripides, Women, and Sexuality*, ed. A. Powell 1990, 76–107. London.

———. 1990b. "The Character-Personality Distinction." In Pelling 1990, 1–31.

———. 1991. "Is There a Concept of the Person in Greek Philosophy?" In Everson 1991, 166–93.

———. 1996a. *Personality in Greek Epic, Tragedy, and Philosophy: The Self in Dialogue*. Oxford.

———. 1996b. "Mind and Madness in Greek Tragedy." *Apeiron* 29:249–67.

———. 2000. "The Body's Fault?: Plato's *Timaeus* on Psychic Illness." In M. R. Wright 2000, 59–84.

Gill, M. L. 2003. "Plato's *Phaedrus* and the Method of Hippocrates." *Modern Schoolman* 80:295–314.

Gillespie, C. M. 1912. "The Use of εἶδος and ἰδέα in Hippocrates." *CQ* 6:179–203.

Ginouvès, R., et al., eds. 1994. *L'eau, la santé et la maladie dans le monde grec: actes du colloque organisé à Paris (CNRS et Fondation Singer-Polignac) du 25 au 27 novembre 1992 par le Centre de recherche "Archéologie et systèmes d'information" et par l'URA 1255 "Médecine grecque."* Athens.

Gleason, M. 1990. "The Semiotics of Gender: Physiognomy and Self-Fashioning in the Second Century C.E." In Halperin, Winkler, and Zeitlin 1990, 389–415.

———. 1995. *Making Men: Sophists and Self-Presentation in Ancient Rome*. Princeton.

———. 1999. "Truth Contests and Talking Corpses." In Porter 1999a, 287–313.

Gocer, A. 1999. "*Hesuchia*, A Metaphysical Principle in Plato's Moral Psychology." In "Recognition, Remembrance, and Reality: New Essays on Plato's Epistemology and Metaphysics," ed. M. L. McPherran, 17–36. Special issue: *Apeiron* 32.

Goff, B. 1990. *The Noose of Words: Readings of Desire, Violence, and Language in Euripides' "Hippolytos."* Cambridge.

Golder, H. 1996. "Making a Scene: Gesture, Tableau, and the Tragic Chorus." *Arion* 4:1–19.

Goldhill, S. 1995. *Foucault's Virginity: Ancient Erotic Fiction and the History of Sexuality.* Cambridge.

Goldhill, S., and R. Osborne, eds. 2006. *Rethinking Revolutions through Ancient Greece.* Cambridge.

Gomperz, H. 1932. "ΑΣΩΜΑΤΟΣ." *Hermes* 67:155–67.

Gomperz, T., ed. and trans. 1910. *Die Apologie der Heilkunst. Eine griechische Sophistenrede des fünften vorchristlichen Jahrhunderts.* 2nd ed. Leipzig.

Good, B. J., and M. J. DelVecchio Good. 1981. "The Meaning of Symptoms: A Cultural Hermeneutic Model for Clinical Practice." In *The Relevance of Social Science for Medicine,* ed. L. Eisenberg and A. Kleinman, 165–96. Dordrecht.

Gorrini, M. E. 2005. "The Hippocratic Impact on Healing Cults: The Archaeological Evidence in Attica." In van der Eijk 2005a, 135–56.

Gosling, J.C.B., and C.C.W. Taylor. 1982. *The Greeks on Pleasure.* Oxford.

Gould, J. 1978. "Dramatic Character and 'Human Intelligibility' in Greek Tragedy." *PCPS* 24:43–67.

Gourevitch, D. 1983. "L'aphonie hippocratique." In Lasserre and Mudry 1983, 297–305.

Gourevitch, D., and M. Gourevitch. 1979. "Histoire d'Io." *L'évolution psychiatrique* 44:263–79.

Graf, F. 1992. "An Oracle against Pestilence from a Western Anatolian Town." *ZPE* 92:267–79.

———. 1997. *Magic in the Ancient World.* Trans. F. Philip. Cambridge, Mass. [*La magie dans l'Antiquité gréco-romaine: idéologie et pratique.* Paris, 1994.]

Graham, D. W. 1984. "Aristotle's Discovery of Matter." *Archiv für Geschichte der Philosophie* 66:37–51.

———. 1987. "The Paradox of Prime Matter." *Journal of the History of Philosophy* 25:475–90.

———. 1999. "Empedocles and Anaxagoras: Responses to Parmenides." In Long 1999a, 159–80.

———. 2006. *Explaining the Cosmos: The Ionian Tradition of Scientific Philosophy.* Princeton.

Greenberg, N. 1962. "Euripides' *Orestes*: An Interpretation." *HSCP* 66:157–92.

Greene, E. 1996. "Sappho, Foucault, and Women's Erotics." *Arethusa* 29:1–14.

Greenwood, L.H.G. 1953. *Aspects of Euripidean Tragedy.* Cambridge.

Gregory, J. W. 1977. "Euripides' *Heracles.*" *YCS* 25:259–75.

Grensemann, H., ed. and trans. 1968a. *Die hippokratische Schrift "Über die heilige Krankheit."* Berlin.

———, ed. and trans. 1968b. *Hippokrates. Über Achtmonatskinder. (De octimestri partu.) Über das Siebenmonatskind. <Unecht>.* CMG I 2.1. Berlin.

———. 1975. *Knidische Medizin.* Teil I. Berlin.

———. 1982. *Hippokratische Gynäkologie. Die gynäkologischen Texte des Autors C nach den pseudohippokratischen Schriften "De muliebribus"* I, II und *"De sterilibus."* Wiesbaden.

———. 1987. *Knidische Medizin.* Teil II. Stuttgart.

Griffiths, E. M. 2002. "Euripides' *Herakles* and the Pursuit of Immortality." *Mnemosyne* 55:641–56.

Grmek, M. D., ed. 1980. *Hippocratica: actes du Colloque hippocratique de Paris, 4–9 septembre 1978.* Paris.

———. 1987. "Les *indicia mortis* dans la médecine gréco-romaine." In *La mort, les morts et l'au-delà dans le monde romain: actes du colloque de Caen, 20–22 novembre 1985*, ed. F. Hinard, 129–44. Paris.

———. 1989. *Diseases in the Ancient Greek World.* Trans. M. Muellner and L. Muellner. Baltimore. [*Les maladies à l'aube de la civilisation occidentale: recherches sur la réalité pathologique dans le monde grec préhistorique, archaïque, et classique.* Paris, 1983.]

———. 1991. "Ideas on Heredity in Greek and Roman Antiquity." *Physis* 28:11–34.

Groß, A. K. 1970. "Götterhand und Menschenhand im homerischen Epos." *Gymnasium* 77:365–75.

Grosz, E. 1994. *Volatile Bodies: Toward a Corporeal Feminism.* Bloomington, Ind.

———. 2005. *Time Travels: Feminism, Nature, Power.* Durham.

Guardasole, A. 2000. *Tragedia e medicina nell'Atene del V secolo a.C.* Naples.

Gundert, B. 1992. "Parts and Their Roles in Hippocratic Medicine." *Isis* 83:453–65.

———. 2000. "Soma and Psyche in Hippocratic Medicine." In J. P. Wright and Potter 2000, 13–35.

Guthrie, W.K.C. 1957. "Aristotle as a Historian of Philosophy: Some Preliminaries." *JHS* 77:35–41.

———. 1962–69. *A History of Greek Philosophy.* 3 vols. Cambridge.

Hadot, P. 1995. *Philosophy as a Way of Life: Spiritual Exercises from Socrates to Foucault.* Trans. M. Chase. Cambridge, Mass. [Expanded edition of *Exercices spirituels et philosophie antique.* 2nd ed. Paris, 1987.]

Hainsworth, B. 1993. *The Iliad: A Commentary.* Vol. 3: *Books 9–12.* Cambridge.

Hall, T. S. 1974. "Idiosyncrasy: Greek Medical Ideas of Uniqueness." *Sudhoffs Archiv* 58:283–302.

Halleran, M. R. 1986. "Rhetoric, Irony, and the Ending of Euripides' *Herakles*." *ClAnt* 5:171–81.

Halliday, W. R. 1913. *Greek Divination: A Study of Its Methods and Principles.* London.

Halliwell, S. 1990. "Traditional Greek Conceptions of Character." In Pelling 1990, 32–59.

Halperin, D. 1990. "The Democratic Body: Prostitution and Citizenship in Classical Athens." In *One Hundred Years of Homosexuality: And Other Essays on Greek Love*, 88–112. London.

Halperin, D., J. J. Winkler, and F. I. Zeitlin, eds. 1990. *Before Sexuality: The Construction of Erotic Experience in the Ancient Greek World.* Princeton.

Hamilton, R. 1985. "Slings and Arrows: The Debate with Lycus in the *Heracles*." *TAPA* 115:19–25.

Hankinson, R. J. 1991. "Greek Medical Models of Mind." In Everson 1991, 194–217.

———. 1992. "Doing without Hypotheses: The Nature of *Ancient Medicine*." In López Férez 1992, 55–67.

———. 1995a. "Pollution and Infection: An Hypothesis Still-born." *Apeiron* 28:25–65.

———. 1995b. "The Growth of Medical Empiricism." In Bates 1995, 60–83.

———. 1998a. *Cause and Explanation in Ancient Greek Thought.* Oxford.

———. 1998b. "Magic, Religion and Science: Divine and Human in the Hippocratic Corpus." *Apeiron* 31:1–34.

———, ed. and trans. 1998c. *Galen, On Antecedent Causes.* Cambridge.

———. 2006. "Body and Soul in Greek Philosophy." In *Persons and Their Bodies: Rights, Responsibilities, Relationships*, ed. M. J. Cherry, 35–56. Dordrecht.

Hanson, A. E. 1975. "Hippocrates: *Diseases of Women* I." *Signs* 1:567–84.

———. 1990. "The Medical Writers' Woman." In Halperin, Winkler, and Zeitlin 1990, 309–38.

———. 1991. "Continuity and Change: Three Case Studies in Hippocratic Gynecological Therapy and Theory." In Pomeroy 1991, 73–110.

———. 1992a. "The Logic of the Gynecological Prescriptions." In López Férez 1992, 235–50.

———. 1992b. "Conception, Gestation, and the Origin of Female Nature in the *Corpus Hippocraticum*." *Helios* 19:31–71.

———. 1995. "Uterine Amulets and Greek Uterine Medicine." *Medicina nei secoli* 7:281–99.

———. 1996. "Fragmentation and the Greek Medical Writers." In *Collecting Fragments/ Fragmente Sammeln*, ed. G. W. Most, 289–314. Göttingen.

———. 2007. "The Hippocratic *Parthenos* in Sickness and Health." In *Virginity Revisited: Configurations of the Unpossessed Body*, ed. B. MacLachlan and J. Fletcher, 40–65. Toronto.

Hanson, M., ed. and trans. 1999. *Hippocrates, On Head Wounds*. CMG I.4.1. Berlin.

Haraway, D. 1988. "Situated Knowledges: The Science Question in Feminism and the Privilege of Partial Perspective." *Feminist Studies* 14:575–99.

Harries, H. 1891. *Tragici Graeci qua arte usi sint in describenda insania*. Kiel.

Harrison, E. L. 1960. "Notes on Homeric Psychology." *Phoenix* 14:63–80.

Hartigan, K. V. 1987. "Euripidean Madness: Herakles and Orestes." *G & R* 34:126–35.

Havelock, E. 1972. "The Socratic Self as It Is Parodied in Aristophanes' *Clouds*." *YCS* 22:1–18.

Hawhee, D. 2004. *Bodily Arts: Rhetoric and Athletics in Ancient Greece*. Austin.

Hawley, R. 1998. "The Male Body as Spectacle in Attic Drama." In Foxhall and Salmon 1998a, 83–99.

Heeßel, N. P. 2004. "Diagnosis, Divination and Disease: Towards an Understanding of the *rationale* behind the Babylonian *Diagnostic Handbook*." In Horstmanshoff and Stol 2004, 97–116.

Heiberg, I. L., ed. 1927. *Hippocratis opera*. CMG I.1. Leipzig.

Heidegger, M. 1992. *Parmenides*. Trans. A. Schuwer and R. Rojcewicz. Bloomington, Ind. [*Parmenides*. Frankfurt am Main, 1982.]

Heidel, W. A. 1910. "Περὶ φύσεως: A Study of the Conception of Nature among the Pre-Socratics." *Proceedings of the American Academy of Arts and Sciences* 14:79–133.

Heinimann, F. 1945. *Nomos und Physis. Herkunft und Bedeutung einer Antithese im griechischen Denken des 5. Jahrhunderts*. Basel.

Henrichs, A. 1975. "Two Doxographical Notes: Democritus and Prodicus on Religion." *HSCP* 79:93–123.

———. 1976. "The Atheism of Prodicus." *Cronache ercolanesi* 6:15–21.

———. 1979. "'Thou Shalt Not Kill a Tree': Greek, Manichaean and Indian Tales." *Bulletin of the American Society of Papyrologists* 16:85–108.

———. 1996. "Dancing in Athens, Dancing on Delos: Some Patterns of Choral Projection in Euripides." *Philologus* 140:48–62.

Hershkowitz, D. 1998. *The Madness of Epic: Reading Insanity from Homer to Statius*. Oxford.

Herter, H. 1950. "Böse Dämonen im frühgriechischen Volksglauben." *Rheinisches Jahrbuch für Volkskunde* 1:112–43. Reprinted in Herter 1975, 43–75.

Herter, H. 1957. "Σῶμα bei Homer." In *Charites. Studien zur Altertumswissenschaft*, ed. K. Schauenburg, 206–17. Bonn. Reprinted in Herter 1975, 91–105.

———. 1975. *Kleine Schriften*. Munich.

Hirzel, R. 1914. *Die Person. Begriff und Name derselben im Altertum*. Munich.

Hoessly, F. 2001. *Katharsis. Reinigung als Heilverfahren. Studien zum Ritual der archaischen und klassischen Zeit sowie zum Corpus Hippocraticum*. Göttingen.

Holmes, B. 2007. "The *Iliad*'s Economy of Pain." *TAPA* 137:45–84.

———. 2008. "Euripides' Heracles in the Flesh." *ClAnt* 27:231–81.

———. Forthcoming (a). "Marked Bodies (Gender, Race, Class, Age, Disability, Disease)." In *A Cultural History of the Human Body*, vol. 1: *Ancient Greece to Early Christianity*, ed. D. Garrison. Oxford.

———. Forthcoming (b). "Body, Soul, and Medical Analogy in Plato." In *When Worlds Elide*, ed. J. P. Euben and K. Bassi. Lanham, Md.

Holt, P. 1981. "Disease, Desire, and Deianeira: A Note on the Symbolism of the *Trachiniae*." *Helios* 8:63–73.

Hooker, J. T. 1987. "Homeric φίλος." *Glotta* 65:44–65.

———. 1988. "*Odyssey* and *Iliad*: Folly and Delusion." *Ziva antika* 38:5–9.

Hopkins, A., and M. Wyke, eds. 2005. *Roman Bodies: Antiquity to the Eighteenth Century*. London.

Horden, P. 1999. "Pain in Hippocratic Medicine." In *Religion, Health and Suffering*, ed. J. Hinnells and R. Porter, 295–315. London.

Horky, P. S. 2006. "The Imprint of the Soul: Psychosomatic Affection in Plato, Gorgias, and the 'Orphic' Gold Tablets." *Mouseion* 6:371–86.

Horstmanshoff, H.F.J. 1990. "The Ancient Physician: Craftsman or Scientist?" *JHM* 45:176–97.

———. 2004. "'Did the God Learn Medicine?': Asclepius and Temple Medicine in Aelius Aristides' *Sacred Tales*." In Horstmanshoff and Stol 2004, 325–42.

Horstmanshoff, H.F.J., and R. M. Rosen. 2003. "The *Andreia* of the Hippocratic Physician and the Problem of Incurables." In Rosen and Sluiter 2003, 95–114.

Horstmanshoff, H.F.J., and M. Stol, eds. 2004. *Magic and Rationality in Ancient Near Eastern and Graeco-Roman Medicine*. Leiden.

Huffman, C. A., ed. and trans. 1993. *Philolaus of Croton: Pythagorean and Presocratic*. Cambridge.

Humphreys, S. C. 1996. "From Riddle to Rigour: Satisfactions of Scientific Prose in Ancient Greece." In *Proof and Persuasion: Essays on Authority, Objectivity and Evidence*, ed. S. Marchand and E. Lunbeck, 3–24. Brepols.

———. 1999. "From a Grin to a Death: The Body in the Greek Discovery of Politics." In Porter 1999a, 126–46.

Hunter, V. 1992. "Constructing the Body of the Citizen: Corporal Punishment in Classical Athens." *Echos du monde classique* 36:271–91.

Hussey, E. 1990. "The Beginnings of Epistemology: From Homer to Philolaus." In *Epistemology*, ed. S. Everson, 11–38. Cambridge.

———. 2006. "Parmenides on Thinking." In R. King 2006, 13–30.

Hutchinson, G. O. 2004. "Euripides' Other *Hippolytus*." *ZPE* 149:15–28.

Ierodiakonou, K. 2005. "Empedocles on Colour and Colour Vision." *OSAP* 29:1–37.

Ingenkamp, H. G. 1983. "Das στοχάσασθαι des Arztes (*VM*, 9)." In Lasserre and Mudry 1983, 257–62.

Innocenti, P. 1970. "Nota sul termine εἶδος nel 'Corpus' Omerico e in Esiodo." *Atti e memorie dell'Accademia Toscana di scienze e lettere, La Colombaria* 35:1–26.

Inwood, B., ed. and trans. 2001. *The Poem of Empedocles.* 2nd ed. Toronto.

Ioannidi, H. 1992. "La sensation-perception dans le *corpus* hippocratique." In López Férez 1992, 69–73.

Ireland, S., and F.L.D. Steel. 1975. "Φρένες as an Anatomical Organ in the Works of Homer." *Glotta* 53:183–95.

Irwin, T. 1983. "Euripides and Socrates." *CP* 78:183–97.

———. 1995. *Plato's Ethics.* 2nd ed. Oxford.

Isaac, B. 2004. *The Invention of Racism in Classical Antiquity.* Princeton.

Jaeger, W. 1944. *Paideia: The Ideals of Greek Culture; The Conflict of Cultural Ideals in the Age of Plato*, trans. G. Highet, from the German manuscript. Oxford.

———. 1947. *The Theology of the Early Greek Philosophers.* Trans. E. S. Robinson, from the German manuscript. Oxford.

———. 1957. "Aristotle's Use of Medicine as Model of Method in His Ethics." *JHS* 77:54–61.

Jahn, T. 1987. *Zum Wortfeld "Seele-Geist" in der Sprache Homers.* Munich.

Jandolo, M. 1967. "Manifestazioni somatiche delle psicosi in Ippocrate." *Rivista di storia della medicina* 11:45–48.

Janko, R. 1992. *The Iliad: A Commentary.* Vol. 4: *Books 13–16.* Cambridge.

———. 2001. "The Derveni Papyrus (Diagoras of Melos, *Apopyrgizontes Logoi?*): A New Translation." *CP* 96:1–32.

Johansen, T. 2000. "Body, Soul, and Tripartition in Plato's *Timaeus.*" *OSAP* 19:87–111.

Johnston, S. I. 1995. "Defining the Dreadful: Remarks on the Greek Child-Killing Demon." In Meyer and Mirecki 1995, 361–87.

Joly, R. 1960. *Recherches sur le traité pseudo-hippocratique du régime.* Paris.

———. 1966. *Le niveau de la science hippocratique: contribution à la psychologie de l'histoire des sciences.* Paris.

———, ed. and trans. 1970. *Hippocrate, De la génération; De la nature de l'enfant; Des maladies IV; Du fœtus de huit mois.* CUF t. 11. Paris.

———, ed. and trans. 1972. *Hippocrate, Du régime des maladies aiguës; Appendice; De l'aliment; De l'usage des liquides.* CUF t. 6.2. Paris.

———, ed. 1977. *Corpus Hippocraticum: actes du Colloque hippocratique de Mons (22–26 septembre 1975).* Mons.

———, ed. and trans. 1978. *Hippocrate, Des lieux dans l'homme; Du système des glandes; Des fistules—Des hémorroïdes; De la vision; Des chairs; De la dentition.* CUF t. 13. Paris.

Joly, R., and S. Byl, ed. and trans. 2003. *Hippocrate, Du régime.* 2nd ed. *CMG* I.2.4. Berlin.

Jonas, H. 1966. *The Phenomenon of Life: Toward a Philosophical Biology.* New York.

Jones, W.H.S., ed. and trans. 1923a. *Hippocrates.* Vol. 1. Cambridge, Mass.

———, ed. and trans. 1923b. *Hippocrates.* Vol. 2. Cambridge, Mass.

———, ed. and trans. 1931. *Hippocrates.* Vol. 4. Cambridge, Mass.

———. 1946. *Philosophy and Medicine in Ancient Greece.* Baltimore.

———, trans. 1947. *The Medical Writings of Anonymous Londinensis.* Cambridge.

Jörgensen, O. 1904. "Das Auftreten der Götter in den Büchern ι–μ der *Odyssee.*" *Hermes* 39:357–82.

Jori, A. 1996. *Medicina e medici nell'antica Grecia: saggio sul "Perì téchnes" ippocratico.* Naples.

——. 2002. "Il caso, la fortuna e il loro rapporto con la malattia e la guarigione nel *Corpus Hippocraticum.*" In Thivel and Zucker 2002, 197–228.

Jouan, F. 1970. "Le *Prométhée* d'Eschyle et l'*Héraclès* d'Euripide." *REA* 72:317–31.

Jouan, F., and H. van Looy, eds. 1999–2003. *Euripide, Fragments.* CUF t. 8.1–4. Paris.

Jouanna, J. 1961. "Présence d'Empédocle dans la *Collection Hippocratique.*" *Bullétin de l'Association Guillaume Budé* 20:452–63.

——. 1965. "Rapports entre Mélissos de Samos et Diogène d'Apollonie à la lumière du traité hippocratique *De Natura Hominis.*" *REA* 67:306–23.

——. 1974. *Hippocrate: pour une archéologie de l'école de Cnide.* Paris.

——. 1983a. "Médecine et protection: essai sur une archéologie philologique des formes de pensée." In Lasserre and Mudry 1983, 21–39.

——. 1983b. "Le sommeil médecin (Sophocle, *Philoctète* v. 859 ἀλεὴς ὕπνος)." In *Théâtre et spectacles dans l'Antiquité: actes du Colloque de Strasbourg, 5–7 novembre 1981,* 49–62. Leiden.

——, ed. and trans. 1983c. *Hippocrate. Maladies II.* CUF t. 10.2. Paris.

——. 1984. "Rhétorique et médecine dans la *Collection hippocratique*: contribution à l'histoire de la rhétorique au Vᵉ siècle." *REG* 97:26–44.

——. 1987. "Médecine hippocratique et tragédie grecque." In *Anthropologie et théâtre antique: actes du colloque international de Montpellier, 6–8 mars 1986.* Cahiers du GITA 3:109–31.

——. 1988a. "La maladie sauvage dans la *Collection hippocratique* et la tragédie grecque." *Métis* 3:343–60.

——, ed. and trans. 1988b. *Hippocrate, Des vents; De l'art.* CUF t. 5.1. Paris.

——. 1990a. "La maladie comme agression dans la *Collection hippocratique* et la tragédie grecque: la maladie sauvage et dévorante." In Potter, Maloney, and Desautels 1990, 39–60.

——, ed. and trans. 1990b. *Hippocrate, De l'ancienne médecine.* CUF t. 2.1. Paris.

——. 1992. "La naissance de la science de l'homme chez les médecins et les savants à l'époque d'Hippocrate: problèmes de méthode." In López Férez 1992, 91–111.

——, ed. and trans. 1996. *Hippocrate, Airs, eaux, lieux.* CUF t. 2.2. Paris.

——. 1998. "L'interprétation des rêves et la théorie micro-macrocosmique dans le traité hippocratique *Du régime*: sémiotique et mimesis." In *Text and Tradition: Studies in Ancient Medicine and Its Transmission Presented to Jutta Kollesch,* ed. K. D. Fischer, D. Nickel, and P. Potter, 161–74. Leiden.

——. 1999. *Hippocrates.* Trans. M. DeBevoise. Baltimore. [*Hippocrate.* Paris, 1992.]

——, ed. and trans. 2000. *Hippocrate, Epidémies V et VII.* CUF t. 4.3. Paris.

——. 2001. "Air, miasme et contagion à l'époque d'Hippocrate et survivance des miasmes dans la médecine posthippocratique (Rufus d'Éphèse, Galien et Palladios." In *Air, miasmes et contagion: les épidémies dans l'Antiquité et au Moyen Âge,* ed. S. Bazin-Tacchella, D. Quéruel, and É. Samama, 9–28. Langres.

——, ed. and trans. 2002. *Hippocrate, La nature de l'homme. 2nd* ed. CMG I.1.3. Berlin.

——, ed. and trans. 2003. *Hippocrate, La maladie sacrée.* CUF t. 2.3. Paris.

——. 2007a. "La théorie de la sensation, de la pensée et de l'âme dans le traité hippocratique du *Régime*: ses rapports avec Empédocle et le *Timée* de Platon." *AION: Annali dell'Istituto Universitario Orientale di Napoli: Sezione filologico-letteraria* 29:9–38.

————. 2007b. "Aux racines de la mélancolie: la médecine grecque est-elle mélancolique?" In *De la mélancolie*, ed. J. Clair and R. Kopp, 11–51. Paris.

Jouanna, J., and P. Demont. 1981. "Le sens d'ἰχώρ chez Homère (*Iliade* V, v. 340 et 416) et Eschyle (*Agamemnon*, v. 1480) en relation avec les emplois du mot dans la *Collection hippocratique*." *REA* 83:197–209.

Jourdain-Annequin, C. 1985. "Héraclès *latris* et *doulos*: sur quelques aspects du travail dans le mythe heroïque." *Dialogues d'histoire ancienne* 11:487–538.

Joyce, R. A. 2005. "Archaeology of the Body." *Annual Review of Anthropology* 34:139–58.

Just, R. 1985. "Freedom, Slavery, and the Female Psyche." *History of Political Thought* 6:169–88.

————. 1989. *Women in Athenian Law and Life*. London.

Justesen, P. 1928. *Les principes psychologiques d'Homère*. Copenhagen.

Kahn, C. 1960. *Anaximander and the Origins of Cosmology*. New York.

————. 1985. "Democritus and the Origins of Moral Psychology." *AJP* 106:1–31.

Kallet, L. 1999. "The Diseased Body Politic, Athenian Public Finance, and the Massacre at Mykalessos (Thucydides 7.27–29)." *AJP* 120:223–44.

Kamerbeek, J. 1948. "On the Conception of ΘΕΟΜΑΧΟΣ in Relation with Greek Tragedy." *Mnemosyne* 4:271–83.

Katz, J. T., and K. Volk. 2000. "'Mere Bellies'?: A New Look at *Theogony* 26–8." *JHS* 120:122–31.

Katz, M. A. 1989. "Sexuality and the Body in Ancient Greece." *Métis* 4:155–79.

Keil, F. C., et al. 1999. "Mechanism and Explanation in the Development of Biological Thought: The Case of Disease." In *Folkbiology*, ed. D. L. Medin and S. Atran, 285–319. Cambridge, Mass.

Kennedy, G. A. 1991. *On Rhetoric: A Theory of Civic Discourse*. New York.

Kerferd, G. B. 1981. *The Sophistic Movement*. Cambridge.

————. 1985. "Gorgias and Empedocles." In Montoneri and Romano 1985, 595–605.

King, H. 1988. "The Early Anodynes: Pain in the Ancient World." In *The History of the Management of Pain: From Early Principles to Present Practice*, ed. R. D. Mann, 51–62. Carnforth and Park Ridge, N.J. Rev. version in H. King 1998, 114–31.

————. 1994. "Producing Woman: Hippocratic Gynaecology." In *Women in Ancient Societies: An Illusion of the Night*, ed. L. J. Archer, S. Fischler, and M. Wyke, 102–14. Basingstoke.

————. 1998. *Hippocrates' Woman: Reading the Female Body in Ancient Greece*. London.

King, R.A.H., ed. 2006. *Common to Body and Soul: Philosophical Approaches to Explaining Living Behaviour in Greco-Roman Antiquity*. Berlin.

Kingsley, P. 1995. *Ancient Philosophy, Mystery, and Magic: Empedocles and Pythagorean Tradition*. Oxford.

Kinnier Wilson, J. V., and E. H. Reynolds. 1990. "Translation and Analysis of a Cuneiform Text Forming Part of a Babylonian Treatise on Epilepsy." *Medical History* 34:185–98.

Kirk, G. S. 1990. *The Iliad: A Commentary*. Vol. 2: *Books 5–8*. Cambridge.

Kirk, G. S., J. E. Raven, and M. Schofield. 1983. *The Presocratic Philosophers*. 2nd ed. Cambridge.

Kitto, H.D.F. 1955. "The Dance in Greek Tragedy." *JHS* 75:36–41.

Kleinman, A. 1988. *The Illness Narratives: Suffering, Healing, and the Human Condition*. New York.

Klibansky, R., E. Panofsky, and F. Saxl. 1964. *Saturn and Melancholy: Studies in the History of Natural Philosophy, Religion, and Art.* New York.

Knappett, C. 2006. "Beyond Skin: Layering and Networking in Art and Archaeology." *Cambridge Archaeological Journal* 16:239–51.

Knox, B.M.W. 1952. "The *Hippolytus* of Euripides." *YCS* 13:3–31.

Koller, H. 1958. "Σῶμα bei Homer." *Glotta* 37:276–81.

Kollesch, J. 1991. "Darstellungsformen der medizinischen Literatur im 5. und 4. Jahrhundert. v. Chr." *Philologus* 135:177–83.

Kosak, J. C. 2004. *Heroic Measures: Hippocratic Medicine in the Making of Euripidean Tragedy.* Leiden.

Kotansky, R. 1995. "Greek Exorcistic Amulets." In Meyer and Mirecki 1995, 243–77.

Kovacs, D., ed. and trans. 1994–2002. *Euripides.* 6 vols. Cambridge, Mass.

———. 1996. *Euripidea altera.* Leiden.

———. 2002. "Rationalism, Naïve and Malign, in Euripides' *Orestes*." In *Vertis in usum: Studies in Honor of Edward Courtney,* ed. J. F. Miller, C. Damon, and K. S. Myers, 277–86. Leipzig.

———. 2003. *Euripidea tertia.* Leiden.

Kraus, C. S. 1998. "Dangerous Supplements: Etymology and Genealogy in Euripides' *Heracles*." *PCPS* 44:137–57.

Kroeker, E. 1938. *Der Herakles des Euripides.* Gießen.

Kudlien, F. 1968. "Early Greek Primitive Medicine." *Clio Medica* 3:305–36.

———. 1973. "The Old Greek Concept of 'Relative Health.'" *Journal of the History of Behavioral Sciences* 9:53–59.

Kühlewein, H., ed. 1894–1902. *Hippocratis opera quae feruntur omnia.* 2 vols. Leipzig.

Kuntz, M. 1994. "The Prodikean 'Choice of Heracles': A Reshaping of Myth." *Classical Journal* 89:163–81.

Kuriyama, S. 1999. *The Expressiveness of the Body and the Divergence of Greek and Chinese Medicine.* New York.

Kurke, L. 1999. *Coins, Bodies, Games, and Gold: The Politics of Meaning in Archaic Greece.* Princeton.

Lacan, J. 1977. "The Mirror Stage as Formative of the Function of the I as Revealed in Psychoanalytic Experience." In *Écrits: A Selection,* trans. A. Sheridan, 1–7. New York. ["Le stade du miroir comme formateur de la fonction du Je." *Revue française de psychanalyse* 4 (1949): 449–55.]

Laín Entralgo, P. 1970. *The Therapy of the Word in Classical Antiquity.* Trans. L. J. Rather and J. M. Sharp. New Haven. [*La curacion por la palabra en la antigüedad clasica.* Madrid, 1958.]

———. 1975. "Quaestiones hippocraticae disputatae tres." In Bourgey and Jouanna 1975, 305–19.

Laks, A. 1999. "Soul, Sensation, and Thought." In Long 1999a, 250–70.

———. 2002. "'Philosophes présocratiques': remarques sur la construction d'une catégorie de l'historiographie philosophique." In Laks and Louguet 2002, 17–38.

———. 2006. *Introduction à la "philosophie présocratique."* Paris.

———, ed. and trans. 2008. *Diogène d'Apollonie.* 2nd ed. Sankt Augustin.

Laks, A., and C. Louguet, eds. 2002. *Qu'est-ce que la philosophie présocratique?/What Is Presocratic Philosophy?* Villeneuve-d'Ascq.

Lambek, M. 1998. "Body and Mind in Mind, Body and Mind in Body: Some Anthropological Interventions in a Long Conversation." In Lambek and Strathern 1998b, 103–23.

Lambek, M., and A. Strathern. 1998a. "Introduction. Embodying Sociality: Africanist-Melanesianist Comparisons." In Lambek and Strathern 1998b, 1–25.

————, eds. 1998b. *Bodies and Persons: Comparative Perspectives from Africa and Melanesia.* Cambridge.

Lami, A., ed. and trans. 2007. "[Ippocrate], *Sui disturbi virginali*: testo, traduzione e commento." *Galenos* 1:15–59.

Lanata, G. 1967. *Medicina magica e religione popolare in Grecia fino all'età di Ippocrate.* Rome.

————. 1968. "Linguaggio scientifico e linguaggio poetico: note al lessico del 'de morbo sacro.'" *QUCC* 5:22–36.

Langholf, V. 1983. "Symptombeschreibungen in *Epidemien* I und III und die Struktur des *Prognostikon*." In Lasserre and Mudry 1983, 109–20.

————. 1990. *Medical Theories in Hippocrates: Early Texts and the "Epidemics."* Berlin.

————. 1997–2004. "Zeichenkonzeptionen in der Medizin der griechischen und römischen Antike." In *Semiotik. Ein Handbuch zu den zeichentheoretischen Grundlagen von Natur und Kultur*, ed. R. Posner, K. Robering, and T. A. Sebeok, 912–21. Berlin, 1997–2004.

Langslow, D. R. 1999. "The Language of Poetry and the Language of Science: The Latin Poets and 'Medical Latin.'" In *Aspects of the Language of Latin Poetry*, ed. J. N. Adams and R. G. Mayer, 183–225. Oxford.

Laqueur, T. 1990. *Making Sex: Body and Gender from the Greeks to Freud.* Cambridge, Mass.

Larmour, D.H.J., P. A. Miller, and C. Platter, eds. 1998. *Rethinking Sexuality: Foucault and Classical Antiquity.* Princeton.

Larock, V. 1930. "Les premières conceptions psychologiques des Grecs." *RBPh* 9:377–406.

Laser, S. 1983. *Medizin und Körperpflege.* Göttingen.

Laskaris, J. 1999. "Archaic Healing Cults as a Source for Hippocratic Pharmacology." In Garofalo et al. 1999, 1–12.

————. 2002. *The Art Is Long: "On the Sacred Disease" and the Scientific Tradition.* Leiden.

Lasserre, F., and P. Mudry, eds. 1983. *Formes de pensée dans la collection hippocratique: actes du IVᵉ Colloque international hippocratique, Lausanne, 21–26 septembre 1981.* Geneva.

Lateiner, D. 1986. "The Empirical Element in the Methods of Early Greek Medical Writers and Herodotus: A Shared Epistemological Response." *Antichthon* 20:1–20.

————. 1995. *Sardonic Smile: Nonverbal Behavior in Homeric Epic.* Ann Arbor.

Latour, B. 1999. *Pandora's Hope: Essays on the Reality of Science Studies.* Cambridge, Mass.

Lawrence, S. E. 1998. "The God That Is Truly God and the Universe of Euripides' *Heracles*." *Mnemosyne* 51:129–46.

Le Blay, F. 2005. "Microcosm and Macrocosm: The Dual Direction of Analogy in Hippocratic Thought and the Meteorological Tradition." In van der Eijk 2005a, 251–69.

Leder, D. 1990. *The Absent Body.* Chicago.

Lee, K. H. 1982. "The Iris-Lyssa Scene in Euripides' *Heracles*." *Antichthon* 16–18:44–53.

Lefkowitz, M. 1987. "Was Euripides an Atheist?" *Studi di filologia classica* 5:149–66.

———. 1989. "'Impiety' and 'Atheism' in Euripides' Dramas." *CQ* 39:70–82.

———. 2002. "Apollo in the *Orestes*." *Studi di filologia classica* 20:46–53.

Leftwich, G. V. 1995. "Polykleitos and Hippokratic Medicine." In *Polykleitos, the Doryphoros, and Tradition*, ed. W. G. Moon, 38–51. Madison.

Lesher, J. H. 1991. "Xenophanes on Inquiry and Discovery: An Alternative to the 'Hymn to Progress' Reading of Fr. 18." *AncPhil* 11:229–48.

———, ed. and trans. 1992. *Xenophanes of Colophon, Fragments*. Toronto.

———. 1994. "The Emergence of Philosophical Interest in Cognition." *OSAP* 12:1–34.

Lesky, A. 1961. "Göttliche und menschliche Motivierung im homerischen Epos." In *Sitzungsberichte der Heidelberger Akademie der Wissenschaften, Philosophisch-Historische Klasse*, Abhandlung 4.

———. 1966. "Decision and Responsibility in the Tragedy of Aeschylus." *JHS* 86:78–85.

Leszl, W. 2006. "Aristoteles on the Unity of Presocratic Philosophy: A Contribution to the Reconstruction of the Early Retrospective View of Presocratic Philosophy." In *La costruzione del discorso filosofico nell'età dei Presocratici/The Construction of Philosophical Discourse in the Age of the Presocratics*, ed. M. M. Sassi, 355–80. Pisa.

———. 2007. "Democritus' Works: From Their Titles to Their Contents." In Brancacci and Morel 2007, 11–76.

Lichtenthaeler, C. 1963. *Quatrième série d'études hippocratiques* (VII–X). Geneva.

LiDonnici, L. R., trans. 1995. *The Epidaurian Miracle Inscriptions*. Atlanta.

Lidz, J. W. 1995. "Medicine as Metaphor in Plato." *Journal of Medicine and Philosophy* 20:527–41.

Lienau, C., ed. and trans. 1973. *Hippokrates. Über Nachempfängnis, Geburtshilfe und Schwangerschaftsleiden*. CMG I.2.2. Berlin.

Lincoln, B. 1975. "Homeric λύσσα: 'Wolfish Rage.'" *Indogermanische Forschung* 80:98–105.

Lingis, A. 2000. *Dangerous Emotions*. Berkeley.

Lloyd, G.E.R. 1963. "Who Is Attacked in *On Ancient Medicine*?" *Phronesis* 8:108–26. Reprinted with a new introduction in Lloyd 1991a, 49–69.

———. 1964. "The Hot and the Cold, the Dry and the Wet in Greek Philosophy." *JHS* 84:92–106.

———. 1966. *Polarity and Analogy: Two Types of Argumentation in Early Greek Thought*. Cambridge.

———. 1967. "Popper versus Kirk: A Controversy in the Interpretation of Greek Science." *British Journal for the Philosophy of Science* 18:21–38. Reprinted with a new introduction in Lloyd 1991a, 100–120.

———. 1975a. "Alcmaeon and the Early History of Dissection." *Sudhoffs Archiv* 59:113–47. Reprinted with a new introduction in Lloyd 1991a, 164–93.

———. 1975b. "The Hippocratic Question." *CQ* 25:171–92. Reprinted with a new introduction in Lloyd 1991a, 194–223.

———. 1979. *Magic, Reason, and Experience: Studies in the Origin and Development of Greek Science*. Cambridge.

———. 1983. *Science, Folklore, and Ideology: Studies in the Life Sciences in Ancient Greece*. Cambridge.

———. 1987. *The Revolutions of Wisdom: Studies in the Claims and Practice of Ancient Greek Science*. Berkeley.

———. 1990. *Demystifying Mentalities*. Cambridge.

———. 1991a. *Method and Problems in Greek Science*. Cambridge.

———. 1991b. "The Invention of Nature." In Lloyd 1991a, 417–34.

———. 1992. "The Transformations of Ancient Medicine." *BHM* 66:114–32. Reprinted in Lloyd 2006, chap. 1.

———. 1996. *Adversaries and Authorities: Investigations into Ancient Greek and Chinese Science*. Cambridge.

———. 2002a. *The Ambitions of Curiosity: Understanding the World in Ancient Greece and China*. Cambridge.

———. 2002b. "Le pluralisme de la vie intellectuelle avant Platon." In Laks and Louguet 2002, 39–53. English trans.: Lloyd 2006, chap. 10.

———. 2003. *In the Grip of Disease: Studies in the Greek Imagination*. Oxford.

———. 2004. *Ancient Worlds, Modern Reflections: Philosophical Perspectives on Greek and Chinese Science and Culture*. Oxford.

———. 2005. *The Delusions of Invulnerability: Wisdom and Morality in Ancient Greece, China and Today*. London.

———. 2006. *Principles and Practices in Ancient Greek and Chinese Science*. Aldershot.

Lloyd, G.E.R., and N. Sivin. 2002. *The Way and the Word: Science and Medicine in Early China and Greece*. New Haven.

Lloyd, M. 1992. *The Agon in Euripides*. Oxford.

Lloyd-Jones, H. 1983. *The Justice of Zeus*. 2nd ed. Berkeley.

Lock, M. 2007. "Medical Anthropology: Intimations for the Future." In *Medical Anthropology: Regional Perspectives and Shared Concerns*, ed. F. Saillant and S. Genest, 267–88. Malden, Mass.

Long, A. A. 1966. "Thinking and Sense-Perception in Empedocles: Mysticism or Materialism?" *CQ* 16:256–76.

———, ed. 1999a. *The Cambridge Companion to Early Greek Philosophy*. Cambridge.

———. 1999b. "The Scope of Early Greek Philosophy." In Long 1999a, 1–21.

Longrigg, J. 1963. "Philosophy and Medicine: Some Early Interactions." *HSCP* 67:147–75.

———. 1985. "Elements and After: A Study in Presocratic Physics of the Second Half of the Fifth Century." *Apeiron* 19:93–115.

———. 1989. "Presocratic Philosophy and Hippocratic Medicine." *History of Science* 27:1–39.

———. 1999. "Presocratic Philosophy and Hippocratic Dietetic Theory." In Garofalo et al. 1999, 43–50.

Lonie, I. M. 1965a. "The Cnidian Treatises of the Corpus Hippocraticum." *CQ* 15:1–30.

———. 1965b. "The Hippocratic Treatise Περὶ διαίτης ὀξέων." *Sudhoffs Archiv* 49:50–79.

———. 1977. "A Structural Pattern in Greek Dietetics and the Early History of Greek Medicine." *Medical History* 21:235–60.

———. 1978. "Cos versus Cnidus and the Historians: Parts I and II." *History of Science* 16:42–75, 77–92.

———, trans. 1981. *The Hippocratic Treatises "On Generation," "On the Nature of the Child," "Diseases IV."* Berlin.

———. 1983. "Literacy and the Development of Hippocratic Medicine." In Lasserre and Mudry 1983, 145–61.

Lonsdale, S. H. 1990. *Creatures of Speech: Lion, Herding, and Hunting Similes in the "Iliad."* Stuttgart.

López Férez, J. A., ed. 1992. *Tratados hipocráticos: estudios acerca de su contenido, forma e influencia; actas del VIIe Colloque international hippocratique, Madrid, 24–29 de septiembre de 1990*. Madrid.

Loraux, N. 1979. "La gloire et la mort d'une femme." *Sorcières* 18:51–57.

———. 1986. "Le corps vulnérable d'Arès." In "Corps des dieux," ed. C. Malamoud and J.-P. Vernant, 335–54. Special issue: *Le temps de la réflexion 7*.

———. 1987. *Tragic Ways of Killing a Woman*. Trans. A. Forster. Cambridge, Mass. [*Façons tragiques de tuer une femme*. Paris, 1985.]

———. 1995. *The Experiences of Tiresias: The Feminine and the Greek Man*. Trans. P. Wissing. Princeton. [*Les expériences de Tirésias: le féminin et l'homme grec*. Paris, 1989.]

———. 1997. "Un absent de l'histoire?: le corps dans l'historiographie thucydidéenne." *Métis* 12:223–67.

———. 1998. *Mothers in Mourning, with the essay "Of Amnesty and Its Opposite."* Trans. C. Pache. Ithaca. [*Les mères en deuil*. Paris, 1990; "De l'amnistie et de son contraire." In *Usages de l'oubli*, ed. Y. Yerushalmi, 23–47. Paris, 1988.]

Lorenz, H. 2003. "Ancient Theories of Soul." In *The Stanford Encyclopedia of Philosophy (Winter 2003 Edition)*, ed. E. N. Zalta. URL = http://plato.stanford.edu/archives/in2003/entries/ancient-soul/>.

Lowenstam, S. 1981. *The Death of Patroklos: A Study in Typology*. Königstein.

Luppe, W. 2005. "Zu Daten und Reihenfolge der beiden Hippolytos-Dramen des Euripides." *ZPE* 151:11–14.

Luschnig, C.A.E. 1988. *Time Holds the Mirror: A Study of Knowledge in Euripides' "Hippolytus."* Leiden.

Lynn-George, M. 1993. "Aspects of the Epic Vocabulary of Vulnerability." *Colby Quarterly* 29:197–221.

———. 1996. "Structures of Care in the *Iliad*." *CQ* 46:1–26.

MacDowell, D. M. 1961. "Gorgias, Alkidamas, and the Cripps and Palatine Manuscripts." *CQ* 11:113–24.

———. 1982. *Gorgias, Encomium of Helen*. London.

MacKenzie, M. M. 1981. *Plato on Punishment*. Berkeley.

Mackie, C. 1997. "Achilles' Teachers: Chiron and Phoenix in the *Iliad*." *G & R* 44:1–10.

———. 2001. "The Earliest Jason: What's in a Name?" *G & R* 48:1–17.

MacKinney, L. 1964. "The Concept of Isonomia in Greek Medicine." In *Isonomia. Studien zur Gleichheitsvorstellung im griechischen Denken*, ed. J. Mau and E. G. Schmidt, 79–88. Berlin.

Magdelaine, C. 1997. "Microcosme et macrocosme dans le *Corpus hippocratique*: réflexions sur l'homme et la maladie." In *Littérature et médecine: articles*, ed. J.-L. Cabanès, 11–39. Talence.

Mainoldi, C. 1987. "Sonno e morte in Grecia antica." In *Rappresentazioni della morte*, ed. R. Raffaelli, 9–46. Urbino.

Major, R. H. 1957. "How Hippocrates Made His Diagnoses." *International Record of Medicine* 170:479–85.

Maloney, G. 1983. "Contributions hippocratiques à l'étude de l'*Orestie* d'Eschyle." In Lasserre and Mudry 1983, 71–76.

Maloney, G., P. Potter, and W. Frohn. 1979. *Répartition des œuvres hippocratiques par genres littéraires*. Québec.

Manetti, D. 1973. "Valore semantico e risonanze culturali della parola φύσις (*De genitura, De natura pueri, De morbis IV*)." *La parola del passato* 28:426–44.

———. 1999. "Aristotle and the Role of Doxography in the Anonymous Londiniensis (Pbrlibr Inv. 137)." In van der Eijk 1999a, 95–141.

Manetti, D., and A. Roselli, eds. and trans. 1982. *Ippocrate, Epidemie: libro sesto*. Florence.

Manetti, G. 1993. *Theories of the Sign in Classical Antiquity*. Trans. C. Richardson. Bloomington, Ind. [*Le teorie del segno nell'antichità classica*. Milan, 1987.]

———. 1994. "Indizi e prove nella cultura greca: forza epistemica e criteri di validità dell'inferenza semiotica." *Quaderni storici* 85:19–42.

Mansfeld, J. 1971. *The Pseudo-Hippocratic Tract Peri hebdomadōn: Ch. 1–11 and Greek Philosophy*. Assen.

———. 1975. "Alcmaeon: 'Physikos' or Physician?" In *Kephalaion: Studies in Greek Philosophy and Its Continuation Offered to Professor C. J. de Vogel*, 26–38. Assen.

———. 1980. "Theoretical and Empirical Attitudes in Early Greek Scientific Medicine." In Grmek 1980, 371–92.

Mansfeld, J. 1985. "Aristotle and Others on Thales, or the Beginnings of Natural Philosophy (with Some Remarks on Xenophanes)." *Mnemosyne* 38:109–29. Reprinted in *Studies in the Historiography of Greek Philosophy*, 126–46. Assen, 1990.

———. 1999. "Sources." In Long 1999a, 22–44.

Manuli, P. 1980. "Fisiologia e patologia del femminile negli scritti ippocratici dell'antica ginecologia greca." In Grmek 1980, 393–408.

———. 1983. "Donne mascoline, femmine sterili, vergini perpetue: la ginecologia greca tra Ippocrate e Sorano." In *Madre materia: sociologia e biologia della donna greca*, ed. S. Campese, P. Manuli, and G. Sissa, 147–92. Turin.

Marelli, C. 1983. "Place de la *Collection hippocratique* dans les théories biologiques sur le sommeil." In Lasserre and Mudry 1983, 331–33.

Marg, W. 1976. "Kampf und Tod in der *Ilias*." *Würzburger Jahrbücher für die Altertumswissenschaft* 2:7–19.

Marganne, M. H. 1988. "De la physiognomonie dans l'Antiquité gréco-romaine." In *Rhétoriques du corps*, ed. P. Dubois and Y. Winkin, 13–24. Brussels.

Martin, Agnes. 1992. *Writings/Schriften*. Ed. D. Schwarz. Stuttgart.

Martin, Alain, and O. Primavesi, eds. 1999. *L'Empédocle de Strasbourg (P. Strasb. gr. Inv. 1665–1666)*. Berlin.

Martin, D. B. 2004. *Inventing Superstition: From the Hippocratics to the Christians*. Cambridge, Mass.

Martinez, D. G. 1995. " 'May She Neither Eat Nor Drink': Love Magic and Vows of Abstinence." In Meyer and Mirecki 1995, 335–59.

Marzullo, B. 1986–87. "Hippocr. *Progn*. 1 Alex. (*Prooemium*)." *Museum Criticum* 21–22:199–254.

———. 1999. "Il 'dolore' in Ippocrate." *QUCC* 92:123–28.

Mastronarde, D. 1986. "The Optimistic Rationalist in Euripides: Theseus, Jocasta, Teiresias." In *Greek Tragedy and Its Legacy: Essays Presented to D. J. Conacher*, ed. M. Cropp, E. Fantham, and S. E. Scully, 201–11. Calgary.

———. 1990. "Actors on High: The Skene Roof, the Crane, and the Gods in Attic Drama." *ClAnt* 9:247–94.

———, ed. 1994. *Euripides, Phoenissae*. Cambridge.

———. 2002. "Euripidean Tragedy and Theology." *Seminari Romani di cultura greca* 5:17–49.

Mattes, M. 1970. *Der Wahnsinn im griechischen Mythos und in der Dichtung bis zum Drama des fünften Jahrhunderts*. Heidelberg.

Mauri, A. 1990. "Funzione e lessico della follia guerriera nei poemi omerici." *Acme* 43:51–62.

Maurizio, L. 1995. "Anthropology and Spirit Possession: A Reconsideration of the Pythia's Role at Delphi." *JHS* 115:69–86.

Mauss, M. 1966. *Sociologie et anthropologie.* 3rd ed. Paris.

———. 1979. "Body Techniques." In *Sociology and Psychology: Essays,* trans. B. Brewster, 95–123. London. ["Les techniques du corps." In Mauss 1966, 365–86.]

———. 1985. "A Category of the Human Mind: The Notion of Person; the Notion of Self" (trans. W. D. Halls). In *The Category of the Person: Anthropology, Philosophy, History,* ed. M. Carrithers, S. Collins, and S. Lukes, 1–25. Cambridge. ["Une catégorie de l'esprit humain: la notion de personne, celle de 'moi.'" In Mauss 1966, 333–62.]

Mawet, F. 1979. *Recherches sur les oppositions fonctionnelles dans le vocabulaire homérique de la douleur (autour de πῆμα-ἄλγος).* Brussels.

McDermott, E. 2000. "Euripides' Second Thoughts." *TAPA* 130:239–59.

McKeown, N. 2002. "Seeing Things: Examining the Body of the Slave in Greek Medicine." In *Representing the Body of the Slave,* ed. T.E.J. Wiedemann and J. F. Gardner, 29–40. London.

McMullin, E. 1965. "Introduction: The Concept of Matter." In *The Concept of Matter in Greek and Medieval Philosophy,* ed. E. McMullin, 1–23. Notre Dame.

Mejer, J. 2006. "Ancient Philosophy and the Doxographical Tradition." In *A Companion to Ancient Philosophy,* ed. M. L. Gill and P. Pellegrin, 20–33. Malden, Mass.

Merkelbach, R. 1975. "Nachträge zur Archilochos." *ZPE* 16:220–22.

Merleau-Ponty, M. 1962. *The Phenomenology of Perception.* Trans. C. Smith. London. [*Phénomènologie de la perception.* Paris, 1945.]

———. 1968. *The Visible and the Invisible.* Trans. A. Lingis. Evanston. [*Le visible et l'invisible.* Paris, 1964.]

Meskell, L. M. 1996. "The Somatization of Archaeology: Institutions, Discourses, Corporeality." *Norwegian Archaeological Review* 29:1–16.

Mesturini, A. M. 1981. "Magia e medicina in un frammento del *Bellerofonte* di Euripide." *Annali della Facoltà di lettere e filosofia: Università di Genova* 1:35–56.

Métraux, G. 1995. *Sculptors and Physicians in Fifth-Century Greece.* Montréal.

Meyer, M., and P. Mirecki, eds. 1995. *Ancient Magic and Ritual Power.* Leiden.

Michelini, A. 1987. *Euripides and the Tragic Tradition.* Madison.

Michler, M. 1962. "Die praktische Bedeutung des normativen Physis-Begriffes in der hippokratischen Schrift *De fracturis-De articulis.*" *Hermes* 90:385–401.

Mikalson, J. D. 1991. *Honor Thy Gods: Popular Religion in Greek Tragedy.* Chapel Hill.

Miller, G. L. 1990. "Literacy and the Hippocratic Art: Reading, Writing, and Epistemology in Ancient Greek Medicine." *JHM* 45:11–40.

Miller, H. W. 1944. "Medical Terminology in Tragedy." *TAPA* 75:156–67.

———. 1945. "Aristophanes and Medical Language." *TAPA* 76:74–84.

———. 1949. "*On Ancient Medecine* and the Origin of Medicine." *TAPA* 80:187–202.

———. 1952. "*Dynamis* and *Physis* in *On Ancient Medicine.*" *TAPA* 83:184–97.

———. 1953. "The Concept of the Divine in *De morbo sacro.*" *TAPA* 84:1–15.

———. 1955. "*Technē* and Discovery in *On Ancient Medicine.*" *TAPA* 86:51–62.

———. 1959. "The Concept of *Dynamis* in *De victu.*" *TAPA* 90:147–64.

Mills, S. 1997. *Theseus, Tragedy and the Athenian Empire.* Oxford.

Mitsis, P. 1988. *Epicurus' Ethical Theory: The Pleasures of Invulnerability.* Ithaca.

Moline, J. 1975. "Euripides, Socrates and Virtue." *Hermes* 103:45–67.

Monsacré, H. 1984. *Les larmes d'Achille: le héros, la femme et la souffrance dans la poésie d'Homère.* Paris.

Montiglio, S. 2000. *Silence in the Land of Logos.* Princeton.

Montoneri L., and F. Romano, eds. 1985. "Gorgia e la sofistica: atti del convegno internazionale (Lentini-Catania, 12–15 dic. 1983)." Special issue: *Siculorum Gymnasium* 38.

Montserrat, D., ed. 1998. *Changing Bodies, Changing Meanings: Studies on the Human Body in Antiquity.* London.

Moreau, A. 1989. "Transes douloureuses dans le théâtre d'Eschyle: Cassandre et Io." In *Transe et théâtre: actes de la table ronde internationale, Montpellier, 3–5 mars 1988.* Cahiers du GITA 4:103–14.

Most, G. W. 1999. "The Poetics of Early Greek Philosophy." In Long 1999a, 332–62.

Motte, A. 1984. "Le necessaire, le naturel et l'agir humain selon Démocrite." In Benakēs 1984, 339–45.

Mourelatos, A.P.D. 1986. "Quality, Structure and Emergence in Later Pre-Socratic Philosophy." *Proceedings of the Boston Area Colloquium in Ancient Philosophy* 2:127–94.

Mullarkey, J. C. 1994. "Duplicity in the Flesh: Bergson and Current Philosophy of the Body." *Philosophy Today* 38:339–55.

Müller, C. W. 1993. "Euripides, *Bellerophontes* fr. 292N²." *Rheinisches Museum* 136:116–21.

Müri, W. 1936. "ΠΕΡΙ ΑΡΧΑΙΗΣ ΙΗΤΡΙΚΗΣ ΚΑΡ. 9." *Hermes* 71:467–69.

Murnaghan, S. 1988. "Body and Voice in Greek Tragedy." *Yale Journal of Criticism* 1:23–43.

Murray, P. 1981. "Poetic Inspiration in Early Greece." *JHS* 101:87–100.

Musitelli, S. 1968. "Riflessi di teorie mediche nelle 'Baccanti' di Euripide." *Dioniso* 42:93–114.

Naddaf, G. 2005. *The Greek Concept of Nature.* Albany.

Nagler, M. N. 1990. "Odysseus: The Proem and the Problem." *ClAnt* 9:335–56.

Nehamas, A. 1998. "A Fate for Socrates' Reason: Foucault on the Care of the Self." In *The Art of Living: Socratic Reflections from Plato to Foucault,* 157–88. Berkeley.

Nehring, A. 1947. "Homer's Descriptions of Syncopes." *CP* 42:106–21.

Nestle, W. 1938. "Hippocratica." *Hermes* 73:1–38.

Nickel, R. 2002. "Euphorbus and the Death of Achilles." *Phoenix* 56:215–33.

Niebyl, P. 1969. "Venesection and the Concept of the Foreign Body: A Historical Study in the Therapeutic Consequences of Humoral and Traumatic Concepts of Disease." Ph.D. dissertation, Yale University. New Haven.

Nightingale, A. 2004. *Spectacles of Truth in Classical Greek Philosophy: Theoria in Its Cultural Context.* Cambridge.

Nilsson, M. P. 1941. "The Immortality of the Soul in Greek Religion." *Eranos* 39:1–16.

Noussia, M. 1999. "The Profession of the Physician (Solon fr. 1,57–66 Gent.-Pr.² = 13,57–66 W.²)." *Eikasmos* 10:9–20.

Nussbaum, M. 1972. "ΨΥΧΗ in Heraclitus, I and II." *Phronesis* 17:1–16, 153–70.

———. 1994. *The Therapy of Desire: Theory and Practice in Hellenistic Ethics.* Princeton.

———. 2001. *The Fragility of Goodness: Luck and Ethics in Greek Tragedy and Philosophy.* 2nd ed. Cambridge.

Nutton, V. 1983. "The Seeds of Disease: An Explanation of Contagion and Infection from the Greeks to the Renaissance." *Medical History* 27:1–34. Reprinted in *From Democedes to Harvey: Studies in the History of Medicine,* chap. 11. London, 1988.

Nutton, V. 1992. "Healers in the Medical Marketplace: Towards a Social History of Graeco-Roman Medicine." In *Medicine in Society: Historical Essays*, ed. A. Wear, 15–58. Cambridge.

———. 1995. "The Medical Meeting Place." In van der Eijk, Horstmanshoff, and Schrijvers 1995, 3–25.

———. 2002. "Ancient Medicine: Asclepius Transformed." In *Science and Mathematics in Ancient Greek Culture*, ed. C. J. Tuplin and T. E. Rihll, 242–55. Oxford.

———. 2004. *Ancient Medicine*. London.

Obbink, D. 1996. *Philodemus, On Piety*. Oxford.

Oberhelman, S. 1990. "The Hippocratic Corpus and Greek Religion." In *The Body and the Text: Comparative Essays in Literature and Medicine*, ed. B. Clarke and W. Aycock, 141–60. Lubbock, Tex.

O'Brien-Moore, A. 1924. *Madness in Ancient Literature*. Weimar.

Onians, R. B. 1954. *The Origins of European Thought about the Body, the Mind, the Soul, the World, Time, and Fate*. 2nd ed. Cambridge.

Orsini, M. L. 1956. "La cronologia dell'*Encomio di Elena* di Gorgia e le *Troiane* di Euripide." *Dioniso* 19:82–88.

Ortner, S. B. 1974. "Is Female to Male as Nature Is to Culture?" In *Women, Culture and Society*, ed. M. Z. Rosaldo and L. Lamphere, 67–87. Stanford.

Osborne, R. 2007. "Tracing Cultural Revolution in Classical Athens." In *Debating the Athenian Cultural Revolution*, ed. R. Osborne, 1–26. Cambridge.

Osler, M. J. 2000. "The Canonical Imperative: Rethinking the Scientific Revolution." In *Rethinking the Scientific Revolution*, ed. M. J. Osler, 3–22. Cambridge.

Owen, G.E.L. 1960. "Eleatic Questions." *CQ* 10:84–102.

Padel, R. 1981. "Madness in Fifth-Century (B.C.) Athenian Tragedy." In *Indigenous Psychologies: The Anthropology of the Self*, ed. P. Heelas and A. Lock, 105–31. London.

———. 1983. "Women: Model for Possession by Greek Daemons." In *Images of Women in Antiquity*, ed. A. Cameron and A. Kuhrt, 3–19. Detroit.

———. 1990. "Making Space Speak." In Winkler and Zeitlin 1990, 336–65.

———. 1992. *In and Out of the Mind: Greek Images of the Tragic Self*. Princeton.

———. 1995. *Whom Gods Destroy: Elements of Greek and Tragic Madness*. Princeton.

Padilla, M. 1992. "The Gorgonic Archer: Danger of Sight in Euripides' *Heracles*." *Classical World* 86:1–12.

Pagel, W. 1939. "Prognosis and Diagnosis: A Comparison of Ancient and Modern Medicine." *Journal of the Warburg Institute* 2:382–98.

Palmer, J. 2003. "On the Alleged Incorporeality of What Is in Melissus." *AncPhil* 23:1–10.

———. 2004. "Melissus and Parmenides." *OSAP* 26:19–54.

Papadopoulou, T. 1999. "Subjectivity and Community in Greek Tragedy: The Example of Euripides' *Heracles*." In Patsalidis and Sakellaridou 1999, 297–307.

———. 2004. "Herakles and Hercules: The Hero's Ambivalence in Euripides and Seneca." *Mnemosyne* 57:257–83.

———. 2005. *Heracles and Euripidean Tragedy*. Cambridge.

Parke, H. W. 1967. *The Oracles of Zeus: Dodona, Olympia, Ammon*. Cambridge, Mass.

Parker, H. N. 1997. "The Teratogenic Grid." In *Roman Sexualities*, ed. J. Hallett and M. B. Skinner, 47–65. Princeton.

Parker, R. 1983. *Miasma: Pollution and Purification in Early Greek Religion*. Oxford.

———. 1998. "Pleasing Thighs: Reciprocity in Greek Religion." In *Reciprocity in Ancient Greece*, ed. C. Gill, N. Postlethwaite, and R. Seaford, 105–25. Oxford.

Parry, H. 1969. "Euripides' *Orestes*: The Quest for Salvation." *TAPA* 100:337–53.

Patsalidis, S., and E. Sakellaridou, eds. 1999. (*Dis*) *Placing Classical Greek Theatre*. Thessaloniki.

Pearcy, L. T. 1992. "Diagnosis as Narrative in Ancient Literature." *AJP* 113:595–616.

Pearson, A. C. 1909. "Phrixus and Demodice: A Note on Pindar, *Pyth*. IV. 162f." *Classical Review* 23:255–57.

Pease, A. S. 1911. "The Omen of Sneezing." *CP* 6:429–43.

Peixoto, M.C.D. 2001. "L'innocence du corps, l'ambiguïté de l'âme: le rapport corps/âme chez Démocrite." In *Les anciens savants: études sur les philosophies préplatoniciennes*, ed. P.-M. Morel and J.-F. Pradeau, 191–209. Strasbourg.

Pelliccia, H. 1995. *Mind, Body, and Speech in Homer and Pindar*. Göttingen.

Pelling, C., ed. 1990. *Characterization and Individuality in Greek Literature*. Oxford.

Pendrick, G. J., ed. and trans. 2002. *Antiphon the Sophist: The Fragments*. Cambridge.

Peponi, A. E. 2002. "Mixed Pleasures, Blended Discourses: Poetry, Medicine, and the Body in Plato's *Philebus* 46–47c." *ClAnt* 21:135–60.

Perilli, L. 1991. "Il lessico intellettuale di Ippocrate: σημαίνειν e τεκμαίρεσθαι." *Lexicon philosophicum* 5:153–79.

———. 1994. "Il lessico intellettuale di Ippocrate: l'estrapolazione logica (ἐκδιηγεῖσθαι, ἐλπίζειν, λογίζεσθαι, συμβάλλεσθαι)." *Aevum antiquum* 7:59–99.

Pickard-Cambridge, A. 1968. *The Dramatic Festivals of Athens*. 2nd ed. Oxford.

Pigeaud, J. 1976. "Euripide et la connaissance de soi: quelques réflexions sur Hippolyte 73 à 82 et 373 à 430." *Les études classiques* 44:3–24.

———. 1977. "Qu'est-ce qu'être malade?: quelques réflexions sur le sens de la maladie dans *Ancienne Médecine*." In Joly 1977, 196–219.

———. 1980. "Quelques aspects du rapport de l'âme et du corps dans le *Corpus hippocratique*." In Grmek 1980, 417–32.

———. 1983. "Remarques sur l'inné et l'acquis dans le *Corpus hippocratique*." In Lasserre and Mudry 1983, 41–55.

———. 1987. *Folie et cures de la folie chez les médecins de l'Antiquité gréco-romaine*. Paris.

———. 1988. "Le style d'Hippocrate ou l'écriture fondatrice de la médecine." In *Les savoirs de l'écriture en Grèce ancienne*, ed. M. Detienne, 305–29. Lille.

———. 1990. "La maladie a-t-elle un sens chez Hippocrate?" In Potter, Maloney, and Desautels 1990, 17–38.

———. 1999. *Poésie du corps*. Paris.

———. 2006. *La maladie de l'âme: étude sur la relation de l'âme et du corps dans la tradition médico-philosophique antique*. 3rd ed. Paris.

Piqueux, A. 2006. "Le corps comique sur les vases 'phlyaques' et dans la comédie attique." *Pallas* 71:27–55.

Plambök, G. 1964. "Dynamis im Corpus Hippocraticum." *Akademie der Wissenschaften und der Literatur, Mainz: Abhandlungen der Geistes- und Sozialwissenschaftlichen Klasse* 2:59–110.

Polack, H., ed. 1976. *Textkritische Untersuchungen zu der hippokratischen Schrift "Prorrhetikos I."* Hamburg.

Pollan, M. 2008. *In Defense of Food: An Eater's Manifesto*. New York.

Pomeroy, S. B., ed. 1991. *Women's History and Ancient History*. Chapel Hill.

Popper, K. 1969. "Back to the Presocratics." In *Conjectures and Refutations: The Growth of Scientific Knowledge*, 136–65. London.

Porter, J. I. 1993. "The Seductions of Gorgias." *ClAnt* 12:267–99.

Porter, J. I., ed. 1999a. *Constructions of the Classical Body*. Ann Arbor.

———. 1999b. Introduction. In Porter 1999a, 1–18.

———. 2005. "Foucault's Ascetic Ancients." *Phoenix* 59:121–32.

Porter, J. I., and M. Buchan. 2004. Introduction. In "Before Subjectivity?: Lacan and the Classics," ed. J. I. Porter and M. Buchan, 1–19. Special issue: *Helios* 31.

Potter, P., ed. and trans. 1980. *Hippokrates. Über die Krankheiten III. CMG* I.2.3. Berlin.

———, trans. 1988a. *Hippocrates*. Vol. 5. Cambridge, Mass.

———, trans. 1988b. *Hippocrates*. Vol. 6. Cambridge, Mass.

———. 1990. "Some Principles of Hippocratic Nosology." In Potter, Maloney, and Desautels 1990, 237–53.

———, ed. and trans. 1995. *Hippocrates*. Vol. 8. Cambridge, Mass.

Potter, P., G. Maloney, and J. Desautels, eds. 1990. *La maladie et les maladies dans la Collection hippocratique: actes des VIᵉ Colloque international hippocratique, Québec du 28 septembre au 3 octobre 1987*. Québec.

Pozzi, D. C. 1994. "Deianeira's Robe: Diction in Sophocles' *Trachiniae*." *Mnemosyne* 47:577–85.

Preiser, G. 1976. *Allgemeine Krankheitsbezeichnungen im Corpus Hippocraticum. Gebrauch und Bedeutung von Nousos und Nosema*. Berlin.

Prioreschi, P. 1992. "Supernatural Elements in Hippocratic Medicine." *JHM* 47:389–404.

Procopé, J. F. 1989. "Democritus on Politics and the Care of the Soul." *CQ* 39:307–31.

———. 1990. "Democritus on Politics and the Care of the Soul: Appendix." *CQ* 40:21–45.

Prost, F., and J. Wilgaux, eds. 2006. *Penser et représenter le corps dans l'Antiquité: actes du colloque international de Rennes, 1–4 septembre 2004*. Rennes.

Psichari, J. 1908. "Sophocle et Hippocrate: à propos du Philoctète à Lemnos." *Revue de philology* 32:95–128.

Pucci, P. 1980. *The Violence of Pity in Euripides' "Medea."* Ithaca.

———. 2005. "Euripides' Heaven." In *The Soul of Tragedy: Essays on Athenian Drama*, ed. V. Pedrick and S. M. Oberhelman, 49–71. Chicago.

Rabinowitz, N. 1986. "Female Speech and Female Sexuality: Euripides' *Hippolytos* as Model." In "Rescuing Creusa: New Methodological Approaches to Women in Antiquity," ed. M. B. Skinner, 127–40. Special issue: *Helios* 13.

Radici Colace, P. 1992. "Il controllo del futuro dalla medicina magico-sacrale all'esperienza laica di Ippocrate." *Messana* 13:79–86.

Rawlings, H. R. 1975. *A Semantic Study of Prophasis to 400 B.C.* Wiesbaden.

Reale, G. 1970. *Melisso: testimonianze e frammenti*. Florence.

Reckford, K. 1974. "Phaedra and Pasiphae: The Pull Backward." *TAPA* 104:307–28.

Redfield, J. 1985. "Le sentiment homérique du Moi." *Le genre humain* 12:93–111.

———. 1994. *Nature and Culture in the "Iliad": The Tragedy of Hector*. Expanded ed. Durham.

Reeve, C.D.C. 2000. "The Role of TEXHN in Plato's Conception of Philosophy." *Proceedings of the Boston Area Colloquium in Ancient Philosophy* 16:207–22.

Regenbogen, O. 1930. "Eine Forschungsmethode antiker Naturwissenschaft." *Quellen und Studien zur Geschichte der Mathematik, Astronomie und Physik* I 2:131–82. Reprinted in *Kleine Schriften*, 141–94. Munich, 1961.

Rehm, R. 2002. *The Play of Space: Spatial Transformation in Greek Tragedy*. Princeton.

Reinhardt, K. 1957. "Die Sinneskrise bei Euripides." *Die neue Rundschau* 68:615–46. English trans.: "The Intellectual Crisis in Euripides." In *Euripides*, ed. J. Mossman, 16–46. Oxford, 2003.

Renehan, R. 1979. "The Meaning of ΣΩΜΑ in Homer: A Study in Methodology." *California Studies in Classical Antiquity* 12:269–82.

———. 1980. "On the Greek Origins of the Concepts Incorporeality and Immateriality." *GRBS* 21:105–38.

———. 1985. "Review Article: A New Commentary on Euripides." *CP* 80:143–75.

———. 1992. "The Staunching of Odysseus' Blood: The Healing Power of Magic." *AJP* 113:1–4.

Rey, R. 1995. *The History of Pain*. Trans. L. E. Wallace, J. A. Cadden, and S. W. Cadden. Cambridge, Mass. [*Histoire de la douleur*. Paris, 1993.]

Rheinberger, H.-J. 1997. *Toward a History of Epistemic Things: Synthesizing Proteins in the Test Tube*. Stanford.

Richardson, N. J., ed. 1974. *The Homeric Hymn to Demeter*. Oxford.

Richert, R. A., and P. L. Harris. 2006. "The Ghost in My Body: Children's Developing Concept of the Soul." *Journal of Cognition and Culture* 6:409–27.

Richlin, A. 1991. "Zeus and Metis: Foucault, Feminism, Classics." *Helios* 18:160–80.

———. 1993. "Not before Homosexuality: The Materiality of the *Cinaedus* and the Roman Law against Love between Men." *Journal of the History of Sexuality* 3:523–73.

———. 1997. "Towards a History of Body History." In *Inventing Ancient Culture: Historicism, Periodization and the Ancient World*, ed. M. Golden and P. Toohey, 16–35. New York.

———. 1998. "Foucault's *History of Sexuality*: A Useful Theory for Women?" In Larmour, Miller, and Platter 1998, 138–70.

Riedweg, C. 1990. "The 'Atheistic' Fragment from Euripides' *Bellerophontes* (286N²)." *ICS* 15:39–53.

Riese, W. 1944. "The Structure of the Clinical History." *BHM* 16:437–49.

Ritter, E. K. 1965. "Magical-Expert (=Āšipu) and Physician (=Asû): Notes on Two Complementary Professions in Babylonian Medicine." In *Studies in Honor of Benno by University of Chicago, Oriental Institute, Landsberger on His Seventy-Fifth Birthday*, 299–321. Chicago.

Rivier, A. 1958. "Euripide et Pasiphaé." In *Lettres d'occident: de l'Iliade à l'Espoir; études et essais offerts à André Bonnard*, 51–74. Neuchâtel.

———. 1960. "L'élément démonique chez Euripide jusqu'en 428." In *Euripide: sept exposés et discussions*, 45–86. Fondation Hardt, Entretiens sur Antiquité classique 6. Geneva.

Robert, F. 1975. "La prognose hippocratique dans les livres V et VII des 'Épidémies.'" In *Le monde grec: pensée, littérature, histoire, documents; hommages à Claire Préaux*, ed. J. Bingen, G. Cambier, and G. Nachtergael, 257–70. Brussels.

Robinson, D. 1990. "Homeric φίλος: Love of Life and Limbs, and Friendship with One's θυμός." In *Owls to Athens: Essays on Classical Subjects Presented to Sir Kenneth Dover*, ed. E. M. Craik, 97–108. Oxford.

Robinson, T. M. 2000. "The Defining Features of Mind-Body Dualism in the Writings of Plato." In J. P. Wright and Potter 2000, 37–55.

Rodgers, V. A. 1969. "Σύνεσις and the Expression of Conscience." *GRBS* 10:241–54.

Rohde, E. 1925. *Psyche: The Cult of Souls and Belief in Immortality among the Greeks*. Trans. W. B. Hillis, from the 8th ed. New York. [*Psyche. Seelencult und Unsterblichkeitsglaube der Griechen*. Freiburg, 1894.]

Rohdich, H. 1968. *Die Euripideische Tragödie. Untersuchungen zu ihrer Tragik.* Heidelberg.

Roscher, W. H. 1898. "Die 'Hundekrankheit' (κύων) der Pandareostöchter und andere mythische Krankheiten." *Rheinisches Museum* 53:169–204.

———. 1900. *Ephialtes. Eine pathologisch-mythologische Abhandlung über die Alpträume und Alpdämonen des klassischen Altertums.* Leipzig. English trans. as *Pan and the Nightmare.* Trans. A. V. O'Brien. New York, 1972.

———, ed. 1913. *Die hippokratische Schrift von der Siebenzahl in ihrer vierfachen Uberlieferung.* Paderborn.

Roselli, A. 1990. "On Symptoms of Diseases: Some Remarks about the Account of Symptoms in *Diseases* II and *Internal Affections.*" In Potter, Maloney, and Desautels 1990, 159–70.

Rosen, R. M., and I. Sluiter, eds. 2003. *Andreia: Studies in Manliness and Courage in Classical Antiquity.* Leiden.

Ross, W. D. 1958. *Aristotle's Metaphysics.* 2 vols. Rev. ed. Oxford.

Rousselle, A. 1980. "Observation féminine et idéologie masculine: le corps de la femme d'après les médicins grecs." *Annales (Économies, sociétés, civilisations)* 35:1089–1115.

———. 1988. *Porneia: On Desire and the Body in Antiquity.* Trans. F. Pheasant. Oxford. [*Porneia: de la maîtrise du corps à la privation sensorielle, IIe–IVe siècles de l'ère chrétienne.* Paris, 1983.]

Russell, D. C. 2005. *Plato on Pleasure and the Good Life.* Oxford.

Ruttenberg, H. S. 1986. "Plato's Use of the Analogy between Justice and Health." *Journal of Value Inquiry* 20:145–56.

Ryzman, M. 1993. "Heracles' Destructive Impulses: A Transgression of Natural Laws (Sophocles' *Trachiniae*)." *RBPh* 71:69–79.

Salazar, C. F. 2000. *The Treatment of War Wounds in Graeco-Roman Antiquity.* Leiden.

Salem, J. 2007. "Perception et connaissance chez Démocrite." In Brancacci and Morel 2007, 125–42.

Salowey, C. A. 2002. "Herakles and Healing Cult in the Peloponnesos." In *Peloponnesian Sanctuaries and Cults: Proceedings of the Ninth International Symposium at the Swedish Institute at Athens, 11–13 June 1994,* ed. R. Hägg, 171–77. Stockholm.

Samuelsen, H. 2004. "Illness Transmission and Proximity: Local Theories of Causation among the Bissa in Burkina Faso." *Medical Anthropology* 23:89–112.

Sassi, M. M. 2001. *The Science of Man in Ancient Greece.* Trans. P. Tucker. Chicago. [*La scienza dell'uomo nella Grecia antica.* Turin, 1988.]

Saunders, K. B. 1999. "The Wounds in *Iliad* 13–16." *CQ* 49:345–63.

———. 2004. "Frölich's Table of Homeric Wounds." *CQ* 54:1–17.

Scarborough, J. 1970. "Diphilus of Siphnos and Hellenistic Medical Dietetics." *JHM* 25:194–201.

———. 1983. "Theoretical Assumptions in Hippocratic Pharmacology." In Lasserre and Mudry 1983, 307–25.

Scarry, E. 1985. *The Body in Pain: The Making and Unmaking of the World.* New York.

Scheper-Hughes, N., and M. Lock. 1987. "The Mindful Body: A Prolegomenon to Future Work in Medical Anthropology." *Medical Anthropology Quarterly* 1:6–41.

Schibli, H. S., ed. 1990. *Pherekydes of Syros.* Oxford.

Schiefsky, M. 2005a. *Hippocrates, On Ancient Medicine.* Leiden.

———. 2005b. "*On Ancient Medicine* on the Nature of Human Beings." In van der Eijk 2005a, 69–85.

Schlesier, R. 1983. "Daimon und Daimones bei Euripides." *Saeculum* 34:267–79.

———. 1985. "*Héraclès* et la critique des dieux chez Euripide." *Annali della Scuola Normale Superiore di Pisa: Classe di lettere e filosofia* 15:7–40.

———. 1993. "Mixture of Masks: Maenads as Tragic Models." In *Masks of Dionysus*, ed. T. H. Carpenter and C. A. Faraone, 89–114. Ithaca.

Schoenfeldt, M. C. 1999. *Bodies and Selves in Early Modern England: Physiology and Inwardness in Spenser, Shakespeare, Herbert, and Milton.* Cambridge.

Schofield, M. 1991. "Heraclitus' Theory of the Soul and Its Antecedents." In Everson 1991, 13–34.

Schubert, C. 1996. "Menschenbild und Normwandel in der klassischen Zeit." In *Médecine et morale dans l'Antiquité*, ed. J. Jouanna and H. Flashar, 121–55. Fondation Hardt, Entretiens sur l'Antiquité classique 43. Geneva.

Scodel, R. 1984. "Tantalus and Anaxagoras." *HSCP* 88:13–24.

———. 2002. "Homeric Signs and Flashbulb Memory." In *Epea and Grammata: Oral and Written Communication in Ancient Greece*, ed. I. Worthington and J. M. Foley, 99–116. Leiden.

Scott, D. 1999. "Platonic Pessimism and Moral Education." *OSAP* 17:15–36.

Scurlock, J. 1999. "Physician, Exorcist, Conjurer, Magician: A Tale of Two Healing Professionals." In *Mesopotamian Magic: Textual, Historical, and Interpretive Perspectives*, ed. T. Abusch and K. van der Toorn, 69–79. Gröningen.

Seaford, R. 2004. *Money and the Early Greek Mind: Homer, Philosophy, Tragedy.* Cambridge.

Sebeok, T. A. 1976. *Contributions to the Doctrine of Signs.* Bloomington, Ind.

Sedley, D. 1992. "Empedocles' Theory of Vision and Theophrastus' *De sensibus*." In *Theophrastus: His Psychological, Doxographical, and Scientific Writings*, ed. W. W. Fortenbaugh and D. Gutas, 20–31. New Brunswick, N.J.

———. 1999. "Parmenides and Melissus." In Long 1999a, 113–33.

———. 2000. "The Ideal of Godlikeness." In Fine 2000, 791–810.

Segal, C. P. 1962. "Gorgias and the Psychology of the *Logos*." *HSCP* 66:99–155.

———. 1970. "Shame and Purity in Euripides' *Hippolytus*." *Hermes* 98:278–99.

———. 1971. *The Theme of the Mutilation of the Corpse in the "Iliad."* Leiden.

———. 1978. "Pentheus and Hippolytus on the Couch and on the Grid: Psychoanalytic and Structuralist Readings of Greek Tragedy." *Classical World* 72:129–48.

———. 1988. "Confusion and Concealment in Euripides' *Hippolytus*: Vision, Hope, and Tragic Knowledge." *Métis* 3:263–82.

Segvic, H. 2000. "No One Errs Willingly: The Meaning of Socratic Intellectualism." *OSAP* 19:1–45.

Serghidou, A. 1997. "Corps héroïque et expérience du moi servile dans la tragédie." *Echos du monde classique* 16:391–420.

Serres, M. 1995. *Genesis.* Trans. G. James and J. Nielson. Ann Arbor. [*Genèse.* Paris, 1982.]

Shapiro, H. A. 1993. *Personifications in Greek Art: The Representation of Abstract Concepts, 600–400 B.C.* Zürich.

Sharples, R. W. 1983. " 'But Why Has My Spirit Spoken with Me Thus?': Homeric Decision-Making." *G & R* 30:1–7.

Siebert, G. 1981. "*Eidōla*: le problème de la figurabilité dans l'art grec." In *Méthodologie iconographique: actes du colloque de Strasbourg, 27–28 avril 1979*, ed. G. Siebert, 63–73. Strasbourg.

Siegel, R. E. 1964. "Clinical Observation in Hippocrates: An Essay on the Evolution of the Diagnostic Art." *Mount Sinai Journal of Medicine* 31:285–303.

Silverman, K. 1983. *The Subject of Semiotics*. New York.

Simon, B. 1978. *Mind and Madness in Ancient Greece: The Classical Roots of Modern Psychiatry*. Ithaca.

Sindzingre, N., and A. Zempléni. 1992. "Causality of Disease among the Senufo." In *The Social Basis of Health and Healing in Africa*, ed. S. Feierman and J. M. Janzen, 315–38. Berkeley.

Singer, P. N. 1992. "Some Hippocratic Mind-Body Problems." In López Férez 1992, 131–43.

Sissa, G. 1990a. *Greek Virginity*. Trans. A. Goldhammer. Cambridge, Mass. [*Le corps virginal: la virginité féminine en Grèce ancienne*. Paris, 1987.]

———. 1990b. "Maidenhood without Maidenhead: The Female Body in Ancient Greece." In Halperin, Winkler, and Zeitlin 1990, 339–64.

———. 1999. "Sexual Bodybuilding: Aeschines against Timarchus." In Porter 1999a, 147–68.

Skoda, F. 1994. "L'eau et le vocabulaire de la maladie." In Ginouvès et al. 1994, 249–64.

Slatkin, L. 1991. *The Power of Thetis: Allusion and Interpretation in the "Iliad."* Berkeley.

———. 2004. "Measuring Authority, Authoritative Measures: Hesiod's *Works and Days*." In *The Moral Authority of Nature*, ed. L. Daston and F. Vidal, 25–49. Chicago.

Slings, S. R. 1975. "Three Notes on the New Archilochus Papyrus." *ZPE* 18:170.

Smith, J. Z. 1978. "Towards Interpreting Demonic Powers in Hellenistic and Roman Antiquity." *Aufstieg und Niedergang der römischen Welt* 2.16.1:425–39. Berlin.

Smith, W. D. 1965. "So-Called Possession in Pre-Christian Greece." *TAPA* 96:403–26.

———. 1966. "Physiology in the Homeric Poems." *TAPA* 97:547–56.

———. 1967. "Disease in Euripides' *Orestes*." *Hermes* 95:291–307.

———. 1979. *The Hippocratic Tradition*. Ithaca.

———. 1980. "The Development of Classical Dietetic Theory." In Grmek 1980, 439–48.

———. 1982. "Erasistratus's Dietetic Medicine." *BHM* 56:398–409.

———. 1983. "Analytical and Catalogue Structure in the *Corpus Hippocraticum*." In Lasserre and Mudry 1983, 277–84.

———. 1989. "Notes on Ancient Medical Historiography." *BHM* 63:73–109.

———, ed. and trans. 1990. *Hippocrates, Pseudepigraphic Writings*. Leiden.

———. 1992. "Regimen, κρῆσις, and the History of Dietetics." In López Férez 1992, 263–71.

———, ed. and trans. 1994. *Hippocrates*. Vol. 7. Cambridge, Mass.

Snell, B. 1953. *The Discovery of the Mind: The Greek Origins of European Thought*. Trans. T. G. Rosenmeyer. Cambridge, Mass. [English trans. from *Die Entdeckung des Geistes. Studien zur Entstehung des europäischen Denkens bei den Griechen*. 2nd ed., Hamburg, 1948. Revised 4th ed., Göttingen, 1975.]

———. 1964. *Scenes from Greek Drama*. Berkeley.

Solmsen, F. 1950. "Tissues and the Soul: Philosophical Contributions to Physiology." *PhR* 59:435–68. Reprinted in Solmsen 1968–82, 1:502–35.

———. 1955. "Antecedents of Aristotle's Psychology and Scale of Beings." *AJP* 76:148–64. Reprinted in Solmsen 1968–82, 1:588–604.

———. 1957. "The Vital Heat, the Inborn Pneuma and the Aether." *JHS* 77:119–23. Reprinted in Solmsen 1968–82, 1:605–11.

———. 1961. "Greek Philosophy and the Discovery of the Nerves." *Museum Helveticum* 18:169–97. Reprinted in Solmsen 1968–82, 1:536–82.

———. 1968–82. *Kleine Schriften.* 3 vols. Hildesheim.

———. 1973. "'Bad Shame' and Related Problems in Phaedra's Speech (Eur. *Hipp.* 380–388)." *Hermes* 101:420–25. Reprinted in Solmsen 1968–82, 3:64–69.

———. 1984. "Φρήν, καρδία, ψυχή in Greek Tragedy." In *Greek Poetry and Philosophy: Studies in Honour of Leonard Woodbury,* ed. D. E. Gerber, 265–74. Chico, Calif.

Sontag, S. 1978. *Illness as Metaphor.* New York.

Sorabji, R. 2003. "The Mind-Body Relation in the Wake of Plato's *Timaeus.*" In *Plato's "Timaeus" as Cultural Icon,* ed. G. J. Reydams-Schils, 152–62. Notre Dame.

Souilhé, J. 1919. *Étude sur le terme δύναμις dans les dialogues de Platon.* Paris.

Sourvinou-Inwood, C. 2003. *Tragedy and Athenian Religion.* Lanham, Md.

Spatafora, G. 1999. *I moti dell'animo in Omero.* Rome.

Spatharas, D. 2002. "Gorgias' *Encomium of Helen* and Euripides' *Troades.*" *Eranos* 100:166–74.

Spelman, E. V. 1982. "Woman as Body: Ancient and Contemporary Views." *Feminist Studies* 8:109–31.

Stafford, E. 2000. *Worshipping Virtues: Personification and the Divine in Ancient Greece.* London.

Stalley, R. 1981. "Mental Health and Individual Responsibility in Plato's *Republic.*" *Journal of Value Inquiry* 15:109–24.

———. 1996. "Punishment and the Physiology of the *Timaeus.*" *CQ* 46:357–70.

Starobinski, J. 1974. "L'épée d'Ajax." In *Trois fureurs,* 9–71. Paris.

Stehle, E. 2002. "The Body and Its Representations in Aristophanes' *Thesmophoriazousai*: Where Does the Costume End?" *AJP* 123:369–406.

Stewart, A. 1997. *Art, Desire, and the Body in Ancient Greece.* Cambridge.

Stinton, T.C.W. 1976. "'Si credere dignum est': Some Expressions of Disbelief in Euripides and Others." *PCPS* 22:60–89.

Stol, M. 1993. *Epilepsy in Babylonia.* Gröningen.

Strange, S. K. 1985. "The Double Explanation in the *Timaeus.*" *AncPhil* 5:25–39. Reprinted in Fine 2000, 399–417.

Stratton, G. M. 1917. *Theophrastus and the Greek Physiological Psychology before Aristotle.* London.

Striker, G. 1987. "Origins of the Concept of Natural Law." *Proceedings of the Boston Area Colloquium in Ancient Philosophy* 2:79–94.

Sullivan, S. D. 1983. "Love Influences *Phrenes* in Greek Lyric Poetry." *Symbolae osloenses* 58:15–22.

———. 1987. "Πραπίδες in Homer." *Glotta* 65:182–93.

———. 1988. *Psychological Activity in Homer: A Study of Phren.* Ottawa.

———. 1994a. "'Self' and Psychic Entities in Early Greek Epic." *Eos* 82:5–16.

———. 1994b. "The Removal of Psychic Entities in Early Greek Poetry." *Eos* 82:189–99.

———. 1995. "What's There in a Heart?: *Kradiē* in Homer and the *Homeric Hymns.*" *Euphrosyne* 23:9–25.

———. 1996. "The Psychic Term ἦτορ: Its Nature and Relation to Person in Homer and the *Homeric Hymns.*" *Emerita* 64:11–29.

Sutton, D. F. 1975. "A Series of Vases Illustrating the Madness of Lycurgus." *Rivista di studi classici* 23:356–60.

Tambornino, John. 2002. *The Corporeal Turn: Passion, Necessity, Politics.* Lanham, Md.

Tambornino, Julius. 1909. *De antiquorum daemonismo.* Gießen.

Taussig, M. T. 1993. *Mimesis and Alterity: A Particular History of the Senses.* New York.

———. 2003. "Viscerality, Faith, and Skepticism: Another Theory of Magic." In *Magic and Modernity: Interfaces of Revelation and Concealment,* ed. B. Meyer and P. Pels, 272–306. Stanford.

Taylor, C.C.W. 1967. "Pleasure, Knowledge and Sensation in Democritus." *Phronesis* 12:6–27.

———, trans. 1999a. *The Atomists: Leucippus and Democritus.* Toronto.

———. 1999b. "The Atomists." In Long 1999a, 181–204.

———. 2007. "Democritus and Lucretius on Death and Dying." In Brancacci and Morel 2007, 77–86.

Taylor, J. S. 2005. "Surfacing the Body Interior." *Annual Review of Anthropology* 35:741–56.

Temkin, O. 1949. "Medicine and the Problem of Moral Responsibility." *BHM* 23:1–20.

———. 1953. "Greek Medicine as Science and Craft." *Isis* 44:213–25.

———. 1963. "The Scientific Approach to Disease: Specific Entity and Individual Sickness." In Crombie 1963, 629–47.

Theodorou, Z. 1993. "Subject to Emotion: Exploring Madness in *Orestes.*" *CQ* 43:32–46.

Thivel, A. 1975. "Le 'divin' dans la *Collection hippocratique.*" In Bourgey and Jouanna 1975, 57–76.

———. 1981. *Cnide et Cos?: essai sur les doctrines médicales dans la collection hippocratique.* Paris.

———. 1985. "Diagnostic et pronostic à l'époque d'Hippocrate et à la nôtre." *Gesnerus* 42:479–97.

———. 2000. "L'évolution du sens de δίαιτα." In *La lengua científica griega: orígenes, desarrollo e influencia en las lenguas modernas europeas,* ed. J. A. López-Férez, 25–37. Madrid.

Thivel, A., and A. Zucker, eds. 2002. *Le normal et le pathologique dans la Collection hippocratique: actes du Xème Colloque internationale hippocratique, Nice, 6–8 octobre 1999.* Nice.

Thomas, R. 1993. "Performance and Written Publication in Herodotus and the Sophistic Generation." In *Vermittlung und Tradierung von Wissen in der griechischen Kultur,* ed. W. Kullmann and J. Althoff, 225–44. Tübingen.

———. 2000. *Herodotus in Context: Ethnography, Science, and the Art of Persuasion.* Cambridge.

Tigerstedt, E. N. 1970. "*Furor poeticus:* Poetic Inspiration in Greek Literature before Democritus and Plato." *Journal of the History of Ideas* 31:163–78.

Tortora, G. 1983. "'Νοῦς' e 'Καιρός' nell'etica democritea." In *Democrito: Dall'atomo alla città,* ed. G. Casertano, 103–34. Naples.

———. 1984. "Φύσις and διδαχή in Democritus' Ethical Conception (B33 D–K)." In Benakēs 1984, 387–97.

Tracy, T. J. 1969. *Physiological Theory and the Doctrine of the Mean in Plato and Aristotle.* The Hague.

Treherne, P. 1995. "The Warrior's Beauty: The Masculine Body and Self-Identity in Bronze-Age Europe." *Journal of European Archaeology* 3:105–44.

Tsagarakis, O. 1977. *Nature and Background of Major Concepts of Divine Power in Homer*. Amsterdam.

Untersteiner, M. 1939. "Il concetto di δαίμων in Omero." *Atene e Roma* 16:93–134.

———. 1953. "Un aspetto dell'essere melissiano." *Rivista critica di storia della filosofia* 8:597–606.

van der Eijk, P. J. 1997. "Towards a Rhetoric of Ancient Scientific Discourse: Some Formal Characteristics of Greek Medical and Philosophical Texts (Hippocratic Corpus, Aristotle)." In *Grammar as Interpretation: Greek Literature in Its Linguistic Contexts*, ed. E. J. Bakker, 77–129. Leiden.

———, ed. 1999a. *Ancient Histories of Medicine: Essays in Medical Doxography and Historiography in Classical Antiquity*. Leiden.

———. 1999b. "Historical Awareness, Historiography and Doxography in Greek and Roman Medicine." In van der Eijk 1999a, 1–31.

———, ed. and trans. 2000–2001. *Diocles of Carystus*. 2 vols. Leiden.

———. 2004. "Divination, Prognosis and Prophylaxis: The Hippocratic Work 'On Dreams' (*De victu* 4) and Its Near Eastern Background." In Horstmanshoff and Stol 2004, 187–218.

———, ed. 2005a. *Hippocrates in Context: Papers Read at the XIth International Hippocrates Colloquium, University of Newcastle upon Tyne, 27–31 August 2002*. Leiden.

———. 2005b. *Medicine and Philosophy in Classical Antiquity: Doctors and Philosophers on Nature, Soul, Health and Disease*. Cambridge.

van der Eijk, P. J., H. F. J. Horstmanshoff, and P. H. Schrijvers, eds. 1995. *Ancient Medicine in Its Socio-Cultural Context*. 2 vols. Amsterdam.

van Groningen, B. 1958. "Les traités hippocratiques." In *La composition littéraire archaïque grecque: procédés et réalisations*, 247–55. Amsterdam.

van Wees, H. 2004. *Greek Warfare: Myths and Realities*. London.

van Wolputte, S. 2004. "Hang on to Your Self: Of Bodies, Embodiment, and Selves." *Annual Review of Anthropology* 33:251–69.

Vasquez, P. R. 1972. "Literary Convention in Scenes of Madness and Suffering in Greek Tragedy." Ph.D. dissertation, Columbia University, New York.

Vegetti, M. 1976. Introduzione. *Opere di Ippocrate*, 21–89. 2nd ed. Turin.

———. 1983. "Metafora politica e immagine del corpo negli scritti ippocratici." In Lasserre and Mudry 1983, 459–69.

———. 1996. "Iatròmantis: previsione e memoria nella Grecia antica." In *Il signori della memoria e dell'oblio*, ed. M. Bettini, 65–81. Florence.

———. 1998. "Empedocle: 'medico e sofista' (*Antica Medicina* 20)." *Elenchos* 19:347–59.

———. 1999. "Culpability, Responsibility, Cause: Philosophy, Historiography, and Medicine in the Fifth Century." In Long 1999a, 271–89.

Vermeule, E. 1979. *Aspects of Death in Early Greek Art and Poetry*. Berkeley.

Vernant, J.-P. 1983. *Myth and Thought among the Greeks*. Trans. J. Lloyd, with J. Fort. Boston. [*Mythe et pensée chez les Grecs: études de psychologie historique*. Rev. ed. Paris, 1985.]

———. 1988a. "Tensions and Ambiguities in Greek Tragedy." In Vernant and Vidal-Naquet 1988, 29–48. [First published in English in *Interpretation: Theory and Practice*. Ed. C. Singleton, 105–21. Baltimore, 1969. Reprinted in Vernant and Vidal-Naquet 1972–86, 1:21–40.]

Vernant, J.-P. 1988b. "Intimations of the Will in Greek Tragedy." In Vernant and Vidal-Naquet 1988, 49–84. ["Ébauches de la volonté." In Vernant and Vidal-Naquet 1972–86, 1:43–74.]

———. 1989. *L'individu, la mort, l'amour: soi-même et l'autre en Grèce ancienne.* Paris.

———. 1991a. *Mortals and Immortals: Collected Essays.* Ed. F. I. Zeitlin. Princeton.

———. 1991b. "Mortals and Immortals: The Body of the Divine." In Vernant 1991a, 27–49. ["Mortels et immortels: le corps divin." In Vernant 1989, 7–39.]

———. 1991c. "A 'Beautiful Death' and the Disfigured Corpse in Homeric Epic." In Vernant 1991a, 50–74. ["La belle mort et le cadavre outragé." In Vernant 1989, 41–79.]

———. 1991d. "*Panta kala*: From Homer to Simonides." In Vernant 1991a, 84–91. ["*Pánta kála*: d'Homère à Simonide." In Vernant 1989, 91–101.]

———. 1991e. "From the 'Presentification' of the Invisible to the Imitation of Appearance." In Vernant 1991a, 151–63. ["De la présentification de l'invisible à l'imitation de l'apparence." In *Mythe et pensée chez les Grecs: études de psychologie historique,* 339–51. Rev. ed. Paris, 1985.]

Vernant, J.-P., and P. Vidal-Naquet. 1972–86. *Mythe et trágedie en Grèce ancienne.* 2 vols. Paris.

———. 1988. *Myth and Tragedy in Ancient Greece.* Trans. J. Lloyd. New York. [Translation of Vernant and Vidal-Naquet 1972–86.]

Verrall, A. W. 1905. *Essays on Four Plays of Euripides: Andromache, Helen, Heracles, Orestes.* Cambridge.

Versnel, H. S. 1987. "What Did Ancient Man See When He Saw a God?: Some Reflections on Greco-Roman Epiphany." In *Effigies dei: Essays on the History of Religions,* ed. D. van der Plas, 42–55. Leiden.

Vian, F. 1965. "Mélampous et les Proitides." *REA* 67:25–30.

Villard, L. 2006. "Vocabulaire et représentation de la douleur dans la *Collection hippocratique.*" In Prost and Wilgaux 2006, 61–78.

Villari, E. 2003. "La physiognomonie comme technè." In *Ars et ratio: sciences, art, et métiers dans la philosophie hellénistique et romaine; actes du colloque international organisé à Créteil, Fontenay et Paris du 16 au 18 octobre 1997,* ed. C. Lévy, B. Besnier, and A. Gigandet, 89–101. Brussels.

Vivante, P. 1955. "Sulla designazione del corpo in Omero." *Archivio glottologico italiano* 40:39–50.

———. 1983. "On Homer *Il.* 1, 46–47." *Eranos* 81:1–6.

Vlastos, G. 1945. "Ethics and Physics in Democritus (Part One)." *PhR* 54:578–92. Reprinted in Vlastos 1995, 1:328–40.

———. 1946. "Ethics and Physics in Democritus (Part Two)." *PhR* 55:53–64. Reprinted in Vlastos 1995, 1:340–50.

———. 1947. "Equality and Justice in Early Greek Cosmologies." *CP* 42:156–78. Reprinted in Vlastos 1995, 1:57–88.

———. 1950. "The Physical Theory of Anaxagoras." *PhR* 59:31–57. Reprinted in Vlastos 1995, 1:303–27.

———. 1952. "Theology and Philosophy in Early Greek Thought." *Philosophical Quarterly* 2:97–123. Reprinted in Vlastos 1995, 1:3–31.

———. 1953a. "*Isonomia.*" *AJP* 74:337–66. Reprinted in Vlastos 1995, 1:89–111.

———. 1953b. "Review of J. E. Raven, *Pythagoreans and Eleatics.*" *Gnomon* 25:29–35. Reprinted in Vlastos 1995, 1:180–88.

———. 1975. *Plato's Universe.* Seattle.

———. 1995. *Studies in Greek Philosophy*. 2 vols. Princeton.

von Fritz, K. 1943. "ΝΟΟΣ and ΝΟΕΙΝ in the Homeric Poems." *CP* 38:79–93.

———. 1945. "ΝΟΥΣ, ΝΟΕΙΝ, and Their Derivatives in Pre-Socratic Philosophy (Excluding Anaxagoras). Part I: From the Beginnings to Parmenides." *CP* 40:223–42.

———. 1946. "ΝΟΥΣ, ΝΟΕΙΝ, and Their Derivatives in Pre-Socratic Philosophy (Excluding Anaxagoras). Part II: The Post-Parmenidean Period." *CP* 41:12–34.

von Staden, H. 1975. "Experiment and Experience in Hellenistic Medicine." *BICS* 22: 178–99.

———. 1989. *Herophilus: The Art of Medicine in Early Alexandria*. Cambridge.

———. 1990. "Incurability and Hopelessness: The *Hippocratic Corpus*." In Potter, Maloney, and Desautels 1990, 75–112.

———. 1992a. "Spiderwoman and the Chaste Tree: The Semantics of Matter." *Configurations* 1:23–56.

———. 1992b. "Women and Dirt." *Helios* 19:7–30.

———. 1992c. "Affinities and Elisions: Helen and Hellenocentrism." *Isis* 83:578–95.

———. 1992d. "The Mind and Skin of Heracles: Heroic Diseases." In *Maladie et maladies: histoire et conceptualisation; mélanges en l'honneur de Mirko Grmek*, ed. D. Gourevitch, 131–50. Geneva.

———. 1992e. "The Discovery of the Body: Human Dissection and Its Cultural Contexts in Ancient Greece." *Yale Journal of Biology and Medicine* 65:223–41.

———. 1996. "'In a Pure and Holy Way': Personal and Professional Conduct in the Hippocratic Oath?" *JHM* 51:404–37.

———. 1998. "*Dynamis*: The Hippocratics and Plato." In *Philosophy and Medicine*, ed. K. J. Boudouris, 262–79. Alimos, Greece.

———. 1999a. "Reading the Agonal Body: The Hippocratic Corpus." In *Medicine and the History of the Body: Proceedings of the 20th, 21st, and 22nd International Symposium on the Comparative History of Medicine; East and West*, ed. Y. Otsuka, S. Sakai, and S. Kuriyama, 287–94. Tokyo.

———. 1999b. "Celsus as Historian?" In van der Eijk 1999a, 251–94.

———. 2002. "῾Ως ἐπὶ τὸ πολύ: 'Hippocrates' between Generalization and Individualization." In Thivel and Zucker 2002, 23–43.

———. 2007a. "Purity, Purification, and Katharsis in Hippocratic Medicine." In *Katharsiskonzeptionen vor Aristoteles*, ed. M. Vöhler and B. Seidensticker, 21–51. Berlin.

———. 2007b. "*Physis* and *Technē* in Greek Medicine." In *The Artificial and the Natural: An Evolving Polarity*, ed. B. Bensaude-Vincent and W. R. Newman, 21–49. Cambridge, Mass.

———. 2008. "'The *Oath*,' the Oaths, and the Hippocratic Corpus." In *La science médicale antique: nouveaux regards; études réunies en l'honneur de Jacques Jouanna*, ed. V. Boudon-Millot, A. Guardasole, and C. Magdelaine, 425–66. Paris.

Vust-Mussard, M. 1970. "Remarques sur les livres I et III des *Épidémies*: les histoires de malades et le pronostic." *Études de lettres* 3:65–76.

Wallace, R. W. 1994. "Private Lives and Public Enemies: Freedom of Thought in Classical Athens." In *Athenian Identity and Civic Ideology*, ed. A. L. Boegehold and A. C. Scafuro, 127–55. Baltimore.

Warren, C.P.W. 1970. "Some Aspects of Medicine in the Greek Bronze Age." *Medical History* 14:364–77.

Warren, J. 2002. *Epicurus and Democritean Ethics: An Archaeology of "Ataraxia."* Cambridge.

Warren, J. 2007a. "Democritus on Social and Psychological Harm." In Brancacci and Morel 2007, 87–104.

———. 2007b. "Anaxagoras on Perception, Pleasure, and Pain." *OSAP* 33:19–54.

Webster, T.B.L. 1954. "Personification as a Mode of Greek Thought." *Journal of the Warburg and Courtauld Institutes* 17:10–21.

———. 1957. "Some Psychological Terms in Greek Tragedy." *JHS* 77:149–54.

Weil, S. 2005. "The *Iliad*, or the Poem of Force." In S. Weil and R. Bespaloff, *War and the "Iliad,"* 1–37, trans. M. McCarthy. New York. [*L'Iliade, ou le poème de la force*. Paris, 1989.]

Weiss, G. 1999. *Body Images: Embodiment as Intercorporeality*. New York.

Wellmann, M. 1930. "Die ps. hippokratische Schrift Περὶ ἀρχαίης ἰητρικῆς." *Sudhoffs Archiv* 23:299–305.

Wesoly, M. 1987. "'To Correct the Argument of Melissus' (*"De. Nat. Hom."* 1): An Allusion to Gorgias?" *Eos* 75:13–19.

West, M. L. ed. 1978. *Hesiod, Works and Days*. Oxford.

———, ed. and trans. 2003. *Greek Epic Fragments*. Cambridge, Mass.

Wickkiser, B. 2008. *Asklepios, Medicine, and the Politics of Healing in Fifth-Century Greece*. Baltimore.

Wilamowitz-Moellendorff, U. von, ed. 1909. *Euripides. Herakles*. 2nd ed. Berlin.

Wildberg, C. 1999–2000. "Piety as Service, Epiphany as Reciprocity: Two Observations on the Religious Meaning of the Gods in Euripides." In Cropp, Lee, and Sansone 1999–2000, 235–56.

———. 2006. "Socrates and Euripides." In *A Companion to Socrates*, ed. S. Ahbel-Rappe and R. Kamtekar, 21–35. Malden, Mass.

Wilford, F. A. 1965. "Δαίμων in Homer." *Numen* 12:217–32.

Wilkins, J. 2005. "The Social and Intellectual Context of *Regimen II*." In van der Eijk 2005a, 121–33.

Willcock, M. M. 1970. "Some Aspects of the Gods in the *Iliad*." *BICS* 17:1–10.

Williams, B. 1993. *Shame and Necessity*. Berkeley.

Willink, C. W. 1968. "Some Problems of Text and Interpretation in the *Hippolytus*." *CQ* 18:11–43.

———. 1983. "Prodikos, 'Meteorosophists' and the 'Tantalos' Paradigm." *CQ* 33:25–33.

———. 1986. *Euripides, Orestes*. Oxford.

Winkler, J. J. 1990a. "Phallos Politikos: Representing the Body Politic in Athens." *differences* 2:29–45.

———. 1990b. *The Constraints of Desire: The Anthropology of Sex and Gender in Ancient Greece*. New York.

Winkler, J. J., and F. I. Zeitlin, eds. 1990. *Nothing to Do with Dionysus?: Athenian Drama in Its Social Context*. Princeton.

Winnington-Ingram, R. P. 1960. "*Hippolytus*: A Study in Causation." In *Euripide: sept exposés et discussions*, 171–97. Fondation Hardt, Entretiens sur l'Antiquité classique 6, Geneva.

———. 1969. "Euripides: *Poiētēs Sophos*." *Arethusa* 2:127–42.

Withington, E. T., ed. and trans. 1928. *Hippocrates*. Vol. 3. Cambridge, Mass.

Wittern, R., ed. and trans. 1974. *Die hippokratische Schrift "De morbis I."* Hildesheim.

———. 1987. "Diagnostics in Classical Greek Medicine." In *History of Diagnostics: Proceedings of the 9th International Symposium on the Comparative History of Medicine—East and West*, ed. Y. Kawakita, 69–89. Osaka.

———. 1998. "Gattungen im Corpus Hippocraticum." In *Gattungen wissenschaftlicher Literatur in der Antike,* ed. W. Kullmann, J. Althoff, and M. Asper, 17–36. Tübingen.

Woerther, F. 2008. "Music and the Education of the Soul in Plato and Aristotle: Homeopathy and the Formation of Character." *CQ* 58:89–103.

Wohl, V. 1998. *Intimate Commerce: Exchange, Gender, and Subjectivity in Greek Tragedy.* Austin.

———. 2002. *Love among the Ruins: The Erotics of Democracy in Classical Athens.* Princeton.

Wohlberg, J. 1968. "The Palace-Hero Equation in Euripides." *Acta Antiqua Academiae Scientiarum Hungaricae* 16:149–55.

Woodford, S. 1966. "*Exemplum virtutis*: A Study of Heracles in Athens in the Second Half of the Fifth Century B.C." Ph.D. dissertation, Columbia University, New York.

Woodruff, P. 2002. "Natural Justice?" In Caston and Graham 2002, 195–204.

Woolf, R. 2000. "Callicles and Socrates: Psychic (Dis)harmony in the *Gorgias.*" *OSAP* 18:1–40.

Worman, N. 1997. "The Body as Argument: Helen in Four Greek Texts." *ClAnt* 16:151–203.

———. 1999. "The Ties That Bind: Transformations of Costume and Connection in Euripides' *Heracles.*" *Ramus* 28:89–107.

———. 2000. "Infection in the Sentence: The Discourse of Disease in Sophocles' *Philoctetes.*" *Arethusa* 33:1–36.

———. 2002. *The Cast of Character: Style in Greek Literature.* Austin.

Wright, J. P., and P. Potter, eds. 2000. *Psyche and Soma: Physicians and Metaphysicians on the Mind-Body Problem from Antiquity to Enlightenment.* Oxford.

Wright, M. 2006. "*Orestes*, a Euripidean Sequel." *CQ* 56:33–47.

Wright, M. R. 1990. "Presocratic Minds." In *The Person and the Human Mind: Issues in Ancient Modern Philosophy,* ed. C. Gill, 207–25. Oxford.

———, ed. and trans. 1995. *Empedocles: The Extant Fragments.* 2nd ed. London.

———, ed. 2000. *Reason and Necessity: Essays on Plato's "Timaeus."* Swansea.

Wyke, M., ed. 1998. *Gender and the Body in the Ancient Mediterranean.* Malden, Mass.

———, ed. 1999. *Parchments of Gender: Deciphering the Bodies of Antiquity.* Oxford.

Young, I. M. 1980. "Throwing like a Girl: A Phenomenology of Feminine Body Comportment, Motility, and Spatiality." *Human Studies* 3:137–56. Reprinted in Young 2005, 27–45.

———. 2005. *On Female Body Experience: Throwing Like a Girl and Other Essays.* New York.

Yunis, H. 1988. *A New Creed: Fundamental Religious Beliefs in the Athenian Polis and Euripidean Drama.* Göttingen.

Zeitlin, F. I. 1980. "The Closet of Masks: Role-Playing and Myth-Making in the *Orestes* of Euripides." *Ramus* 9:51–77.

———. 1990. "Thebes: Theater of Self and Society in Athenian Drama." In Winkler and Zeitlin 1990, 130–67.

———. 1996. *Playing the Other: Gender and Society in Classical Greek Literature.* Chicago.

INDEX LOCORUM

physiognomy, 184
Pigeaud, J., 166, 168n.88
Pindar, 30, 45
plague: gods of, 44, 48–49, 80; healers and interpreters of, 79, 80nn.166, 167; in the *Iliad*, 44, 48–49; in Thucydides, 26–27
Plato, 45; *Alcibiades* I, 6, 207–8; *Apology*, 89, 206–7; the care of the soul in, 206–11, 277n.4; *Crito*, 208; concept of disease, 131, 139, 209–10; and the history of dualism, 28–29, 30n.104, 31, 227; *Gorgias*, 174, 200–1; inspiration in, 69n.118; *Laws*, 90, 91, 98, 181–82; *Phaedo*, 194, 201–2; *Phaedrus*, 135, 180; *Philebus*, 28, 104, 119n.141, 215; *Protagoras*, 208, 209, 210, 215n.77; the *psukhē* in, 28, 31, 182, 188n.165, 201–2, 205–6, 206–11; and psychic struggle, 223n.104; and Pythagoreanism, 31; relationship to medicine, 135, 179–82, 191, 205–6, 208–9; *Republic*, 48, 162, 179–80, 193–94, 205–6, 226, 270n.162; *Sophist*, 90–91; *Symposium*, 200n.27; *Timaeus*, 24, 27–28, 139, 187–88, 275. *See also* analogy, medical
pleasure (*hēdonē*), 188n.165; ancient theories of, 112–14; as bodily, 201–2; as a cause of (bodily) disease, 198–200, 202–3, 220–21; in the *Philebus*, 105; physiology of, 199; and psychic disease, 221; and *terpsis*, 222. *See also* desire; *erōs*
Plutarch: on Anaxagoras, 84–85, 89; concept of disease, 1–2; on Democritus, 201, 219–20, 221
Podalirius, 79, 81n.169, 82–83
Pollan, M., 135n.57
Popper, K., 9, 18n.61
Porter, J., 5, 7–8n.25, 212n.67, 215n.75
possession, 53n.43, 67–69, 187n.161, 243–44
Potter, P., 176n.116
pre-symptoms, 1–2, 15, 178–79
prognosis: in Babylonian medicine, 55–56n.55, 80n.164; and bodily zones of meaning, 151; and diagnosis, 125; evaluation in, 151–53; and the physician's reputation, 150–51n.7; positivist views of, 153–54; skepticism about, 142, 147; symptoms in, 150–59
proof, 11–12, 106–7, 119n.142, 125, 127–28, 141, 173
prophasis ([manifest, external] cause), 130n.34, 146
psukhē (soul), 4; care of, 183, 204–5, 207–9, 223–25, 226, 278; as a cause of disease, 202–4, 218–20; diseases of, 209–25, 257–59;

276–78; and dreaming, 197n.15; early concepts of, 6, 29–32, 35, 61; and ethical subjectivity, 32, 37, 195; in Heraclitus, 31, 37n.129, 117; as a life-force, 37, 160; in the medical texts, 160, 183, 190–91n.172; in Plato, 28, 31, 182, 188n.165, 201–2, 205–6, 206–11; and the *sōma*, 6–7, 34–35, 104n.83, 190–91, 195–96, 201–2, 208–9, 225–27, 275
psychoanalysis, 5, 7–8n.25, 19n.64, 20n.68, 190
Pythagoreanism: care of the self in, 25n.86, 195n.9; and Empedocles, 25n.86, 31n.107, 116n.132; and healing, 204n.38; and Plato, 31; on the soul, 30, 31

rationality: definitions of, 11n.35
regimen, 79n.161, 82n.174, 165–66, 177–80, 185n.150, 189–91, 198–99
Renehan, R., 30–31n.106, 32n.111
retrospective diagnosis, 234n.32
Rheinberger, H.-J., 18
rhetoric: in medicine, 10, 120, 142, 174
Robinson, D., 263–64
Rohde, E., 30

Sack of Troy, 82–83
Sappho: symptoms of *erōs* in, 44
Scarry, E., 12–13, 74–75, 115n.126, 119n.141
Schiefsky, M., 167n.87, 169n.91, 170n.95
Sedley, D., 105nn.87, 90
seers. *See* divination
self, the: care of, 5, 26, 177–82, 189–91, 195, 206–8, 276–78. See also *psukhē*
Serres, M., 64n.9
Siegel, R., 9
signs: inference from, 11, 12, 108n.99, 119, 126–28; of the tongue, 154–55n.23. *See also* abduction; symptom
sleep. See *hupnos*
Smith, W., 67n.110, 177n.121, 231–32n.19
Snell, B., 5–9, 17, 28, 29–30, 32, 35, 45–46, 262n.134
Socrates: in the *Clouds*, 89, 92–93, 117; as a historical figure, 37n.129, 194, 206, 209; in Xenophon, 189, 190–91n.172, 210n.63
sōma (body): ancient philosophical concepts of, 102; in Aristotle, 102n.77, 103n.78; as a battlefield, 137–38; in the Cologne Epode, 35; corruptibility of, 28, 105–6; *dunamis* of, 155; early concepts of, 5–6, 29–36; in Empedocles, 104; in Gorgias, 102, 211; in the *Heracles*, 265–66; in Hesiod, 35; in Homer, 5–6, 29–30, 32–34; and human nature, 86,